RESPIRATORY CARE
of the **Newborn**
and **Child**

RESPIRATORY CARE

of the **Newborn**
and **Child**

SECOND EDITION

CLAIRE A. ALOAN, M.S., R.R.T.
Lincare, Inc.
Syracuse, New York

THOMAS V. HILL, M.S., R.R.T.
Kettering College of Medical Arts
Kettering, Ohio

With Fourteen Additional Contributors

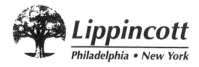
Lippincott
Philadelphia • New York

Acquisitions Editor: Andrew Allen
Assistant Editor: Holly Collins
Project Editor: Tom Gibbons
Production Manager/Managing Editor: Helen Ewan
Production Coordinator: Kathryn Rule
Design Coordinator: Kathy Kelley-Luedtke
Indexer: Maria Coughlin

2nd Edition

Library of Congress Cataloging-in-Publications Data

Respiratory care of the newborn and child / [edited by] Claire A. Aloan,
   Thomas V. Hill; with fourteen additional contributors. — 2nd ed.
      p.   cm.
   Rev. ed. of: Respiratory care of the newborn / Claire A. Aloan.
   c 1987.
   Includes bibliographical references and index.
   ISBN 0-397-54925-3 (pbk. : alk. paper)
   1. Respiratory therapy for children.   2. Respiratory therapy for newborn infants.
3. Pediatric respiratory diseases.   I. Aloan, Claire A.   II. Hill, Thomas V.
III. Aloan, Claire A. Respiratory care of the newborn.
   [DNLM: 1. Respiratory Tract Diseases — in infancy & childhood.
2. Respiratory Tract Diseases — therapy.   WS 280 R43345 1997]
RJ434.A46   1997
618.92'2 — dc21
DNLM/DLC
for Library of Congress   96-39478
                                                                       CIP

Care has been taken to confirm the accuracy of the information presented and to describe generally accepted practices. However, the authors, editors, and publisher are not responsible for errors or omissions or for any consequences from application of the information in this book and make no warranty, express or implied, with respect to the contents of the publication.

The authors, editors and publisher have exerted every effort to ensure that drug selection and dosage set forth in this text are in accordance with current recommendations and practice at the time of publication. However, in view of ongoing research, changes in government regulations, and the constant flow of information relating to drug therapy and drug reactions, the reader is urged to check the package insert for each drug for any change in indications and dosage and for added warnings and precautions. This is particularly important when the recommended agent is a new or infrequently employed drug.

Some drugs and medical devices presented in this publication have Food and Drug Administration (FDA) clearance for use in restricted research settings. It is the responsibility of the health care provider to ascertain the FDA status of each drug or device planned for use in their clinical practice.

9 8 7 6 5 4 3 2 1

Contributors

Claire A. Aloan, MS, RRT
Area Health Care Manager
Lincare, Inc.
Syracuse, New York

Laura Hooker Beveridge, MEd, RRT, RCP
Director of Clinical Services
Augusta Health Alliance/Lincare
Augusta, Georgia

Beverly J. Ervin, MSA, RRT, RCP
Pulmonary Health/Diagnostic
    Coordinator
Respiratory Care Department
The Children's Medical Center
Dayton, Ohio

Robert R. Fluck, Jr., MS, RRT
Associate Professor and Clinical
    Coordinator
Cardiorespiratory Sciences
SUNY–Health Science Center
Syracuse, New York

Earl Fulcher, Jr., MAE, RRT
Director of Clinical Education
Respiratory Therapy Program
Athens Area Technical Institute
Athens, Georgia
Neonatal Respiratory Therapist
Gwinnet Womens Pavilion
Lawrenceville, Georgia

Doug Hansell, BS, RRT
ECMO Program Coordinator
Respiratory Care Services
Brenner Children's Hospital
    and North Carolina Baptist
    Hospitals, Inc.
Winston-Salem, North Carolina

Kim V. Hill, MS, RRT
Program Associate
Respiratory Therapy Review
    Seminars
Kettering, Ohio

Thomas V. Hill, MS, RRT, Perinatal/Pediatric Specialist
Professor and Chairman
Department of Respiratory Care
Kettering College of Medical Arts
Kettering, Ohio

M. Dee Johnson, MS, RRT, CPFT, Perinatal/Pediatric Specialist
Professor, Director of Clinical
    Education
Respiratory Care Department
Kettering College of Medical Arts
Kettering, Ohio

James J. Lawson, RRT
Respiratory Therapist
Department of Respiratory Care
Kettering Medical Center
Kettering, Ohio

Jackie L. Long, MEd, RRT
Associate Dean for Health
  Sciences
Massachusetts Bay Community
  College
Wellesley Hills, Massachusetts

Ruth J. Messinger, MSW
Coordinator, Social Work and
  Community Education
Strong Center for Developmental
  Disabilities
Department of Pediatrics
University of Rochester Medical
  Center
Rochester, New York

Patrick J. Roth
Respiratory Therapy Team Leader
Respiratory Care
Children's Medical Center
Dayton, Ohio

Garth Rubins, RRT
Respiratory Therapist
Children's Medical Center
Dayton, Ohio

**Barbara G. Wilson,
  MEd, RRT**
Research Associate
Pediatric Critical Care and Respi-
  ratory Care Services
Duke University Medical Center
Durham, North Carolina

**Beth A. Zickefoose,
BS, RRT, Perinatal-Pediatric
Specialist**
Assistant Professor
Respiratory Care Program
Sinclair Community College
Dayton, Ohio

Preface to the Second Edition

Since publication of the first edition of *Respiratory Care of the Newborn*, both the art and the science of respiratory care of these special patients have grown by leaps and bounds. Advances in perinatal medicine have improved the ability to recognize high-risk pregnancies, prenatal ultrasound evaluation of the fetus has become commonplace, and the importance of proper prenatal nutrition and medical care has been recognized. Our ability to sustain the life of extremely premature infants with aggressive care has increased. We now have high-tech approaches available to treat disorders of the respiratory and cardiac systems—modalities such as extracorporeal membrane oxygenation, surfactant replacement, and high-frequency ventilation. At the same time, we have recognized the importance not only of maintaining life but also of seeking high-quality, life-long outcomes for the survivors of our neonatal intensive care units.

This edition varies from the previous edition in two primary ways. The first is that it incorporates changes that have taken place in the practice of respiratory care of newborns, including new research findings, treatment approaches, and specialized equipment for the assessment and care of the newborn. The second change is the addition of information necessary for assessment and care of the child with respiratory disease, focusing on conditions most often seen by the perinatal-pediatric respiratory care practitioner.

Respiratory Care of the Newborn and Child is intended to be used as a textbook for respiratory care students and as a reference book for those currently involved in respiratory care of newborns and children—both respiratory care practitioners and nurses. It builds upon an understanding of the anatomy and physiology of the respiratory and cardiac systems and a knowledge of basic respiratory care procedures and equipment. It is not intended to serve as a comprehensive manual but rather as a *clinical* text and reference. The major content of the book is directly related to the evaluation and management of the newborn and child with respiratory disease or with some other disorder that compromises the respiratory system.

Quality patient care seems to flow from a team approach in which physicians, nurses, and respiratory care practitioners work closely together, each lending their special expertise to the management of the infant and child. Toward that end, this book includes several subjects that, although of primary interest to the respiratory care practitioner, are also important to other members of the team as they treat children with cardiopulmonary disorders.

Respiratory Care of the Newborn and Child begins with a discussion of the development of the fetus and of the transition from fetal to neonatal life, which forms the basis for understanding the problems that may arise in the newborn period. Evaluation of the newborn is addressed from several aspects, including those that alert us to possible problems prenatally, physical assessment techniques vital to the minute-to-minute care of the newborn, various types of laboratory and radiologic assessment, and non-invasive monitoring techniques such as transcutaneous monitors and oximetry. Disorders that commonly (and not so commonly) appear in the newborn period are reviewed, including primary respiratory disease, cardiovascular disorders, and congenital anomalies. Assessment of the child with respiratory disease and pulmonary disorders in children are included in order to provide the perinatal-pediatric practitioners with a complete understanding of the care of these young patients. Techniques used to treat these various disorders are reviewed, including oxygen therapy, approaches to mechanical ventilation and positive pressure, bronchial hygiene, airway care, and resuscitation. The book concludes with the presentation of specialized therapies, such as surfactant replacement, high-frequency ventilation, extracorporeal membrane oxygenation, transport of the infant and child, and the provision of respiratory care to the patient well enough to be transferred to his or her home.

It is our hope that this second edition of *Respiratory Care of the Newborn and Child* will continue to provide the members of the health care team with some of the information they need in order to deliver skilled, competent, and compassionate care to these very special patients and their families.

Claire A. Aloan

Thomas V. Hill

Acknowledgments

Special thanks to those who have inspired and nurtured me, both personally and professionally, and who have supported me without reserve:

To Roger, for your unending love and support.

To my very special kids, Virginia Ann and Michael Paul, who keep me focused on the important things.

To Tom, for taking on the second edition and, as usual, doing an outstanding job.

And to Dad, who continues to be my biggest fan.

Claire A. Aloan

Acknowledgments

This book is possible only because of the contributions and efforts of many. I give special thanks to those who inspired and encouraged me:

To my wife, Kim, for your unlimited love, support, and encouragement.

To Claire, for providing the first edition as a strong foundation.

To all of the contributing authors, for your expertise and talents.

To Connie Valeri, for your contributions to Chapter 13.

To my colleagues and students at Kettering College of Medical Arts, for allowing me to pursue this project.

To Andrew Allen, Holly Collins, Tom Gibbons, and the staff of Lippincott-Raven, for your assistance, encouragement, and patience.

And to Virginia and John Hill, for teaching me to keep moving forward, and accept nothing but the best from myself.

Thomas V. Hill

Contents

Part V   **SPECIAL PROCEDURES**

Part VI   **PSYCHOSOCIAL INTERACTIONS**

RESPIRATORY CARE
of the **Newborn**
and **Child**

Part 1
From Fetus to Neonate

Chapter 1

Gestational Development

OBJECTIVES

Having completed this chapter, the reader will be able to:

1 Describe the sequence of events that occurs in the normal development of the pulmonary system.

2 Discuss the five phases of lung development.

3 Explain the significance of pulmonary surfactants and their relationship to gestational age.

4 Discuss the use of the L/S ratio, the shake test, and SPC levels to predict fetal maturity and lung function.

5 Explain the intrinsic and extrinsic factors that may influence the rate of fetal lung maturation.

6 Describe the anatomy and function of the placenta.

7 Describe the fetal circulation.

8 List the factors that contribute to elevated pulmonary vascular resistance in the fetus.

KEY TERMS

canalicular period	L/S ratio
chorionic villi	placenta
cotyledon	pseudoglandular period
ductus arteriosus	pulmonary surfactant
ductus venosus	shake test
embryonic period	terminal air sac period
foramen ovale	umbilical artery
intervillous space	umbilical vein

■ DEVELOPMENT OF THE PULMONARY SYSTEM

The lung develops as a single bud off the anterior portion of the foregut at approximately 3 weeks of gestation and branches into primitive right and left lungs shortly afterward. Development then continues by both single budding and irregular branching. Cartilage appears at the 4th week,

3

with distinct rings in the trachea by the 7th week. By week 6, the embryo has a tracheobronchial tree with 18 segmental bronchi. Pulmonary arteries and veins develop along with the branching airways. By week 16, the conducting airways of the tracheobronchial tree are present in miniature form, but respiratory bronchioles have not yet developed.

By the 24th week, respiratory bronchioles, alveolar ducts, alveoli, pulmonary vessels, and lymphatic vessels have begun to develop. The alveoli are still rudimentary. By the 26th week, formation of the alveolar—capillary unit is sufficient to allow extrauterine life, although many capillaries still are not in contact with air spaces. By weeks 27 to 28, there are more alveolar sacs and more capillaries in contact with them, allowing for better gas-exchange potential. The connective tissue spaces between terminal gas-exchange units remain quite large, making lung compliance low and allowing for accumulation of fluid and air (interstitial emphysema). The large interstitial space also widens the distance for diffusion of gases from alveoli to capillaries, thus impeding gas exchange. From this point forward, new alveolar growth is rapid. By weeks 34 to 36, the alveoli are mature in form. The alveoli continue to develop after birth in both number and size. Whereas growth in the number of alveoli is usually completed by the age of 8 years, the alveoli increase in size until adulthood. The growth and development of the pulmonary structures are summarized in Table 1-1.

Stages of Lung Development

Lung development has been described in five stages (Table 1-2), although it occurs as a continuous, uninterrupted process from the beginning of fetal development through adulthood. The first four stages occur during intrauterine life. The fifth stage, the postnatal stage, continues into adulthood. The intrauterine stages consist of the embryonic period, the pseudoglandular period, the canalicular period, and the terminal air sac period. The **embryonic period** extends from conception through the first 6 weeks of gestation. During this period, development of the proximal air-

TABLE 1-1 Sequential Development of the Pulmonary System

GESTATIONAL AGE	DEVELOPMENT
24 days	Primitive lung bud appears
26–28 days	Lung bud divides into beginnings of two mainstem bronchi
By 6 weeks	Segmental bronchi are formed
By 12 weeks	Major lobes are differentiated
16 weeks	Respiratory bronchioles are differentiated
24 weeks	Alveolar sacs are formed
25–26 weeks	Alveolar–capillary surface is capable of sustaining extrauterine life
28–29 weeks	Terminal air sacs are lined with mature Type II cells from which surfactant is released
30–33 weeks	New alveolar units appear rapidly
34–36 weeks	Mature alveolar structures are evident

TABLE 1-2 Stages of Lung Development

PERIOD	AGE	ACTIVITY
Embryonic	4–6 weeks of gestation	Development of proximal airways
Pseudoglandular	7–16 weeks of gestation	Development of conducting airways
Canalicular	17–24 weeks of gestation	Development of acinus
Terminal Air Sac	24 weeks–birth	Development of gas exchange units
Postnatal	Birth–8 years	Increase in alveolar number and size
	8 years–adulthood	Increase in alveolar size

ways is the major event, ending with the appearance of the segmental bronchi. The **pseudoglandular period** is from 7 to 16 weeks, during which the conducting airways are formed by branching of the bronchial buds. The lungs have a glandular appearance and cilia begin to form in the airways. Cartilage and glands also develop during this period. The **canalicular period** occurs from 17 to 24 weeks. This period is characterized by the development of the acinus, or the gas-exchange portion of the lung. The relative amount of connective tissue decreases and the lungs become more highly vascularized. The last stage of intrauterine lung development, the **terminal air sac period**, occurs from 24 weeks until term. In this period, the alveolar duct system becomes more extensive and the alveolar surface area increases through the development of the alveolar sacs. The distance between the alveolar epithelium and capillaries decreases, making it more feasible for gas exchange to occur. At birth, the lungs contain approximately 55 million alveoli with a surface area of approximately 10 square meters.[5]

The postnatal stage begins at birth and continues into adulthood. During the first 8 years, the lungs grow because of an increase in both the number and size of the alveoli. After that point, lung growth takes place primarily due to an increase in the size of the alveoli. The adult lungs contain approximately 300 million alveoli with a surface area of 70 square meters.

■ SURFACTANT DEVELOPMENT

Pulmonary surfactants are a mixture of phospholipids and proteins and are responsible for altering the surface tension at the alveolar level. These surfactants are secreted by Type II alveolar cells (also called Type II pneumocytes). The major surfactant is phosphatidyl choline, commonly called lecithin. Without an adequate supply of surfactant, alveoli tend to collapse on expiration (atelectasis), making the lungs very stiff and noncompliant. The occurrence of noncompliant lungs caused by immature surfactant production in the newborn is called hyaline membrane disease (HMD) or respiratory distress syndrome (RDS). Lecithin and sphingomyelin, two pulmonary surfactants produced by the fetus and secreted into the amniotic fluid, have been found to change in concentration during gestation and correlate well with the development of lung maturity.

Sphingomyelin and Lecithin

Sphingomyelin is a pulmonary surfactant found in amniotic fluid in fairly constant amounts with advancing gestation. Beginning at about 18 weeks of gestation, sphingomyelin concentrations rise slowly to a peak at 30 weeks and then decline to term. Lecithin concentrations also rise from about 18 weeks and reach a peak at 38 weeks. Lecithin may be produced by several metabolic pathways. The surge in production at 34 weeks represents synthesis of lecithin by a more mature and stable pathway, which coincides with fetal lung maturity (Fig. 1-1).

Assessment of Lung Maturity

The production of these two types of surfactants and their secretion into amniotic fluid can be detected by chemical analysis of amniotic fluid obtained from amniocentesis. Amniotic fluid may also be obtained by vaginal examination in a mother with premature rupture of membranes and by gastric aspirate from the infant in the delivery room. The relationship or ratio of lecithin concentration to sphingomyelin concentration (**L/S ratio**) is calculated and used as an estimate of fetal lung maturity.[3] An L/S ratio of greater than 2.0 predicts mature lungs and is rarely associated with respiratory distress. If the L/S ratio is less than 1.0, severe lung immaturity is present and respiratory distress syndrome is likely. If the L/S ratio is between 1.0 and 2.0, respiratory distress syndrome may or may not develop. The incidence and the severity of respiratory distress correlate with the L/S ratio and with factors such as low birth weight and birth asphyxia. Although other methods of estimating fetal lung maturity have been described, L/S ratio testing continues to be the most commonly used method.[2]

The **shake test** is another procedure that attempts to determine lung maturity.[7] Samples of amniotic fluid are mixed with alcohol and shaken, forming bubbles at the surface. The samples are then allowed to stand while the stability of the bubbles is observed. A complete ring of bubbles at the surface after 15 minutes indicates that the L/S ratio is 2.0 or greater, predictive of fetal lung maturity. If bubbles are absent, pulmonary

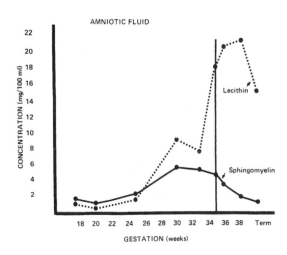

FIGURE 1-1 Lecithin and sphingomyelin levels in amniotic fluid during gestational development. (Avery GB: Neonatology: Pathophysiology and Management of the Newborn, 2nd ed, p 109. Philadelphia, JB Lippincott, 1981)

immaturity is likely. The absence of bubbles is not as specific as a low L/S ratio. Because this test is simple to perform, it may be used as a screening test. A positive test, determined by the presence of stable bubbles, indicates maturity and should not require further testing. In the absence of bubbles, an L/S ratio should be performed.

Another method used to predict lung maturity is direct measurement of the level of saturated phosphatidylcholine (SPC) in amniotic fluid. Torday reported that SPC levels of more than 500 ug/dL are associated with a much lower incidence of HMD than levels of less than 500 ug/dL.[8]

Under certain conditions, the L/S ratio may not correlate well with gestational age, although it will still be predictive of pulmonary maturity. Some conditions may accelerate the maturation of the lungs, whereas others may delay maturation. Thus, an L/S ratio of 2.0 or greater, which would usually indicate a gestational age greater than 34 weeks, may occur in a fetus who is less than 34 weeks but who has accelerated lung maturation. This accounts somewhat for the occurrence of relatively mild or no respiratory distress in some infants of low gestational age. Conditions that may be associated with accelerated maturation of the lungs include toxemia, maternal hypertension, severe diabetes, maternal infection, prolonged rupture of the membranes, and placental insufficiency. Conditions associated with delayed maturation of the lungs include mild diabetes, fetal Rh disease, and smaller identical twins.

Other variables may affect the accuracy of the L/S ratio measurement: if there is maternal bleeding into the amniotic fluid, for example, the L/S ratio will tend to read falsely low. Meconium in the amniotic fluid may also affect the results, with both false-negative and false-positive results possible.

Acceleration of Lung Maturation

Maturation of the lungs through the induction of surfactant production has been shown to be accelerated by the administration of corticosteroids.[6] This finding has encouraged the administration of corticosteroids to the mother before delivery if the fetus is known to have immature lungs. Betamethasone and dexamethasone have been used and should be given at least 48 hours, but not more than 7 days, before delivery to be effective. Additionally, only gestational ages of less than 34 weeks are affected by this therapy, with the most significant results occurring between 30 and 32 weeks of gestation. The use of these drugs does not entirely prevent the development of RDS, but both the incidence and the severity of RDS have been shown to be reduced with no apparent adverse effects on the newborn.[1,4]

■ FETAL CIRCULATION

The **placenta** is the nutrient, gas-exchange, and waste removal organ for the fetus. It provides direct contact between the circulation of the mother and the circulation of the fetus while keeping the two blood supplies separate. Segments called **cotyledons**, which contain fetal vessels, chorionic villi, and an intervillous space, comprise the placenta. The **chorionic villi** are fingerlike projections of tissue that invade the uterine wall at the site of implantation of the placenta. These villi contain the fetal capillaries. The spaces formed in the uterine wall by the villi are surrounded by maternal blood. These blood-filled areas are the **intervillous spaces** and the site of exchange of nutrient, gaseous, and waste substances between the maternal and fetal blood. The surface area for exchange provided by this system increases throughout pregnancy to meet the needs of the growing fetus.

Maternal blood is supplied to the placenta by the uterine arteries, and oxygenated blood from these arteries surrounds the villi. Fetal blood enters the placenta through two **umbilical arteries** in the umbilical cord, and these vessels branch and terminate in capillaries within each villus. After exchange has taken place, fetal blood returns to the fetus through a single **umbilical vein**, and maternal blood drains back into the venous system.

As a gas-exchange organ, the placenta acts to allow diffusion of oxygen from the maternal arterial blood into the fetal circulation and to allow diffusion of carbon dioxide from the fetus into the maternal circulation, subsequently to be returned to the lungs by way of the maternal venous system.

In the fetal circulation (Fig. 1-2), blood that has supplied fetal tissues, thus giving up oxygen and acquiring carbon dioxide, enters the placenta

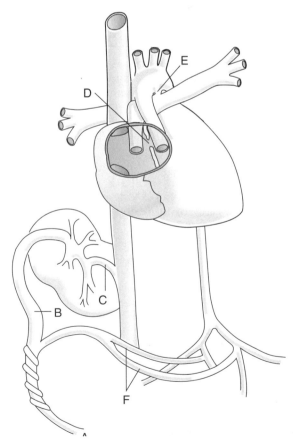

FIGURE 1-2 Fetal circulation. (**A**) Placenta, (**B**) umbilical vein, (**C**) ductus venosus, (**D**) foramen ovale, (**E**) ductus arteriosus, (**F**) umbilical arteries.

by way of the umbilical arteries. Once it has exchanged with the maternal circulation, fetal blood leaves the placenta by way of the umbilical vein, now richer in oxygen and lower in carbon dioxide. Thus, in the fetus, the umbilical vein carries the highest oxygen concentration. Average oxygen saturation in the umbilical vein is about 80%, equivalent to a PO_2 of about 29 mm Hg.

Some of the blood in the umbilical vein supplies the fetal liver, with the remaining blood being diverted through the **ductus venosus** into the inferior vena cava. The inferior vena cava already contains some blood that is returning from the lower part of the body after having supplied the tissues there, and it is thus low in oxygen. The mixing of oxygenated blood from the umbilical vein and deoxygenated blood from the tissues results in an oxygen saturation of about 67% in the inferior vena cava.

This blood then returns by way of the inferior vena cava to the heart, where it enters the right atrium. At this point, there is some mixing with deoxygenated blood from the superior vena cava, which drains the upper part of the body, resulting in a slight drop in oxygen saturation to about 62%. Most of the blood from the inferior vena cava, however, is diverted directly from the right atrium into the left atrium through an opening called the **foramen ovale**. The left atrium also receives some blood from the pulmonary veins. This blood now proceeds from the left atrium to the left ventricle and is ejected into the ascending aorta, where it supplies the coronary arteries and the vessels of the head and the upper extremities of the left side of the body. Thus, blood that is relatively rich in oxygen supplies the brain and heart of the fetus, the organs that use the most oxygen.

Blood returning to the heart from the superior vena cava enters the right atrium, flows into the right ventricle, and is ejected into the pulmonary artery. This blood is relatively low in oxygen, with a saturation of about 52%. Once it has entered the pulmonary artery, most of the blood is diverted into the descending aorta through the **ductus arteriosus**. This blood supplies the lower part of the body and the umbilical arteries. Only about 10% of the blood ejected from the right ventricle passes into the pulmonary circulation. Since pulmonary vascular resistance is much higher than systemic vascular resistance, the blood takes the path of lower resistance through the ductus arteriosus. There is no need to provide a large supply of blood to the pulmonary circulation since the fetal lung is filled with fluid and does not play a role in gas exchange. The pulmonary vascular resistance in the fetus is high because of several factors: the pulmonary vessels are kinked and tortuous and the fluid filling the alveoli exerts pressure against them, and the very low PO_2 leads to hypoxic vasoconstriction of these vessels.

In summary, there are several unique features of the fetal circulation. The placenta serves as the organ of gas exchange. The umbilical vein serves to return oxygenated blood from the placenta to the fetus. The ductus venosus diverts some of this blood into the inferior vena cava. Blood returning to the right atrium through the inferior vena cava is selectively diverted to the left atrium through an opening called the foramen ovale, which allows blood relatively rich in oxygen to be supplied to the brain and heart. Blood entering the right heart from the superior vena cava, which is low in oxygen, enters the pulmonary artery, where most of the blood is diverted to the descending aorta through the ductus arteriosus, a vessel that connects the pulmonary artery and the descending aorta. Blood from the descending aorta supplies the lower part of the body and also supplies the umbilical arteries, which will return blood to the placenta to pick up oxygen and remove carbon dioxide.

▬ REFERENCES

1. Collaborative group on antenatal steroid therapy. Effect of antenatal dexamethasone administration on the prevention of respiratory distress syndrome. Am J Obstet Gynecol 141:276, 1981.
2. Dubin SB: Assessment of fetal lung maturity by laboratory methods. Clin Lab Med 12(3):603, 1992.
3. Gluck L, Kulovich MV, Borer RC Jr: Estimates of fetal lung maturity. In Nesbitt REL (ed): Clinics in Perinatology, vol 1. Philadelphia, WB Saunders, March 1974.
4. Kattner E, Metze B, Waiss E, Obladen M. Accelerated lung maturation following maternal steroid treatment in infants born before 30 weeks gestation. J Perinatal Med 20(6):449, 1992.
5. Langston C, Thurlback WM: Conditions altering normal lung growth and development. In Thibeault DW, Gregory GA: Neonatal Pulmonary Care, 2nd ed. Norwalk CT, Appleton-Century-Crofts, 1986.
6. Liggins GC, Howie RN: A controlled trial of antepartum glucocorticoid treatment for prevention of the respiratory distress syndrome in premature infants. Pediatrics 50:515, 1972.
7. Platzker A, Tooley W et al: Prediction of the idiopathic respiratory distress syndrome by a rapid new test for pulmonary surfactant in amniotic fluid. Clin Res 20:283, 1972.
8. Torday JS: Tests for pulmonary surfactant. In Cloherty JP, Stark AR: Manual of Neonatal Care, 2nd ed. Boston, Little, Brown, 1985.

▬ BIBLIOGRAPHY

Dancis J: Fetomaternal interactio. In Avery GB (ed): Neonatology: Pathophysiology and Management of the Newborn, 2nd ed. Philadelphia, JB Lippincott, 1981.

Gluck L: Fetal lung development. In The Surfactant System and the Neonatal Lung, Mead Johnson Symposium on Perinatal and Developmental Medicine no. 14, 1978.

Murray JF: The Normal Lung: The Basis for Diagnosis and Treatment of Pulmonary Disease, 2nd ed. Philadelphia, WB Saunders, 1986.

Richmond B, Galgocyz M: Development of the cardiorespiratory system. In Lough MD, Williams TJ, Rawson JE (eds): Newborn Respiratory Care. Chicago, Year Book Medical Publishers, 1979.

▬ SELF-ASSESSMENT QUESTIONS

1. At what point in gestation are the lungs first capable of supporting extrauterine life?
   a. 14 weeks
   b. 18 weeks
   c. 23 weeks
   d. 26 weeks

2. During the first 8 years of life, the lungs grow because of an increase in
   a. the size of the alveoli
   b. the number of alveoli
   c. the number of terminal bronchioles
   d. a and b

3. Pulmonary surfactants are produced in the lungs by
   a. alveolar macrophages
   b. Type II alveolar cells
   c. goblet cells
   d. Type I alveolar cells

4. The lecithin/sphingomyelin (L/S) ratio is used to estimate
   a. gestational age
   b. volume of amniotic fluid
   c. fetal lung maturity
   d. birth weight

5. Administration of _____ to mothers in premature labor has been effective in stimulating pulmonary maturity and reducing the severity of respiratory distress of the newborn.
   a. betamethasone
   b. dexamethasone
   c. terbutaline
   d. a and b

6. The _____ is the nutrient, gas-exchange, and waste removal organ for the fetus.
   a. lung
   b. liver
   c. umbilical cord
   d. placenta

7. The umbilical cord contains _____ arteries and _____ veins.
   a. 1, 2
   b. 2, 1
   c. 1, 1
   d. 2, 2

8. In the fetal circulation, blood returning to the right atrium from the inferior vena cava is diverted into the left atrium through the
   a. ductus venosus
   b. ductus arteriosus
   c. foramen ovale
   d. tricuspid valve

9. In the fetal circulation, approximately _____% of the blood passes through the pulmonary circulation.
   a. 10
   b. 30
   c. 50
   d. 70

10. The average oxygen saturation in the umbilical vein is
    a. 20%
    b. 40%
    c. 60%
    d. 80%

Chapter 2

Fetal–Neonatal Transition

OBJECTIVES

Having completed this chapter, the reader will be able to:

1 Describe the chemical and sensory factors that stimulate respiration at birth.

2 Discuss the mechanisms that are responsible for the removal of fetal lung liquid.

3 Describe the establishment of functional residual capacity in the newborn.

4 Discuss the pressure gradients involved in initial respiratory efforts.

5 Describe the changes that occur in the circulatory system at birth.

6 Discuss the factors that influence the transition from fetal to neonatal circulation at birth.

7 List the factors that contribute to a decrease in pulmonary vascular resistance and closure of the ductus arteriosus at birth.

8 Describe the role of prostaglandins and oxygen tensions in circulatory transition.

9 Compare fetal and adult hemoglobin function.

10 Discuss the significance of the presence of fetal hemoglobin.

KEY TERMS

2,3-DPG	prostaglandin synthetase
ligamentum arteriosum	pulmonary vascular resistance
oxyhemoglobin dissociation curve	transient fetal asphyxia
P50	

The transition from fetus to neonate is probably the greatest challenge the human body faces throughout life. In the first minutes of extrauterine life, the newborn must activate his or her central and autonomic nervous systems, replace the liquid in the lungs with air, establish the pulmonary circulation, and change the direction of blood flow through the heart and great vessels. The fact that this transition occurs without complication in almost all newborns is truly amazing when we consider all that must be accomplished and the implications of problems in the transition.

12

INITIATION OF RESPIRATION

It is now known that intrauterine breathing movements occur commonly in the human fetus. Respiratory movements occur from 30% to 65% of the time and only during the rapid eye movement (REM) stage of sleep.[1,3] The placenta assumes the role of exchanging oxygen and carbon dioxide so fetal breathing is not essential to sustain life. It is proposed that these attempts at ventilation provide exercise for the respiratory muscles.[2] The factors that stimulate the infant to initiate respiration at birth are probably both chemical and sensory in nature; the relative roles of various factors are unclear.

During the normal birth process, placental circulation is impaired. Since the placenta provides for gas exchange, **transient fetal asphyxia** (hypoxia, hypercapnia, and respiratory acidosis) results. These chemical factors, through their effects on chemoreceptors, provide a strong stimulus to breathe. Prolonged asphyxia, which results in metabolic acidosis as well as in the previously listed chemical changes, tends to depress rather than to stimulate respiration.

Sensory stimuli may also play an important role in the initiation of respiration. The fetus is enveloped in a warm, wet atmosphere in utero. The sudden departure from this environment into the relatively cool, dry air of the delivery room stimulates nerve endings in the skin and causes subsequent transmission of impulses to the respiratory center in the brain. In addition, handling of the newborn infant provides tactile stimulation, which may also contribute to the first efforts at breathing.

The lung in utero is normally filled with fluid. The volume of fetal lung liquid is approximately 30 mL/kg of body weight and is roughly equal to the functional residual capacity (FRC) of the newborn. Although secretion of this liquid decreases for several days before spontaneous delivery, the fluid must be replaced with air since the lungs replace the placenta as the organ of gas exchange after the infant is delivered. There are three primary mechanisms by which fetal lung fluid is removed: compression of the thorax during delivery, absorption into the pulmonary capillaries, and clearance by the pulmonary lymphatic system. Each of these mechanisms removes approximately one third of the fetal lung liquid.

During normal vaginal delivery, the thoracic cage is greatly compressed as the fetus passes through the birth canal. This squeezing of the chest cage helps to eject some of the fluid from the lungs. As much as one third of the total lung fluid may be squeezed out during passage through the birth canal. Infants born by cesarean section do not experience this compression and may be more likely to have difficulty in clearing lung fluid, resulting in the transient tachypnea syndrome. Many infants born by cesarean section do not develop this problem because they apparently clear lung fluid adequately through the remaining two mechanisms: absorption into the pulmonary capillaries and clearance by the pulmonary lymphatic system.

Because of the very negative pressures created in the pleural space during the first breaths, a pressure gradient is established from the alveoli to the interstitial space, favoring movement of fluid out of the alveoli. In addition, the opening of the alveoli stretches the alveolar walls and enlarges the normal alveolar wall openings or pores, allowing fluid easier exit from the alveoli into the interstitial space. The large increase in pulmonary blood flow that occurs after birth also helps to remove fluid from the lungs. In the normal-term infant, fluid removal to the interstitial space is complete within several breaths, although it may take several hours to remove excess fluid from the interstitial space by means of the capillaries and lymphatics.

After birth, the chest cage recoils, which may passively introduce some air into the lungs. As the newborn infant receives stimuli from the chemical and sensory changes associated with birth, he or she initiates nerve impulses to the muscles of respiration, resulting in an expansion of thoracic volume and a decrease in intrathoracic pressure. Thus, a pressure gradient is established, allowing air to flow into the lungs. To overcome the surface tension of the alveoli and the viscosity of the remaining lung fluid, the newborn infant must often generate negative intrathoracic pressures of 60 to 80 cm H_2O. The volume of the first breath varies from infant to infant, averaging about 40 mL. Not all of this air is exhaled after the first inspiration, with approximately 20 to 30 mL remaining in the lungs as the infant begins to establish FRC.

Subsequent breaths will require lower transpulmonary pressures, as more and more alveoli remain inflated after each breath. Figure 2-1 illustrates the pressure volume relationships in the newborn lung during the first three breaths. Note that following the first breath, lower pressure gradients are required to achieve alveolar filling. The opening of alveoli occurs serially, so that each alveolus becomes fully inflated before the next one opens. A normal FRC is usually established within the first few hours after birth. This sequence represents the normal course of events and requires the presence of surfactant in sufficient quantities to prevent alveolar collapse at the end of expiration. In infants who are born prematurely or who for other reasons have insufficient surfactant, the alveoli collapse and the infant cannot establish a normal FRC. This means that the effort to inflate the lungs with each succeeding breath does not decrease, thus accounting for the respiratory distress seen in these infants.

▰ TRANSITION TO NEONATAL CIRCULATION

The unique aspects of the fetal circulation were described in Chapter 1. After birth, several events occur that cause the circulation to change from the fetal to the neonatal (or *adult*) circulatory pathway. As with the initiation of respiration and removal of lung fluid, these changes occur very rapidly following delivery and are not sequential. The transition from fetal to newborn circulation is summarized in Table 2-1.

Closure of the Foramen Ovale

Once the infant has been delivered, the umbilical cord is clamped, thus removing the infant from the placental circulation. This results in less blood flow returning to the right atrium and decreases the pressure in the right side of the heart. In addition, the placenta is a low-pressure circuit. Loss of this low-pressure outlet for aortic blood flow results in increased pressure in the left side of the heart. Following birth, pulmonary vascular resistance falls as a result of the increase in PA_{O_2} and decrease in PA_{CO_2} that accompany the initiation of alveolar ventilation. As pulmonary vascular resistance decreases, pulmonary perfusion increases greatly, and a

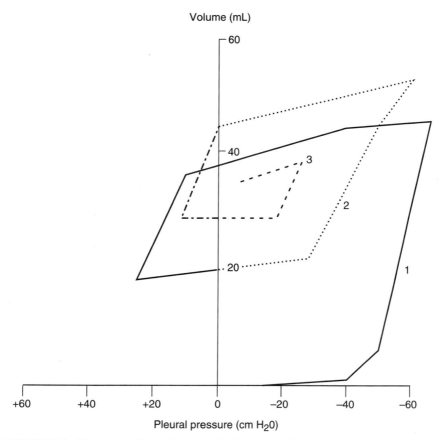

FIGURE 2-1 First three breaths after birth in an infant. Note the high pressure required for the first inflation (60 cm H20) and the decrease in inflation pressure with succeeding breaths. Also note that a functional residual capacity is established at the end of the first expiration and increases with subsequent breaths.

much greater volume of blood is returned to the left atrium through the pulmonary veins, further increasing the pressure in the left side of the heart. This difference in pressure between the right and left sides results in functional closure of the foramen ovale, which is essentially a flap valve. When the pressure in the left side is greater than the pressure in the right side, the flap closes. If these pressures are reversed, the flap opens. Functional closure of the foramen ovale occurs almost immediately after birth. Anatomic closure does not occur for weeks or months after birth and the foramen ovale may remain patent throughout adult life. Should the pressure in the right side of the heart become elevated, the foramen ovale may reopen and allow for shunting of blood from the right side of the heart to the left side without passing through the pulmonary circulation.

Pulmonary Vascular Resistance
The major event that alters pressure on the right side of the heart is **pulmonary vascular resistance,** or resistance to outflow from the right ventricle. Normally, pulmonary vascular resistance falls abruptly at birth for

TABLE 2-1 Transition to Neonatal Circulation

EVENT	CAUSE
Closure of foramen ovale	Increased pressure in left atrium
Decreased pulmonary vascular resistance	Unkinking of pulmonary capillaries
	Increased P_{O_2}
	Decreased P_{CO_2}
Closure of ductus arteriosus	Decreased pulmonary vascular resistance
	Increased P_{O_2}
	Decreased prostaglandin level
Closure of ductus venosus	Clamping of umbilical cord
	Closure of umbilical vein

several reasons. As the fluid is removed from the alveoli, there is less pressure on the pulmonary vessels. As the alveoli expand, they exert traction on the pulmonary vessels, helping to straighten them. As the infant begins to breathe, oxygen tensions rise and the hypoxic vasoconstriction of pulmonary vessels seen in the fetus is reversed. Carbon dioxide tensions fall, also helping to reverse vasoconstriction. Thus, we can see that a number of factors may contribute to an elevated pulmonary vascular resistance in the newborn: failure to remove lung fluid adequately; failure to inflate the lungs adequately; hypoxia; and hypercapnia. If pulmonary vascular resistance does not fall, the infant is likely to continue to use fetal circulatory pathways rather than perfusing the pulmonary capillary bed. This makes it very difficult to oxygenate the infant because there is little blood coming in contact with air spaces.

Ductus Arteriosus

Constriction and closure of the ductus arteriosus occur for several reasons. The decrease in pulmonary vascular resistance allows a much greater portion of the blood ejected from the right ventricle to enter the pulmonary circulation, thus decreasing the blood flow through the ductus. Unlike the foramen ovale, the ductus arteriosus does not close functionally immediately at birth. During the first few hours of life, the ductus remains open and ductal blood flow, although greatly reduced, continues. The direction of flow will usually be from the aorta (left side) to the pulmonary artery (right side) since, as previously discussed, the pressures on the left or systemic side of the circulation become much greater than the pressures on the right or pulmonary side immediately after birth.

Over the next several hours, the ductus begins to constrict, primarily in response to elevated oxygen tensions. This is the opposite response from the pulmonary circulation: hypoxia causes vasoconstriction in the pulmonary vascular bed, whereas elevated oxygen causes vasoconstriction of the ductus arteriosus. Conversely, hypoxia will result in failure of the ductus to constrict. Anatomic closure of the ductus arteriosus is usually complete by 3 weeks of age. Following complete constriction, the ductus arteriosus becomes a ligament (the **ligamentum arteriosum**).

The premature infant may have some difficulty in constriction and closure of the ductus arteriosus because the capacity to respond to elevated oxygen tensions is not well developed. This is probably related to the levels of prostaglandins in the ductus of the premature infant. Prostaglandins E1 and E2 are responsible for keeping the ductus open during fetal life. In the premature infant, they may continue to do so. The enzyme complex responsible for the formation of prostaglandins is called **prostaglandin synthetase**. Prostaglandin synthetase inhibitors, by decreasing the activity of this enzyme complex, can help to decrease the levels of prostaglandins and thus promote constriction of the ductus arteriosus. Indomethacin is a prostaglandin synthetase inhibitor commonly used with good success in infants with a patent ductus arteriosus. Conversely, in infants with congenital heart disease who are dependent upon a ductus arteriosus for survival, prostaglandins have been administered intravenously to keep the ductus open until surgical repair can be performed. This situation will be discussed further in Chapter 11.

Ductus Venosus

The ductus venosus closes anatomically within 3 to 7 days after birth. There is very little blood flow after closure of the umbilical circulation. The mechanism of closure of this vessel is unknown.

▬FETAL HEMOGLOBIN

Fetal hemoglobin differs from adult hemoglobin in its affinity for oxygen. The relationship between oxygen and hemoglobin is represented by the **oxyhemoglobin dissociation curve** (Fig. 2-2), which relates partial pressure of oxygen to the hemoglobin saturation (%). In other words, for any given partial pressure of oxygen (PO_2), a hemoglobin saturation can be predicted. Fetal hemoglobin has a greater affinity for oxygen than does adult hemoglobin, which means that at any given PO_2, fetal hemoglobin will have a higher oxygen saturation than adult hemoglobin. This is often expressed as a shift of the curve to the left. Another way of expressing this relationship is in terms of the P_{50}, which is the partial pressure of oxygen at which the hemoglobin will be 50% saturated. The P_{50} of adult blood is normally 27 mm Hg. Fetal blood has a P_{50} that is 6 to 8 mm Hg lower than that of the normal adult. This means that fetal hemoglobin binds oxygen more readily and releases it less readily.

The major reason for the difference in oxygen affinity of adult and fetal hemoglobin is related to inorganic phosphate, 2,3-diphosphoglycerate (**2,3-DPG**). When 2,3-DPG binds to hemoglobin, it reduces the affinity of hemoglobin for oxygen. In other words, it shifts the curve to the right or increases the P_{50}. Fetal hemoglobin cannot bind 2,3-DPG as well as adult hemoglobin can and, thus, it has a greater affinity for oxygen.

In the newborn, therefore, the ability to bind and release oxygen is related both to the level of fetal hemoglobin present and to the amount of 2,3-DPG in the blood. The level of 2,3-DPG rises throughout gestation and is similar at term to that of adults. It then falls for the first several days after birth, rising again to values exceeding those at birth by the end

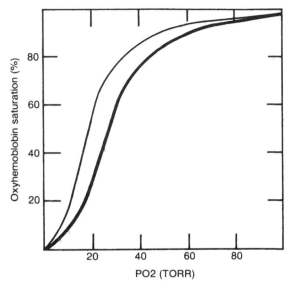

FIGURE 2-2   The oxygen dissociation curve for normal adult blood and, to the left, the dissociation curve for fetal blood, demonstrating an increase in the affinity of fetal hemoglobin for oxygen and a decrease in the release of oxygen.

of the first week of life. Fetal hemoglobin is high in the term newborn and diminishes gradually over the first year of life, causing the oxyhemoglobin dissociation curve to shift gradually to the right, toward its normal position in the adult. The P_{50} value usually increases to the adult level by 6 months of age. This shift differs for premature infants, who have lower 2,3-DPG values and higher fetal hemoglobin levels. The shift in the curve (rise in P_{50}) for premature infants is much more gradual than that for term infants, which means that for any given PO_2 level, the premature infant will usually have less oxygen available for release at the tissue level.

▬REFERENCES

1. Boddy K, Mantell CD: Observations of fetal breathing movements transmitted through maternal abdominal wall. Lancet 2:1219, 1972.
2. Burgess WR, Chernick V. Respiratory Therapy in Newborn Infants and Children, 2nd ed. New York, Thieme, 1986.
3. Nelson N: Physiology of transition. In Avery GB, Fletcher MA, MacDonald MG: Neonatology: Pathophysiology and Management of the Newborn, 4th ed. Philadelphia, JB Lippincott, 1994.

▬BIBLIOGRAPHY

Avery ME, Fletcher BD: The Lung and Its Disorders in the Newborn Infant, 3rd ed. Philadelphia, WB Saunders, 1974.
Burgess WR, Chernick V: Respiratory Therapy in Newborn Infants and Children, 2nd ed. New York, Thieme, 1986.

Escobedo MB: Fetal and neonatal cardiopulmonary physiology. In Schreiner RL, Kisling JA (eds): Practical Neonatal Respiratory Care. New York, Raven, 1982.

Nelson N: Physiology of transition. In Avery GB, Fletcher MA, MacDonald MG: Neonatology: Pathophysiology and Management of the Newborn, 4th ed. Philadelphia, JB Lippincott, 1994.

Sanderson RG: Anatomy, embryology, and physiology. In Sanderson R, Kurth CL (eds): The Cardiac Patient: A Comprehensive Approach, 2nd ed. Philadelphia, WB Saunders, 1983.

▬ SELF-ASSESSMENT QUESTIONS

1. At birth, the onset of respiration is stimulated by
   a. hypoxia
   b. hypercapnia
   c. respiratory acidosis
   d. all of the above

2. Fetal lung fluid is removed by all of the following mechanisms *except*
   a. compression of the chest cage
   b. positive pressure in the airway
   c. absorption by pulmonary capillaries
   d. clearance by pulmonary lymphatics

3. After inspiration during the first breath, the infant does not exhale all of the inhaled volume. This helps in establishing the
   a. residual capacity
   b. tidal volume
   c. functional residual capacity
   d. expiratory reserve volume

4. During the first breath, intrathoracic pressure gradients reach
   a. 20—30 cm H_2O
   b. 40—50 cm H_2O
   c. 60—80 cm H_2O
   d. 90—100 cm H_2O

5. The foramen ovale closes when the pressure in the left side of the heart _____ the pressure in the right side of the heart.
   a. equals
   b. exceeds
   c. falls below
   d. approaches

6. Functional closure of the foramen ovale occurs _____ after birth.
   a. immediately
   b. 4—6 hours
   c. 2—3 days
   d. 1—2 weeks

7. Closure of the ductus arteriosus occurs because of all of the following *except*
   a. decreased pulmonary vascular resistance
   b. increased PO_2
   c. decreased prostaglandin level
   d. increased PCO_2

8. During fetal life, prostaglandins E1 and E2 are responsible for keeping the _____ open.
   a. foramen ovale
   b. ductus venosus
   c. ductus arteriosus
   d. crista dividens

9. Fetal hemoglobin differs from adult hemoglobin in that fetal hemoglobin contains a _____ level of 2,3-DPG.
   a. lower
   b. higher
   c. equal

10. When compared with the adult, at any given PO_2 level, the premature infant will have _____ oxygen available for release at the tissue level.
    a. more
    b. less
    c. the same amount of

Part 2
Assessment of the Newborn and Child

Chapter 3

Prenatal and Perinatal History

OBJECTIVES

Having completed this chapter, the reader will be able to:

1 Discuss the effects of maternal age on pregnancy risk.

2 Describe the features of pregnancy-induced hypertension.

3 List conditions related to uteroplacental insufficiency.

4 Describe the possible consequences of uteroplacental insufficiency.

5 Explain the possible effects of maternal diabetes on fetal development in general and on lung maturation in particular.

6 Discuss the effects of maternal alcohol, drug, and tobacco use on the fetus.

7 Describe the possible effects of maternal infection with rubella, toxoplasmosis, herpes, cytomegalovirus, hepatitis, HIV, and syphilis on the fetus.

8 List anatomic abnormalities that may increase fetal risk.

9 Describe the risks associated with multiple-gestation pregnancies.

10 List problems associated with placental function that may influence fetal outcomes.

11 Describe the risks associated with premature rupture of fetal membranes.

12 Discuss the possible effects of postmaturity.

13 List the major consequences of high-risk pregnancy.

14 Describe the major problems associated with prematurity.

15 Discuss the types of intrauterine growth retardation and the problems that this development may cause.

16 List the features and common complications of fetal asphyxia.

17 Describe the use of ultrasound imaging, urinary estriol levels, chorionic villus sampling, and amniocentesis in the assessment of the fetus.

18 Differentiate between stress and nonstress testing and identify abnormal results of each type of test.

19 Describe the process and stages of normal labor.

20 Discuss the significance of dystocia, cord prolapse, and abnormal fetal presentation to the fetus.

21 Describe the ways in which the fetus may be monitored during labor and delivery.

22 List the types of fetal heart rate patterns that may occur and discuss the significance of each pattern.

KEY TERMS

abruptio placentae
amniocentesis
breech presentation
complete breech
discordant twins
dystocia
early deceleration
eclampsia
effacement
estriol
fetal alcohol syndrome
fetal asphyxia
first stage of labor
footling breech
frank breech
gravida
infant of diabetic mother (IDM)
intrauterine growth retardation
  (IUGR)
intraventricular hemorrhage (IVH)
late deceleration
macrosomic
multiparous

nonstress testing
oligohydramnios
oxytocin challenge test
placenta previa
postmaturity
pre-eclampsia
pregnancy-induced hypertension
prematurity
presentation
primigravida
primiparous
prolapsed cord
premature rupture of membranes
  (PROM)
second stage of labor
stress testing
third stage of labor
transverse lie
twin transfusion syndrome
ultrasound
uteroplacental insufficiency
variable deceleration
vertex presentation

▬ THE HIGH-RISK MOTHER

Many factors lead to the classification of a high-risk pregnancy, including maternal age and parity; history of previous births; use of drugs, tobacco, and alcohol; maternal disease, and anatomic problems of the mother.

Maternal Age and Parity

Neonatal morbidity and mortality are affected by maternal age, with infants of both young and older women being at increased risk. The highest risk occurs if the mother is younger than 16 years of age or older than 40. The upper age limit is lower if it is a woman's first pregnancy. Parity refers to the number of pregnancies a woman has had and the number of live-born children and stillbirths she has delivered. The term *gravida* is used to refer to pregnancy. A woman who is pregnant for the first time is referred to as a **primigravida**. The term *para* refers to completion of pregnancy resulting in a potentially viable infant (more than 20 weeks of gestation). Thus, a woman who delivers for the first time is a primipara or **primiparous**, sometimes abbreviated as primip. This term is used regardless of the outcome of the pregnancy, so that whether birth results in a live or stillborn infant or whether one or more infant is delivered, the woman who delivers for the first time is a primipara. A woman who has delivered more than once is referred to as **multiparous**. In recording a maternal history, the letters "G" and "P" followed by numerals may be used to describe the number of pregnancies or gravida status (G) and the number of deliveries or parity (P). Using this system, the designation G1 P1 would indicate that a woman had one pregnancy which resulted in a potentially viable infant. Grand multiparity (*e.g.*, more than five previous pregnancies) is also associated with increased risk to the fetus.

History of Previous Births

If a mother had difficulty with previous pregnancies, she will be considered to be at high risk. Some of these previous problems include cesarean section, miscarriage, premature or postmature birth, fetal or neonatal death, an infant of high or low birth weight, and an infant requiring either intrauterine or neonatal blood transfusion.

Pregnancy-Induced Hypertension and Uteroplacental Insufficiency

Many maternal diseases are also associated with increased risk to the fetus. One of the more common is **pregnancy-induced hypertension** (PIH), which refers to any hypertension that develops during pregnancy. The severity of PIH ranges from mild hypertension requiring only careful observation to severe hypertension that threatens the life of both mother and fetus. In order to standardize the terminology used to describe PIH, the American College of Obstetricians and Gynecologists (ACOG) established definitions to be used in determining the diagnosis and severity of PIH (Table 3-1). Maternal hypertension may lead to decreased placental blood flow, resulting in **uteroplacental insufficiency** (UPI). Other causes of hypertension, such as renal disease, essential hypertension, or diabetes, may also result in UPI. In addition, UPI may occur with postmaturity, maternal cyanotic heart disease, and chronic hypoxia associated with maternal pulmonary disease. It is more likely to occur in elderly primigravidas and should be suspected when third trimester bleeding or **oligohydramnios** (deficient amount of amniotic fluid) occurs. The decrease in

TABLE 3-1   Definitions of Pregnancy-Induced Hypertension

Pregnancy-induced hypertension	BP $\geq$ 140 mm Hg systolic or $\geq$ 90 mm Hg diastolic after 20th week of gestation or rise of 30 mm Hg systolic or 15 mm Hg diastolic from prepregnant or 2nd trimester measurements of BP
Pre-eclampsia	Hypertension or rise of 30 mm Hg systolic or 15 mm Hg diastolic accompanied by proteinuria, edema, or both*
Severe pre-eclampsia	BP $\geq$ 160/110 mm Hg accompanied by proteinuria and/or edema
Eclampsia	Hypertension accompanied by seizures or coma unrelated to underlying neurologic conditions

*$\geq$ 300 mg of protein in 24-hour urine collection, or $\geq$ 2+ protein on urine dipstick on two samples collected at least 6 hours apart.

(Gant NF, Gilstrap LC: Hypertension in pregnancy. ACOG Tech Bull 219, 1996.)

intervillous blood flow associated with maternal vascular disease results in a limitation of gas and nutrient exchange across the placenta, which may lead to reduced growth of the fetus (**intrauterine growth retardation, IUGR**), intrauterine fetal death, chronic intrauterine asphyxia, or the passage of meconium into the amniotic fluid, with the subsequent possibility of meconium aspiration into the lungs of the fetus.[24]

If UPI is suspected, assessment of placental function should be performed using urinary estriol levels and evaluation of fetal heart rate patterns during fetal movement or during induced contractions. In addition, fetal lung maturity should be assessed, usually by determining the L/S ratio of amniotic fluid. Delivery of the immature fetus is avoided whenever possible. If UPI appears to be severe, however, as indicated by both falling estriol levels and abnormal fetal heart rate responses, intervention may be necessary even with an immature fetus because the fetal prognosis is very poor under these circumstances.

Maternal Diabetes Mellitus

Maternal diabetes mellitus (DM) is also associated with increased fetal risk. Some of the more common problems occurring in **infants of diabetic mothers (IDMs)** include prematurity, stillbirth, congenital anomalies such as congenital heart disease, and birth injury due to very large (**macrosomic**) infants. In addition, diabetes predisposes the mother to the development of hypertension, with the consequent possibility of UPI. The classic IDM is described as a fat, plethoric, large infant; but maternal diabetes may also result in diminished fetal growth due to placental insufficiency.

White has classified diabetes in pregnancy (Table 3-2), and this classification helps to predict fetal outcome.[29] Class A diabetes in pregnancy is characterized by mild diabetes that is controlled by diet alone, and these mothers tend to have infants that are large for their gestational age but do not usually have other problems. Class B mothers tend to have classic large infants, while Class C through F mothers are more likely to deliver infants who are of normal size or small for gestational age.

It has also been shown that maternal DM influences maturation of the fetal lungs, most likely because of the inhibiting effect of increased insulin levels on the development of the enzymes necessary for the synthesis of the phospholipid component of surfactant.[22] Less severe classes of diabetes are associated with delayed maturation of the lungs, whereas chronic intrauterine stress associated with severe DM may accelerate lung maturation.[12] This means that many of the infants seen in the nursery born to diabetic mothers are large yet premature, with lungs that are even less mature than gestational age would predict. Thus, respiratory distress syndrome is likely to occur in these infants and is an important cause of perinatal morbidity and mortality in the IDM.

Although earlier studies established a much higher rate of respiratory distress in IDMs when compared with infants of nondiabetic mothers of the same gestational age,[26] more recent studies have shown no significant difference in the incidence of respiratory distress among these two groups.[16] The decrease in the incidence of respiratory distress in IDMs is most likely due to increased emphasis on tight control of maternal diabetes.[22] In addition, IDMs tend to have increased susceptibility to infection, partly because of their prematurity but possibly related to the

TABLE 3-2   **Classification of Diabetes in Pregnancy**

	AGE AT ONSET	DURATION OF DISEASE	VASCULOPATHY
Gestational diabetes (GDM)*	During pregnancy	—	None
Class A**	Any	Variable	None
Class B***	>20 yrs old	<10 yrs	None
Class C	<20 yrs old	10–19 yrs	None
Class D	<10 yrs old	>20 yrs	None
Class F	Any	Variable	Diabetic nephropathy
Class H	Any	Variable	Cardiopathy
Class R retinopathy	Any	Variable	Proliferative

*GDM may be insulin dependent or non-insulin dependent.

**Class A diabetics are non-insulin dependent.

***Class B through R diabetics are insulin dependent.

(White P: Classification of obstetric diabetes. Am J Obstet Gynecol 130:228, 1978.)

increased incidence of urinary tract infections in the diabetic mother. They are also likely to manifest hypoglycemia, hypocalcemia, and hyperbilirubinemia in the neonatal period.[8]

Alcohol, Drugs, and Tobacco

The maternal use of alcohol, drugs, and tobacco is also associated with increased risk to the fetus. Smoking more than one pack of cigarettes per day is associated with an increased risk of spontaneous abortion and low birth weight, with their coinciding problems. Although acute alcohol consumption before delivery may cause withdrawal symptoms such as tremors and seizures in the newborn, it does not result in fetal abnormality. Chronic alcohol consumption during pregnancy is much more ominous, often resulting in the **fetal alcohol syndrome**, which is characterized by low birth weight, fetal wasting, and various developmental disorders including abnormal brain development and cardiac anomalies.[5]

Other drugs consumed by the mother may affect the fetus. Those that most commonly affect respiration are the sedative drugs, including those given during labor, which may result in depression of respiration in the newborn. Maternal narcotic addiction may result in withdrawal symptoms in the infant, including tremors, dyspnea, cyanosis, convulsions, and death and may also cause IUGR.[11]

Maternal Infections

Maternal infections, transmitted to the infant in utero or during delivery, may also result in increased risk of abnormal fetal outcome. Although many infectious processes may compromise the fetus, the most notable examples include rubella, toxoplasmosis, herpes, cytomegalovirus, syphilis, human immunodeficiency virus (HIV), and hepatitis. The TORCH acronym (T = toxoplasma, O = others, R = rubella, C = cytomegalovirus, H = herpes simplex virus) was introduced in the 1970s as a diagnostic approach in infants with suspected congenital infection.[20]

Rubella infection is associated with a wide range of outcomes, including intrauterine death and severe multiple organ-system disease. Most commonly, though, rubella infection results in no obvious neonatal disease, although most of these symptom-free neonates will develop later evidence of infection. Common disorders seen in infants born with effects of rubella infection include cardiac defects, cataracts, and deafness. Rubella infection is also associated with IUGR. The most serious outcomes are usually associated with infection early in pregnancy.[23]

Toxoplasmosis is caused by a protozoa (*Toxoplasma gondii*) that may be acquired from consumption of contaminated raw or undercooked meat or from oral contact with contaminated cat feces or soil. Maternal infection is difficult to diagnose because it rarely causes symptoms more specific than swelling of the lymph glands. Congenital infection may result in various fetal outcomes, including inflammation of the eye, anemia, convulsions, jaundice, splenomegaly and hepatomegaly, hydrocephalus, and pneumonia. Varying degrees of sight loss, including blindness, and retarded psychomotor development are not uncommon.[1]

Cytomegalovirus (CMV) infection, like toxoplasmosis, is difficult to recognize in the adult. Infection of the fetus may result in a broad spectrum of neonatal disorders, including bleeding disorders, central nervous system (CNS) disorders that may cause apnea or seizures, hyperbilirubinemia, and pneumonia. IUGR may also occur.[25]

Herpes simplex virus occurs in two strains, called types 1 and 2. Type 2 is sexually transmitted and infects the genitalia. The infant usually acquires herpes infection during birth by contact with infected genital secretions or by vertical transmission from the mother to the fetus following rupture of the membranes. Recognition of maternal disease is often difficult because the infection does not always result in noticeable symptoms. Disease in the neonate falls into one of two classes: disseminated or localized.[21] Disseminated disease affects almost every organ system, including the lungs, and is associated with a high mortality rate. Localized disease most commonly affects the CNS, eyes, and skin and is much less likely to cause death. Since infection is rarely acquired in the presence of intact membranes, cesarean section is recommended in the presence of active genital infection to avoid perinatal infection of the newborn.

Maternal syphilis, a sexually transmitted disease caused by the spirochetal bacteria *Treponema pallidum*, is relatively easy to detect using antibody testing of maternal blood. Unfortunately, clinical manifestations of this disease are often overlooked, and many women (specifically, those most likely to harbor this infection) do not avail themselves of prenatal care and thus of the opportunity for blood testing for syphilis. Clinical features of congenital syphilis include intrauterine death, prematurity, hepatitis, hyperbilirubinemia, hepatosplenomegaly, CNS abnormalities, skin lesions, bone disorders, and, occasionally, pneumonia.[25]

It is estimated that from 1 to 8 of every 1000 pregnant women in the United States carry the HIV virus that causes acquired immunodeficiency syndrome (AIDS).[17] Asymptomatic HIV infection does not appear to alter the course of a pregnancy. Clinical maternal AIDS infection exposes the fetus to a greater risk of hepatitis, CMV, toxoplasmosis, and tuberculosis.[6,30] Transmission of HIV to the fetus is probably more common in women with symptomatic AIDS.[18]

Neonatal hepatitis B virus (HBV) infections are acquired at the time of delivery as a result of exposure of the infant to maternal blood. Most of these infants will be asymptomatic, although they may develop persistent infection and become chronic carriers of HBV.[19] The long-term consequences of neonatal HBV are unknown, although it is suspected that these infants are at risk of developing chronic liver disease.

Anatomic Abnormalities

Maternal anatomic abnormalities such as a small bony pelvis, uterine malformations, and incompetent cervix may increase fetal risk. The risk of birth trauma is increased if the bony pelvis is small, and cesarean section delivery may be necessary. Uterine malformations and incompetent cervix may increase the risk of premature delivery of the infant.

▬OTHER RISK FACTORS

Several other factors may increase fetal risk, including multiple gestation, problems with the placenta, premature rupture of the membranes, and postmaturity.

Multiple Gestation

Perinatal mortality is increased among twins, with identical twins (splitting of a single fertilized egg) having higher risk than fraternal twins (fertilization of two eggs). The most common event affecting multiple gestation pregnancies is prematurity. In addition, problems of the placenta and cord occur more frequently, as does IUGR. In some twin births, one placenta is considerably smaller than the other, and the twin supported by this placenta is markedly smaller. This occurrence is referred to as **discordant twins**, and the birth weights may differ by as much as 1000 grams. Abnormal fetal presentation, particularly breech, is also more common in twins.

Another problem that sometimes occurs in multiple-gestation pregnancies is the **twin transfusion syndrome**, also called the intrauterine parabiotic syndrome, in which the circulation of the fetuses are connected. This allows for transfer of blood from one fetus to the other, resulting in one twin with polycythemia and one with anemia. The polycythemic (recipient) twin may have congestive heart failure caused by volume overload and is also more susceptible to increased bilirubin levels because there are more red cells available for hemolysis. The anemic (donor) twin may suffer from IUGR and be in shock at delivery due to acute and dramatic blood loss to the other twin.

Congenital anomalies occur twice as frequently in twins compared to single births,[28] perhaps due to the same factors that caused twinning to occur. The anomalies may include cardiac defects, cleft lip and palate, tracheoesophageal fistula, and conjoined twins.

Placental Problems

Problems that affect the placenta include abnormal implantation, referred to as **placenta previa**, and abnormal separation, called **abruptio placentae** or placental abruption. Normally, the placenta is implanted in the upper wall of the uterus; in placenta previa, it is implanted in the lower wall. Three types of placenta previa occur: in total placenta previa, the placenta completely covers the cervical opening of the uterus; in partial placenta previa, the cervix is partially occluded by the placenta; and in low implantation, the cervix is not occluded at all, although the placenta is implanted very close to the cervical opening. The major problems resulting from placenta previa are an increased incidence of premature labor and early separation of the placenta, since the lower uterine segment thins and the cervix dilates during the early stages of labor. Early placental separation reduces fetal–maternal gas exchange and may result in fetal asphyxia.

Placenta previa can be identified by ultrasound examination, although many previas diagnosed during the second trimester of pregnancy will migrate upward and not cause problems at term. The most common symptom of placenta previa is painless, bright red vaginal bleeding not accompanied by uterine contractions that occurs after 8 weeks' gestation. Maternal and fetal hemorrhage may occur, although the greatest risk to the fetus is premature delivery. If severe bleeding is present, emergency cesarean section is performed because of the risk of extreme blood loss to the mother and fetus. In less severe cases, the mother is stabilized and carefully observed, with assessments of fetal condition performed frequently. If possible, delivery is postponed until fetal lung maturity is established.

Abruptio placentae involves premature separation of a normally implanted placenta. When the placenta separates at its margin, referred to as marginal abruption, bleeding occurs along the uterine wall and ultimately presents as vaginal bleeding, although in some instances, bleeding is confined to the uterine cavity and may be concealed. Bleeding may also occur in the central portion of the placenta, but this does not usually result in vaginal bleeding and is thus more difficult to recognize. Onset of placental separation may also be accompanied by severe pain, uterine contractions, nausea, and maternal hypotension, depending on the amount of blood loss. Both types of abruption increase the incidence of fetal asphyxia and premature delivery, as well as fetal hemorrhage and shock. As with placenta previa, management of abruptio placentae involves weighing the risk to the mother and fetus of severe blood loss against the complications of premature delivery.

Premature Rupture of Membranes

Premature rupture of membranes (PROM) increases the likelihood of fetal infection, especially pneumonia. Generally, rupture is considered premature if it occurs more than 24 hours before delivery of the infant. Early rupture with prolonged labor further increases the risk of fetal infection. PROM is more likely to occur in premature infants than in full-term infants. At this point, the relative risks of infection versus premature delivery must be considered. If the risk of infection appears high, as judged by maternal fever or infected amniotic fluid, acceleration of fetal lung maturity with steroids followed by delivery of the fetus may be indicated.

Postmaturity

An infant delivered after the 42nd week of gestation is defined as **postmature**. Placental function begins to decline after term, and these infants are often small for gestational age with signs of wasting. Physical signs of postmaturity include dry, cracked skin; long nails; excessive scalp hair; and loose skin, caused by loss of subcutaneous fat. Postmature infants also may have meconium staining of the skin, nails, and umbilical cord. This decline in placental function, in addition to diminished fetal growth, predisposes the postmature infant to intrauterine asphyxia and death. These infants do not tolerate the stress of labor well, since labor interferes with an already malfunctioning placental circulation. Assessment of the postmature fetus may involve amniocentesis, urinary estriol testing, and stress testing to determine placental function. Meconium staining of fluid, oligohydramnios, poor response to stress testing, and falling estriol levels may all indicate that placental function is impaired and that delivery, either by induction of labor or by cesarean section, is indicated.

▀CONSEQUENCES OF INCREASED FETAL RISK

The major consequences to the fetus who is determined to be at risk because of any of these factors include prematurity, IUGR, and asphyxia.

Prematurity

Prematurity is defined as delivery before the end of the 37th week of gestation. Although most premature infants are of low birth weight, not all low–birth-weight infants are premature. Thus, classification of prematurity by gestational age rather than by birth weight is appropriate.

Premature infants have the highest infant mortality rate, which is inversely proportional to gestational age (*i.e.*, the lower the gestational age, the higher the mortality). The major problem of prematurity is with the respiratory system. The surface area for gas exchange develops rapidly during the last weeks of gestation, as does the mature form of pulmonary surfactant. Both of these are necessary for adequate extrauterine respiratory function. Impaired gas exchange caused by inadequate surfactant is referred to as hyaline membrane disease (HMD) or respiratory distress syndrome (RDS) and is discussed in Chapter 9. In addition to respiratory problems, premature infants have difficulties in absorbing nutrients from the digestive tract; problems with thermoregulation due to an increased rate of heat loss; poor defenses against infection; poor tissue perfusion due to immature capillary development; and an increased incidence of hemorrhage, particularly into and around the ventricles of the brain (**intraventricular hemorrhage [IVH]**). The most common disorders occurring in the premature infant are thus HMD, asphyxia, and infection.

Intrauterine Growth Retardation

IUGR is also referred to as small for gestational age (SGA) or small-for-dates. These terms do not imply anything about the maturity of the infant, nor do they identify the cause of the diminished growth rate of the fetus. The type of growth retardation that occurs depends on when the factors causing diminished growth occur during pregnancy. If the insult occurs early in pregnancy, when fetal growth occurs primarily because of formation of new cells, growth retardation will manifest as hypoplasia. In this type of growth retardation, described as hypoplastic IUGR, fewer new cells are formed and organs are small and underweight. Infants with hypoplastic IUGR have uniform reduction of head and body size, with all measurements of fetal growth (head circumference, body weight, and body length) falling below the tenth percentile. This is usually a result of insults beginning early in pregnancy or occurring throughout pregnancy, such as chronic maternal malnutrition or intrauterine infection. These infants appear small but proportionate, with skin that may be slightly thickened. They are usually quite active and often have major congenital malformations.

Later in pregnancy, fetal growth occurs primarily as a result of increase in the size of cells rather than number. Growth retardation then causes underweight organs with a normal number of cells that are reduced in size and is referred to as hypotrophic IUGR. The growth of the brain tends to be normal if the insult occurs late in pregnancy. These infants often appear to have an oversized head, although they actually have normal-sized heads and undergrown bodies. They often have loose, dry skin, little subcutaneous fat, and sparse scalp hair and appear more active than expected for their birth weight. The most common causes of this type of IUGR are disorders that interfere with placental blood flow, such as pregnancy-induced hypertension and maternal renal disease.

Growth-retarded infants may have several problems during the newborn period. They are often chronically hypoxic in utero; they thus have difficulty withstanding the stress of labor and often develop asphyxia. Intrauterine hypoxia also predisposes these infants to meconium aspiration, which is apparently due to hypoxic stimulation of meconium release by the fetus and reflex gasping respirations in utero. Hypoglycemia occurs frequently and these infants have more difficulty than appropriately sized infants in the conservation of body heat. Cerebral edema occurs more commonly due to chronic intrauterine asphyxia and birth asphyxia.

Most infants with IUGR are term infants who are small for gestational age. These infants have a higher mortality than do appropriately grown term infants, but not as high as low–birth-weight preterm infants, who have the highest mortality rates. Mortality rates are also affected by the type of IUGR (hypoplastic or hypotrophic) and by associated congenital defects.

Asphyxia

Fetal asphyxia is most commonly associated with impaired maternal blood flow to the placenta, and it results in hypoxia, hypercarbia, and both metabolic and respiratory acidosis. Fetal heart rate monitoring and scalp blood sampling are helpful in the assessment of fetal asphyxia. The passage of meconium-stained amniotic fluid also suggests fetal asphyxia, and meconium aspiration may occur. Other signs of asphyxia include oligohydramnios and reduced fetal breathing and body movements. Hypoxemia associated with asphyxia may result in several types of brain injury, including cerebral edema and necrosis, intraventricular hemorrhage, and subarachnoid hemorrhage. The conditions commonly associated with prematurity, IUGR, and asphyxia are listed in Table 3-3.

▰FETAL ASSESSMENT

When a fetus is determined to be at risk, several methods of assessment may be useful, including ultrasound imaging of the fetus, measurement of maternal urinary estriol levels, amniocentesis, nonstress testing, and stress or oxytocin challenge testing.

TABLE 3-3 Conditions Associated With Prematurity, IUGR, and Asphyxia

---

Prematurity

Abruptio placentae	Placenta previa
Diabetes	PROM
Incompetent cervix	Pregnancy-induced hypertension
Multiple gestation	

IUGR

Advanced diabetes	Intrauterine infection
Alcohol consumption	Malnutrition
Cigarette smoking	Multiple gestation
Chronic renal disease	Single umbilical artery
Essential hypertension	Pregnancy-induced hypertension

Asphyxia

Abnormal fetal presentation	Placenta previa
Abruptio placentae	Postmaturity
Cord prolapse	Prematurity
Hypertension	Pulmonary disease
Meconium staining	Prolonged labor
Multiple gestation	Single umbilical artery
	Pregnancy-induced hypertension

Ultrasound Imaging

Ultrasound imaging involves transmission of high-frequency sound waves from a scanner in contact with the maternal abdominal wall. The sound waves are reflected back from the various organs and tissues, creating a visual image that can be converted to a permanent photographic record. In addition to still photographic images, a "moving picture" can be generated, called real-time imaging, which allows the observation of fetal movement and the assessment of fetal heart and respiratory activity.[9] One of the most helpful uses of ultrasound imaging is in estimating fetal age, particularly when the date of conception is uncertain or when the mother's weight gain or fetal growth does not correlate closely with the estimated fetal age. The ultrasound estimate of fetal age during the first 12 weeks is determined by measuring the crown–rump length. After 12 weeks, the biparietal diameter (BPD) of the fetal skull and fetal femur length become the most accurate estimates of fetal age, with a predictive accuracy of 7 days at 16 weeks' gestation, increasing to 21 days at 40 weeks.[4] Ultrasound examination of the fetus is also helpful in the evaluation of multiple gestation, fetal position, and location of the placenta and in monitoring fetal growth during the course of the pregnancy. Many congenital anomalies can also be detected by ultrasound examination, including abnormalities of the brain, heart and cardiovascular system, thorax, abdomen, and urinary tract.

Urinary Estriol
Estriol is a steroid that is processed in the fetal liver and then transferred across the placenta and excreted in maternal urine. Estriol levels normally increase throughout pregnancy with advancing gestational age, especially in the third trimester. The patterns of excretion are evaluated and compared with normal patterns for the estimated gestational age of the fetus. If the estriol levels are normal or consistently elevated, placental function is assumed to be normal. A falling estriol level is a poor prognostic sign, often preceding fetal death. A chronically low estriol level may indicate chronic uteroplacental insufficiency or an inaccurate estimation of gestational age. If the estriol level is falling or chronically low, further testing is usually indicated.[13]

Alpha Fetoprotein Measurement
Alpha fetoprotein (AFP) is the main serum protein of the developing fetus. Discontinuity of the fetal skin, as occurs in spina bifida or anencephaly, allows AFP to leak from exposed tissues into the amniotic fluid. From there, AFP passes across the fetal membranes and placenta into the maternal circulation, where its level can be easily measured.[14] Elevated maternal serum levels of AFP may indicate the presence of a neural tube defect in the fetus, and although elevated AFP levels are not diagnostic alone, more extensive testing is indicated. Measurement of maternal serum AFP is used as a screening test for neural tube defects, particularly in older mothers.

Amniocentesis
Amniocentesis involves the withdrawal of a sample of amniotic fluid through the maternal abdominal wall. Assessment of amniotic fluid for fetal lung maturity through measurement of the L/S ratio is discussed in Chapter 1. Additionally, amniotic fluid may be examined for bilirubin concentration, creatinine levels, and cellular abnormalities.

Bilirubin is a byproduct of the breakdown of red blood cells. In maternal–fetal Rh incompatibility (fetal erythroblastosis), hemolysis occurs at an excessive rate and increased amounts of bilirubin are present in the amniotic fluid. Bilirubin concentrations measured in amniotic fluid can be compared against normal values and the severity of disease estimated.[3] Severe disease may require intrauterine blood transfusion of the fetus or interruption of the pregnancy. Milder disease can be monitored with repeated amniocentesis for bilirubin levels.

Creatinine levels in amniotic fluid increase throughout pregnancy with advancing gestational age. In uncomplicated pregnancies, creatinine levels may be used to assess fetal maturity. Unfortunately, creatinine levels are not reliable in many high-risk situations, such as pregnancy-induced hypertension, diabetes, and Rh disease.[27]

The amniotic fluid also contains cells that have been shed by the developing fetus. These cells can be examined to determine the presence of genetically transmitted disorders, such as Down's syndrome. In addition, the sex of the fetus can be determined from cellular examination, which may be of consequence in sex-linked inherited disorders such as hemophilia.

Chorionic Villus Sampling

Chorionic villus sampling (CVS) is a method of obtaining placental tissue for prenatal assessment of the fetus that provides an alternative to amniocentesis. Under ultrasonic visualization, a catheter is inserted through the mother's cervix and directed into the placenta. Tissue is then aspirated through the catheter into a syringe. This fetal tissue can provide information regarding fetal chromosomal defects.

Nonstress Testing

Nonstress testing is based on the association of changes in fetal heart rate with fetal movement. Fetal heart rate is recorded externally through the maternal abdominal wall. A normal pattern consists of acceleration (increases) of the fetal heart rate during fetal movement and is described as a reactive test. If this does not occur, the pattern is considered abnormal and is described as a nonreactive test. Nonstress testing is a very useful screening test because it does not involve administration of any drugs and is harmless to the mother and fetus. If a normal pattern is recorded, the fetus is not at significant risk for asphyxia and there is probably no need for further testing. In the presence of a nonreactive test, the test may be repeated later that day or early the next day. Following two consecutive nonreactive tests, stress testing may be indicated.[7]

Stress Testing

Stress testing, also called **oxytocin challenge testing** (OCT), is used to assess the ability of the placenta to remain functional during uterine contractions, and thus the ability of the fetus to withstand the stresses of labor and delivery. As with the nonstress test, fetal heart rate is recorded externally. In addition, uterine contractions are recorded externally through a pressure-sensitive device strapped to the abdominal wall. After measurement of fetal heart rate in the resting state, oxytocin is administered. Oxytocin (Pitocin, Syntocinon) stimulates contraction of the uterus and is administered in increasing dosages until uterine contractions occur. The fetal heart rate is monitored during this process. A negative (normal) test occurs if the fetal heart rate is stable and is very reassuring. A positive (abnormal) test occurs if the fetal heart rate decelerates after the onset of uterine contractions (late deceleration pattern); this pattern is associated with uteroplacental insufficiency and may indicate fetal jeopardy.[24] Stress testing is not usually performed in women with placenta previa or vaginal bleeding, or in any woman at high risk for premature labor.

▬LABOR AND DELIVERY

Labor begins with the onset of uterine contractions and ends with the delivery of the placenta. It is usually divided into three stages. In the **first stage of labor**, contractions are widely spaced. The uterine wall begins to differentiate into a thick upper segment and a thin lower segment; the upper segment supplies most of the force of contraction, thus helping to apply the force necessary for descent of the fetus into the birth canal. Cervical **effacement** (thinning of the cervical wall and incorporation into the uterine wall) occurs and the cervix dilates. As dilation progresses to completion, the **second stage of labor** begins. Fetal descent occurs primarily during this stage, due to uterine contractions and increased abdominal pressure caused by voluntary contractions of abdominal muscles by the mother. The face and shoulders of the fetus rotate to accommodate the dimensions of the birth canal. In a normal vaginal delivery, the head presents first with the face down, then the shoulders, and, rapidly, the rest of the body. The cord is cut and the infant begins extrauterine life. The **third stage of labor** involves separation of the placenta from the uterine wall and continued contractions until the placenta is delivered.

Dystocia

Dystocia refers to difficult or prolonged labor. The first stage of labor may last for many hours, but the second stage should not last for more than an hour or two. It is normally longer in primiparas. If labor is abnormally prolonged, early placental separation is more likely, thus reducing the surface area for gas exchange to the fetus and predisposing the fetus to asphyxia. In addition, compression of the cord is more likely, which also reduces gas exchange and contributes to the development of asphyxia.

Cord Prolapse

Prolapse of the umbilical cord occurs when the cord advances through the cervical opening and is compressed between fetal and maternal parts. Visible prolapse occurs when the cord can be seen in advance of the fetus through the cervical opening, and occult prolapse occurs when cord compression is evident but the cord cannot be visualized. Some compression of the cord occurs commonly during labor and delivery and is usually harmless; however, if cord compression is prolonged, oxygen delivery to the fetus is compromised and severe asphyxia is likely. Fetal heart rate monitoring reveals a pattern of variable decelerations (*i.e.*, decelerations not related to uterine contractions) during cord compression and is thus a useful monitoring procedure in cord prolapse. Cord prolapse is more likely to occur in abnormal fetal presentations, such as breech or transverse lie; with multiple gestation; and in premature rupture of the membranes.

Fetal Presentation

The normal presentation of the fetus is head first, called the **vertex presentation**. This occurs in almost all deliveries. Several abnormal types of presentations may occur, all of which present an increased risk to the fetus. The most common abnormal presentation is **breech**, which has several variations. **Frank breech** occurs when the buttocks present first; **complete breech** involves presentation of both the buttocks and the lower extremities; and **footling breech** or incomplete breech involves presentation of the lower extremities first.

Breech deliveries carry a much higher mortality than vertex deliveries because of the increased risk of trauma and asphyxia. Trauma most commonly occurs to the infant's head due to sustained pressure from contractions and may result in intracranial bleeding with subsequent permanent brain damage or death. Compression of a prolapsed cord is much more common in breech presentation and may result in fetal asphyxia. In addition, breech presentation is more common in the presence of placenta previa, which may further increase the risk of asphyxia. Face and shoulder presentations may also occur, which may prolong labor, since fetal passage through the birth canal is difficult in this position. A shoulder presentation occurs when the fetus is in a **transverse** position rather than a vertical position. Fetal passage is impaired and labor prolonged. If the position of the fetus cannot be corrected, cesarean section may be performed to avoid fetal asphyxia and excessive trauma to the mother.

Membranes
Rupture of membranes may occur spontaneously during labor or may be artificially performed by the obstetrician. Membranes may also rupture well before the onset of labor, leading to increased risk of fetal infection. When the membranes rupture, the amniotic fluid should be examined carefully. Foul-smelling, discolored amniotic fluid may be indicative of an infectious process, whereas meconium passage into the amniotic fluid may cause discoloration of the fluid or obvious observation of meconium itself in the fluid.

Fetal Monitoring
Fetuses who have been identified as high risk should be monitored closely during labor and delivery. A significant number of vulnerable fetuses are not identified in advance as high risk; these fetuses tolerate the stress of labor poorly. Thus, fetal monitoring has become commonplace for most deliveries, regardless of previous assessment of fetal risk. The most common method used to monitor the fetus during labor is fetal heart rate (FHR) monitoring. Before rupture of the membranes, external monitoring must be used. This procedure is the same as that used in stress testing during pregnancy. After rupture of the membranes, direct fetal monitoring can be employed, which involves placement of a monitoring electrode directly on the fetal presenting part (usually the scalp) to record fetal heart rate, and placement of a pressure-monitoring device directly into the uterus to record uterine contractions. This method is more accurate than external monitoring. Accelerations of FHR during labor are reassuring. The three most significant deceleration patterns observed during fetal heart rate monitoring are early deceleration, late deceleration, and variable deceleration (Fig. 3-1).[15]

Early deceleration (Type I) means that FHR decreases at the same time that uterine contractions occur and returns to normal (120 to 160 beats/min) between contractions. This is thought to be due to stimulation of the vagus nerve following compression of the head and does not seem to have any clinical significance or to be associated with any increase in abnormal fetal outcomes.

Late deceleration (Type II) means that FHR decreases after the onset of a contraction and returns to normal after the contraction has ended. Thus, the deceleration lags behind the uterine contractions. This is believed to be due to impaired maternal blood flow to the placenta and is associated with uteroplacental insufficiency. It is often associated with fetal asphyxia and low Apgar scores. Administration of oxygen to the mother may help to correct this, as well as attention to maternal hemodynamic status.

Variable deceleration (Type III) means that there is no relationship between uterine contractions and decreases in fetal heart rate. This is the most common deceleration pattern and is believed to be caused by com-

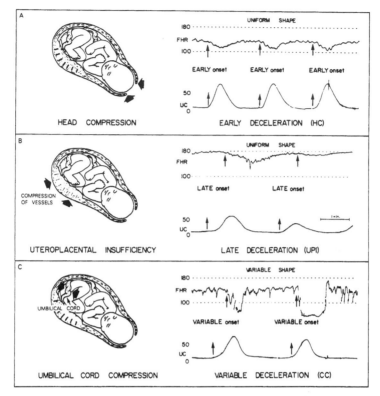

FIGURE 3-1   Fetal heart rate patterns. (Avery GB: Noeonatology: Pathophysiology and Management of the Newborn, 2nd ed, p 123. Philadelphia, JB Lippincott, 1981)

pression of the umbilical cord by fetal parts. Most fetuses can tolerate short periods of cord compression, but longer periods usually result in asphyxia. Changes in maternal position often help to alleviate this problem.

Fetal Scalp Monitoring

Another method of monitoring fetal status during labor is the sampling and analysis of fetal capillary blood.[2] A blood sample is drawn from the presenting fetal part (usually the scalp) and the pH of the blood is measured. Normally, fetal blood pH falls somewhat during labor owing to the transient effects of contractions on maternal–fetal gas exchange. The pH at the beginning of labor is usually about 7.35, falling to 7.25 as the second stage of labor progresses. If the pH falls below 7.20, fetal distress is likely.

There are two types of situations that cause the pH to fall. Interference with placental blood flow inhibits the removal of carbon dioxide from the fetus, resulting in increased serum carbon dioxide levels and decreased pH (respiratory acidosis). This probably accounts for the normal drop in pH seen during routine deliveries. If, however, interference with blood flow is prolonged, oxygen levels supplied to the fetus will drop to dangerously low levels. The fetus will no longer be able to carry out metabolism through normal aerobic pathways and will revert to secondary pathways operative in the absence of oxygen (anaerobic metabolism). One of the end products of the anaerobic pathway is lactic acid, which builds up in the fetal blood and produces lactic acidosis, accounting for the severe drops in pH seen in fetal asphyxia.

Fetal scalp blood sampling and analysis are usually reserved for those cases in which the fetus has demonstrated an abnormal response to labor, such as a late deceleration pattern, or in which the fetus is known to be at high risk of asphyxia for various reasons previously discussed.

Monitoring of fetal scalp pH by means of an electrode attached to the scalp has been proposed. This would allow continuous monitoring of the infant during the later stages of delivery.[14]

■REFERENCES

1. Alford CA, Stagno S, Reynolds DW: Congenital toxoplasmosis: Clinical, laboratory and therapeutic considerations, with special reference to subclinical disease. Bull NY Acad Med 50:160, 1974.
2. Beard RW, Morris ED, Clayton SG: pH of fetal capillary blood as an indicator of the condition of the fetus. J Obstet Gynaecol Br Commonw 74:812, 1967.
3. Bowman JM, Pollack JM: Amniotic fluid spectrophotometry and early delivery in the management of erythroblastosis fetalis. Pediatrics 35:815, 1965.
4. Campbell S, Newan GB: Growth of the fetal biparietal diameter during normal pregnancy. Br J Obstet Gynaecol 78:513, 1971.
5. Clarren SK, Smith DK: The fetal alcohol syndrome. N Engl J Med 298:1063, 1978.
6. Cotton P: Medicine's arsenal in battling "dominant dozen," other AIDS-associated opportunistic infections. JAMA 266:1664, 1991.
7. Everston L, Paul RH: Antepartum fetal heart disease testing: The nonstress test. Am J Obstet Gynecol 132:895, 1978.
8. Fletcher AB: The infant of the diabetic mother. In Avery GB (ed): Neonatology: Pathophysiology and Management of the Newborn, 2nd ed. Philadelphia, JB Lippincott, 1981.
9. Fox HE, Hohler CW: Fetal evaluation by real-time imaging. Clin Obstet Gynecol 20:339, 1977.
10. Gant NF, Gilstrap LC: Hypertension in pregnancy. ACOG Tech Bull 219, 1996.
11. Giacoia GP, Yaffe SJ: Drugs and the perinatal patient. In Avery GB (ed): Neonatology: Pathophysiology and Management of the Newborn, 2nd ed. Philadelphia, JB Lippincott, 1981.
12. Gluck L, Kulovich MV: Lecithin/sphingomyelin ratios in amniotic fluid in normal and abnormal pregnancy. Am J Obstet Gynecol 115:539, 1973.
13. Greene JW, Beargie RA: The use of urinary estriol excretion studies in the assessment of the high-risk pregnancy. Pediatr Clin North Am 17:43, 1970.
14. Greene MF: Fetal assessment. In Cloherty JP, Stark AR: Manual of Neonatal Care, 2nd ed. Boston, Little, Brown, 1985.
15. Hon EH: An Atlas of Fetal Heart Rate Patterns. New Haven, Harty Press, 1968.
16. Hunter DJ, Burrows RF, Mohide PT, Whyte RK: Influence of maternal insulin-dependent diabetes mellitus on neonatal morbidity. Can Med Assoc 149:47, 1993.
17. Killam AP: The impact of maternal illness. In Avery GB, Fletcher MA, MacDonald MG (eds): Neonatology: Pathophysiology and Management of the Newborn, 4th ed. Philadelphia, JB Lippincott, 1994.
18. MacGregor SN: Human immunodeficiency virus in pregnancy. Clin Perinatol 18:33, 1991.
19. Modlin JF: Perinatal viral infections and toxoplasmosis. In Cloherty JP, Stark AR: Manual of Neonatal Care, 2nd ed. Boston, Little, Brown, 1985.
20. Nahmias AJ: The TORCH complex. Hospital Practice 9:65, 1974.
21. Nahmias AJ, Visintine AM: Herpes simplex. In Remington JS, Klein JO (eds): Infectious Diseases of the Fetus and Newborn Infant. Philadelphia, WB Saunders, 1976.
22. Ogata ES. Carbohydrate homeostasis. In Avery GB, Fletcher MA, MacDonald MG (eds): Neonatology: Pathophysiology and Management of the Newborn, 4th ed. Philadelphia, JB Lippincott, 1994.

23. Peckham GS: Clinical and laboratory study of children exposed in utero to maternal rubella. Arch Dis Child 47:571, 1972.
24. Quilligan EJ, Nochimson DJ, Freeman RK: Management of the high-risk pregnancy. In Avery GB (ed): Neonatology: Pathophysiology and Management of the Newborn, 2nd ed. Philadelphia, JB Lippincott, 1981.
25. Reynolds DW, Stagno S, Alford CA: Chronic congenital and perinatal infections. In Avery GB (ed): Neonatology: Pathophysiology and Management of the Newborn, 2nd ed. Philadelphia, JB Lippincott, 1981.
26. Robert MF, Neff RK, Hubbell JP, Taeusch HW, Avery ME: Association between maternal diabetes and the respiratory distress syndrome in the newborn. N Engl J Med 294:357, 1976.
27. Roopnarinesingh S: Amniotic fluid creatinine in normal and abnormal pregnancies. Obstet Gynaecol Br 77:785, 1970.
28. Stark AR: Twins. In Cloherty JP, Stark AR: Manual of Neonatal Care, 2nd ed. Boston, Little, Brown, 1985.
29. White P: Classification of obstetric diabetes. Am J Obstet Gynecol 130:228, 1978.
30. Working group on HIV testing of pregnant women and newborns: HIV infection, pregnant women, and newborns: A policy proposal for information and testing. JAMA 264:2416, 1990.

▬ BIBLIOGRAPHY

Harrison MR, Golbs MS, Filly RA: The Unborn Patient: Prenatal Diagnosis and Treatment. Orlando, FL, Grune and Stratton, 1984.
Harvey CJ: Critical Care Obstetrical Nursing. Gaithersburg, MD, Aspen, 1991.
Hon EH, Koh KS: Management of labor and delivery. In Avery GB (ed): Neonatology: Pathophysiology and Management of the Newborn, 2nd ed. Philadelphia, JB Lippincott, 1981.
Korones SB: High-Risk Newborn Infants, 3rd ed. St Louis, CV Mosby, 1981.
Lubchenco LO: The High Risk Infant. Philadelphia, WB Saunders, 1976.
Quilligan EJ, Nochimson DJ, Freeman RK: Management of the high-risk pregnancy. In Avery GB (ed): Neonatology: Pathophysiology and Management of the Newborn, 2nd ed. Philadelphia, JB Lippincott, 1981.

▬ SELF-ASSESSMENT QUESTIONS

1. Which of the following factors does *not* increase the risk of neonatal morbidity and mortality?
   a. increasing maternal age
   b. maternal drug abuse
   c. placenta previa
   d. vertex presentation

2. Infants of diabetic mothers are at increased risk of
   a. hypocalcemia
   b. hypoglycemia
   c. infection
   d. all of the above

3. The most common event affecting multiple pregnancies is
   a. abruptio placentae
   b. prematurity
   c. oligohydramnios
   d. infection

4. When the placenta implants in the lower uterine wall and completely covers the cervical opening, this is described as
   a. abruptio placentae
   b. partial placenta previa
   c. total placenta previa
   d. low implantation

5. Onset of abruptio placentae may be accompanied by
   a. uterine contractions
   b. vaginal bleeding
   c. severe pain
   d. all of the above

6. The greatest risk to the postmature fetus is
   a. declining placental function
   b. meconium aspiration
   c. infection
   d. falling estriol levels

7. Fetal asphyxia may result in
   a. hypoxia
   b. metabolic alkalosis
   c. hypocarbia
   d. respiratory alkalosis

8. The ultrasound estimate of fetal age during the first 12 weeks of gestation is determined by measuring the
   a. biparietal diameter
   b. crown–rump length
   c. femur length
   d. all of the above

9. Decreases in maternal urinary estriol levels may indicate
   a. maternal hypotension
   b. abnormal presentation
   c. maternal diabetes
   d. uteroplacental insufficiency

10. Decreases in fetal heart rate during uterine contractions that return to normal between contractions are referred to as
    a. Type I decelerations
    b. Type II decelerations
    c. Type III decelerations
    d. Type IV decelerations

Chapter 4

Physical Examination of the Newborn

OBJECTIVES

Having completed this chapter, the reader will be able to:

1 Describe the Apgar scoring system.
2 Interpret Apgar scores and suggest appropriate treatment.
3 Describe the criteria used in the assessment of gestational age and the assessment of appropriateness of intrauterine growth.
4 Describe the normal respiratory rate and pattern of a newborn.
5 State the normal range for heart rate for the newborn.
6 List the most common causes of newborn tachycardia and bradycardia.
7 Describe the use of the apical impulse in the evaluation of the newborn.
8 Recognize normal blood pressure ranges for the newborn.
9 Describe temperature assessment in the newborn.
10 List and describe the most common signs of respiratory distress in the newborn.
11 Describe normal breath sounds in the newborn.
12 Discuss the difficulties associated with auscultation of the newborn.
13 Recognize the significance of abnormalities in breath sounds.
14 Describe the procedure for examination of the head, face, and neck of the newborn.
15 Describe the procedure for examination of the abdomen, skin, and extremities of the newborn.

KEY TERMS

acrocyanosis	rales
apnea	rhonchi
Colorado intrauterine growth curve	scarf sign
heel-to-ear sign	see-saw respirations
New Ballard Score	square window
periodic breathing	tachypnea

THE APGAR SCORING SYSTEM

Evaluation of the newborn begins as soon as the infant is delivered. While standard care procedures following delivery are being performed, including bulb suction of the upper airway, drying and warming of the infant, and cutting and clamping of the cord, a preliminary assessment is done. The most important observation is the infant's heart rate. Additionally, the infant's respiratory effort, skin color, and response to handling and stimulation are evaluated. These parameters are incorporated into a standardized evaluation system developed by Dr. Virginia Apgar in the 1950s, commonly referred to as the Apgar score, which allows rapid evaluation of a depressed infant and of the severity of the depression.[1] The infant is scored in five categories at 1 minute and 5 minutes after delivery. (These scores are traditionally recorded in the infant's chart as "Apgars 8 and 10," for example, meaning that the infant had a score of 8 at 1 minute and 10 at 5 minutes.) The scores range from 0 (no points in any category) to 10 (2 points in each of five categories). The five parameters scored in this system include heart rate, respiratory effort, muscle tone, reflex irritability, and skin color. The scoring in each category is described in Table 4-1.

The following system may be helpful in remembering the five categories of the Apgar system:

A: Appearance (skin color)

P: Pulse (heart rate)

G: Grimace (reflex irritability)

A: Activity (muscle tone)

R: Respiration (respiratory effort)

The 1-minute score is especially useful in identifying the infant who needs immediate intervention. An Apgar score of 2 or less indicates a severely depressed infant who requires immediate resuscitation, including ventilatory assistance (see Resuscitation of the Neonate in Chapter 20). If

TABLE 4-1   Apgar Scoring System Criteria

CATEGORY	0 POINTS	1 POINT	2 POINTS
Heart rate	Absent	Under 100	Over 100
Respiratory effort	Absent	Irregular, weak, or gasping	Crying infant, vigorous breathing
Muscle tone	Flaccid, limp	Some flexion of extremities	Active flexion of extremities, good motion, resistance to extension
Reflex irritability	Unresponsive	Frown or grimace when stimulated	Active movement, crying, cough, or sneeze
Skin color	Totally cyanotic, or pale or gray	Acrocyanosis (cyanotic hands and feet with pink body)	Completely pink

the score is between 3 and 6, the infant may need some assistance, usually requiring stimulation and oxygen. Infants with scores of 7 or more are considered stable and require only routine care and close observation.

The 5-minute score is useful in assessing the infant's recovery from depression and the effectiveness of any previous interventions. If the infant remains depressed at 5 minutes, with a score less than 6, major depression is present and the infant should be under special care. These infants are at high risk of developing major complications of the newborn period, including respiratory distress, aspiration syndromes, and hypoglycemia. They will usually need intravenous fluids and oxygen, and many will require ventilatory assistance.

▬ESTIMATION OF GESTATIONAL AGE

Soon after admittance to the nursery, the infant's gestational age is assessed. One common system used for estimating gestational age is that developed by Dubowitz and co-workers in the early 1970s, commonly referred to as the Dubowitz score.[3] This system involves the scoring of 10 external characteristics and 11 neuromuscular signs. As a result of the need for increasing the accuracy of estimates of gestational age in very low-birth-weight infants, the **New Ballard Score** (NBS) was introduced in 1991,[2] extending the range and accuracy of age assessment to within 1 week.[4] The NBS, shown in Figure 4-1, condenses the Dubowitz scoring system to seven physical and six neurologic criteria and is particularly useful for neonates who are intubated and heavily monitored, since it does not require lifting the infant.

Various investigators and hospitals have modified the systems used for estimation of gestational age, but all are based on evaluation of one or more of the external and neurologic criteria that have been defined for gestational age, and which are summarized in Table 4-2.[3,7]

External Criteria

Vernix. At birth, the infant is covered with a grayish white, cheeselike substance composed of sebaceous gland secretions, lanugo, and shed epithelial cells referred to as vernix caseosa. The amount of vernix covering the infant decreases with advancing gestational age, so that the preterm infant is covered with vernix, the term infant has very little vernix, usually only in the body creases, and the post-term infant has no vernix at all.

Skin. The skin becomes thicker and less transparent with increasing gestational age, so that the preterm infant's skin is thin (almost transparent), the term infant's skin is pale with few visible vessels, and the post-term infant's skin may be thick and soft and begin peeling and cracking after birth. The skin in the early preterm Caucasian infant appears dark red in color, gradually fading to pink, then to pale pink over the entire body, becoming generally pale with pink ears, lips, palms, and soles by term. The skin color of African-American and Asian infants should be evaluated by examination of the ears, lips, palms, and soles of the feet.

Nails. Nails are present and cover the nail bed in any viable infant. Post-term infants may have especially long fingernails.

Neuromuscular Maturity

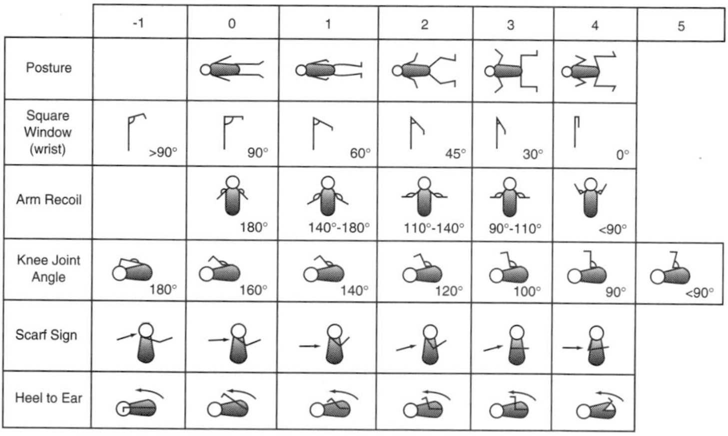

	-1	0	1	2	3	4	5
Posture							
Square Window (wrist)	>90°	90°	60°	45°	30°	0°	
Arm Recoil		180°	140°-180°	110°-140°	90°-110°	<90°	
Knee Joint Angle	180°	160°	140°	120°	100°	90°	<90°
Scarf Sign							
Heel to Ear							

Physical maturity

Skin	sticky friable transparent	gelatinous red, translucent	smooth pink, visible veins	superficial peeling and/or rash, few veins	cracking pale areas rare veins	parchment deep cracking no vessels	leathery cracked wrinkled	
Lanugo	none	sparse	abundant	thinning	bald areas	mostly bald		
Plantar Surface	heel – toe 40–50 mm:-1 <40 mm:-2	>50 mm no crease	faint red marks	anterior transverse crease only	creases ant. 2/3	creases over entire sole		
Breast	Imperceptible	barely perceptible	flat areola no bud	stippled areola 1–2 mm bud	raised areola 3–4 mm bud	full areola 5–10 mm bud		
Eye/Ear	lids fused loosely:-1 tightly:-2	lids open pinna flat stays folded	sl. curved pinna; soft: slow recoil	well-curved pinna; soft but ready recoil	formed and firm instant recoil	thick cartilage ear stiff		
Genitals male	scrotum flat, smooth	scrotum empty faint rugae	testes in upper canal rare rugae	testes descending few rugae	testes down good rugae	testes pendulous deep rugae		
Genitals female	clitoris prominent labia flat	prominent clitoris small labia minora	prominent clitoris enlarging minora	majora and minora equally prominent	majora large minora small	majora cover clitoris and minora		

Maturity Rating

score	weeks
-10	20
-5	22
0	24
5	26
10	28
15	30
20	32
25	34
30	36
35	38
40	40
45	42
50	44

FIGURE 4-1   New Ballard scoring system. (Ballard JL, Khoury JC, Wedig K, Wang L, Eilers-Walsman BL, Lipp R: New Ballard Score, expanded to include extremely premature infants. J Pediatr 119:417, 1991)

TABLE 4-2   Criteria for Assessment of Gestational Age

CRITERIA	CHANGES AS GESTATION ADVANCES
External Criteria	
Vernix	Decreases
Skin thickness	Increases
Skin transparency	Decreases
Skin color	Changes from dark red to pale with pink extremities during gestation
Plantar creases	Increases
Breast tissue	Increases
Pinna	Increased incurving
Ear cartilage	Increases
Lanugo	Decreases
Genitalia (female)	Clitoris becomes less prominent, and labia majora increase in size to cover clitoris
Genitalia (male)	Testes descend into scrotal sacs, rugae appear late in gestation
Neurologic Criteria	
Posture	Initial hypotonia changes to frog-leg position, then to flexion of all extremities, with recoil of extremities following extension at term
Popliteal angle	Decreases as muscle tone increases
Ankle dorsiflexion	Angle diminishes toward zero as joint becomes more flexible
Square window	Wrist angle same as ankle dorsiflexion
Heel to ear	Changes from little or no flexion of knee with heel very close to ear, to increasing flexion
Scarf sign	Resistance increases to infant's hand around neck to opposite shoulder
Head lag	Head initially lags behind trunk as supine infant is pulled erect by arms; becomes more in line with trunk as gestation advances
Ventral suspension	Infant suspended in prone position will be hypotonic initially, then begin flexion of extremities and lift head even with and eventually above back with extremities fully flexed

Sole (Plantar) Creases. Creases develop on the soles of the feet during gestation, beginning with the ball of the foot and proceeding toward the heel. An infant of about 32 weeks' gestation will have one or two anterior creases. By 37 weeks, the creases should be present over about two thirds of the sole, and by 40 weeks the entire sole is covered. The post-term infant has deeper creases.

Breast Tissue and Areola. The areola develops at about 34 weeks, with a palpable nodule of breast tissue present after the 36th week. Although the volume of the breast depends on nutrition and fat deposition, the development of the areola is affected only by gestational age.

Ears. Before 33 weeks' gestation, the pinna (external ear) is flat with very little incurving of the edge. At 33 or 34 weeks' gestation, the upper pinna begins incurving, and by 38 weeks the upper two thirds of the pinna is completely curved. This curving extends to the lobe by 39 or 40 weeks. Additionally, ear cartilage development proceeds throughout gestation. Before 32 weeks' gestation, there is little cartilage and the ears are soft, fold easily, and remain folded. By 36 weeks, they recoil from folding, and by term they are firm and erect and recoil instantly.

Hair. Preterm infants tend to have very fine hair that mats. In term infants, the hairs tend to lie flat in single strands. A receding hairline may be present in post-term infants.

Lanugo. Early in gestation, fine body hair (lanugo) is present over the entire body. As gestation progresses it disappears first from the face, then the trunk and extremities. By term, it is usually inconspicuous or present only in small amounts on the upper back.

Genitalia. Maturity of the external genitalia is one of the more reliable physical indicators of gestational age.[2] The clitoris is prominent in the female at 30 to 32 weeks. The labia majora are widely separated and the labia minora protruding. As gestation proceeds, the labia majora increase in size until they completely cover the clitoris by term. In the male, the testes gradually descend toward the scrotum during gestation. At 30 weeks, they can be palpated in the inguinal canal. By 37 weeks they are located high in the scrotal sacs and by 40 weeks should be completely descended. Rugae (folds or wrinkles) begin to appear at about 36 weeks and cover the entire scrotum by 40 weeks.

Neurologic Signs

Posture and Extremities. Before 30 weeks' gestation, the infant will tend to be hypotonic with arms and legs extended. By 34 weeks, flexion of the legs occurs, resulting in the "frog-leg" position, but the arms remain extended. By 36 to 38 weeks, both arms and legs should be flexed, but the infant will not recoil the extremities if they are extended. By 38 to 40 weeks, the infant should recoil the extremities after extension.

Flexion Angles. The popliteal angle is measured by placing the infant's knee to the chest and attempting to extend the leg. As muscle tone develops during gestation, the angle formed when the leg is extended as far as possible becomes smaller and smaller. Ankle and wrist angles are signs of joint flexibility and diminish toward zero as term approaches. The test for wrist flexion is often referred to as **square window** and involves flexing the hand onto the forearm and measuring the angle formed at the wrist. Ankle dorsiflexion is measured by flexing the foot onto the anterior leg and measuring the angle formed at the ankle. Premature infants tend to have less flexible joints than do term infants.

Muscle Tone. Heel-to-ear and scarf sign are signs related to muscle tone that are evaluated in the New Ballard scoring system. The **heel-to-ear sign** involves placing the infant's foot as near to the head as possible and observing how close it comes and also the degree of flexion of the knee. The very preterm infant will have little or no flexion and the examiner will be able to place the heel very close to the ear. The knee becomes increasingly flexed as gestation proceeds. The **scarf sign** involves trying to put the infant's hand around the neck and around the opposite shoulder. Resistance to this maneuver increases with advancing gestational age.

Once gestational age has been estimated, a comparison can be made between the growth of the infant being evaluated and appropriate growth for the estimated gestational age. One common method of comparing normal and actual growth is the **Colorado intrauterine growth curve**. These curves plot gestational age against birth weight, length, and head circumference. An example of a Colorado growth curve for birth weight and gestational age is shown in Figure 4-2. These curves are based on data obtained for infants born in Colorado from 1948 to 1961.[8] Infants who score between the 10th and 90th percentiles on the Colorado curve are considered appropriate for gestational age (AGA); those scoring below the 10th percentile are small for gestational age (SGA), or intrauterine growth retarded (IUGR); and those scoring above the 90th percentile are large for

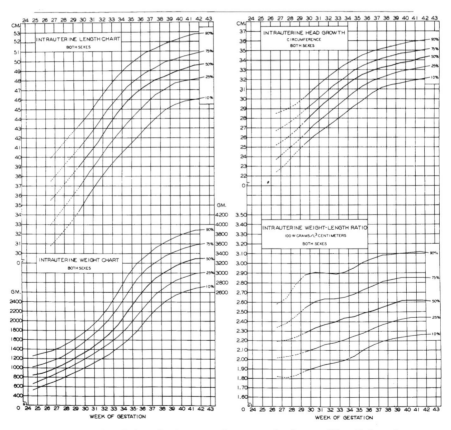

FIGURE 4-2   The Colorado intrauterine growth charts. The Colorado curves give percentiles of intrauterine growth for weight, length, and head circumference. (Lubchenco LO, Hansman C, Boyd E: Peadiatrics 37:403, 1966. Copyright © American Academy of Pediatrics, 1966)

gestational age (LGA). As previously discussed, identification of each of these groups is important in determining which infants are at high risk, and what those particular risks might be.

▬ VITAL SIGNS

Normal values for respiratory rate, heart rate, blood pressure, and temperature for newborn infants are shown in Table 4-3. Interpretation of the vital signs measured during physical examination should be based upon familiarity with the ranges considered normal for newborns.

Respiratory Rate

The normal respiratory rate for a newborn varies between 30 and 60 breaths per minute. Fluctuation of the respiratory rate is normal, and respirations are not necessarily regular, particularly in the preterm infant. **Periodic breathing** is defined as respiration interrupted by short periods of apnea, lasting up to 10 seconds, and which are not associated with any other abnormalities such as cyanosis or bradycardia. This breathing pattern occurs commonly in preterm infants, is not considered pathologic, and does not require treatment. There is very little chest wall movement in the newborn, with most of the respiratory excursion caused by the movement of the diaphragm. Thus, the abdomen rises and falls quite obviously with each inspiration and expiration, and should be observed for a full minute when counting the respiratory rate.

Heart Rate

Heart rate in the newborn is generally determined by auscultation. The normal heart rate fluctuates between 110 and 160 beats per minute; it may be slightly higher in the preterm infant. Transient increases may occur when the infant is agitated. Persistent tachycardia is usually associated with congenital heart defects, particularly if they result in congestive heart failure, or with shock. Bradycardia is usually secondary to significant apnea. In addition to heart rate, palpation of the apical impulse is important in evaluating cardiac status. Palpation of the apical impulse is used to locate the position of the heart. The apical impulse is normally felt at the fifth intercostal space in the midclavicular line. This may also be visible as a localized pulsation. Several abnormalities may result in a shift of the api-

TABLE 4-3 Normal Vital Signs in the Newborn

		NORMAL RANGE
Respiratory rate		30–60 breaths per minute
Heart rate		110–160 beats per minute
Blood pressure	<2000 g	50/35 mm Hg
	2000–3000 g	60/35 mm Hg
	>3000 g	35/40 mm Hg
Temperature (skin)		36.5°C

cal impulse from its normal position, such as with pneumothorax, where the apical impulse will shift away from the affected side.

Blood Pressure

Blood pressure is usually measured with a Doppler apparatus and a blood pressure cuff. The blood pressure cuff must be appropriate for the size of the infant in order to obtain accurate measurements. Usually a cuff of 1 inch width or less is used, although larger infants may require a larger cuff. Blood pressures are often obtained from the leg with the cuff around the thigh, in addition to being obtained from the arm. In low-birth-weight infants, blood pressure averages 50/35 mm Hg. Infants with birth weights about 2000 g have an average blood pressure of 60/35 mm Hg, whereas infants about 3000 g have an average blood pressure of 65/40 mm Hg. Evaluation of peripheral pulses (brachial, radial, femoral) is also valuable in the indirect assessment of blood pressure. Weak peripheral pulses commonly indicate a hypotensive state.

Temperature

An infant's temperature is usually measured in the rectum, in the axilla, or on the skin. Rectal temperature is the best assessment of core temperature. Axillary temperature is usually somewhat lower than rectal temperature but may be falsely high; it is recommended only for routine monitoring in the absence of any problems with thermoregulation. Skin temperatures are helpful because they allow constant measurement and do not interfere with the care of the baby. In addition, the metabolic response of the infant to cold temperatures is sensed and mediated by the skin receptors. In general, continuous monitoring of skin temperature is recommended for infants who require close thermal monitoring and regulation. Skin temperature is usually maintained at about 36.5° Celsius to minimize oxygen consumption, which increases with both elevated and reduced body temperatures.

■ SIGNS OF RESPIRATORY DISTRESS

Five signs commonly appear in the infant with respiratory distress to varying degrees: tachypnea, cyanosis, nasal flaring, expiratory grunting, and retractions. Additionally, periods of apnea and bradycardia may occur.[5] None of these signs is specific for any particular disease or type of disease. Many of these signs occur in both respiratory and cardiac disorders, and some may be associated with disorders of other body systems.

Tachypnea. **Tachypnea** in the newborn is defined as a respiratory rate in excess of 60 breaths per minute, although a rate in excess of 50 breaths per minute should increase the index of suspicion for respiratory or cardiac difficulty. Because of the normal fluctuations in respiratory rate and pattern in the newborn, tachypnea should be determined by several separate counts of respiratory rate for a full minute rather than by a single, isolated measurement.

Cyanosis. Cyanosis, or bluish discoloration, may be localized or generalized, with the latter indicating a more serious problem. A well-lighted environment is essential to the evaluation of cyanosis. Central cyanosis, which involves the mucous membranes, indicates that there is an excessive amount of unsaturated hemoglobin present (in excess of 5 g/dl). Peripheral cyanosis (**acrocyanosis**, or cyanosis of the hands and feet) is common in newborns and is not necessarily a sign of difficulty.

Because of the presence of fetal hemoglobin in the newborn, with its increased affinity for oxygen, cyanosis occurs at a lower partial pressure of oxygen in newborns than in adults. The presence of central cyanosis usually indicates an arterial oxygen tension of less than 40 mm Hg. This is an ominous situation because even a slight drop in the partial pressure of oxygen at this point will result in a sharp decline in hemoglobin saturation and thus in the oxygen-carrying capacity of the blood. Further, because cyanosis is related to the amount of unsaturated hemoglobin present, the anemic infant is unlikely to demonstrate cyanosis even though he or she may be extremely hypoxemic. Thus, the presence of cyanosis is a very serious sign; its absence, however, does not rule out the possibility of a hypoxic infant.

Nasal Flaring. Nasal flaring involves flaring of the nostrils (alae nasi) during inspiration and is believed to be a sign of air hunger. Presumably, the more pressure that must be generated to move air, the higher the degree of flaring. Nasal flaring may be present intermittently and may be barely discernible or very obvious.

Expiratory Grunting. Expiratory grunting is common in the infant with hyaline membrane disease, although it may be seen in other disorders as well. It is believed to be an attempt on the part of the neonate to maintain positive pressure on expiration and prevent alveolar collapse. Grunting results from exhalation against a partially closed glottis (partial Valsalva maneuver) and may vary from mild (audible only with a stethoscope) to severe (audible with the naked ear).

Retractions. Retractions involve inward movement of the chest wall either between the ribs (intercostal), above the clavicles (supraclavicular), or below the rib margins (subcostal). They may also occur at the top (suprasternal) or the bottom (xiphoid) margins of the sternum. Retractions may occur in any age group, but are much more common in the newborn because of the very high compliance of the chest cage. As the infant develops difficulty moving air and generates more pressure in an attempt to increase air movement, the chest wall is drawn in. Initially, with moderate distress, slight subcostal and intercostal retractions occur. As distress increases, retractions become more widespread and obvious, and eventually the retractions at the sternal level (xiphoid retractions) may mimic the appearance of pectus excavatum. As the infant forcefully contracts the diaphragm in an attempt to move more air, the abdomen protrudes. The high negative pressures generated in the chest cage with this diaphragmatic contraction result in the entire anterior chest wall and sternum moving inward, producing a characteristic "**see-saw**" or paradoxical type of respiratory pattern.

The Silverman scoring system (Fig. 4-3) was developed as a method of measuring the degree of respiratory distress and estimating the severity of the underlying lung disease.[10] When evaluating an infant using this scoring system, the higher the score, the more severe the degree of lung disease.

Apnea. **Apnea** in the newborn is defined as periods of absence of respiration for at least 20 seconds, or periods of absence of respiration that are accompanied by bradycardia (generally defined as a heart rate less than 100

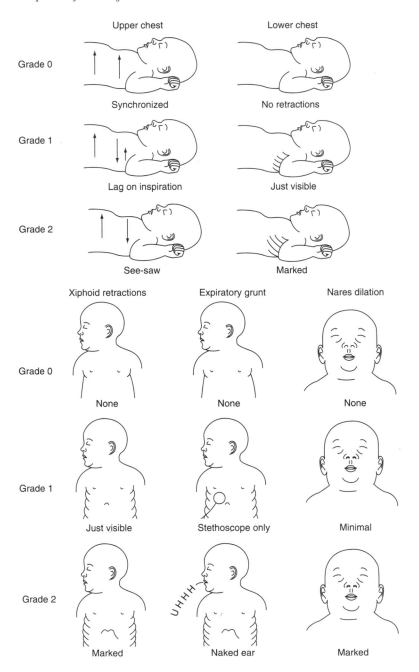

FIGURE 4-3   Silverman scoring system. (Silverman WA, Andersen DH: Silverman score—a system for grading severity of underlying lung disease. Pediatrics 17:1, 1956).

beats/min) or cyanosis, or both. Apnea, which will be discussed in detail later, is associated with many types of disorders, including prematurity, sepsis, cardiorespiratory disease, and central nervous system disorders.

■AUSCULTATION OF THE CHEST

Auscultation of the newborn chest is much less valuable than in any other age group and requires an experienced listener. The newborn chest is very small, and localization of findings with a stethoscope is extremely difficult. Breath sounds are easily transferred from one area of the chest to another. Nevertheless, an experienced neonatal care provider can improve the findings of the physical examination of the infant with careful auscultation.

Three basic types of breath sounds can be distinguished: diminished breath sounds, rales, and rhonchi. Diminished breath sounds in one area of the lung are difficult to appreciate because sounds from unaffected areas may be transmitted to the affected area; however, a difference in air entry between the two lungs may be detected and may be helpful in the recognition of pneumothorax, atelectasis, or lobar emphysema. A generalized decrease in air entry may also be noticed in diseases that result in loss of lung volume, notably hyaline membrane disease.

Rales, which are also called crackles, are described as short, interrupted, nonmusical sounds heard most readily during inspiration. Rales are associated most often with hyaline membrane disease, pulmonary edema, and pneumonia.

Rhonchi are described as changes in pitch of the breath sounds and probably result from a narrowing of the airways by secretions, swelling, foreign matter, or spasm of bronchial smooth muscle. Rhonchi in infants are usually low pitched (sometimes referred to as coarse rhonchi) and are associated with secretions or foreign (aspirated) matter. Very high-pitched rhonchi are referred to as wheezes and are unusual in the newborn period. Infants who subsequently develop bronchopulmonary dysplasia following treatment of hyaline membrane disease may develop wheezing.

■EXAMINATION OF THE HEAD, FACE, AND NECK

The purposes of the remainder of the physical examination are to determine whether any congenital anomalies are present; to what extent gestational age, labor, delivery, analgesics, or anesthetics have affected the infant; and whether the infant has any sign of infection or metabolic disease. During the overall physical examination, the infant should be naked to provide unobstructed observation. Although a thorough exam can be performed in as little as 10 minutes, care must be taken to insure that the child does not get too cold. The room lights should be bright enough to allow detection of skin color and markings, but not so bright as to discourage the infant from opening his or her eyes.

Head

Inspection of the head includes assessment of the shape and size of the head, relative to the rest of the infant's body. The head circumference (occipital frontal circumference, OFC) should be measured and used along with other physical and neurologic criteria to establish gestational age. The shape of the head may have been changed by compression of the skull during passage through the mother's pelvis (molding), and the skull bones may actually override at the suture lines. These changes should correct themselves within a few days.

The ears should be examined for shape, size, position, and the presence of ear canals. Tympanic membranes should be inspected for any signs of infection. The position and bilateral symmetry of the ears should be noted, since infants with some congenital anomalies may present with ears set lower than normal.

Face
Examination of the eyes should include evaluation of the relative size, shape, and position of the eye in its socket and assessment of whether the infant has vision, as evidenced by reaction to light. Hittner and colleagues described a method of assessing gestational age by determining the disappearance of the anterior vascular capsule of the lens, which occurs with increasing gestational age.[6]

The nose should be examined for shape, size, and patency of the nasal passages. It should appear appropriately sized and positioned when viewed from both the lateral and anterior views. Any signs of trauma which may have occurred during delivery should be noted. Air flow through the nose can be detected by holding a strand of thread in front of each nostril and observing fluttering of the thread during breathing.[4]

The mouth should be checked carefully to be sure that the lips, hard palate, and soft palate are intact, and that there are no deciduous teeth present. The size of the tongue and jawbone relative to the mouth should be assessed to determine if either macroglossia (large tongue) or micrognathia (small jaw) are present. These abnormalities commonly occur in infants with Down syndrome. It is also useful to evaluate the presence or absence of the suck and gag reflexes.

Neck
The neck should be inspected for range of motion, goiter, and the presence of cysts.

■ EXAMINATION OF THE ABDOMEN, SKIN, AND EXTREMITIES

Abdomen
The abdominal wall should be inspected for protrusion of abdominal contents, such as omphalocele or gastroschisis, which are described further in Chapter 12.

The position and appearance of the umbilicus should be noted; discoloration or discharge may indicate infection.

Skin
The epidermis, or skin, of the newborn is extremely thin and the oxygenated capillary blood makes it appear very pink. The practitioner should note any unusual markings, pigmentation, rashes, or bruising which may have occurred during delivery. The resiliency of the skin (turgor) and the presence of edema should be noted. Between 25% and 50%

of all term newborns and a higher percentage of premature newborns develop clinical jaundice.[9] The presence of jaundice should be noted, although it will resolve without treatment in many infants.

Extremities

The fingers and toes should be examined for position, size, and number. Abnormalities in shape and number may indicate the presence of other congenital or chromosomal anomalies. The color of the hands and feet should be examined, remembering that in many normal infants, acrocyanosis may persist for several hours following birth. The brachial and femoral pulses should be palpated to assess their strength and symmetry, providing valuable information about the condition of the cardiovascular system.

▬REFERENCES

1. Apgar V: A proposal for a new method of evaluation of the newborn infant. Anesth Analg 32:260, 1953.
2. Ballard JL, Khoury JC, Wedig K, Wang L, Eilers-Walsman BL, Lipp R: New Ballard Score, expanded to include extremely premature infants. J Pediatr 119:417, 1991.
3. Dubowitz LMS, Dubowitz V, Goldberg C: Clinical assessment of gestational age in the newborn infant. J Pediatr 77:1, 1970.
4. Fletcher MA: Physical assessment and classification. In Avery GB, Fletcher MA, MacDonald MG (eds): Neonatology: Pathophysiology and Management of the Newborn, 4th ed. Philadelphia, JB Lippincott, 1994.
5. Guthrie RD, Hodson WA: Clinical diagnosis of pulmonary insufficiency: History and physical. In Thibeault DW, Gregory GA (eds): Neonatal Pulmonary Care. Menlo Park, CA, Addison-Wesley, 1979.
6. Hittner HM, Horsch NJ, Rudolph AJ: Determination of gestational age by examination of anterovascular capsule of lens. Pediatr 91:455, 1977.
7. Korones SB: Significance of the relationship of birth weight to gestational age. In High Risk Newborn Infants, 3rd ed. St. Louis, CV Mosby, 1981.
8. Lubchenco LO, Hansman C, Boyd E: Intrauterine growth in length and head circumference as estimated from live births at gestational ages from 26 to 42 weeks. Pediatrics 37:403, 1966.
9. Odell GB: Bilirubin Neonatal Hyperbilirubinemia. New York, Grune & Stratton, 1982.
10. Silverman WA, Andersen DH. Silverman score—a system for grading severity of underlying lung disease. Pediatrics 17:1, 1956.

▬BIBLIOGRAPHY

Cochran WD: History and physical examination of the newborn. In Cloherty JP, Stark AR (eds): Manual of Neonatal Care, 2nd ed. Boston, Little, Brown, 1985.

Fletcher MA: Physical assessment and classification. In Avery GB, Fletcher MA, MacDonald MG (eds): Neonatology: Pathophysiology and Management of the Newborn, 4th ed. Philadelphia, JB Lippincott, 1994.

▬SELF-ASSESSMENT QUESTIONS

1. A newborn with a heart rate of 120 beats/min, irregular respirations, active flexion of extremities, active movement, and acrocyanosis would have an Apgar score of
   - a. 4
   - b. 6
   - c. 8
   - d. 10

2. The New Ballard Score allows estimation of gestational age to within
   - a. 2 days
   - b. 7 days
   - c. 15 days
   - d. 30 days

3. As a fetus develops in utero, the number of creases on the sole of the foot
   a. increases
   b. decreases
   c. remains the same

4. In the newborn, periodic breathing is defined as periods of apnea which last up to
   a. 2 seconds   c. 20 seconds
   b. 10 seconds   d. 1 minute

5. Palpation of the apical impulse is accomplished by placing the finger in the _____ intercostal space in the _____ line.
   a. second, midaxillary   c. fifth, midaxillary
   b. fifth, midclavicular   d. seventh, midclavicular

6. Which of the following signs of respiratory distress is an attempt by the infant to maintain positive pressure in the airway?
   a. nasal flaring   c. tachypnea
   b. retractions   d. expiratory grunting

7. The Silverman scoring system was developed as a method of measuring the degree of
   a. respiratory distress   c. hypoxemia
   b. tachypnea   d. prematurity

8. Diminished breath sounds over the left side of a newborn's chest may indicate the presence of
   a. hyaline membrane disease   c. bronchopulmonary dysplasia
   b. pneumothorax   d. cystic fibrosis

9. Which of the following terms describes changes in the shape of the infant's skull which may occur during delivery?
   a. mottling   c. lanugo
   b. acrocyanosis   d. molding

10. Only 2% of newborn infants will develop clinical jaundice.
    a. true
    b. false

Chapter 5

Special Problems in the Newborn

OBJECTIVES

Having completed this chapter, the reader will be able to:

1 List the three major components of the thermoregulatory system.

2 Describe the normal thermoregulatory mechanisms in the newborn.

3 List the factors that may interfere with thermoregulation in the newborn.

4 Discuss the mechanisms of heat loss in the newborn, including methods of prevention of each.

5 Describe the response of the newborn to cold stress and to heat stress.

6 Discuss the potential consequences of both cold and heat stress.

7 Explain the concept of neutral thermal environment and discuss its importance in the newborn.

8 Describe temperature assessment and its relationship to maintenance of neutral thermal environment in the newborn.

9 Explain the importance of heating and monitoring temperature when administering oxygen by hood.

10 Describe the problems related to low humidity of environmental gas.

11 Discuss the relationships between respiratory care procedures and thermoregulation.

12 Discuss the origin and conjugation of bilirubin.

13 Describe the factors that may interfere with excretion of conjugated bilirubin in the newborn.

14 Discuss the significance of the enterohepatic shunt.

15 List the reasons for increased bilirubin levels in the newborn.

16 Differentiate between physiologic jaundice and nonphysiologic jaundice in the newborn.

17 List the causes of jaundice.

18 Discuss the factors that increase the risk of kernicterus.

19 Describe the methods used to treat hyperbilirubinemia.

20 Discuss the possible side effects of phototherapy.

21 List the reasons why insensible water loss is higher in the low-birth-weight infant.

22 Discuss the importance of neutral thermal environment maintenance in fluid balance.

23 List factors that can increase or decrease insensible water loss.

24 Describe the features of the immature gastrointestinal tract that reduce absorption of nutrients.

25 Identify the nutritional requirements of the newborn.

26 Discuss the changes that occur in the newborn when infection is present, as compared to the changes in older patients.

27 Describe the features of the immune response that may be deficient in the newborn.

28 List the types of infants who are at high risk of developing infection after birth.

29 List the signs of systemic infection in the newborn.

30 Discuss the methods used to prevent infection.

31 Describe the ways in which the practitioner evaluates the neurologic status of an infant.

32 Differentiate between periodic breathing and apnea.

33 List factors associated with apnea.

34 Describe the types of seizures that occur in the newborn.

35 Differentiate between jitteriness and seizures.

36 List the major causes of seizures in the newborn.

37 Discuss the types of intracranial hemorrhage that occur, including their usual cause, clinical presentation, and consequences.

38 Describe the pathogenesis of intraventricular hemorrhage and explain its relationship to prematurity.

KEY TERMS

bilirubin
chemotaxis
conjugated bilirubin
direct-reacting bilirubin
exchange transfusion
icterus
indirect-reacting bilirubin
insensible water loss
intraventricular hemorrhage
kernicterus
leukocytosis

neutral thermal environment
nonshivering thermogenesis
opsonization
phagocytosis
phototherapy
physiologic jaundice
servocontrol
thermogenesis
thermoregulation
unconjugated bilirubin

▄ THERMOREGULATION

Thermoregulation, or the maintenance of body temperature, poses special problems for the newborn, and particularly for the premature newborn. Because thermoregulation is important in determining oxygen consumption, and because the administration of many respiratory care procedures may influence heat loss or gain, those involved in respiratory care of the newborn need to pay special attention to this area.

Regulatory Mechanisms

Infants are homeothermic organisms, which means that they maintain a fairly constant core temperature over a wide range of environmental temperatures. The production, dissipation, and conservation of heat are all necessary and normal functions of the homeothermic organism. Heat is a normal byproduct of cellular metabolism. To prevent core temperature from rising, heat must be lost (dissipated) at the same rate at which it is produced. If the environmental temperature falls, then the organism must either conserve heat or increase heat production to maintain core temperature. If the environmental temperature rises, the organism must increase heat loss, usually through peripheral vasodilation and sweating mechanisms. This requires a thermoregulatory system with three major components: a sensory system for monitoring temperature (the skin); a central regulatory system to keep core temperature constant (probably located in the hypothalamus); and some method of regulating heat production and heat loss.

The newborn infant has the same homeothermic responses as the adult, although the range of environmental temperatures over which the newborn can maintain a constant temperature is narrower than that for adults.[15,62,63] The reasons for this narrower range include the relatively large surface area to weight ratio in the infant, resulting in an increased rate of heat gain or loss; relatively poor thermal insulation of the infant due to minimal subcutaneous fat; and a small overall mass to hold heat.[34,60] In addition, shivering and sweating, which are major methods of heat gain and loss in the adult, are not well developed in the newborn.

The major receptors for monitoring temperature are located in the skin of the newborn, particularly on the face.[15,45] These sensors detect changes in environmental temperature and respond rapidly to increases in heat retention or loss in order to maintain a constant internal temperature. This internal temperature is regulated through a central regulatory mechanism that is most likely located in the hypothalamus. The function of this central regulator may be altered by such factors as intracranial hemorrhage, birth trauma, asphyxia, and hypoglycemia, usually resulting in a decreased ability to respond to cold stress.[60]

In response to changes in environmental temperature, infants, like adults, must have ways of adjusting heat production (**thermogenesis**) and heat loss. The major mechanisms of heat loss are peripheral vasodilation and evaporative heat loss from sweat and insensible water. The ability to control peripheral blood flow through vasodilation of skin vessels is well developed even in very small infants and represents the most important method of dissipating heat in newborns.[15,33] Term infants have sweat glands, but this is not a very effective method of heat dissipation for them, and preterm infants have essentially no ability to sweat.[32]

Thermogenesis

It has been well demonstrated that increased heat production occurs even in very small premature infants, by both shivering and nonshivering thermogenesis.[59] The major mechanism of heat production in the newborn is through the metabolism of brown fat stores and is referred to as **non-shivering thermogenesis.**[36] This mechanism is impaired in the presence of hypoxemia; thus maintenance of oxygenation in the newborn is important to the maintenance of body temperature.[61] Although shivering and other muscular activities that result in increased heat production do occur, they are much less effective than nonshivering thermogenesis. In general, visible shivering does not occur in newborns unless the environmental temperature is very low. Hey reported that shivering became apparent in infants when the environmental temperature was less than 15°C.[35]

Brown fat, the primary source of nonshivering thermogenesis, is stored in deposits around the heart and great vessels, in the nape of the neck, between the scapulas, around the adrenal glands and kidneys, and surrounding the spinal cord.[16] Brown fat cells appear at 26 to 30 weeks of gestational age and disappear during the weeks following birth. Exposure to low environmental temperature rapidly depletes these stores. Brown fat is richly supplied with sympathetic innervation. In response to cold stress, these nerves release norepinephrine, which is thought to be the principal mediator of nonshivering thermogenesis.[37]

Mechanisms of Heat Loss

The four major mechanisms of heat loss in the newborn are conduction, convection, radiation, and evaporation. These mechanisms are summarized in Table 5-1.

Conduction refers to direct loss to a cooler surface in contact with the body. This is not usually a problem as long as care providers avoid placing infants on cold surfaces without first covering the surface or wrapping the infant. In addition, mattresses should be made of material that is poorly conductive, so that cold temperatures of surfaces below the mattress will not be transmitted through the mattress to the infant.

TABLE 5-1   Mechanisms of Heat Loss

MECHANISM	DEFINITION	PREVENTION
Conduction	Direct heat loss to a cooler surface in contact with body surfaces	1. Avoid placing infant on cold, unprotected surface. 2. Use poorly conductive material for mattress.
Convection	Heat loss to cooler surrounding air	1. Heat environmental air. 2. Avoid drafts. 3. Heat inspired gas when infant is intubated.
Radiation	Loss of heat to cooler solid surfaces that are not in contact with body surfaces, such as the walls of the incubator	1. Avoid cooling of walls of incubator. 2. Keep room temperature high. 3. Use double-walled incubators or a heat shield within the incubator.
Evaporation	Loss of heat when a liquid such as body fluid becomes a gas (water vapor)	1. Increase the relative humidity of the environment. 2. Humidify inspired gas when infant is intubated.

Convection refers to loss of heat from a body surface to cooler surrounding air. The rate of convective heat loss depends on both the temperature of the air and the rate of airflow. Convective heat loss is minimized by maintaining surrounding air temperature and by avoiding drafts. This is easily accomplished by placing the infant inside an incubator (isolette). In the intubated infant, heating the inspired gas will prevent heat loss across the respiratory tract.

Radiation involves the loss of heat to solid surfaces that are not in contact with the body. The rate of radiant heat loss depends on the temperature of the solid surfaces, usually the walls of the incubator. Radiant heat loss will be increased if the room is air conditioned or if the incubator is placed near a window and the incubator walls are cooled. Radiant heat loss can be minimized by keeping room temperature high, using double-walled incubators and heat shields around the infant inside the incubator, and keeping incubators away from cold sources such as windows.

Evaporation is a heat-consuming process that results in heat loss when a liquid, including sweat and insensible water lost from the skin and respiratory tract, becomes a gas (evaporates or becomes water vapor). The rate of evaporation, and thus the rate of heat loss by this process, depends on the humidity of the surrounding air. If the humidity level is low, evaporation will occur at a faster rate and more heat will be lost. This is the major reason why a newborn infant should be dried immediately after delivery. In addition, bathing a newborn should be postponed until the infant is stable. Infants who are having difficulty conserving heat or those at high risk for such difficulty (particularly very small premature infants) may be supplied with increased humidity in their environment. Infants with an endotracheal tube in place must be supplied with adequately humidified gas to prevent both heat and fluid loss.

Response to Cold Stress

When an infant is exposed to cool environmental temperature, the first response is an attempt to conserve body heat. This is achieved by constriction of cutaneous vessels, thus exposing less blood to the mechanisms of heat loss. This peripheral vasoconstriction can lead to anaerobic metabolism and metabolic acidosis. The acidosis may cause pulmonary vasoconstriction, leading to further hypoxemia.[24] Because the infant has a large ratio of body surface area to body weight, the constriction of blood vessels in the skin is not as effective in preventing heat loss in infants as it is in the adult. If this mechanism is not sufficient to prevent heat loss, the infant must generate heat by increased metabolism. The initiation of thermogenesis is through skin thermal sensors, which are activated when skin temperature drops below 35° to 36° C.[37] This occurs before core temperature drops, thus helping to maintain the constant internal temperature of the homeotherm, and can be diminished by increasing the environmental temperature and thus increasing the skin temperature.

Consequences of Cold Stress

As previously discussed, the major mechanism for generating heat in the newborn is metabolism of brown fat. As with all metabolic processes, oxygen is consumed when brown fat metabolism is increased. This increase in oxygen consumption may result in hypoxemia. In addition, lack of adequate oxygen supply may result in metabolic acidosis caused by anaerobic metabolism (anaerobic glycolysis). Anaerobic glycolysis rapidly depletes body stores of glycogen, resulting in hypoglycemia. Infants who are classi-fied as intrauterine growth retardation (see Chapter 3) already have reduced glycogen stores and are thus more susceptible to the development of hypoglycemia when cold-stressed. Additionally, infants who are hypox-emic before exposure to cold are more susceptible to these consequences. They are less able to produce heat from nonshivering thermogenesis and are thus more susceptible to hypothermia. Infants who cannot compensate for cold stress and who become hypothermic (core temperature below nor-mal) are likely to develop severe apnea.[4] Infants who are persistently hypox-emic may therefore require a higher environmental temperature to main-tain body heat.

A further consequence of cold stress relates to the increased caloric demands of thermogenesis. Calories are consumed as heat is produced, resulting in an increased caloric requirement for the infant. If these calo-ries are not replaced, the infant will experience difficulty with normal growth and weight gain.

In summary, cold stress may result in hypoxemia, metabolic acidosis, hypoglycemia, impaired weight gain, hypothermia, and apnea.

Response to Heat Stress

Although exposure to cold air is a more common problem in the care of the newborn, overheating may occur if careful attention is not given to environmental temperature control. This is particularly true if heated gas is added to the infant's environment without monitoring the temperature of the gas. If the infant is overheated, peripheral vasodilation occurs in an attempt to increase heat loss. Increased evaporative loss may also occur from sweating and insensible sources. These heat-dissipating activities may cause increased oxygen consumption, resulting in hypoxemia. In addition, elevated temperatures have been associated with an increased incidence of apneic spells in the newborn.

Neutral Thermal Environment

Neutral thermal environment (NTE) refers to environmental conditions that allow the infant to maintain a normal internal temperature without increasing oxygen consumption. The temperature range required to maintain NTE is widest for full-term infants of normal birth weight. It becomes progressively narrower with decreasing birth weight or gesta-tional age. Very premature infants who are small for gestational age have a very limited range of temperatures over which they can maintain normal core temperature, and they require close control of their environment. These infants have very little body insulation and lose heat more easily than do larger, older infants. The temperature required to maintain NTE also depends on whether the infant is naked or clothed. Obviously, tem-perature maintenance will be more effective in the clothed infant, but crit-ically ill infants often require minimal or no clothing in order for intensive care to be performed adequately.

Full-term infants who are clothed and covered with a light blanket in an open crib can maintain a normal body temperature with minimal oxygen consumption with a room temperature of 24° or 25° C. By contrast, a naked

TABLE 5-2 NTE Temperatures

BIRTHWEIGHT	AGE	NAKED	CLOTHED
1 kg	0 days	35°C	32°C
	30 days	33°C	25°C
2 kg	0 days	34°C	28°C
	30 days	32°C	24°C
3 kg	0 days	33°C	27°C
	30 days	32°C	23°C

All data are for infants in a draft-free environment with a relative humidity of about 50% and with a heat shield placed between the infant and the incubator walls.

(Adapted from Hey EH: Thermoregulation. In Avery GB, Fletcher MA, MacDonald MG [eds]. Neonatology: Pathophysiology and Management of the Newborn, 4th ed. Philadelphia, JB Lippincott, 1994.)

premature newborn weighing 1 kg who is maintained in a double-walled incubator or with a heat shield in a single-walled incubator, with no drafts and with a relative humidity of 50%, will require an average NTE temperature of 35° C on the first day of life. NTE temperatures will be higher in a single-walled incubator without a heat shield and may be reduced if environmental humidity is increased. Average NTE temperatures for infants of several birth weights and ages are summarized in Table 5-2.

Maintenance of NTE

Temperature must be assessed to determine what temperature is required to maintain NTE. The three major methods used for temperature assessment in the newborn are rectal, axillary, and skin temperature measurements. Rectal temperatures give the best estimation of core temperature; however, core temperature is a poor indicator of thermal balance in a cold environment, as the homeotherm will do everything possible to maintain this temperature. Once the core temperature begins to fall, the battle to maintain temperature in the face of cold stress may be nearly lost. Axillary temperatures are not particularly accurate. Brown fat deposits are located in the axillary region, and the increased metabolism of these deposits in the presence of cold stress may cause axillary temperatures to be falsely elevated. In addition, the measurement of temperature in the closed space of the axilla may result in a falsely high temperature value. Since skin temperature sensors, particularly on the face, are responsible for sensing the environmental temperature and mediating the infant's response, measurement of skin temperature provides the best method of temperature assessment. In addition, skin temperature can be monitored continuously, without interfering with care of the infant, which is preferable to intermittent monitoring of temperature at another site. Maintaining the abdominal skin temperature at approximately 36° to 36.5°C will avoid overheating or underheating and associated problems, particularly increased oxygen consumption.[64]

It is important to remember that the major skin temperature sensors of the infant are located on the face. If the rest of the body is well heated but the face is exposed to cold air, the infant will react as if cold-stressed. It is, therefore, necessary to heat the gas supply to an oxygen hood and to monitor the temperature of the hood, keeping it the same temperature as that of the incubator. In addition, the gas flow into the hood should be directed away from the infant's face to avoid convective heat loss.

Incubators, or isolettes (Fig. 5-1), provide four essential functions: isolating the infant from the environment, controlling the infant's body temperature, providing humidity control, and regulating oxygen concentration (although oxygen administration is usually accomplished by other methods). While incubators are quite capable of providing a very stable environment for the infant, they may limit access to the infant when certain patient care activities are performed.

Radiant warmers (Fig. 5-2) provide control of the infant's body temperature and offer the advantage of unlimited access to the patient. For this reason, they are preferred when caring for infants who are critically ill and require frequent attention and intervention. Warmers also allow several people to care for the infant at the same time, such as during resuscitation or other emergency procedures. Air currents from the room can sweep between the heat source and the infant, resulting in convective and evaporative heat loss. The use of plastic wrap (cellophane wrap) over the edges of the warmer surface has been shown to be effective in preventing both convection and evaporative heat loss.[3]

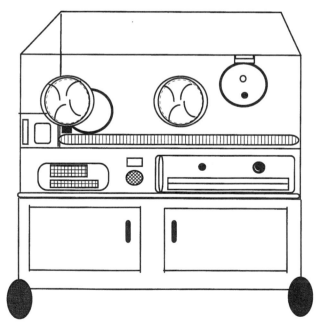

FIGURE 5-1   Incubator, or isolette. (Respiratory Therapy Review Perinatal/Pediatric Study Guide. Kettering, OH, RTS Publishing Company, 1996. Used with permission.)

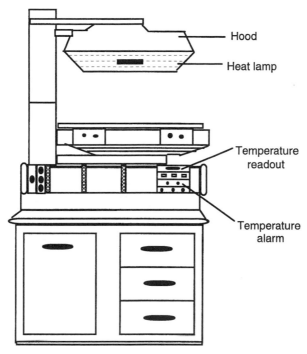

FIGURE 5-2 Radiant warmer. (Respiratory Therapy Review Perinatal/Pediatric Study Guide. Kettering, OH, RTS Publishing Company, 1996. Used with permission.)

Most of the time, temperature control for NTE in the newborn is achieved by **servocontrol**. This means that a temperature sensor is applied to the infant's skin, usually on the abdomen, and the environmental temperature automatically adjusts itself to maintain skin temperature at a preset level, usually between 36° and 36.5° C. This may be achieved using either an incubator or an overhead (radiant) warmer. The sensor is usually attached to the skin of the exposed abdomen with adhesive tape. This may present a problem if the environmental humidity level is low and the evaporative heat loss is high. The skin under the adhesive tape will have low evaporative heat loss and a higher temperature than other areas. The incubator or warmer, however, sees only the temperature of the sensor and turns off and on in response to this temperature. If this temperature is falsely elevated, the infant will experience significant cold stress. This is particularly a problem with a very small premature infant, who has little ability to retain or produce heat and who is being cared for naked under a warmer. Increasing the relative humidity of the ambient air will decrease evaporative heat loss and help to eliminate this problem.[4]

Respiratory Care Procedures and Thermoregulation
It is obvious from this discussion that respiratory care and thermoregulation in the newborn are closely related. Oxygenation and the maintenance of normal temperature are also very directly related. The hypoxemic infant has more difficulty maintaining a normal temperature when cold-

stressed, and cold stress itself results in increased oxygen consumption and consequent hypoxemia. Thus, careful attention to maintenance of adequate environmental temperature and adequate oxygenation is needed.

Oxygen hoods (oxyhoods) are a very common method of delivering oxygen to newborns. It is extremely important to heat the gas that supplies the hood and to monitor the temperature of the gas within the hood. The face is the major temperature-sensing area of the newborn, and the gas surrounding the face must be maintained at the same temperature as the NTE temperature of the incubator or radiant warmer. Underheating of hood gas may result in cold stress of the infant, whereas overheating may result in hyperthermia and its consequences. In addition, the gas supply to the hood should not be directed toward the infant's face.

Infants who are breathing through an endotracheal tube need inspired gas that is heated and humidified to avoid both humidity loss and heat loss from the respiratory tract. Supplying cool gas through an endotracheal tube or, for that matter, a nasopharyngeal tube or nasal prongs may result in cold stress.

Finally, evaporative heat loss may be minimized by supplying humidified gas to the ambient environment, particularly for very small premature infants who are extremely susceptible to heat loss. This is easily accomplished by directing warm, humidified air into the incubator or radiant warmer surface.

▰BILIRUBIN

Formation
Bilirubin is a substance formed from the catabolism of hemoglobin to its heme and globin portions. The heme portion is further broken down to form carbon monoxide (CO) and biliverdin, which is converted by biliverdin reductase to bilirubin. About 75% of bilirubin is derived from the normal destruction of circulating red blood cells. The life span of neonatal red blood cells is shorter than the average adult span of 120 days, so that production of bilirubin in the newborn is higher than in the adult. The remainder is derived from heme catabolism from nonhemoglobin sources and from destruction of immature red blood cell precursors.[43]

Conjugation
The free bilirubin molecule formed in the spleen and liver is a fat-soluble substance and is referred to as **unconjugated** or **indirect-reacting** bilirubin. Because this unconjugated bilirubin is fat soluble and not water soluble, it cannot be excreted in either bile or urine. Additionally, it has a high affinity for both fatty tissue and brain tissue. This bilirubin is transported in the plasma bound to albumin. In the liver, bilirubin is conjugated to form a water-soluble complex, referred to as **conjugated** or **direct-reacting bilirubin**. This water-soluble complex is excreted through the biliary tract and into the gastrointestinal tract. If excess amounts are formed, it may also be excreted through the kidneys in the urine.

The reactions that result in the conjugation of bilirubin require protein carriers to accept the unconjugated bilirubin when it enters the liver and an enzyme to catalyze the conjugation (glucuronyl transferase). A deficiency of either protein carriers or the required enzyme, both of which may occur in premature infants, will result in a decreased ability to form conjugated bilirubin. In addition, oxygen and glucose are required, so that hypoxia and hypoglycemia, which occur commonly in sick newborns, will also decrease the ability to conjugate bilirubin.

Excretion and Enterohepatic Shunt

Once the conjugated bilirubin has entered the gastrointestinal tract through the biliary system, it is either excreted in the feces or converted back to unconjugated bilirubin by the enzyme beta-glucuronidase, which is found in increased amounts in the fetal and newborn small intestine. This fat-soluble bilirubin is then absorbed through the intestinal walls into the portal (liver) circulation and the bloodstream. An additional source of intestinal bilirubin is meconium, which normally contains bilirubin. If meconium passage is delayed (*e.g.*, with intestinal obstruction or delayed feeding), more bilirubin will be absorbed across the intestinal walls. The reabsorption of unconjugated bilirubin through the intestines is referred to as the *enterohepatic shunt* and contributes significantly to the amount of bilirubin present in the newborn.[43]

Jaundice

Jaundice is the most common and one of the most distressing problems that can occur in newborns.[43] An increase in serum bilirubin occurs in almost all newborns, for several reasons: they have more circulating red cells per unit of body weight than do adults and newborn red cells have a shorter life span. The rate of bilirubin production decreases postnatally but is still about twice as high as the normal adult rate at 2 weeks of age.[11] In addition, the enterohepatic shunt previously described results in more absorption of bilirubin in the neonate than in the adult, owing to an absence of bacterial flora and an increased activity of beta-glucuronidase in the newborn.[14]

Research on newborn monkeys also suggests that ligandin, the predominant protein that binds bilirubin for conjugation in the liver, may be deficient in the first few days after birth, resulting in decreased uptake of bilirubin by the liver.[38] Glucuronyl transferase activity necessary for conjugation in the liver has also been demonstrated to be insufficient in monkeys. Activity of this enzyme increases postnatally, coinciding with the normal decrease in serum bilirubin levels. This enzyme is also decreased in activity in premature infants.[27] Finally, the ability of the newborn liver to excrete bilirubin is less than that of the adult, which may play a role if the bilirubin load is very high, as it might be in hemolytic disease of the newborn, causing an increase in conjugated bilirubin in the serum.

In about one half of newborns, the serum bilirubin is high enough to produce visible jaundice (clinical jaundice or **icterus**) within the first week of life. Serum bilirubin must be greater than 4 mg/100 mL for this to occur. In most instances, this is considered a normal event and is referred to as **physiologic jaundice**. There are, however, many nonphysiologic causes of jaundice, and a distinction must be made between those cases that require further investigation and those that do not. Bilirubin levels generally peak in term infants between 3 and 4 days of age, and in preterm infants between 5 and 6 days of age, so that the appearance and rate of rise of bilirubin levels may be a helpful guide. Guidelines for the assumption of physiologic jaundice are listed in Table 5-3. If any of these conditions are not met, an underlying cause for the jaundice should be sought, including factors known to influence bilirubin levels and underlying disease or abnormality in the infant.

Causes of Jaundice

Factors that have been shown to influence serum bilirubin levels are listed in Table 5-4. Certain ethnic groups, including people of East Asia and Greece and Native Americans, have higher average bilirubin values.[26,58] African Americans have lower average bilirubin levels.[43] Some maternal drugs, including oxytocin, may alter bilirubin levels.[43] Early feedings tend to decrease bilirubin levels, probably because of a decrease in the enterohepatic shunt.[71] Delayed cord clamping may increase red cell and blood volume and thus cause an increase in bilirubin.[56] Infants of diabetic mothers and infants who have experienced asphyxia and hypoxia have an increased incidence and severity of jaundice.[22] Vitamin E, an antioxidant that prevents damage to red blood cell membranes and hemolysis and is often administered to preterm infants in an effort to prevent side effects of oxygen therapy (retrolental fibroplasia and bronchopulmonary dysplasia), decreases serum bilirubin levels.[28] Finally, phenolic detergents that may be used as disinfectants to clean surfaces in the nursery have been associated with increased bilirubin, probably due to inhibition of glucuronyl transferase, and should not be used.[20,74]

Diseases and disorders that may result in jaundice include those that increase the bilirubin load and those that decrease the ability of the liver to clear bilirubin. The bilirubin load is increased by hemolytic disease, most notably Rh and ABO incompatibility; by extravascular blood (hematomas, hemorrhage), which results in increased breakdown of the extravasated cells and increased bilirubin production; by polycythemia (*e.g.*, from twin-to-twin or materno-fetal transfusion); and by an increase in the enterohepatic shunt (*e.g.*, secondary to intestinal obstruction). The ability of the liver to clear bilirubin may be influenced by inherited disorders, by biliary obstruction, and by infections, including bacterial sepsis, congenital syphilis, and the TORCH infections.

TABLE 5-3   Guidelines for the Assumption of Physiologic Jaundice

1. The infant is otherwise well.

2. The jaundice first appears after 24 hours of age.

3. The jaundice lasts less than 1 week in the term infant, or less than 2 weeks in the preterm infant.

4. The total serum bilirubin is less than 13 mg/100 mL in the term infant, or less than 15 mg/100 mL in the preterm infant.

5. The level of conjugated serum bilirubin does not exceed 1.5 mg/100 mL.

6. The serum bilirubin concentration is not rising more than 5 mg/100 mL/day.

(From Maisels MJ: Neonatal jaundice. In Avery GB [ed]: Neonatology: Pathophysiology and Management of the Newborn, 2nd ed. Philadelphia, JB Lippincott, 1981.)

TABLE 5-4 Factors That Influence Serum Bilirubin Levels

INCREASE SERUM BILIRUBIN	DECREASE SERUM BILIRUBIN
Ethnicity	Ethnicity
Maternal drugs	Maternal drugs
oxytocin	phenobarbital
epidural anesthesia	aspirin
Delayed cord clamping	heroin
Low birthweight	alcohol
Prematurity	Early feedings
Diabetic mother	Maternal cigarette smoking
Phenolic detergents (used to clean nursery surfaces)	Vitamin E administration
Hemolytic disease	
Extravascular blood	
Polycythemia	
Enterohepatic shunt	
Inherited disorders	
Biliary obstruction	
Infection	
Vitamin K administration	

Kernicterus

Any of these disorders may result in hyperbilirubinemia and may lead to its most serious consequence, kernicterus. **Kernicterus**, or bilirubin encephalopathy, occurs when unconjugated bilirubin is deposited in brain cells, resulting in varying degrees of impaired perceptual, intellectual, or motor function or in deafness. As a general rule, kernicterus occurs when the serum bilirubin exceeds 20 mg/100 mL in term infants, 15 mg/100 mL in preterm infants, and 10 to 12 mg/100 mL in very small preterm infants (less than 1500 g), but many factors may alter the values.

For bilirubin to be deposited in brain cells, it must be unbound. Normally, unconjugated bilirubin is carried in the blood bound to albumin. Bound bilirubin cannot leave the plasma and is therefore not a problem. In the term infant, bilirubin levels of higher than 20 mg/100 mL generally exceed the binding ability of the plasma. This is not a fixed number, however, and the bilirubin level varies greatly with many factors. Obviously, the albumin level itself is an important factor.

In addition, binding capacity is decreased in the presence of acidosis and hypothermia. Some drugs and other substances can displace bilirubin from albumin. Fetal albumin has a decreased binding capacity compared to adult albumin, so that binding capacity increases with increasing gestational age and with increasing postdelivery age, up to about 5 months of age.

Lucey has described several factors that increase the likelihood of kernicterus in the low-birth-weight infant, including birth weight of less than

1500 g, hypothermia, asphyxia (either prenatally or postnatally), hypoal-buminemia, septicemia, meningitis, drugs that affect binding ability, and serum bilirubin of greater than 10 mg/100 mL.[41]

Treatment of Hyperbilirubinemia

The major methods used to treat hyperbilirubinemia are phototherapy, exchange transfusion, and drug administration. Phototherapy involves the use of blue light to decompose bilirubin by photo-oxidation, forming non-toxic byproducts that are water soluble and can be excreted by the kidneys. **Exchange transfusion** is the classic treatment for neonatal jaundice and involves the actual removal of bilirubin by removing the infant's blood and replacing it with whole blood transfusions. In addition, administration of albumin before or during exchange transfusion may be helpful. Phenobarbital can also be used because it accelerates normal excretion pathways through the liver; however, it is generally considered to be a slower method of treatment. Wennberg and colleagues have reported success with the use of this drug prenatally by administering it to mothers of fetuses with Rh disease, resulting in a slower rate of rise of bilirubin post-natally and in fewer infants requiring exchange transfusion.[70]

The major considerations in the use of exchange transfusion or pho-totherapy are based on the actual serum bilirubin level, the birth weight of the infant, the rate of rise of bilirubin, and the presence of factors known to increase the risk of kernicterus, such as acidosis, hypoxia, hypothermia, and hypoalbuminemia. In general, all infants with a serum bilirubin level of 20 mg/100 mL or greater should be transfused, whereas infants with levels of less than 5 mg/100 mL require no treatment. Guide-lines commonly used for the management of term and low-birth-weight infants with hyperbilirubinemia are presented in Tables 5-5 and 5-6.

Phototherapy

In 1958, Cremer and colleagues observed that exposure of infants to sun-light or blue fluorescent lights reduced serum bilirubin levels.[18] Since that time, **phototherapy** has become the most common treatment of jaundice in the newborn. Phototherapy involves the placement of the infant "under the lights" to prevent or treat moderate hyperbilirubinemia. This form of

---

TABLE 5-5   Treatment of Hyperbilirubinemia in Full-Term Infants

	BILIRUBIN LEVEL IN MG/DL	
TREATMENT	*No Hemolysis and Infant Doing Well*	*Hemolysis Likely or Infant Is Sick*
Phototherapy	17–22	13–15
Interrupt or modify nursing, with or without phototherapy	17–22	Usually not indicated
Exchange transfusion	25–29	17–22

(Adapted from Maisels MJ: Jaundice. In Avery GB, Fletcher MA, MacDonald MG [eds]. Neonatology: Pathophysiology and Management of the Newborn, 2nd ed. Philadelphia: JB Lippincott, 1994.)

TABLE 5-6 Treatment of Hyperbilirubinemia in Low-Birth-Weight Infants

	BILIRUBIN LEVEL IN MG/DL	
BIRTH WEIGHT (G)	*Phototherapy*	*Exchange Transfusion*
<1500	5–8	13–16
1500–1999	8–12	16–18
2000–2499	11–14	18–20

(Adapted from Maisels MJ: Jaundice. In Avery GB, Fletcher MA, MacDonald MG [eds]. Neonatology: Pathophysiology and Management of the Newborn, 2nd ed. Philadelphia: JB Lippincott, 1994.)

treatment also reduces the need for exchange transfusion. Blue light is more effective than white light, although less is known about its side effects. Phototherapy results in the breakdown of bilirubin into more water-soluble products that can be excreted in bile, feces, and urine. It also enhances the excretion of unconjugated bilirubin itself. This technique has been used for more than 20 years without the occurrence of apparent serious side effects such as an increased metabolic rate (increasing caloric requirements, oxygen consumption, and carbon dioxide production), hyperthermia, increased water loss through the skin and gastrointestinal system, premature aging of retinal cells, and "sunburn."[37,43] Eye shields are used to protect the infant's eyes from potential damage, and a plastic shield (such as the "roof" of the incubator) should be placed between the lights and the infant to protect the skin. Fluid balance should be monitored closely and fluid replacement increased as needed.

Exchange Transfusion
Exchange transfusion involves the removal of twice the infant's calculated blood volume and the replacement of this volume, usually with whole blood. The two major indications for this procedure are to prevent or treat hyperbilirubinemia and to correct the anemia of severe erythroblastosis. The need for transfusion of the infant with hemolytic disease can be predicted by following the rate of rise of the bilirubin. These infants are at risk for developing hydrops fetalis, which is characterized by massive edema, pleural effusions, and ascites. Factors that predispose these infants to this disorder include severe anemia and decreased serum protein levels. In addition to treatment of hyperbilirubinemia and anemia, these infants should be treated for asphyxia, acidosis, hypoglycemia, and hypothermia, since any or all of these disorders may precipitate heart failure or cardiovascular collapse. Mechanical ventilation with positive end expiratory pressure (PEEP) is frequently required to treat associated pulmonary edema.

Pharmacologic Treatment
Drug therapy of neonatal hyperbilirubinemia is directed toward accelerating the normal metabolic pathways for bilirubin clearance, inhibiting the enterohepatic circulation of bilirubin, and interfering with bilirubin formation by either blocking the breakdown of heme or inhibiting hemolysis.[43] The most commonly used agent is phenobarbital, which has been shown to be effective in lowering serum bilirubin levels during the first

week of life when given to the mother, infant, or both.[42,65] Combining phenobarbital with phototherapy does not lower serum bilirubin levels more rapidly than phototherapy alone.[66] The major side effects of phenobarbital therapy are lethargy and slow feeding.

■FLUID BALANCE

Although fluid balance is important to critically ill patients in all age groups, there are some special considerations in the newborn. The amount of body water and the distribution of body water vary with gestational age and change after birth. Total body water (TBW) is approximately 94% of the body weight at 12 weeks' gestation and decreases to approximately 78% at term. Extracellular water decreases from 59% of body weight at 24 weeks to about 44% at term, while intracellular water increases from 27% to 34% of body weight during the same period.[7] Fluid management must allow for this variation. Fluid overloading, particularly in the low-birth-weight infant in the first days postnatally, may be associated with congestive heart failure with patent ductus arteriosus (PDA) and necrotizing enterocolitis.[5,6] **Insensible water loss** (IWL) is the loss of water from the skin and respiratory tract. About 30% of IWL occurs through the respiratory tract in expired gas, with the remaining 70% occurring through the skin. Additionally, IWL is relatively greater in the low-birth-weight infant because of increased skin permeability, larger body surface area per unit of body weight, and high skin blood flow in relation to weight. The high respiratory rate in these infants may also account for some of the increased IWL.[48]

The factors that influence IWL are listed in Table 5-7. Ambient temperature must be closely monitored because a temperature elevation of as little as 1°C above the NTE temperature range has been shown to increase IWL through increased evaporative heat loss.[6] Use of radiant warmers and phototherapy, as previously described, also increase IWL.[49,72] Using a heat shield, increasing the relative humidity of the environment, and humidifying inspired gases may decrease IWL.[8,23,32]

TABLE 5-7   Factors That Influence Insensible Water Loss (IWL)

INCREASE IWL	DECREASE IWL
Prematurity	Humidification of inspired gases
Increased ventilation rate or volume	Plexiglas heat shields
Elevated ambient temperature	Thin plastic blankets
Skin breakdown or injury	Topical agents
Radiant warmer	Semipermeable membrane (artificial skin)
Phototherapy	
Increased motor activity	
Crying	

▬NUTRITION

Nutrition is defined as the ingestion of the materials needed for the body's metabolic requirements, including growth, replacement, and energy production. Good nutrition is an essential element of the care of any infant and implies a diet that provides for normal growth, development, and body composition. In addition to promoting good health, proper nutrition has also been effective in inhibiting disease. Ideal nutritional management includes monitoring and assessing the infant's growth pattern. Body weight, length, and head circumference can be measured and plotted on various growth curves to estimate the appropriateness of size and weight gains. Serum electrolytes, calcium, phosphorus, albumin, and hemoglobin should also be monitored to prevent dietary deficiencies.

In premature infants, the gastrointestinal tract has a tremendous ability to adapt and grow, despite the fact that it too may be slightly immature. The challenges faced by the premature gastrointestinal tract include poor carbohydrate absorption because of lactase deficiency and fat malabsorption due to the small size of the bile acid pool and the lack of pancreatic lipase. Suck and swallow reflexes do not generally develop until the 34th week of gestation and may be absent or ineffective in premature infants. Enteral feeding beyond the level that provides calories and nutrients may stimulate intestinal growth and development.

The nutritional requirements of newborns are listed in Table 5-8. These requirements should be monitored closely and adjusted according to the individual needs and challenges of each infant. Infants with ineffective sucking reflexes or who do not tolerate oral feedings can receive nutritional supplements by other means. Nasogastric, orogastric, and gastrostomy tubes have been used successfully to feed premature and term infants. Total parenteral nutrition (TPN), the provision of all calories and essential nutrients by the intravenous route, is helpful in managing the nutritional requirements of critically ill infants. The problems facing the cardiovascular and respiratory systems often overwhelm the caregivers, but close attention to adequate nutrition can contribute greatly to the success of the medical care of these special patients.

▬IMMUNITY AND INFECTION IN THE NEWBORN

The immune response serves three major functions in the human body: defense against microorganisms, removal of worn-out cells to maintain homeostasis, and recognition and destruction of mutant cells.[9] In respiratory care, we are primarily concerned with the prevention and treatment of infection, and thus our major concern with the immune system lies in its ability or inability to protect the infant from pathogenic organisms. The newborn has an immune system that is both immature in its development and inexperienced in responding to pathogens.[10] Newborns are therefore susceptible to infections, and respiratory care providers need to be sensitive to prevention and recognition of infection.

Immune Mechanisms

The immune response has many components, including nonspecific responses such as phagocytosis and the inflammatory response, and specific responses of the T cells (cell-mediated response) and B cells (humoral

TABLE 5-8   Nutritional Requirements for Newborns

NUTRIENT	AMOUNT
Water	140–150 mL/kg/day
Calories	100–120 kcal/kg/day
Protein	7%–16% of calories
Fat	35%–55% calories
Carbohydrates	35%–65% of calories

(Adapted from Fletcher AB: Nutrition. In Avery GB, Fletcher MA, MacDonald MG [eds]: Neonatology: Pathophysiology and Management of the Newborn, 4th ed. Philadelphia: JB Lippincott, 1994.)

response) of the immune system. Abnormalities or deficiencies of any or all parts of this system may affect both the infant's ability to defend against infection and the care provider's ability to recognize an infectious process.

The inflammatory response in newborns is not well developed. Fever in the older child or adult is most commonly present with infection, but the febrile response is not well developed in the neonate. Thus, the presence or absence of elevated temperature is not a reliable indicator of infection in this population. Instability or lability of temperature may be a warning sign, however. Increases in white blood cell count (**leukocytosis**) and increased erythrocyte sedimentation rate, used to monitor infection in older patients, are similarly poor indicators in the newborn. An increase in bands (non-segmented neutrophils) is more significant and helpful in the diagnosis of neonatal infection. In addition, bacterial infection may activate the clotting system, eventually leading to disseminated intravascular coagulation (DIC). The monitoring of clotting factors and other components of the clotting system may be helpful in predicting infection.

Chemotaxis involves the movement of phagocytic cells toward a foreign stimulus such as an invading bacteria or virus. Chemotaxis is present in the newborn but is diminished when compared to the adult response.[46] **Phagocytosis**, which involves the ingestion of foreign particles by specific scavenger cells, may also be deficient. Various studies have shown that neonatal leukocytes may have abnormal phagocytic ability under varying conditions, although there is conflicting evidence as to whether this occurs in all newborns.[25,47]

To prepare virulent particles for phagocytosis, specific antibodies and the complement system are necessary. This process, called **opsonization**, is relatively deficient in the term newborn and more so in the preterm infant. Immunoglobulin M is probably important in the opsonization of many infectious agents, but this immunoglobulin does not cross the placenta. This may account for the relatively high incidence of gram-negative infections in the newborn population. The complement system plays a major role in the natural resistance to infection. Many components of this system have been found to be decreased in the newborn period.[10] In addition, the ability of newborn white blood cells to kill bacteria (bactericidal activity) may also be deficient, particularly in sick newborns.[73]

B cells are responsible for the synthesis of antibodies, including IgG, IgA, and IgM. These antibodies are the major defense against pyogenic pathogens such as *Haemophilus influenzae* and the meningococcus. In addition to reacting with antigens such as bacteria, antibodies are important in phagocytosis, chemotaxis, and the release of mediators of the inflammatory response. Levels of these substances are affected by transfer across the placenta and by maturation of the antibody-producing system of the body. Immunoglobulin G is actively transported across the placenta from the mother to the fetus, but other immunoglobulins are not. At birth, the infant has almost exclusively IgG, with little or no IgA or IgM. Immunoglobulin G is passively acquired from the mother, and the newborn cannot form sufficient quantities of this substance, which has a relatively short life. Thus, IgG levels decline during the first few months after birth, resulting in a condition referred to as physiologic hypogammaglobulinemia. After birth, the infant begins to produce increasing amounts of IgM, reaching adult levels by 1 year of age, and IgA, reaching adult levels by 10 years of age.[10]

Systemic Infection

Although localized infections such as skin lesions, conjunctivitis, and gastroenteritis do occur in the newborn, systemic infections are far more serious and difficult to recognize and treat. Signs and symptoms are often very subtle and nonspecific. Because of deficiencies in the immune response, the newborn cannot localize infections very well, and systemic infection occurs commonly. The deficiencies of the immune system also predispose the infant to more serious infections such as those caused by gram-negative organisms. Respiratory care providers should be aware of the risk factors that increase the likelihood of infection and of the signs and symptoms that may indicate infection. A high index of suspicion may help to identify infections in their early stages, when treatment is more effective. In addition, care providers should be constantly vigilant in their attempts to avoid introducing or spreading infection in the nursery.

Systemic infections of the newborn include sepsis, meningitis, and pneumonitis, all of which present in the same general manner and may occur at the same time. The initial approach to these problems is essentially the same. Infants who are at high risk of developing systemic infections include those born after premature rupture of the membranes (or more than 24 hours between membrane rupture and delivery of the infant); infants who required resuscitation at birth; any premature infant; infants with meconium aspiration; and infants born to mothers with fever, known infection, or amnionitis. Foul-smelling amniotic fluid following membrane rupture may be an indication of infection.

Signs of systemic infection are nonspecific and may include respiratory distress, apneic spells, and cyanosis even without obvious involvement of the pulmonary system. Other signs include unstable temperature, jaundice, difficulty feeding, lethargy, vomiting, and irritability. The presence of any of these signs in the high-risk infant indicates that diagnostic procedures should be performed, including Gram stain and culture and sensitivity testing of both blood and spinal fluid, along with a chest radiograph. Sputum sampling may also be helpful if pneumonitis is present. Complete blood count may be supportive of a diagnosis of infection, particularly if the white blood cell count is less than 5000/mm^3 or bands are greater than

2000/mm^3. A declining platelet count or an absolute decrease in platelets below 100,000/mm^3 also supports a diagnosis of systemic infection.[13]

Once a systemic infection is suspected, cultures should be drawn and antibiotic therapy begun immediately with broad-spectrum antibiotics to cover both gram-positive and gram-negative possibilities. Combinations of ampicillin and kanamycin or ampicillin and gentamycin are commonly used. *Escherichia coli*, Group B beta-hemolytic streptococcus, and *Staphylococcus aureus* are some of the more common agents that may be responsible for these infections.

Prevention of Infection

Prevention of infection is extremely important in the newborn, particularly the premature newborn with other disorders such as respiratory distress syndrome. Handwashing is the single most important and effective method of preventing the introduction and spread of infection and should be performed before and after every contact with an infant in the intensive care nursery. The initial washing should employ an iodophor preparation and should last at least 2 minutes. The effectiveness of iodophors is primarily related to the length of time they are applied. Vigorous scrubbing, although often used, is probably unnecessary. Handwashing between contacts requires about 15 seconds.

Other activities that will help to prevent nosocomial infections include the use of cover gowns by all personnel or visitors in street clothing and by any person who holds an infant. Personnel with acute febrile illness, or any highly contagious infection, should stay away from the nursery. Strict attention to aseptic technique is mandatory during invasive procedures such as endotracheal suctioning, arterial puncture, and heel sticks. Skin puncture sites must be thoroughly cleansed. Sterile technique should be used for cutdowns and catheterizations. Standard cleaning procedures for equipment should be followed and surveillance procedures established to insure their success. In general, incubators and other "housing" devices should be changed weekly and thoroughly cleaned when changed. Sterile water should be discarded after 24 hours. Oxygen hoods and equipment used for humidification and ventilation should be changed daily.

■ INTRACRANIAL HEMORRHAGE

Intracranial hemorrhage in the newborn is often related to asphyxia and hypoxia, and respiratory care providers need to be aware of the need to respond quickly to insults that may result in either of these sequelae. In addition, infants with intracranial disorders often present with various respiratory difficulties, and the respiratory care practitioner should recognize these potential signs of difficulty.

Evaluation of Neurologic Status

Although a thorough neurologic evaluation is the province of the neonatologist, all personnel involved in the care of sick premature newborns should be aware of the potential indicators of neurologic dysfunction, including changes in level of alertness, diminished cranial nerve function, changes in motor function, and decreased sensory response, as well as the more obvious indicators such as apneic spells and seizures.

A decrease from the normal level of alertness of an infant may be one of the first signs of central nervous system disorder. The clinician should be aware of what the normal alert state of the infant is in order to determine deviations from normal. Infants of less than 28 weeks' gestation are generally not alert, whereas a distinct change in the level of alertness occurs after this time.[57] Infants over 28 weeks' gestational age can be aroused from sleep and will remain awake for several minutes; they may also experience spontaneous periods of increased alertness. By 32 weeks, frequent alert states occur without stimulation, and the infant begins to exhibit roving eye movements. By 37 weeks, alertness is further increased and vigorous crying often occurs during awake periods. Term infants have additional ability to engage in periods of attention to specific stimuli.

Cranial nerve function may be evaluated by checking vision, pupillary reaction, hearing, and sucking and swallowing ability. Infants under 28 weeks blink when exposed to bright light.[57] By 32 weeks, infants exhibit the "dazzle reflex," described as the behavior of closing the eyes to bright light for as long as the light persists.[69] By 37 weeks, infants will turn their eyes toward a soft light, and by term they will exhibit visual following, which is the major definitive sign of cerebral function in newborns.[57] Pupillary reaction to light is not consistently present until 32 weeks, although it may appear as early as 29 weeks.[55] Fixed and dilated pupils are associated with hypoxic or ischemic brain injury and with intraventricular hemorrhage in newborns.[69] Hearing deficit is very difficult to evaluate in the newborn. Infants of 28 weeks will usually exhibit a startle response to a loud noise, whereas infants of more advanced gestational age may respond more subtly with such responses as changes in activity or respiratory pattern or widening of the eyes.[57,69] The complex series of activities necessary for sucking and swallowing, which are mediated by several cranial nerves, are present by 28 weeks. Infants of this age tire easily with oral feeding, however, and it may place them in a dangerous position and should be avoided. By 32 to 34 weeks, feeding should present no problem. Depression of the central nervous system associated with many disorders may disturb the ability to suck.

Motor function is evaluated by observing tone and posture, motility, muscle power, deep tendon reflexes (biceps, knee and ankle jerks), plantar response, and primary neonatal reflexes such as the Moro reflex and palmar grasp. All of these must be evaluated in relationship to the normal response for the infant's gestational age. For example, a generalized decrease in tone is expected at 28 weeks but not at term. Infants of 32 weeks may normally have decreased upper extremity tone but not lower extremity tone. Generalized hypotonia occurs in central nervous system disturbance, including hypoxic-ischemic encephalopathy and intracranial hemorrhage, although hypertonia may also occur.[69] Transillumination to detect increased intracranial fluid, skull radiographs, electroencephalograms, and CT and radionuclide brain scans may be helpful in evaluating neurologic status. Evaluation of the cerebrospinal fluid for red and white blood cells and protein is also beneficial.

Periodic Breathing and Apnea
Periodic breathing and apneic spells both occur commonly in the premature newborn. While apneic spells may be associated with central nervous system disorders, other causes may need to be excluded.

The classic pattern of periodic breathing, seen in 25% to 50% of premature infants, involves a pattern of apnea for 5 to 10 seconds, followed by ventilation at a rate of 50 to 60 breaths per minute, with an overall respiratory rate between 30 and 40 per minute.[2] There are no changes in heart rate, color, or temperature during the periods of apnea and only minor and inconsistent variations in blood gas values.[17,53,54] The occurrence of this pattern of breathing is highly related to the level of maturity, with the least mature infants exhibiting the most pronounced pattern of periodic breathing. The incidence of this pattern declines dramatically after 36 weeks of gestational age.[69] Periodic breathing probably results from immature development of the system that regulates respiration centrally.

True apneic spells in the newborn are defined as apnea of more than 20 seconds duration or apnea associated with bradycardia and cyanosis. At least 25% of premature infants in some nurseries have been shown to exhibit apneic spells.[19] This probably represents an exaggeration of the normally poor control of respiration seen in the premature newborn in response to some stress or insult. Thus, apnea and periodic breathing can be seen as variations on a continuum of abnormal regulation of respiration.

The most common factor associated with frequent apnea is extreme prematurity. Hypoxemia, either secondary to pulmonary disease or precipitated by airway obstruction, is also commonly associated with apnea. Primary central nervous system disorders may predispose the infant to apnea, and apnea may be one manifestation of seizure disorder. Metabolic disorders that disturb CNS metabolism, such as hypoglycemia, hypocalcemia, acidosis, and severe hyperbilirubinemia, may also be associated with an increased incidence of apnea.[69]

Treatment of apnea involves prompt recognition through the use of monitors and alarms, treatment of the underlying disorder whenever possible, and continuous positive airway pressure (CPAP) or theophylline therapy, or both, when necessary. The etiology and treatment of apnea of prematurity will be discussed further in Chapter 9.

Seizures

Seizures are another manifestation of central nervous system disorder. Unlike the older child, the newborn does not usually exhibit well-organized, generalized seizures, and premature newborns are even less "well organized" than term newborns. The presentation of seizure may be very subtle and the recognition very difficult. Because seizures are very often related to significant underlying disease, recognition of their occurrence is very important, and care providers should become familiar with the more common modes of presentation.

The most common type of seizure in the newborn, particularly in the very premature infant, presents in a manner that may be readily overlooked. Eye deviation or jerking, eyelid blinking or fluttering, drooling or sucking, tonic limb posturing, or apnea may all occur. "Rowing" or "swimming" movements of the upper extremities may also be present and, less commonly, "pedaling" movements of the lower extremities. Full-term infants with anoxic brain damage are more likely to exhibit multifocal clonic seizures, in which clonic movements (characterized by alternate contraction and relaxation of muscles) occur in one limb and then migrate to another body part, without any particular ordering of the involved areas. Focal clonic seizures may also occur, with well-localized clonic movements, although these do not necessarily indicate localized disease in the newborn. Premature infants with intraventricular hemorrhage are most likely to exhibit generalized tonic seizures (sustained muscle contraction), often associated with noisy, snoring respirations, various abnormalities of gaze or eye movement, or clonic movements of a limb. Finally, seizures may be myoclonic, with single or multiple jerks of flexion of upper or lower extremities, or both.[69]

Jitteriness is another sign associated with central nervous system disorder in newborns; it should not be confused with seizure. Jitteriness is rarely seen outside the newborn period and is a movement disorder characterized by tremors and occasional clonus. The major differences between jitteriness and seizure include lack of abnormal gaze or eye movement with jitteriness, no stimulus sensitivity with seizures but extreme stimulus sensitivity with jitteriness, dominance of tremor in jitteriness and clonic jerking in seizure, and response of tremor to flexion of extremity in jitteriness but not in seizures.[69]

Etiology of Seizures

The most common causes of seizures in the newborn are related to complications of the perinatal period, including hypoxic or ischemic brain damage, cerebral contusion from obstetric trauma, and intracranial hemorrhage. Of these, hypoxic–ischemic encephalopathy is the most common, usually resulting from perinatal asphyxia. Cerebral trauma is most commonly associated with difficult delivery of a large, full-term infant, whereas intracranial hemorrhage may be associated with either birth trauma or hypoxia, or both. Other causes of seizures include metabolic disturbances, infection, developmental disorders (most commonly of the cerebral cortex), and maternal addiction to narcotics or barbiturates.

Causes Other Than Intracranial Hemorrhage

The most common metabolic disturbance associated with seizures is hypoglycemia (blood glucose less than 20 mg/100 mL in premature infants, or less than 30 mg/100 mL in full-term infants). In addition to seizures, these infants usually are jittery, stuporous, and hypotonic and may exhibit apneic spells. Hypocalcemia (serum calcium less than 7 mg/100 mL) may occur within the first 2 to 3 days of life, often in association with hypoxic–ischemic brain injury following asphyxic insult. It is unclear whether seizure in this setting is secondary to hypocalcemia or anoxic brain injury. Hypocalcemia occurring later in the first week is more likely to be etiologic in seizure production. Infections related to seizures include bacterial meningitis and the TORCH group of infections. Maternal addiction to narcotics or barbiturates results in passive fetal addiction and the development of withdrawal symptoms in the first 2 or 3 days of life.[12,75] Seizures are infrequently associated with addiction, with jitteriness and irritability occurring much more commonly.

Types of Intracranial Hemorrhage

Intracranial hemorrhage is a relatively common occurrence in premature newborns and is related primarily to asphyxia in this group. In term infants, hemorrhage is more likely to be associated with trauma. Four major types of hemorrhage occur: subdural hemorrhage secondary to trauma, periventricular–intraventricular hemorrhage secondary to asphyxia, subarachnoid hemorrhage related to both trauma and asphyxia, and intercerebellar hemorrhage, which is probably secondary to asphyxia.

SUBDURAL HEMORRHAGE

Subdural hemorrhage may result from tears in various vessels. The most serious consequences result when infratentorial hemorrhage occurs, causing rapid and lethal compression of the brain stem. The infant with such hemorrhage usually has severe disturbance from birth, with stupor or coma, eye deviation, unequal pupils with disturbed response to light, and rapid respiration, progressing to coma, fixed and dilated pupils, ataxic respirations, and respiratory arrest. Rupture of superficial cerebral veins may also occur, resulting in subdural hemorrhage with few clinically significant consequences.

PRIMARY SUBARACHNOID HEMORRHAGE

Primary subarachnoid hemorrhage occurs when there is hemorrhage into the subarachnoid space that is not the result of extension of a subdural or intraventricular hemorrhage. This occurs commonly but is usually not of major clinical significance.

INTRAVENTRICULAR HEMORRHAGE

Periventricular–intraventricular hemorrhage, commonly referred to as **intraventricular hemorrhage** (IVH), classically involves hemorrhage into the subependymal germinal matrix, which then bursts through into the ventricular system. Some of these hemorrhages, however, remain subependymal. The lesion begins in the capillaries of the periventricular vascular network.[30] This disturbance is almost invariably associated with prematurity, with the highest risk associated with the lowest gestational age.[67] In two studies of premature infants of less than 32 weeks' gestation or less than 1500 g birth weight, 40% to 50% had documented IVH.[1,52]

Two major consequences are associated with IVH: rapid deterioration, which is usually associated with massive hemorrhage (conversely, massive hemorrhage does not always result in rapid deterioration); and a much slower, more subtle progression, which Volpe and Koenigsberger have referred to as saltatory deterioration because of its halting progression.[69] Rapid deterioration usually occurs within 24 to 48 hours after a major episode of asphyxia.[31] The infant's condition evolves rapidly from stupor and hyperventilation, proceeding to coma and respiratory arrest, with fixed pupils, eye deviation, flaccid quadriparesis, and occasional tonic seizures and decerebrate posturing. CT scan of the brain reveals major hemorrhage, and severe hydrocephalus or death usually ensues. By contrast, saltatory deterioration may go unnoticed, with some of the signs mentioned previously occurring at various times, and with most infants surviving, a few with hydrocephalus.[69]

Pathogenesis of IVH. Prematurity predisposes the infant to IVH for several reasons. First, the subependymal germinal matrix is present in the preterm infant but not in the term infant. This matrix provides very poor support for the vessels passing through it. Second, vascular autoregulation is not good in premature infants, so that increases in vascular pressure with resuscitation and fluid infusion may result in vessel rupture.[39,68] Periventricular vessels in premature infants are thin and fragile. Third, the anatomy of the periventricular vessels involves a sharp U-turn of the blood vessels, which predisposes to venous stasis, congestion, and, thus, increased intravascular pressure and consequent rupture of vessels.[69] Asphyxia may increase the incidence of this occurrence by causing circulatory failure and increased venous congestion, by directly injuring the vascular endothelium, or by impairing vascular autoregulation.[40,51]

INTERCEREBELLAR HEMORRHAGE

Intercerebellar hemorrhage (ICH) has been demonstrated to occur with relative frequency in small premature infants. In two studies of infants younger than 32 weeks and 1500 g birth weight, 15% to 25% had major ICH.[29,44] There was a strong association between ICH and IVH, and it is postulated that ICH may be an extension of IVH.[21] Clinically, ICH is associated with perinatal asphyxia, respiratory distress syndrome, or both. It usually results in rapid deterioration and death, with apnea, bradycardia, decreasing hematocrit, and blood in the cerebrospinal fluid. The onset varies over the first weeks of life, with death occurring within 12 to 36 hours of onset, very much like severe IVH. The pathogenesis remains unclear, although some relationship to mask CPAP has been demonstrated.[50]

■REFERENCES

1. Ahmann PA, Lazzara A, Dykes FD et al: Intraventricular hemorrhage: Incidence and outcome. Ann Neurol 4:186, 1978.
2. Avery ME, Fletcher BD: The Lung and Its Disorders in the Newborn Infant, 3rd ed. Philadelphia, WB Saunders, 1974.
3. Baumgart S, Engle WD, Fox WW, Polin, RA: Effect of heat shielding on convective and evaporative heat losses and on radiant heat transfer in the premature infant. J Pediatrics 99:948, 1981.
4. Belgaumkar TK, Scott KE: Effects of low humidity on small premature infants in servo-control incubators. Biol Neonate 26:348, 1975.
5. Bell EF, Warburton D, Stonestreet BS, Oh W: High-volume fluid intake predisposes premature infants to necrotizing enterocolitis. Lancet 2:90, 1979.
6. Bell EF, Warburton D, Stonestreet BS, Oh W: Randomized trial comparing high and low volume maintenance fluid administration in low birth weight infants with reference to congestive heart failure secondary to patent ductus arteriosus. N Engl J Med 302:598, 1980.
7. Bell EF, Oh W: Fluid and electrolyte management. In Avery GB, Fletcher MA, MacDonald MG (eds): Neonatology: Pathophysiology and Management of the Newborn, 4th ed. Philadelphia, JB Lippincott, 1994.
8. Bell EF, Weinstein MR, Oh W: Heat balance in premature infants: Comparative effects of convectively heated incubator and radiant warmer, with and without plastic heat shield. J Pediatr 96:460, 1980.
9. Bellanti JA: Immunology II. Philadelphia, WB Saunders, 1978.
10. Bellanti JA, Boner AL: Immunology of the fetus and newborn. In Avery GB (ed): Neonatology: Pathophysiology and Management of the Newborn, 2nd ed. Philadelphia, JB Lippincott, 1981.
11. Bertoletti AL, Stevenson DK, Ostrander CR, Johnson JD: Pulmonary excretion of carbon monoxide in the human infant as an index of bilirubin production: 1. Effects of gestational age and postnatal age and some common neonatal abnormalities. J Pediatr 94:952, 1979.
12. Bleyer WA, Marshall RE: Barbiturate withdrawal syndrome in a passively addicted infant. JAMA 221:185, 1972.
13. Borer RC, Wall PM, Rothfelder BS: Bacterial Infection in the Newborn. Ann Arbor, University of Michigan, 1977.

14. Brodersen R, Herman LS: Intestinal reabsorption of unconjugated bilirubin: A possible contributing factor in neonatal jaundice. Lancet 1:1242, 1962.
15. Bruck K: Temperature regulation in the newborn infant. Biol Neonate 3:65, 1961.
16. Burgess WR, Chernick V: Respiratory Therapy in Newborn Infants and Children, 2nd ed. New York, Thieme, 1986.
17. Chernick V, Heldrich F, Avery ME: Periodic breathing of premature infants. J Pediatr 64:330, 1964.
18. Cremer RJ, Perryman PW, Richards DH. Influence of light on the hyperbilirubinemia of infants. Lancet 1:1094, 1958.
19. Daily WJR, Klaus M, Meyer HBP: Apnea in premature infants: Monitoring, incidence, heart rate changes, and an effect of environmental temperature. Pediatrics 43:510, 1969.
20. Daum F, Cohen MI, McNamara H: Experimental toxicologic studies on a phenol detergent associated with neonatal hyperbilirubinemia. J Pediatr 89:853, 1976.
21. Donat JF, Okasaki H, Kleinberg F: Cerebellar hemorrhage in newborn infants. Am J Dis Child 133:441, 1979.
22. Drew JH, Barrie J, Horacek I, Kitchen WH: Factors influencing jaundice in immigrant Greek infants. Arch Dis Child 53:49, 1978.
23. Fanaroff AA, Wald M, Gruber HS, Klaus MH: Insensible water loss in low birth weight infants. Pediatrics 50:236, 1972.
24. Fant M, Cloherty JP: Temperature control. In Cloherty JP, Stark AR (eds): Manual of Neonatal Care, 2nd ed. Boston, Little, Brown, 1985.
25. Froman ML, Stiehm ER: Impaired opsonic activity but normal phagocytosis in low birth-weight infants. N Engl J Med 281:926, 1969.
26. Gartner LM, Lee K-S: Jaundice and liver disease. In Behrman RE (ed): Neonatal Perinatal Medicine. St. Louis, CV Mosby, 1977.
27. Gartner LM, Lee K-S, Vaisman S et al: Development of bilirubin transport and metabolism in the newborn rhesus monkey. J Pediatr 90:513, 1977.
28. Gross SJ: Vitamin E and neonatal bilirubinemia. Pediatrics 64:321, 1979.
29. Grunnett ML, Shields WD: Cerebellar hemorrhage in the premature infant. J Pediatr 88:605, 1976.
30. Hambleton G, Wigglesworth JS: Origin of intraventricular hemorrhage in the preterm infant. Arch Dis Child 51:651, 1976.
31. Harrison VC, Heese H de V, Klein M: Intracranial hemorrhage associated with hyaline membrane disease. Arch Dis Child 43:116, 1968.
32. Hey EN, Katz G: Evaporative water loss in the new-born baby. J Physiol 200:605, 1969.
33. Hey EN, Katz G: The range of thermal insulation in the tissues of the newborn baby. J Physiol 207:667, 1970.
34. Hey EN, Katz G, O'Connell B: The total thermal insulation of the newborn baby. J Physiol 207:683, 1970.
35. Hey EH: Thermoregulation. In Avery GB, Fletcher MA, MacDonald MG (eds): Neonatology: Pathophysiology and Management of the Newborn, 4th ed. Philadelphia, JB Lippincott, 1994.
36. Hull D: Brown adipose tissue. Br Med Bull 22:92, 1966.
37. Korones SB: High-Risk Newborn Infants: The Basis for Intensive Nursing Care, 3rd ed. St. Louis, CV Mosby, 1981.
38. Levi AJ, Gatmaitan Z, Adias I: Deficiency of hepatic organic anion-binding protein, impaired organic anion uptake by liver and "physiologic jaundice" in newborn monkeys. N Engl J Med 283:1136, 1970.
39. Lou HC, Lassen NA, Friis-Hansen B: Impaired autoregulation of cerebral blood flow in the distressed newborn. J Pediatr 94:118, 1979.
40. Lou HC, Lassen NA, Tweed WA et al: Pressure passive cerebral blood flow and breakdown of the blood–brain barrier in experimental fetal asphyxia. Acta Paediatr Scand 68:57, 1979.
41. Lucey JF: The unsolved problem of kernicterus in the susceptible low birth weight infant. Pediatr 49:646, 1972.
42. Maisels MJ. Neonatal jaundice. In: Sinclair JC, Bracken MB (eds): Effective Care of the Newborn Infant. Oxford, Oxford University Press, 1992.
43. Maisels MJ: Jaundice. In Avery GB, Fletcher MA, MacDonald MG (eds): Neonatology: Pathophysiology and Management of the Newborn, 4th ed. Philadelphia, JB Lippincott, 1994.
44. Martin R, Roessman U, Fanaroff A: Massive intracerebellar hemorrhage in low birth weight infants. J Pediatr 89:290, 1976.

45. Mestyan I, Jarai GB, Feket M: Surface temperature versus deep body temperature and the metabolic response to cold of hypothermic premature infants. Biol Neonate 7:230, 1964.
46. Miller ME: Chemotactic function in the human neonate: Humoral and cellular function. Pediatr Res 5:487, 1971.
47. Miller ME: Phagocytosis in the newborn infant: Humoral and cellular factors. J Pediatr 74:255, 1969.
48. Oh W: Fluid and electrolyte management. In Avery GB (ed): Neonatology: Pathophysiology and Management of the Newborn, 2nd ed. Philadelphia, JB Lippincott, 1981.
49. Oh W, Karecki H: Phototherapy and insensible water loss in the newborn infant. Am J Dis Child 124:230, 1972.
50. Pape KE, Armstrong DL, Fitzhardinge PM: Central nervous system pathology associated with mask ventilation in the very low birth-weight infant: A new etiology for intracerebellar hemorrhage. Pediatrics 58:473, 1976.
51. Pape KE, Wigglesworth JS: Haemorrhage, Ischaemia and the Perinatal Brain. Philadelphia, JB Lippincott, 1979.
52. Papile L, Burstein J, Burstein R et al: Incidence and evolution of subependymal hemorrhage: A study of infants with birth weights less than 1500 gm. J Pediatr 92:529, 1978.
53. Rigatto H, Brady JP: Periodic breathing and apnea in preterm infants: Evidence for hypoventilation possibly due to central respiratory depression: I. Pediatrics 50:202, 1972.
54. Rigatto H, Brady JP: Periodic breathing in preterm infants: Hypoxia as a primary event: II. Pediatrics 50:219, 1972.
55. Robinson RJ: Assessment of gestational age by neurologic examination. Arch Dis Child 41:437, 1966.
56. Saigal S, O'Neill A, Surainder Y et al: Placental transfusion and hyperbilirubinemia in the premature. Pediatrics 49: 406, 1972.
57. Saint-Anne Dargassies S: Neurological maturation of the premature infant of 28–41 weeks gestational age. In Falkner F (ed): Human Development. Philadelphia, WB Saunders, 1966.
58. Saland J, McNamara H, Cohen MI: Navajo jaundice: A variant of neonatal hyperbilirubinemia associated with breast feeding. J Pediatr 85:271, 1974.
59. Scopes JW: Metabolic rate and temperature control in the human baby. Br Med Bull 22:88, 1966.
60. Scopes JW: Thermoregulation in the newborn. In Avery GB (ed): Neonatology: Pathophysiology and Management of the Newborn, 2nd ed. Philadelphia, JB Lippincott, 1981.
61. Scopes JW, Ahmed I: Range of critical temperatures in sick and premature newborn babies. Arch Dis Child 41: 417, 1966.
62. Silverman WA, Blanc WA: The effects of humidity on survival of newly born premature infants. Pediatrics 20: 477, 1957.
63. Silverman WA, Fertig JW, Berger AP: The influence of the thermal environment upon the survival of newly born premature infants. Pediatrics 22:876, 1958.
64. Silverman WA, Sinclair JC, Agate FJ: The oxygen cost of minor changes in heat balance of small newborn infants. Acta Paediatr Scand 55:294, 1966.
65. Valaes T, Harvey-Wilkes K: Pharmacologic approaches to the prevention and treatment of neonatal hyperbilirubinemia. Clin Perinatol 17:245, 1990.
66. Valdes OS, Maurer HM, Shumway CN et al: Controlled clinical trials of phenobarbital and/or light in reducing neonatal hyperbilirubinemia in a predominantly Negro population. J Pediatrics 79:1015, 1971.
67. Volpe JJ: Neonatal intracranial hemorrhage. Clin Perinatol 4:77, 1977.
68. Volpe JJ: Neonatal periventricular hemorrhage: Past, present, and future. J Pediatr 92:693, 1978.
69. Volpe JJ, Koenigsberger R: Neurologic disorders. In Avery GB (ed): Neonatology: Pathophysiology and Management of the Newborn, 2nd ed. Philadelphia, JB Lippincott, 1981.
70. Wennberg RP, Depp R, Heinrichs WL: Indications for early exchange transfusion in patients with erythroblastosis fetalis. J Pediatr 92:789, 1978.
71. Wennberg RP, Schwartz R, Sweet AY: Early versus delayed feeding of low birth weight infants: Effects on physiologic jaundice. J Pediatr 68:800, 1966.
72. Williams PR, Oh W: The effects of radiant warmer on insensible water loss in newborn infants. Am J Dis Child 128:511, 1974.
73. Wright WC Jr, Ank BJ, Herbert J et al: Decreased bactericidal activity of leukocytes of stressed newborn infants. Pediatrics 56:578, 1975.
74. Wysowski DK, Flynt JW, Goldfield M et al: Epidemic neonatal hyperbilirubinemia and the use of phenolic disinfectant detergent. Pediatrics 61:1, 1978.
75. Zelson C, Rubir E, Wasserman E: Neonatal narcotic addiction. Pediatrics 48:178, 1971.

▬SELF-ASSESSMENT QUESTIONS

1. The three major components of the thermoregulatory system are
    I. skin
    II. hypothalamus
    III. method of regulating heat loss
  a. I only
  b. II and III
  c. III only
  d. I, II, and III

2. The major mechanism for heat production in the newborn is
  a. reduced oxygen consumption
  b. metabolism of brown fat
  c. shivering
  d. increased metabolic rate

3. What abdominal skin temperature will avoid overheating or under-heating and problems associated with oxygen consumption in newborns?
  a. 28°C   c. 36°C
  b. 30°C   d. 44°C

4. The reabsorption of unconjugated bilirubin through the intestines is referred to as the
  a. enterohepatic shunt   c. icterus
  b. kernicterus   d. jaundice

5. Which of the following factors will *increase* serum bilirubin levels in the infant?
    I. vitamin K administration
    II. phenolic detergents
    III. vitamin E administration
    IV. early feedings
  a. I only
  b. I and II
  c. III and IV
  d. I, II, III, and IV

6. Which of the following factors *decrease* insensible water loss?
    I. crying
    II. Plexiglas heat shields
    III. semipermeable membrane
  a. I only
  b. II and III
  c. I and III
  d. I, II, and III

7. What is the daily recommended nutritional requirement for water in the newborn?
  a. 10–20 mL/kg
  b. 50–60 mL/kg
  c. 90–100 mL/kg
  d. 140–150 mL/kg

8. Which of the following is a sign of systemic infection in the newborn?
   a. irritability   c. difficulty feeding
   b. apneic spells   d. all of the above

9. Major causes of seizures in the newborn include
   a. hypoxic brain damage
   b. obstetric trauma
   c. cerebral contusion
   d. all of the above

10. The major types of intracranial hemorrhage in the newborn include
    I. subarachnoid
    II. cerebellar
    III. subdural
    IV. periventricular–intraventricular
    a. II and III
    b. I and IV
    c. II, III, and IV
    d. I, II, III, and IV

Chapter 6

History and Physical Assessment of the Child

EARL FULCHER, JR.

OBJECTIVES

Having completed this chapter, the reader will be able to:

1 Obtain an accurate medical history through the use of condition-specific questions.

2 Understand the importance of utilizing certain calming measures during the assessment of the child.

3 Recognize respiratory insufficiency through the use of appropriate observation skills.

4 Understand how palpation and diagnostic percussion of the chest can be used to detect areas of pulmonary disease.

5 Understand how to distinguish between adventitious breath sounds and normal sounds produced in the upper airway.

6 Apply basic physiologic principles in the assessment of the cardiac system of the child.

KEY TERMS

crackles	rhonchi
diagnostic percussion	stridor
digital clubbing	vesicular breath sounds
paradoxical breathing	wheezes
pulsus paradoxus	

▬OBTAINING A MEDICAL HISTORY

A thorough medical history should be obtained for any child who initially presents with dyspnea or signs of respiratory distress. A concise but complete medical history can be obtained in only a few moments and can be vital to the proper assessment and treatment of the child. The history should be acquired from a parent or guardian. The child may also be questioned if he or she has the capacity to relay the necessary information.[24]

The first question that should be asked is whether the patient has ever displayed or been treated for similar symptoms. This one question will often rapidly lead the clinician toward an accurate diagnosis and appropriate treatment plan. The clinician should seek to discover the specific type of care that was administered during previous episodes. The amount of time between hospitalizations or visits to a physician should also be assessed at this time. This information may assist the clinician in determining whether the problem is acute or chronic and what may be triggering recurrent episodes of the same symptoms.

The pediatric clinician should then ask a series of condition-specific questions concerning the child's health. Common conditions that often lead to pulmonary insufficiency in the child are small airway disease, infectious processes, upper airway obstruction, and congenital disorders. There are specific causative agents and risk factors that may predispose children to these pulmonary conditions (Table 6-1).

The child who presents with signs of small airway obstruction should be assessed for the risk factors of asthma or bronchiolitis. The practitioner who suspects asthma needs to determine whether there is a family history of asthma, how often the symptoms reoccur, and the child's reaction after exposure to certain allergens such as pollen and cigarette smoke. A common cold often leads to an asthma exacerbation in children. A history of upper respiratory tract infection (URI) also precedes symptoms of small airway obstruction caused by bronchiolitis. Therefore, a thorough history is often needed to differentiate between asthma and bronchiolitis in the young child when the symptoms were preceded by a URI.[12,15,16] The child with a history of gastroesophageal reflux may be predisposed to reactive airway disease. Whenever aspiration of gastric contents is thought to be the cause of reactive airways, a feeding history should also be obtained.[12,16,20] Other factors which may lead to small airway obstruction include neonatal chronic lung disease and congenital airway malformations such as tracheal esophageal fistula.

Infectious pulmonary processes are often associated with an elevated body temperature and increased sputum production. Therefore, the high-

TABLE 6-1 Common Causes of Pulmonary Insufficiency in Children

SMALL AIRWAY DISEASE	INFECTION	UPPER AIRWAY OBSTRUCTION	CONGENITAL DISORDERS
Asthma	Viral pneumonia	Croup	Cystic fibrosis
Bronchiolitis	Bacterial pneumonia	Foreign body aspiration	Tracheomalacia
GI reflux (reactive airway disease)	Sepsis	Epiglottitis	Immotile cilia syndrome
Neonatal chronic lung disease		Thermal airway burn	Laryngomalacia

est reported temperature should be recorded as well as the use of any antipyretics and antibiotics. Knowing the degree of fever as well its onset and duration may also help the clinician determine whether the causative agent is bacterial or viral. The amount, color, odor, and consistency of sputum needs to be assessed. Parents or guardians of children with infectious pulmonary processes may report feeding difficulties secondary to vomiting caused by thick sputum or mucus. The clinician should also determine whether other family members or the child's peers have recently displayed and been treated for similar symptoms. Many viruses that present as a common cold in the older child or adult may lead to a pulmonary infection in an infant or toddler.[8]

Signs of upper airway obstruction may also be preceded by a history of URI in cases of croup (see Chap. 10). A rapid onset of upper airway obstruction along with a history of high fever and other signs of bacterial infection should lead the clinician to suspect epiglottitis. When epiglottitis is suspected, the clinician should quickly attempt to ascertain whether the child has been vaccinated for *Hemophilus influenzae* type B, the causative agent in epiglottitis.[21] A rapid onset of upper airway obstruction without signs of infection requires the clinician to determine whether the possible cause may be foreign body aspiration or an airway burn. Very hot foods, especially those heated in a microwave oven, may lead to upper airway inflammation and signs of partial airway obstruction in young children.[18]

The child who presents with recurrent episodes of productive cough and chronic respiratory tract infections should be assessed for possible hereditary disorders such as cystic fibrosis and immotile cilia syndrome. Along with a history of repeated pulmonary or sinus infections, the child's parent or guardian should be questioned concerning a family history of similar symptoms and disorders.[5,9,17]

In addition to gathering the above information, the clinician should determine current medications being used by the child. These may include supplemental oxygen, antibiotics, bronchodilators, corticosteroids, antipyretics, theophylline, and cough suppressants. The clinician should also ascertain the child's use of home medical equipment such as apnea monitors, air compressors for nebulizer therapy, and peak flowmeters. This information may assist not only in the assessment of the patient but also in the initial care plan.

■ GENERAL ASSESSMENT

When preparing to assess the child who presents with signs of respiratory insufficiency, it is important to first determine the patient's current emotional state and to evaluate his or her interaction with a parent or guardian. Is a parent or guardian present? Does the child appear frightened? Is the child crying? Did the child just experience an invasive procedure such as venipuncture? Is the child experiencing pain in conjunction with breathing difficulty? The answers to these questions can be quickly acquired from a nurse, physician, or other health care professional who has seen the child prior to the arrival of the respiratory care practitioner.

Shortness of breath, along with the environment of a hospital or clinic, can be very frightening for the young child. Steps that can be taken to ease this fear include having a parent or guardian present during the assessment; sitting or kneeling in front of the child instead of standing; speaking in a soft, calm voice; and using common words and phrases to describe the procedures that will take place. When appropriate, the use of children's adhesive stickers, coloring books, or dolls may also help to calm the frightened child.[24]

The pediatric clinician should immediately begin to assess the patient upon entrance into the patient's room. This initial assessment is done by simply observing the child while using the calming measures listed earlier. The clinician should immediately note whether the child appears to be of appropriate height and weight for his or her age. Failure to thrive is often a sign of chronic conditions in the child.[17,24] The presence of a cough may be a sign that the child is experiencing bronchospasm or airway inflammation.[12] The child's body position may hold clues as to the cause of respiratory distress. The child who is sitting upright with the neck extended in a forward position may be experiencing partial upper airway obstruction.[25] The child's ability to talk *without* frequent pauses can assist the clinician in determining the severity of respiratory insufficiency. Finally, the clinician should quickly note whether the child has any dysmorphic features that may be associated with the symptoms that are present.

■ ASSESSMENT OF THE RESPIRATORY SYSTEM

The entire process of obtaining a medical history, general assessment of the child, and assessment of the respiratory system can usually be completed in only a few minutes. Assessment of the respiratory system may be performed at the same time or immediately after the medical history is obtained. Assessment of the respiratory system includes inspection for signs of increased work of breathing, percussion and palpation of the chest, and auscultation of the chest.

Inspection

The child's respiratory rate and pattern are often indications of the cause and severity of respiratory distress. Upon inspecting the child's respiratory system for signs of increased work of breathing, the level of consciousness should be determined. A child's respiratory rate and pattern will vary significantly during sleep versus awake times and with the level of anxiety or sedation. Therefore, the respiratory rate and pattern should be assessed *before* any other procedure or assessment is performed. Since a child's respiratory rate may vary significantly, the respiratory rate must be counted for one full minute.

The normal respiratory rate of the child decreases with increasing age (Table 6-2). Tachypnea, especially in the sleeping child, should always be cause for concern. Tachypnea may occur as a result of hypoxemia or elevated $PaCO_2$. The clinician must also remember that tachypnea may be a result of fever or metabolic acidosis. Bradypnea may be an indication of low body temperature, heavy sedation, or impending respiratory failure. Kussmaul's breathing, a rapid and deep breathing pattern, may be observed in the pediatric diabetic patient during a ketoacidotic state. A **paradoxical** pattern, with the abdomen moving noticeably outward and the chest inward during inspiration, is often a sign of decreased lung compliance and, possibly, impending respiratory failure.[2]

TABLE 6-2 Normal Respiratory Rates in Children*

AGE	RATE (BREATH PER MIN)
Infant	30–60
Toddler	24–40
Preschooler	22–34
School-aged child	18–30
Adolescent	12–16

*The patient's normal range should always be considered. Also, the child's respiratory rate is expected to increase in the presence of fever or stress.

The ratio of inspiratory time to expiratory time (I:E ratio) should also be noted when assessing the respiratory pattern. Children with a restrictive lung disorder will display a rapid, shallow breathing pattern with an increased I:E ratio while those with an obstructive disorder will display a slow, deep breathing pattern with a decreased I:E ratio. Learning to recognize abnormal breathing rates and patterns is a critical skill that must be acquired by all clinicians caring for the sick child.

During the initial evaluation of the child, the color of the skin, mucous membranes, and nail beds should be assessed. A dusky or mottled color may indicate hypovolemia, shock, or cardiac dysfunction. Cyanosis, a bluish color of the skin and mucous membranes, is defined as greater than 5 g/dL of unsaturated hemoglobin.[6] Cyanosis must be evaluated by looking at the lips and nail beds of a child in a well-lit room. It is possible for a patient to be severely hypoxemic without appearing cyanotic. This could occur in the anemic patient since there is not enough hemoglobin present for cyanosis to appear. Cyanosis may also appear in the child who is severely hypothermic, such as the near-drowning victim (see Chap. 10). The typical cause of cyanosis is arterial hypoxemia secondary to a right-to-left intrapulmonary shunt. Intrapulmonary shunt of a degree that is severe enough to lead to a cyanotic appearance is usually caused by significant atelectasis, lung consolidation, pulmonary edema, or airway obstruction. The PaO_2 will typically be less than 50 torr when cyanosis is present.[6,7] *Therefore, cyanosis should always be considered a late, grave sign of hypoxemia.* Supplemental oxygen therapy or an increase in delivered FIO_2 should be implemented immediately without waiting for confirmation of a low PaO_2 or SaO_2.

Other signs of an increased work of breathing secondary to respiratory insufficiency are diaphoresis, nasal flaring, and retractions. Diaphoresis occurs when the respiratory muscles are performing at their maximum level because of a significant strain placed on them to overcome increased resistive and elastic forces present in the lung. The child who is diaphoretic because of pulmonary insufficiency is usually severely ill and may be on the verge of respiratory failure. Nasal flaring is a compensatory mechanism by the body to decrease airway resistance during times of increased ventilatory requirements. Nasal flaring is most often seen in infants and young children.

Retractions occur when a child begins to breathe with increased effort during respiratory distress. The increased ventilatory efforts cause the intrapleural pressure to become more negative, which leads to an inward pull on the soft tissue around the bony structures of the thorax.[2,22] Retractions are classified by their location and severity. As respiratory distress worsens and ventilatory efforts increase, the amount of inward movement of the soft tissues also increases. Intercostal retractions are the most common and vary in severity with the degree of respiratory distress. Substernal retractions are often present along with intercostal retractions during more severe cases of pulmonary insufficiency. The presence of suprasternal retractions should alert the clinician to the possibility of upper airway obstruction.

The pediatric clinician should also assess the child for **digital clubbing**. Clubbing is defined as an enlargement of the terminal phalanges both on the hands and feet. The exact cause for clubbing is unknown. It is most often associated with chronic conditions of reduced oxygen delivery to the tissues.[13] Clubbing of the digits may be an indication of chronic pulmonary or cardiovascular disorders including cystic fibrosis, severe asthma, pulmonary fibrosis, and congenital heart disease.

Percussion and Palpation of the Chest

The examiner performs palpation of the child's chest by placing his or her hands *lightly* on the patient's chest, ensuring that the fingertips and palms are in contact with the chest. Palpation may be performed with one or both hands, always assuring that each area of one lung is compared with the same area of the opposite lung. The patient is instructed to take slow, deep breaths if possible.

Palpation of the chest may be used to determine the presence of asymmetrical chest movement, tactile fremitus, and tenderness or pain. Asymmetrical chest movement may be noted if both hands are placed on the anterior, upper chest with one hand rising to a greater degree than the other. Asymmetrical chest movement may be an indication of unilateral atelectasis or pneumothorax. Tactile fremitus is usually a sign of accumulation of secretions in the large airways. Tactile fremitus may also be felt on the anterior chest if a large amount of secretions are present in the upper airway. If, during palpation, the child complains of pain or tenderness at the peak of inspiration, this may be indicative of a pleural infection or pneumothorax.[4]

Diagnostic percussion of the chest is performed by placing one or more fingers of one hand between the ribs of the child and then tapping the tips of those fingers with a finger from the other hand, which is held in a crooked and stiff manner (Fig. 6-1). The sound produced by the tapping of the clinician's fingers is then assessed with each area of one lung compared to the same area of the opposite lung.

Diagnostic percussion is typically not useful in the young child or infant since their chest walls are very compliant and small, causing sounds to transmit readily and be similar throughout. Diagnostic percussion may be used to determine the presence of atelectasis or consolidation and air trapping or pneumothorax. The percussion note produced over an atelectatic or consolidated area of the lung will be dull. The percussion note produced over an area of the lung which is hyperinflated or has a pneumothorax present will be hyperresonant.[13,19] One should repeatedly

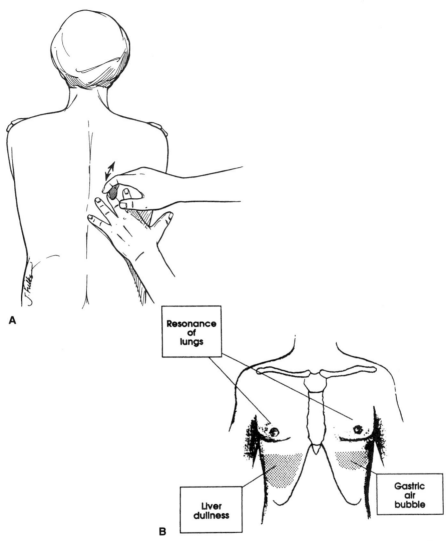

FIGURE 6-1   (*A*) The examiner's middle finger is placed against the posterior chest wall and is struck with the opposite middle finger. (*B*) Percussion notes over the lungs, liver, and gastric air bubble. (Barnes TA: Core Textbook of Respiratory Care Practice, 2nd ed. St Louis, Mosby, 1994.)

perform diagnostic chest percussion on "normal" individuals to gain an understanding of what normal percussion notes sound like prior to evaluating children with possible respiratory disease.

Auscultation of the Chest

Auscultation of the chest is often the primary assessment tool utilized by respiratory care practitioners and other health care professionals in their evaluation of the child with respiratory insufficiency. Auscultation plays an integral role in the assessment of the child and can often lead the clinician toward an accurate diagnosis and proper treatment plan. However, the type of breath sounds heard during auscultation should be used in conjunction with other data and information collected during the assessment of the patient. Breath sounds alone should *not* be used to diagnose and treat the patient.

Auscultation of the chest of a young child or infant presents the clinician with several potential roadblocks which may lead to an inaccurate assessment of breath sounds. The first problem is that an infant or toddler usually will not remain motionless or quiet during auscultation. Vocal sounds or sounds made by the movement of clothing or linen against the stethoscope may be misinterpreted as abnormal sounds. The infant or toddler usually will *not* take a deep inspiration upon command, thereby making the clinician's evaluation that much more difficult. Therefore, the room should be as quiet as possible with the volume on televisions, radios, and video games minimized. The parent or guardian may be asked to assist in this effort. As mentioned in earlier sections, the young child or infant may become frightened during the assessment process and begin crying. The parent or guardian should be encouraged to sit with or hold the child while auscultation is performed. If the child continues to cry despite repeated comfort measures, proper evaluation of breath sounds will be virtually impossible and should be recorded as such.

The size of the stethoscope can be a potential problem, however the adult-sized stethoscope is typically adequate for children from the toddler age and older. A pediatric-sized stethoscope should be used on newborns and infants. The pediatric clinician must be aware of all conditions that may lead to a misinterpretation of breath sounds and learn to minimize their effects.

Auscultation of the child should be performed in a systematic fashion, with each area or segment of one lung immediately compared to the same area of the opposite lung. The clinician should be aware of the location of the segments of the lung when viewing the chest from anterior, posterior, and lateral perspectives (Fig. 6-2). The clinician should then use this knowledge when assessing breath sounds. Auscultation of breath sounds over each area of the lung should be performed during at least two complete respiratory cycles. Only listening during inspiration or for just one breath may cause the clinician to miss potentially important sounds such as end-expiratory wheezing or intermittent crackles.

The breath sounds normally heard over the trachea and large airways are typically described as *bronchial*. Bronchial breath sounds have a smooth, rushing quality that can be heard during inspiration and exhalation. Normal breath sounds that are heard over the periphery of the lung are described as **vesicular breath sounds**. Vesicular sounds are smooth and low in frequency and can only be heard during inspiration as gas enters inflated alveoli. Bronchial breath sounds heard over the periphery of the lung indicate lung consolidation. This occurs because the sound of gas flowing through the small airways is transmitted much easier through dense, consolidated lung tissue than through air-filled alveoli.[19]

Abnormal breath sounds are termed adventitious breath sounds. The nomenclature of adventitious breath sounds has been challenged and changed by some authors in recent years.[4,23] The two adventitious sounds whose meaning has not changed are wheezes and crackles. **Crackles** are the sounds typically heard during inspiration as fluid-filled or deflated alveoli

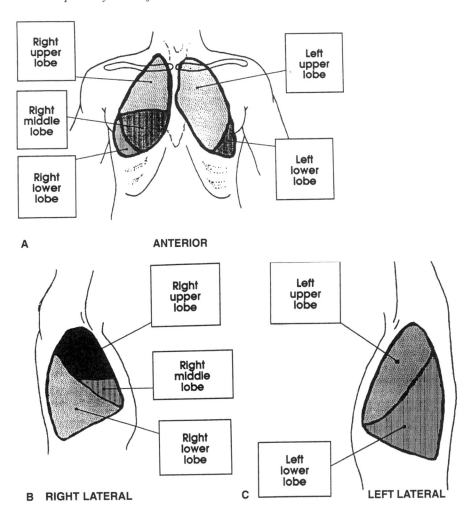

FIGURE 6-2   (*A*) Location of the lobes of the lungs on the anterior thorax. (*B*) Location of the lobes of the right lung on the lateral thorax. (*C*) Location of the lobes of the left lung on the lateral thorax. (Barnes TA: Core Textbook of Respiratory Care Practice, 2nd ed. St Louis, Mosby, 1994.)

reexpand. Crackles, sometimes referred to as rales in clinical medicine, have a popping quality, much like the sound heard as air-filled "bubble" packaging material is squeezed in one's hand. Crackles are only heard during inspiration and are most often associated with atelectasis and pulmonary edema. **Wheezes** are high-pitched, musical sounds which occur during exhalation as gas flows through airways that are partially obstructed by bronchospasm, mucus, or edema. Wheezes are commonly heard in children with asthma or bronchiolitis. The pediatric clinician must be aware of the fact that wheezes are not only caused by bronchospasm.[19] They may also be heard in children with pulmonary edema, foreign body obstruction, airway tumors, and external compression of airways by a vascular ring.[16]

The term **rhonchi** is used by the American Thoracic Society to describe the sounds produced when gas flows through airways that have an excessive amount of secretions present.[3] Rhonchi are low-pitched, rumbling sounds. It has been suggested by some authors that rhonchi should be termed low-pitched wheezes since the sounds are generated in the airways, as are wheezes.[4,13,23] However, *rhonchi* is arguably the term that is used most commonly in clinical medicine. Rhonchi are typically heard in patients who are secreting an increased amount of mucus, such as those with bronchiectasis or pneumonia, or those with an artificial airway in place.

Stridor is a sound produced as gas flows past a partial obstruction during inspiration. It is a high-pitched sound that has a musical quality, much like wheezes. The difference between stridor and wheezes lies at the point of origin. Stridor originates in the upper airway during inspiration, whereas wheezes typically originate in the small airways during exhalation. Using the stethoscope to listen to sounds heard over the larynx as well as over the chest may help the pediatric clinician make this distinction. Stridor will typically be heard at a much greater intensity over the larynx as compared to the chest. When partial upper airway obstruction produces a high-pitched sound during inspiration, it should be termed stridor and *not* an inspiratory wheeze. Stridor is most frequently heard in the pediatric patient with croup, postextubation glottic edema, or foreign body aspiration.

The pediatric clinician must be careful not to confuse other upper airway noises with adventitious breath sounds. The child who has a common cold will have increased nasal secretions. The sound of air flowing past nasal secretions may transmit to the chest, especially in the small child or infant. The sounds produced as a child is snoring or whimpering may also transmit to the lower airways and be heard over the chest. The sucking sounds of an infant drinking from a bottle may be transmitted to the lower airway. Again, the clinician can listen with the stethoscope placed on the child's neck as well as the chest to help distinguish the exact origin of the sound.

When discussing breath sounds, one must also consider the situation in which little or no sound is heard over the chest. This has been termed a silent chest and is a grave sign.[11,14] The quality of air entry during inspiration should always be assessed. This may be termed poor, fair, or good. The child who presents with poor or no air entry is experiencing severe upper or lower airway obstruction. This may occur in the child with severe upper airway edema, foreign body aspiration, or pneumothorax, or during a severe asthma exacerbation. Regardless of the cause, appropriate therapy must be initiated *immediately* or respiratory arrest may occur.

▬ASSESSMENT OF THE CARDIAC SYSTEM

When assessing the cardiac system of the child, clinicians must remember that the cardiac and pulmonary systems work together to provide oxygen to the tissues. Note the following equation:

$$O_2 \text{ delivery to tissues} = \text{Cardiac Output} \times O_2 \text{ Content}$$

Therefore, if the pulmonary system is unable to oxygenate arterial blood sufficiently, the heart will attempt to compensate by increasing cardiac output. The heart will also attempt to increase cardiac output if oxygen content is reduced secondary to anemia.

Cardiac output is defined as the heart rate multiplied by stroke volume. The stroke volume is the volume of blood the heart ejects during each beat. As the stroke volume decreases, as with hypovolemia, the heart rate will increase in order to maintain cardiac output. Stroke volume is assessed by measuring the arterial blood pressure and quality of palpable pulses. A weak, thready pulse is indicative of a decreased cardiac output. As cardiac output decreases, arterial blood pressure will be maintained initially as systemic vascular resistance increases. However, as vascular tone reaches its limits, blood pressure will begin to fall in a linear fashion with the cardiac output. These basic physiologic principles must be applied when assessing the cardiac system of the child.[2,11]

Cardiac performance is usually assessed by evaluating a child's heart rate, blood pressure, and perfusion state. These measurements may all be performed in a noninvasive manner. Normal values for heart rate and blood pressure in the child are listed in Tables 6-3 and 6-4.

Normal heart rates in the child decrease with increasing age. The heart rate may be obtained by palpation of a peripheral pulse, auscultation, or use of an ECG monitor. Often, the young child will not allow the clinician to palpate a pulse for more than a few seconds. The respiratory care practitioner may find it helpful to count the heart rate of an infant or toddler during auscultation of breath sounds. The clinician should assess the rhythm or regularity of the heart rate as well as whether a murmur is present. Murmurs may be heard in some children with congenital heart disease (see Chap. 11).

Sinus tachycardia and sinus bradycardia are the most common dysrhythmias found in the child. Cardiac arrest in the child is usually preceded by respiratory failure or a severe hypoxic event. The child's cardiac system initially responds to hypoxia or hypovolemia by increasing the heart rate. However, if hypoxemia and acidosis persist, as in circulatory shock, the child will become bradycardic. *Bradycardia in the child is a late, grave sign and may indicate impending cardiac arrest.*[1,2] Sinus tachycardia will also occur with fever or during excited or agitated states. The other common dysrhythmia in children is supraventricular tachycardia (SVT), which may require cardioversion. Ventricular fibrillation, severe heart blocks, and other potentially lethal dysrhythmias are uncommon in children.[1,11]

TABLE 6-3   Normal Heart Rates in Children*

AGE	AWAKE HEART RATE (PER MIN)	SLEEPING HEART RATE (PER MIN)
Neonate	100–180	80–160
Infant (6 mo)	100–160	75–160
Toddler	80–110	60–90
Preschooler	70–110	60–90
School-age child	65–110	60–90
Adolescent	60–90	50–90

*Always consider patient's normal range and clinical condition. Heart rate will normally increase with fever or stress.

TABLE 6-4   Normal Blood Pressures in Children*

AGE	SYSTOLIC PRESSURE (MM HG)	DIASTOLIC PRESSURE (MM HG)
Birth (12 hr, <1000 g)	39–59	16–36
Birth (12 hr, 3 kg)	50–70	25–45
Neonate (96 hr)	60–90	20–40
Infant (6 mo)	87–105	53–66
Toddler (2 yr)	95–105	53–66
School age (7 yr)	97–112	57–71
Adolescent (15 yr)	112–128	66–80

*Blood pressure ranges taken from the following sources: *Neonate:* Versmold H et al: Aortic blood pressure during the first 12 hours of life in infants with birth weight 610–4220 g. Pediatrics 67:107, 1981. 10th–90th percentile ranges used. *Others:* Horan MJ (chairman). Task Force on Blood Pressure Control in Children, report of the second task force on blood pressure in children. Pediatrics 79:1, 1987. 50th–90th percentile ranges indicated.

As stated earlier, arterial blood pressure will remain unchanged initially during low cardiac output states. However, as cardiac function continues to worsen or vascular volume is continually depleted, the blood pressure will decrease in a parallel fashion with the cardiac output. Therefore, a significant decrease in arterial blood pressure should be considered a sign of impending circulatory failure. A formula for approximating the lower limit of systolic blood pressure in the child is: 70 + (2 × age in years).[2] The pulse pressure (difference between systolic and diastolic pressures) will also begin to narrow as cardiac output falls. **Pulsus paradoxus** (a decrease in systolic pressure of greater than 8 torr *during* a spontaneous inspiration) may be a sign of a tension pneumothorax or cardiac tamponade.[10]

The child's ability to perfuse vital organs and extremities can be assessed by determining capillary refill, level of consciousness, and urine output. A capillary refill time of greater than 3 seconds is indicative of a low perfusion state. The child who does not respond to his or her parents or is unresponsive to pain may be experiencing decreased cerebral perfusion. Urinary output is directly related to renal perfusion. Normal urine output in children is 1 to 2 mL/kg/hr. A urine output of less than 1 mL/kg/hr is indicative of a low perfusion state.[2,11] The child who has a low cardiac output and decreased renal perfusion may also display edema in the extremities and dependent areas.

■REFERENCES

1. American Heart Association: Textbook of Advanced Cardiac Life Support. Dallas TX, American Heart Association, 1994.
2. American Heart Association and American Academy of Pediatrics: Textbook of Pediatric Advanced Life Support. Dallas TX, American Heart Association, 1988.
3. American Thoracic Society Ad Hoc Committee on Pulmonary Nomenclature: Updated nomenclature for membership reaction. ATS News, 16:8, 1981.
4. Banner AS: Physical examination. In: Dantzker DR, MacIntyre NR, and Bakow ED (eds): Comprehensive Respiratory Care. Philadelphia, WB Saunders, 1995.

5. Cunningham JC, Taussig, LM: How cystic fibrosis is diagnosed. In An Introduction to Cystic Fibrosis for Patients and Families. Bethesda MD, Cystic Fibrosis Foundation, 1991.
6. DesJardins T: Cardiopulmonary Anatomy and Physiology: Essentials for Respiratory Care. Albany NY: Delmar, 1993.
7. Dimaio AM, Singh J: The infant with cyanosis in the emergency room. Pediatr Clin North Am 39(5):987–1006, 1992.
8. Hall CB: Respiratory syncytial virus: What we know now. Contemporary Pediatrics Nov:1–11, 1993.
9. Hardy KA: Advances in our understanding and care of patients with cystic fibrosis. Respiratory Care 38(3):282–289, 1993.
10. Hazinski MF: Cardiovascular disorders. In Hazinski MF (ed): Nursing Care of the Critically Ill Child, 2nd ed. St. Louis, Mosby-Year Book, 1992.
11. Hazinski MF: Children are different. In Hazinski MF (ed): Nursing Care of the Critically Ill Child, 2nd ed. St. Louis, Mosby-Year Book, 1992.
12. Hazinski TA: Bronchial hyperreactivity in infants. Respiratory Care 36(7):735–743, 1991.
13. Hess D, Low GG: Bedside patient assessment. In Barnes TA (ed): Core Textbook of Respiratory Care Practice. Mosby-Year Book, 1994.
14. Kussin PS: Pathophysiology and management of life-threatening asthma. In Branson RD, MacIntyre NR (eds): Adult Asthma. Respir Care Clin 1(2):181–182, 1995.
15. Larsen GL: Asthma in children. New England Journal of Medicine 326(23):1540–1545, 1992.
16. National Institutes of Health: Executive summary: Guidelines for the diagnosis and management of asthma. Publication No. 91-3042A. June 1991.
17. Orenstein DM: Cystic fibrosis. Respiratory Care 36(7):746–756, 1991.
18. Peters SJ: Commentary on thermal epiglottitis after swallowing hot tea. ENA's Nurse Scan Emergency Care 3(3):8–12, 1993.
19. Shapiro BA, Kacmarek RM, Cane RD, Peruzzi WT, Hauptman D: Clinical evaluation of the pulmonary system. In Clinical Application of Respiratory Care, 4th ed. St. Louis, Mosby-Year Book, 1991.
20. Stone CS: Respiratory disorders. In Millonig VL (ed): Pediatric Nurse Practitioner Certification Review Guide, 2nd ed. Potomac MD, Health Leadership Associates, 1994.
21. Valdepena HG, Wald ER, Rose E, Ungkanont K, Casselbrant ML: Epiglottitis and *Haemophilus influenzae* immunization: The Pittsburgh experience—a five-year review. Pediatrics 96(3):424–427, 1995.
22. Walsh MC, Carlo WA, Miller MJ: Respiratory diseases of the newborn. In Carlo WA, Chatburn RL (eds): Neonatal Respiratory Care. Chicago, Year Book Medical, 1988.
23. Wilkins RL, Dexter JR, Smith MP, et al: Lung sound terminology used by respiratory care practitioners. Respiratory Care 34(1):36–40, 1989.
24. Wong DL, Whaley LF: Health history. In Clinical Manual of Pediatric Nursing. St. Louis, CV Mosby, 1990.
25. Zander J, Hazinski MF: Pulmonary disorders. In Hazinski MF (ed): Nursing Care of the Critically Ill Child, 2nd ed. Mosby-Year Book, 1992.

▬ SELF-ASSESSMENT QUESTIONS

1. How would one determine the potential cause of partial upper airway obstruction when obtaining a medical history?

2. Describe different calming measures that can be used during the assessment of the child with respiratory insufficiency.

3. Describe clinical signs and symptoms that may be observed in the child with respiratory insufficiency.

4. List the origin and possible conditions that may lead to the following adventitious breath sounds: crackles, wheezes, rhonchi, and stridor.

5. Define cardiac output and explain how it relates to the assessment of the cardiac system in the child.

Chapter 7

Laboratory and Radiologic Assessment

OBJECTIVES

Having completed this chapter, the reader will be able to:

1 Discuss the advantages and disadvantages associated with the use of arterial lines.

2 Describe the placement of an umbilical artery catheter.

3 Explain the technique used for sampling from an arterial line in the newborn and child.

4 State the preferred site for peripheral artery puncture.

5 Explain the use of transillumination when performing arterial puncture.

6 Describe the technique used for peripheral artery puncture in the newborn and child.

7 Discuss the problems associated with peripheral artery puncture.

8 Discuss the accuracy of arterialized capillary samples.

9 Describe the procedure used for obtaining and preparing capillary samples.

10 Describe normal blood gases in newborns and children.

11 Discuss the features, causes, and treatment of the four major blood gas disturbances.

12 State the normal or acceptable ranges for oxygen tensions in the newborn period.

13 Compare hemoglobin and hematocrit values in the newborn period to those of the normal child and adult.

14 List possible causes of anemia and polycythemia in the newborn.

15 List possible causes and the major consequence of thrombocytopenia.

16 Discuss the use of the white blood cell count in evaluating the newborn and child.

17 Describe the features of the normal chest film in the newborn and child.

18 Describe the use of the radiograph in evaluating tube and catheter position.

KEY TERMS

acidosis	lactic acidosis
alkalosis	lucent
anaerobic metabolism	metabolic acidosis
anemia	metabolic alkalosis
arterialized capillary blood	neutropenia
base deficit	partially compensated
base excess	polycythemia
compensation	respiratory acidosis
disseminated intravascular	respiratory alkalosis
coagulation	thrombocytopenia
erythroblastosis fetalis	uncompensated

▬ BLOOD GASES

Blood gas analysis is indicated in order to obtain information about the oxygenation, ventilation, and acid–base status of the infant or child. Analysis of arterial blood samples remains the most reliable index of oxygenation and ventilation. Some special procedures are used in the newborn and young child, however, so that competence in obtaining and analyzing samples in older patients does not necessarily imply competence in the handling of samples from the newborn and child.

Three basic types of samples are obtained for blood gas analysis: arterial samples from single puncture of a peripheral artery; arterial samples from an arterial line, including an umbilical artery line in the newborn; and arterialized capillary samples. In addition, samples from the umbilical vein are occasionally used in newborns in emergency situations, although these samples are not valid for oxygen tension values.

Peripheral Artery Puncture

Samples may be obtained for blood gas analysis from one of several peripheral arteries, including the radial, brachial, temporal, femoral, and posterior tibial arteries; the femoral artery, however, is not used for blood sampling in the newborn. The radial artery is the preferred site because the vessel is close to the skin, there are no veins or nerves immediately adjacent to the artery, and good collateral circulation to the hand is available through the ulnar artery. The puncture site is determined by palpation of the arterial pulse. Transillumination of the infant's arm, by placing the transilluminator under the back of the wrist, helps to visualize the artery and may be useful if the artery is difficult to locate by palpation. Care should be taken to insure that the light source does not burn the skin. Before obtaining blood from the radial artery, a modified Allen's test should be performed to establish the presence of collateral circulation from the ulnar artery.

A heparinized 1-cc tuberculin syringe is used, with care taken to eject all heparin from the deadspace of the syringe in order to avoid dilutional effects and decreases in pH from excess heparin. Peripheral artery puncture is usually accomplished with a 25- or 26-gauge needle. Alternatively, puncture may be accomplished with a 25-gauge scalp vein butterfly needle, and the blood then withdrawn from the infusion tubing with a heparinized syringe. The practitioner must be careful to follow universal precautions to minimize the risk of contact with the patient's blood. The skin of the infant and the gloved, palpating finger of the sampler should be cleansed with alcohol or iodophor before puncture.

When sampling from the radial artery, the nondominant hand should be used to stabilize the patient's arm. The needle should be inserted at a 30- to 45-degree angle into the direction of arterial blood flow. The bevel of the needle normally faces in the direction of blood flow (up, in the case of the radial artery), although there is some controversy over whether this is necessary. The radial artery of a newborn or child is, of course, quite small, and it is possible to unknowingly advance the needle completely through the artery. If blood is not obtained after initially advancing the needle, slowly withdraw the needle while watching for a flash of blood to enter the needle hub. In most newborns and infants, it may be necessary to aspirate the sample into the syringe, due to the lower range of normal blood pressure. In children with sufficient blood pressure to force the blood into a self-filling syringe, aspiration will not be necessary.

Once a sufficient volume of blood has been obtained, withdraw the needle from the artery and immediately apply direct pressure to the puncture site for 5 minutes. Closely observe the site for any signs of bleeding. Any air bubbles present in the sample should be removed and the sample prepared for analysis.

Complications of peripheral artery puncture, including hematoma formation, infection, hemorrhage, and embolism, are uncommon when proper puncture procedures are followed. The major problem associated with peripheral puncture in infants and children is that it requires considerable disturbance of the patient, which may make the blood gas values quite different from what they would be in the resting state, and therefore of questionable value. If the puncture cannot be accomplished quickly and with minimal discomfort to the patient, it is probably not worthwhile.

Arterial Lines

The placement of an indwelling catheter into a peripheral artery provides undisturbed access for frequent blood gas sampling and continuous monitoring of blood pressure. In critically ill children requiring mechanical ventilation, an arterial line provides essentially unlimited access to the numerous blood gases required to optimize ventilator settings. The complications associated with indwelling catheters are similar to those for arterial puncture, with the additional risk posed by the continuous presence of the catheter in the blood vessel.

Peripheral arteries that have been used include the radial, brachial, and femoral arteries. Arterial lines are most commonly placed by percutaneous catheterization of the artery, although occasionally a surgical cutdown procedure may be required. The artery is located by palpation, and an angiocath (catheter over a needle) is used to puncture the artery. Once the flow of arterial blood has been confirmed, the catheter is advanced over the needle into the lumen of the vessel (Fig. 7-1), and the needle is

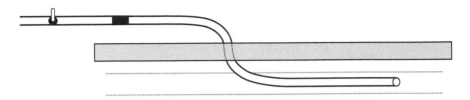

FIGURE 7-1   Catheter inside the artery.

removed. The catheter is secured in place and the site is covered with a sterile surgical dressing to prevent contamination. A very slow, continuous infusion of heparinized isotonic saline is attached to the catheter to prevent clotting. The infusion rate is 1 to 2 mL/h for newborns and 3 mL/h for pediatric patients.[6] A stopcock or similar device is attached to the hub of the catheter to allow removal of blood for blood gas analysis (Fig. 7-2). The limb where the catheter is placed should be immobilized to prevent movement of the catheter.

The most common site at which an arterial line is placed in the newborn is the umbilical artery. Placement of an umbilical artery line allows for frequent sampling without disturbance of the infant; provides valid measurement of all traditional blood gas values, including PO_2, PCO_2, and pH; and allows for continuous blood pressure measurement. Arterial lines may also be placed in a peripheral artery in the newborn if the umbilical artery is not accessible or becomes nonfunctional. Umbilical artery lines are inserted through the umbilicus into one of the two umbilical arteries. After insertion, the position of the catheter should be checked by x-ray study. The tip of the catheter may be placed either at the L3–L4 position (called the low position) or above the diaphragm (T8, called the high position), depending on physician preference. The length of the catheter required to reach either point may be determined from a graph that relates the shoulder-to-umbilicus measurement to various catheter loca-

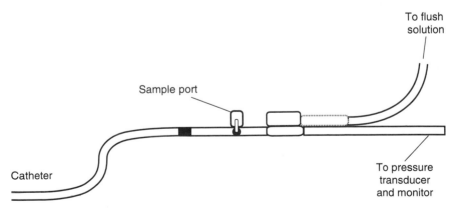

FIGURE 7-2   Stopcock attached to distal end of arterial catheter. The sample port and attachments for the flush solution and pressure transducer are also shown.

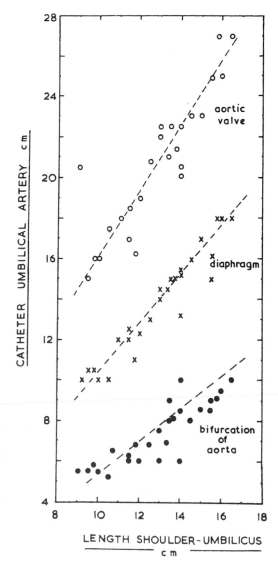

FIGURE 7-3 Relation between the shoulder-to-umbilicus measurement and the length of umbilical artery catheter needed to reach the aortic bifurcation, diaphragm, and aortic valve. (From Dunn PM: Localization of the umbilical catheter by post-mortem measurement. Arch Dis Child 41:69,1966.)

tions (Fig. 7-3).[5] The catheter is secured in place with either suture or umbilical tape attached to both the umbilical stump and the line and is then taped to the abdominal wall (Fig. 7-4).

Although several risks are associated with the use of peripheral arterial lines, properly trained personnel should be able to avoid most of them. Infection may be avoided by maintaining strict attention to sterile technique during catheter insertion and during aspiration of blood from the catheter. An obstructed arterial line should never be flushed because thromboembolism may occur. If the line is obstructed (blood cannot be withdrawn) or if there is any other sign of malfunction, such as diminished perfusion to the extremities, the catheter should be withdrawn and, if necessary, replaced. Hemorrhagic complications may be avoided by pay-

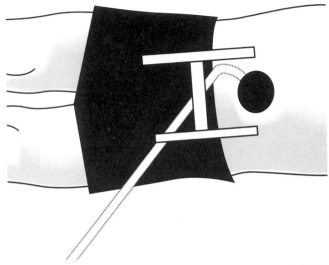

FIGURE 7-4 Method of securing umbilical catheter to the umbilical stump and abdominal wall.

ing careful attention to blood withdrawal procedures and by withdrawing the catheter only part way when it is to be removed and waiting for vasospasm to occur before removing it completely from the artery. Proper technique for infusion of solutions, including the use of filters, will help to avoid the possibility of air embolism.

When obtaining blood from an arterial line for arterial blood gas studies, the following technique should be followed:

1. Attach a sterile syringe to the open port of the stopcock and turn the stopcock off to the infusion fluid (Fig. 7-5A).
2. Withdraw fluid from the line until blood is obtained and fills the tubing (usually 1.5–2 mL). Turn the stopcock to the neutral position (see Fig. 7-5B), which will prevent contamination of the sample with infusion fluid and also prevent blood loss from the patient.
3. Remove and cap this syringe to maintain sterility and set it aside. This fluid and blood will be returned to the patient to minimize blood loss from sampling procedures.
4. Using another sterile syringe that has been heparinized, withdraw the blood sample to be analyzed (see Fig. 7-5C). The amount of blood needed will vary with the type of equipment used for analysis of blood gases, but it is usually 0.5 to 1.0 mL. Remove the sample syringe.
5. Reconnect the syringe with the fluid previously withdrawn. After attaching this syringe to the infusion port, aspirate slightly to remove air from the sampling port and then tap the syringe to make air bubbles rise to the top, so that they will not be infused through the line. Then infuse the fluid slowly, watching the line for any air bubbles that may remain. If a bubble is noted, reaspirate the line, tap the syringe again, and attempt to reinfuse.

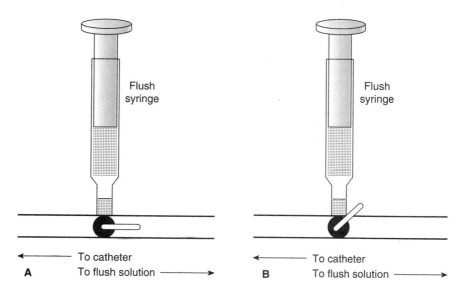

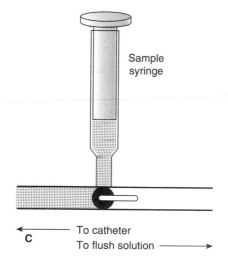

FIGURE 7-5 (*A*) Syringe attached to sample port with the stopcock turned "off" to the infusion fluid. (*B*) Syringe attached to sample port with the stopcock turned to the "neutral" position. (*C*) Sample syringe attached to sample port with the stopcock turned to allow blood to flow into the syringe.

6. Turn the stopcock off to the sampling port and flush the line so that it is clear of blood, making sure that all connections are tight. If the blood pressure waveform is displayed on a monitor, check to see that a clear waveform is present.
7. Prepare the sample for analysis by rolling the syringe to mix the blood and the heparin, by labeling the syringe, and by immersing the syringe in ice water unless analysis is performed immediately.
8. Keep an accurate record of all blood samples withdrawn. Infants and small children who require frequent sampling may require a transfusion to replace the blood volume used for blood gas analysis, and an accurate record of the blood volume withdrawn is very helpful.

Arterialized Capillary Sampling

Peripheral artery puncture requires some skill and cannot be performed frequently on the extremely small vessels of the newborn. For these reasons, capillary blood obtained from the heel of the infant is sometimes used in place of arterial blood. Capillary blood samples may also be drawn from the fingers or toes of older infants and children if arterial puncture is contraindicated.[2] The heel is warmed for several minutes before puncture is performed to "arterialize" the capillary blood. When properly performed, **arterialized capillary blood** ("heel sticks") may provide fairly accurate values for pH and P_{CO_2}.

There is relatively little difference in the arterial and venous values for measurements of pH and P_{CO_2}, in any case. Unfortunately, the same cannot be said for P_{O_2}.[3] The measurement of oxygen tension using capillary samples, however well arterialized, is always risky. Most studies show that there is very poor correlation between capillary and arterial values when the actual arterial P_{O_2} is greater than 60 mm Hg, meaning that an infant who has an acceptable range for capillary oxygen levels might well have an excessively high arterial oxygen level and thus be at risk for the development of retrolental fibroplasia.[1,8] On the other hand, it is possible to have an acceptable capillary oxygen tension when the actual arterial oxygen tension is unacceptably low, allowing the infant to be exposed to dangerously low levels of oxygen and the possible consequences, including brain damage and pulmonary vasoconstriction. A falsely high capillary oxygen tension is usually the result of exposure of the blood to room air during sampling. Capillary samples are not recommended for assessing the oxygenation status of the newborn, although they may be acceptable for monitoring acid–base and ventilatory status using pH and P_{CO_2}. The availability of pulse oximetry has greatly reduced the need for frequent blood gas analysis because of its ability to accurately estimate P_{O_2} both intermittently and continuously.

Arterialized capillary samples are obtained from the lateral heel surface of the infant (Fig. 7-6). The heel is warmed for several minutes before puncture is performed to arterialize the capillary blood. Czervinske recommends warming the heel at 45° C for 5 to 7 minutes before each puncture to improve the consistency of the blood gas results.[2] After adequate warming of the heel with a warm water bath, a warm cloth, or a warming pack, the skin is cleansed with alcohol and punctured with a lancet to a depth of about 3 mm. A quick, stabbing motion should be used, not a slash. The first drop of blood is discarded. The tip of a heparinized capillary sampling tube is placed as close as possible to the puncture site and freely flowing blood is collected in the tube. Every effort should be made to avoid exposing the blood to the atmosphere and to avoid introducing air bubbles into the tube. The foot should not be squeezed to increase blood flow because this may both damage the foot and alter blood gas values. If blood does not flow freely, another puncture should be performed.

Once the capillary tube has been filled, the blood may be aspirated from the tube into a heparinized tuberculin syringe and prepared for analysis. Alternatively, one end of the tube may be sealed, after which a small steel wire is inserted into the open end of the tube. A magnet is passed along the length of the tube to mix the blood and heparin. As with arterial samples, the capillary sample should be iced and analyzed as soon

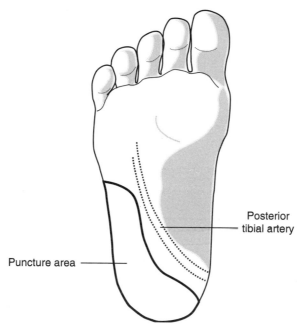

FIGURE 7-6 Diagram of an infant's heel, showing the area where the puncture should be performed.

as possible. Pressure should be applied to the heel as needed to stop blood flow and a dry dressing applied to the site.

Interpretation of Blood Gas Results

The standard values measured from a blood gas analysis include pH, PCO_2, and PO_2. In addition, bicarbonate level is calculated (from its relationship to PCO_2 and pH) and reported. Oxygen saturation may be determined from its relationship to pH, PCO_2, and PO_2 or may be directly measured separately from blood gases using an oximeter. **Base excess**, like bicarbonate, is calculated and represents the amount of acid or base added from metabolic (nonrespiratory) causes. A positive base excess means either an excess of base or a deficit of fixed acid, whereas a negative base excess, also called **base deficit**, means either a deficit of base or an excess of fixed acid.

The normal values for blood gases in the newborn and child (Table 7-1) are similar but not identical to those in the adult population. The pH is normally slightly acidotic (less than 7.4) at birth and rises to the normal or "neutral" value of 7.4 over the first 24 hours of life. The PCO_2 is normally quite high at birth (greater than 50 mm Hg), since the birth process interferes with placental blood flow, and the PO_2 is usually fairly low (less than 55 mm Hg) for the same reason. In the term infant, PO_2 usually rises above 60 mm Hg by the first hour of life. The premature infant may take much longer to reach this level. The PCO_2 usually falls to about 35 mm Hg by 1 hour and remains low. Bicarbonate values are slightly below the "normal" of 24 mEq/L, so that the pH, which results from the relationship between bicarbonate and PCO_2, remains in the normal range (7.35–7.45).

TABLE 7-1 Normal Blood Gas Values for Newborns and Children

	NEWBORN (24 HOURS OF AGE)	CHILDREN
pH	7.30–7.40	7.35–7.45
PaO_2 (mm Hg)	60–80	85–100
$PaCO_2$ (mm Hg)	26–40	35–45
$HCO3^-$ (mEq/L)	18–25	22–26
Base excess	−4–+2	−2–+2

(From Deming DD: Respiratory assessment of neonatal and pediatric patients. In Wilkins RL, Krider SJ, Sheldon RL (eds): Clinical Assessment in Respiratory Care, 3rd ed. St Louis, Mosby-Year Book, 1995.)

Four major classes of acid–base disturbance may be present in the newborn and child as well as in other age groups: respiratory acidosis, metabolic acidosis, respiratory alkalosis, and metabolic alkalosis. In addition, mixed disorders may occur (*e.g.*, mixed respiratory and metabolic acidosis). After the onset of the initial disturbance, the body may attempt **compensation**. The pH is determined by the relationship between bicarbonate and PCO_2. If one rises or falls, the other may move in the same direction as a compensatory mechanism. As long as the relationship between the two values (or the ratio, as it is usually expressed) remains the same, the pH will not change. Thus, to compensate for a disturbance that results in an increase or decrease in one component (bicarbonate or CO_2), the body will attempt to move the other component in the same direction to maintain the ratio. The changes that occur in pH, PCO_2, and HCO_3^- with acid–base disturbances are discussed further and are summarized in Table 7-2.

RESPIRATORY ACIDOSIS
Respiratory acidosis occurs when the PCO_2 rises above the normal value. This will initially result in a decrease in pH (**acidosis**). Over a period of hours or days, the kidneys may compensate for this disturbance by conserving bicarbonate and eliminating hydrogen ions, thus attempting to return the pH toward its normal value. If no compensation has occurred (bicarbonate value is normal), the disturbance is termed **uncompensated** respiratory acidosis. If compensation has occurred to the point where the pH has been returned to the normal range (7.35–7.45), the disturbance is termed fully compensated respiratory acidosis. If compensation has begun (bicarbonate is elevated) but is not complete (pH remains less than 7.35), it is termed **partially compensated** respiratory acidosis. The initial disturbance remains respiratory acidosis, regardless of compensation.

Respiratory acidosis always indicates that ventilation is not adequate to keep up with the metabolic production of carbon dioxide. This may occur in many types of diseases that affect the cardiopulmonary, central nervous, or musculoskeletal system. The usual treatment for respiratory acidosis is to increase the level of ventilation or to reverse the cause of inad-

TABLE 7-2 Acid–Base Disturbances in Newborns and Children

	pH	P_{CO_2}	HCO_3^-
Respiratory acidosis			
Uncompensated	↓	↑	Normal
Partially compensated	↓	↑	↑
Fully compensated	Normal	↑	↑
Respiratory alkalosis			
Uncompensated	↑	↓	Normal
Partially compensated	↑	↓	↓
Fully compensated	Normal	↓	↓
Metabolic acidosis			
Uncompensated	↓	Normal	↓
Partially compensated	↓	↓	↓
Fully compensated	Normal	↓	↓
Metabolic alkalosis			
Uncompensated	↑	Normal	↑
Partially compensated	↑	↑	↑
Fully compensated	Normal	↑	↑

equate ventilation, if possible. In some cases, chronic respiratory acidosis may occur and may not require treatment.

RESPIRATORY ALKALOSIS

Respiratory alkalosis occurs when the P_{CO_2} falls below the normal range. This will initially result in an increase in pH (**alkalosis**). Respiratory alkalosis results from excessive ventilation. As in respiratory acidosis, the kidneys may gradually compensate by altering levels of bicarbonate and hydrogen ion to return the ratio toward normal and thus restore the pH to its normal range. Uncompensated, partially compensated, or fully compensated respiratory alkalosis may occur. The most common cause of respiratory alkalosis in the newborn is mechanical hyperventilation. This may be intentional (*e.g.*, in the treatment of persistent fetal circulation to reverse pulmonary vasoconstriction) or accidental, in which case ventilator settings should be adjusted to decrease minute ventilation. Additionally, an infant who is actively resisting peripheral artery puncture (crying) will usually show a transient respiratory alkalosis. In older children, respiratory alkalosis may occur as the result of hypoxemia, so the practitioner is wise to also evaluate the P_{O_2} and O_2 saturation. Finally, the P_{CO_2} may fall below normal levels in an attempt to compensate for a very low bicarbonate concentration.

METABOLIC ACIDOSIS

Metabolic acidosis occurs when the serum bicarbonate level is decreased. This will initially result in a decreased pH (acidosis). The respiratory system may compensate for this problem quite rapidly by decreasing the P_{CO_2}, thus restoring the relationship between bicarbonate and P_{CO_2} toward normal. As with respiratory disturbances, metabolic acidosis may be uncompensated, partially compensated, or fully compensated. It is rare to see an uncompensated disturbance unless the patient has poor pulmonary function and cannot increase ventilation and decrease CO_2 or is being mechanically ventilated with no ability to increase ventilation.

Metabolic acidosis results from either an addition of fixed acids or a loss of base from the body. A common cause of metabolic acidosis in the newborn is the accumulation of lactic acid. Lactic acid is produced as a byproduct of metabolism that occurs in the absence of oxygen (**anaerobic metabolism**). Thus, **lactic acidosis** occurs any time the tissues are deprived of an adequate supply of oxygen. Inadequate tissue oxygenation may occur from various causes, including low blood oxygen levels, diminished or abnormal hemoglobin, diminished perfusion of tissues, and sepsis. Additionally, an increased rate of anaerobic glycolysis associated with hypothermia contributes to lactic acidosis.

Treatment of metabolic acidosis involves identification of the primary disturbance and attention to the reversal of that disturbance. If, for instance, acidosis is due to hypoxia, oxygen administration or manipulation of ventilator settings is indicated. If acidosis is due to hypothermia, maintenance of a neutral thermal environment is indicated. Circulatory support may be needed if acidosis is due to poor perfusion, and transfusion may be needed if the oxygen-carrying capacity of the blood is too low to supply tissue oxygen needs. Bicarbonate therapy should be reserved for cases of severe or persistent metabolic acidosis and should be administered with caution.

METABOLIC ALKALOSIS

Metabolic alkalosis occurs when the serum bicarbonate level is increased. This will initially result in an increased pH (alkalosis). Metabolic alkalosis may be caused by either a gain of base or a loss of acid. The compensation mechanism for this disturbance would be to retain CO_2, to offset the increase in bicarbonate and to maintain the normal ratio. This compensation mechanism is not adequate to reverse alkalosis, since retained CO_2 results in a strong stimulation to breathe. In other words, it is difficult to decrease ventilation to the point at which sufficient CO_2 is retained to compensate for metabolic alkalosis. This disturbance may occur when gastric acid is lost through vomiting or nasogastric suctioning, as a result of diuretic therapy, or iatrogenically secondary to the administration of excessive bicarbonate.

OXYGENATION STATUS

In addition to evaluating acid–base status, blood gases provide an indication of oxygenation. The Po_2 is only one aspect of oxygenation; adequate and functional hemoglobin must also be present for sufficient oxygen-carrying capacity. Normally, Po_2 is maintained between 50 and 70 mm Hg in the newborn and between 85 and 100 mm Hg in the child. Slightly lower values may be accepted when capillary samples are used, although it must be remembered that oxygen values of capillary samples are not accurate. Frequent monitoring of blood oxygen levels is extremely important in the infant receiving oxygen therapy because excessive oxygen levels may lead to serious complications, including retinopathy of prematurity and bronchopulmonary dysplasia. The use of pulse oximetry to accurately estimate hemoglobin saturation is extremely helpful in monitoring the oxygenation status of the infant and child either intermittently or continuously.

■HEMATOLOGY

The normal ranges of hematology values for newborns and children are shown in Table 7-3.

Hemoglobin and Hematocrit

Normal hemoglobin levels in newborns vary according to sample site and age. In utero, the low Pao_2 present in the fetus stimulates the production of red blood cells and hemoglobin values tend to be higher than adult values (16–19 g %). At birth, the hypoxic stimulus to produce red blood cells decreases with the rising Pao_2 and hemoglobin values fall to lower than adult values (11–13 g %) over the first several weeks of life. There may be some variation, depending on whether a venous or capillary sample is analyzed. Similarly, the hematocrit values for newborns tend to be high (55% to 60%) and to decrease to 30% to 40% during the first weeks. Both hemoglobin and hematocrit levels for premature infants will be lower than those found in full-term babies. Newborns will limit the production of red blood cells until stimulated by a mild "physiologic anemia," which usually occurs at approximately 6 weeks of age.[4] As the infant increases red blood cell production, the hemoglobin and hematocrit levels rise to the adult level and remain there.

Venous hemoglobin levels of less than 13 g % indicate **anemia**, whereas hemoglobin concentrations above 23 g % or hematocrit values above 70% indicate polycythemia. Some infants may be symptomatic at lower levels. Anemia may be due to hemolysis secondary to Rh incompatibility (**erythroblastosis fetalis**), ABO incompatibility, or infection; it may also occur secondary to blood loss either prenatally or postnatally. **Polycythemia** may occur from placental transfusion at birth, from transfusion of blood to the fetus from either the mother or a twin fetus, or from increased production of red blood cells by the stressed fetus (*e.g.*, after chronic intrauterine hypoxia).

Thrombocytes

Platelets (thrombocytes) are blood cells that are vitally important to the coagulation process. A platelet count of less than 100,000/mm³ (**throm-**

TABLE 7-3 Normal Hematology Values for Newborns and Children

	NEWBORNS	CHILDREN
Hemoglobin (g %)	16–19	13–15
Hematocrit (%)	55–60	40–50
Thrombocytes (mm³)	100,000–350,000	150,000–400,000
Leukocytes (mm³)	9,000–30,000	5,000–11,000

bocytopenia) is considered abnormally low and may result from several problems. Thrombocytopenia is often associated with perinatal infection, particularly bacterial sepsis, and the TORCH infections (toxoplasmosis, rubella, cytomegalovirus, and herpes). Some drugs taken by the mother may cause decreased platelet counts, including thiazide diuretics that may be used to treat maternal pre-eclampsia. Symptoms of thrombocytopenia include petechiae and bruising (ecchymoses). The principal hazard of thrombocytopenia is hemorrhage, particularly into the central nervous system.

The syndrome known as **disseminated intravascular coagulation** (DIC) also results in a decreased platelet count. In this syndrome, some stimulus (such as infection) results in clotting in the bloodstream. Platelets and other clotting factors are rapidly consumed by this intravascular coagulation process. DIC syndrome is thus sometimes called consumption coagulopathy and may result in bleeding anywhere in the body. Paradoxically, heparin may help to treat this disease because it interrupts the ongoing coagulation and thus the consumption of platelets and clotting factors.

Leukocytes

The white blood cell (leukocyte) count in the newborn has a wide normal range, with a low value of $9,000/mm^3$ and a high value of $30,000/mm^3$. Initially, the most numerous white blood cell is the polymorphonuclear leukocyte (neutrophil), which averages $11,000/mm^3$. The lymphocyte becomes the most prominent white blood cell during the first week of life and remains so throughout the early childhood years. Band (immature) forms of neutrophils range from 5% to 10% of the total white blood cell count. Elevated bands are associated with infection but may result from other causes. **Neutropenia** (neutrophil count of less than 7800 in the first 60 hours of life or less than 1750 thereafter) is the most useful indicator of infection in the newborn.[7] In addition, abnormalities of neutrophil structure, such as toxic granulation, may be indications of infection. The most common cause of severe neutropenia in the newborn is overwhelming sepsis. Neutropenia may also occur as a primary deficiency not secondary to infection, such as that secondary to maternal neutropenia.

■CHEST RADIOGRAPH

Chest films are invaluable in evaluating the initial cause of cardiorespiratory disturbance and in following the course of treatment. Radiographs illustrating specific respiratory diseases will be presented in later chapters, along with discussions of the pathophysiology and management of these conditions. It is essential, however, to have some understanding of the normal film before discussing changes from the normal.

Normal Chest Film

The normal lung field can be described as **lucent** (Fig. 7-7), meaning that it appears well aerated, or black, on chest x-ray film but that the pulmonary vasculature (blood vessels) can be distinguished from the hilum to the chest wall. The lung fields appear symmetrical and the rib interspaces equal. The overall configuration of the chest is that of a cone or triangle. The diaphragms are well rounded and the costophrenic angles clear. In the lateral film, the ribs appear to slope downward from back to front.

The heart is somewhat difficult to evaluate on the normal neonatal chest film because cardiovascular changes occur rapidly in the first hours and the thymus gland outline, which is prominent in the newborn chest, blends with the cardiac silhouette. The size of the heart is usually evaluated by comparing the transverse diameter of the heart to the transverse diameter of the lungs on an inspiratory film. The heart diameter should not exceed 60% of the lung field diameter. A poor inspiration or an expiratory film will make the heart appear larger.

The mediastinum should be evaluated for midline position, since several conditions can alter its position. Increases in the volume of one hemithorax (*e.g.*, from pneumothorax) will cause the mediastinum to shift away from the affected side, whereas decreases (as with atelectasis) will cause the mediastinum to shift toward the affected side.

As infants become older, it becomes easier to obtain and interpret radiographs of the chest. By the age of 2 to 3 years, children can follow instructions which allow the radiologist to obtain inspiratory and expiratory films. Before this age, right and left lateral decubitus films can be used to obtain the same information as inspiratory and expiratory films.[4] A normal pediatric chest film is shown in Figure 7-8.

Tube and Catheter Position

The x-ray is also useful in evaluating the position of tubes and catheters, in particular the position of endotracheal tubes and umbilical artery and vein catheters. The endotracheal tube position should be evaluated for

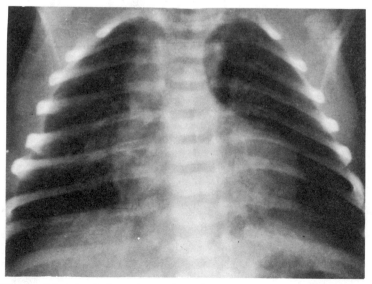

FIGURE 7-7 The normal newborn chest film. (Avery GB: Neonatology: Pathophysiology and Management of the Newborn, 2nd ed, p 463. Philadelphia, JB Lippincott, 1981.)

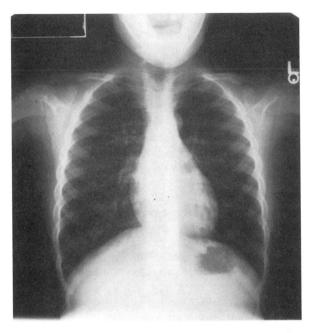

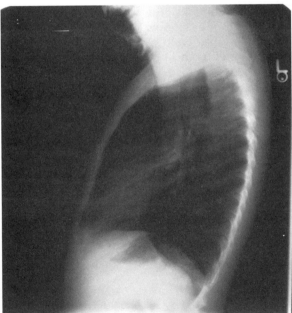

FIGURE 7-8   Posterior-anterior (PA) (*top*) and lateral (*bottom*) chest x-rays from a 6 1/2-year-old child with normal anatomy and physiology. (Courtesy of Children's Medical Center, Dayton, OH.)

placement of the tip of the tube above the carina to insure that endo-bronchial intubation does not occur, and it should be rechecked periodi-cally to assure that the tube has not migrated out of position. The carina is normally located at the level of the fourth thoracic vertebral body. The tip of the tube should be located above this level, at the second or third body. The umbilical artery catheter may be placed high in the descending aorta (between T4 and T11) or low in the abdominal aorta at approxi-mately the level of L4. An umbilical vein catheter usually lies in the infe-rior vena cava just below the entrance into the right atrium or within the right atrium itself (Fig. 7-9).

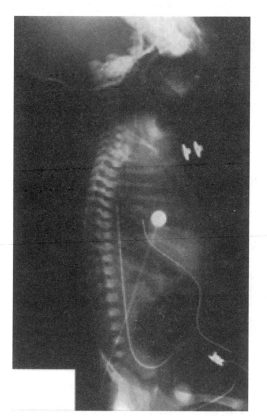
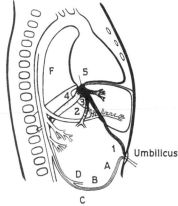

FIGURE 7-9 Lateral radiograph and diagram of the course of umbilical venous and arterial catheters. Umbilical venous catheter enters through umbilicus, passes through *1*, umbilical vein, *2*, portal vein, *3*, ductus venosus, and *4*, inferior vena cava and stops in *5*, right atrium. Umbilical arterial catheter enters through umbili-cus, passes through *A*, umbilical artery, *B*, hypogastric artery, *C*, internal iliac artery, *D*, common iliac artery, and *E*, abdominal aorta and stops in *F*, thoracic aorta. (Wilkins RL, Sheldon RL, Krider SJ: Clinical Assessment in Respiratory Care, 3rd ed. St. Louis, Mosby, 1995.)

■REFERENCES

1. Cassady G: Transcutaneous monitoring in the newborn infant. J Pediatr 103:837, 1983.
2. Czervinske MR: Arterial blood gas analysis and other cardiopulmonary monitoring. In Koff PB, Eitzman D, Neu J (eds): Neonatal and Pediatric Respiratory Care, 2nd ed. St. Louis, Mosby-Year Book, 1993.
3. Courtney SE: Capillary blood gases in the neonate. Am J Dis Child 144:168, 1990.
4. Deming DD: Respiratory assessment of neonatal and pediatric patients. In Wilkins RL, Krider SJ, Sheldon RL (eds): Clinical Assessment in Respiratory Care, 3rd ed. St Louis: Mosby-Year Book, 1995.
5. Dunn PM: Localization of the umbilical catheter by postmortem measurement. Arch Dis Child 41:169, 1966.
6. Levin DL, Mast CP: Arterial catheters. In Levin DL, Morriss FC, Moore GC (eds): A Practical Guide to Pediatric Intensive Care. St. Louis, Mosby-Year Book, 1984.
7. Oski FA: Hematologic problems. In Avery GB (ed): Neonatology: Pathophysiology and Management of the Newborn, 2nd ed. Philadelphia, JB Lippincott, 1981.
8. Schreiner RL et al: Techniques of obtaining arterial blood. In Schreiner RL, Kisling JA (eds): Practical Neonatal Respiratory Care. New York, Raven Press, 1982.

■SELF-ASSESSMENT QUESTIONS

1. What is the most reliable index of oxygenation and ventilation in the newborn and child?
   a. pulse oximetry
   b. arterial blood gas analysis
   c. transcutaneous monitoring
   d. capnography

2. Which is the preferred vessel for arterial puncture in the child?
   a. radial
   b. brachial
   c. femoral
   d. dorsalis pedis

3. Possible complications from the insertion of an indwelling arterial line include
   a. infection
   b. obstruction
   c. hemorrhage
   d. all of the above

4. When properly performed, capillary blood samples can provide accurate values for
   I. $Paco_2$
   II. Pao_2
   III. pH
   a. I only
   b. I and II
   c. II and III
   d. I and III

5. Interpret the following blood gas results: pH = 7.30, $Paco_2$ = 52 mm Hg, Hco_3^- = 25 mEq/L
   a. respiratory acidosis
   b. respiratory alkalosis
   c. metabolic acidosis
   d. metabolic alkalosis

6. Interpret the following blood gas results: pH = 7.51, $Paco_2$ = 47 mm Hg, Hco_3^- = 34 mEq/L
   a. uncompensated respiratory acidosis
   b. partially compensated respiratory alkalosis
   c. uncompensated metabolic acidosis
   d. partially compensated metabolic alkalosis

7. The respiratory system will compensate for a severe metabolic acidosis by
   a. decreasing minute ventilation   c. decreasing tidal volume
   b. increasing minute ventilation   d. increasing $Paco_2$

8. A hemoglobin value of 10% would be interpreted as
   a. hyperglycemia   c. anemia
   b. thrombocytopenia   d. polycythemia

9. What is the effect of disseminated intravascular coagulation (DIC) on platelet count?
   a. increases platelet count
   b. decreases platelet count
   c. DIC has no effect on platelet count

10. When the lung fields appear well aerated, or black, on the x-ray film, their appearance is best described as
    a. opaque   c. lucent
    b. dense   d. reticulogranular

Chapter **8**

Noninvasive Monitoring

M. DEE JOHNSON

OBJECTIVES

Having completed this chapter, the reader will be able to:

1 Describe the methods for direct measurement of respiratory rate in the newborn.

2 Discuss the capabilities of the equipment used in apnea monitoring.

3 Discuss the advantages and disadvantages associated with direct respiratory monitoring techniques.

4 Describe the principles of measurement of pulse oximetry.

5 Describe the selection of the correct sites for measurement of oxygen saturation for the infant and child.

6 Discuss the advantages and disadvantages of the pulse oximeter as the method used to measure oxygen saturation.

7 Describe the principles of measurement of the transcutaneous monitoring of oxygen and carbon dioxide.

8 Describe the monitoring and calibration of the transcutaneous monitor.

9 Discuss the advantages and disadvantages of transcutaneous monitoring with the infant and child.

10 Describe the principles of measurement of capnography.

11 Describe the monitoring and calibration of capnography for the infant and child.

12 Discuss the advantages and disadvantages of capnography with the infant and child.

13 Describe the use of pulmonary function monitoring to assess the infant and child.

14 Describe the methods and desired parameters measured during pulmonary function testing.

15 Discuss the advantages of pulmonary function testing for the infant and child.

16 Describe the cardiac assessment of the infant and child using electrocardiograms and echocardiography.

KEY TERMS

airway resistance
anemometer
capnography
capnometer
distal-diverting
erythema
impedance
light-emitting diode (LED)
lung compliance
nondiverting

noninvasive monitoring
oxygen saturation
pneumogram
pneumotachograph
proximal-diverting
pulse oximetry
situs inversus
transcutaneous
transpulmonary pressure

Noninvasive monitoring of the infant and pediatric patient is important in all areas of acute and chronic care. This type of monitoring involves devices or procedures that do not require entering the body or puncturing the skin. The technology continues to improve, enabling the practitioner to evaluate the patient quickly at the bedside both in and out of the hospital setting. This is because of the response time of the equipment, the size and weight of the apparatus, and the ease of interpretation of data. Most noninvasive measurements can be done on a one-time, intermittent, or continuous basis. Such monitors have the capability of evaluating the partial pressure of oxygen, partial pressure of carbon dioxide, heart rate, respiratory rate, and presence of apnea. The availability of these evaluation methods decreases the need for the practitioner to use the more invasive techniques described in Chapter 7.

■APNEA MONITORING

One of the challenges in the successful monitoring of the neonate is the detection of respirations or, more importantly, the absence of respirations (apnea). It is especially important when the child is unattended or asleep. Methods of direct monitoring of respiration rely on detection of respiratory movement. The infant most likely to require this type of monitoring is one who is premature and has had repeated periods of apnea in the hospital prior to discharge. The premature or full-term infant who has experienced episodes of bradycardia after birth, regardless of the need for resuscitation, will qualify for apnea monitoring. This monitor can also be provided if the physician feels that the infant may be at risk for sudden infant death syndrome (SIDS), as in the case of an infant whose siblings have died from SIDS. The monitoring will be started in the hospital and continue in the home after discharge. All monitors are regulated by the Food and Drug Administration (FDA).

Impedance pneumography is the most common method used to monitor the respiratory rate and assess the breathing pattern in the neonatal or pediatric patient. Impedance pneumography provides for continuous monitoring of respirations utilizing one set of electrodes for both electrocardiographic and respiratory monitoring. This method is both easy and portable. This device, commonly referred to as an apnea monitor, has the ability to measure the presence or lack of both respirations and heart rate. It is considered an indirect method of monitoring when compared with the $PetCO_2$ method, which monitors respirations directly.

Impedance pneumography is the measurement of resistance (impedance) between blood, muscle, fat, and air and an electrical current. Impedance pneumography involves placing two standard electrocardiogram electrodes, which are flat, flexible pads, on either side of the patient's anterior chest such that the pads are located over the midaxillary line (Fig. 8-1). The monitor sends a low-amplitude, high-frequency current through these electrodes. The electrical impedance that the current encounters is affected by the distance between the chest leads, which changes with respiratory motion, and by the type of tissue between the leads. The monitor uses a breath rate detector and an algorithm to calculate respiratory rate from the changing impedance and displays continuous respiratory waveforms.

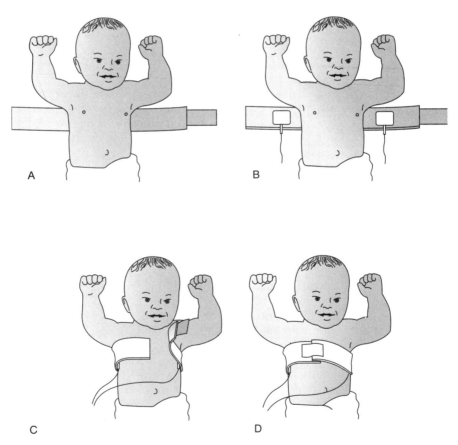

FIGURE 8-1 Application of an impedance pneumography electrode belt. (**A**) Place baby on belt so that belt is aligned with baby's nipples. (**B**) Place electrodes onto belt with Velcro side down. (**C,D**) Wrap belt with electrodes around baby's chest. (**E**) Connect electrodes to SmartMonitor and plug machine into electrical outlet. (Redrawn from Healthdyne.) (*Continues*)

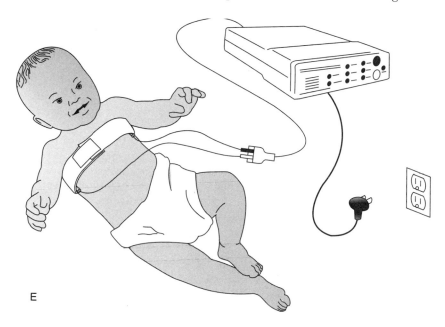

E

FIGURE 8-1   (Continued.)

Impedance pneumography can be used to record results and produce an electrocardiogram (**pneumogram**) that supplies written documentation of the occurrence of apneic periods and cardiac patterns. These results can then be measured and interpreted. The interpretation is compiled by personnel trained in reading pneumograms.

Before the application of the electrodes, all soaps, oil, powder, and lotion should be rinsed from the chest thoroughly. A soft foam belt with Velcro on the ends is placed around the baby's chest and fastened. The electrode pads are secured in place onto the portion of the belt covering the anterior chest (see Fig. 8-1). When placing the belt around the chest, care must be taken to make sure that the belt does not overlap itself in the area of the electrical pads. The belt is secure if the practitioner can place one finger between the belt and the infant's chest. This will enable the machine to obtain a proper reading. Special attention should be taken to assure that the appropriate-sized belt is used and the electrodes are placed properly to obtain a reliable signal.

If the belt becomes soiled, it can be easily cleaned. After removing the electrodes, the belt can be hand washed, rinsed thoroughly, and air dried before replacing it around the infant's chest. Fabric softener should not be used as it will reduce static electricity, thus interfering with the readings of the monitor.

The apnea monitor has advantages when used in the evaluation of respirations and heart rate of the infant. An obvious advantage is that the procedure is noninvasive and painless. Another advantage is that the alarm system is used to detect apnea, bradycardia, and tachycardia. The monitor alarm is normally set for a high heart rate of 150 and a low rate of 100 per minute. The apnea alarm is set by adjusting the time delay control knob to the desired number of seconds. The four possible settings are 10, 15, 20, and 25 seconds. There is an audible and visual alarm system that warns the practitioner if the infant is experiencing a problem.

Most alarms detect abnormalities in respiratory rate, heart rate, battery malfunction, and loose connections or disconnection of the electrodes from the belt. The alarms are easily heard and the practitioner can readily identify the problem by looking for the flashing light on the face of the monitor. The monitor can also be equipped with a remote alarm attachment, which enables the alarm to be placed in a different room from the monitor and still be heard. Most monitors are equipped with a memory, so that the practitioner can trace events as they occurred over a period of time and have them transferred to a written record (pneumogram). The monitor can also be used in conjunction with a pulse oximeter to obtain additional information during periods of apnea.

There are some disadvantages to this device. One disadvantage to impedance pneumography is its sensitivity to body movement and postural changes, which can cause irregular readings. Since infant movement during the sleep cycle is uncontrollable, the results are often altered by the detection of movement or the shifting of the lead position on the chest. Another disadvantage is that the monitor can often become accidentally disconnected. This will cause the alarm to sound and wake the infant from sleep. This is a problem for the infant who is active during sleep and is continually awakened. It is also a problem when it affects the compliance of the parent or the infant's caregiver. One study on the problem of compliance with home use stated that 23.1% of mothers reported using the monitor 12 or fewer hours per day and that 10.8% believed their infants did not need a monitor.[1] This can cause a problem when a continuous reading is desirable for evaluation and repeated disconnects interrupt the sleep pattern.

Another problem with the monitor is that it may detect cardiogenic oscillations and artifacts from patient motion and count them as true respirations. In addition, apnea caused by an upper airway obstruction may not be detected because the chest cage movement is continuous in some infants. Impedance pneumography measures changes in chest wall configuration, not the effectiveness of ventilation. There are also a frequent number of false apnea alarms caused by poor electrode placement, abdominal breathing, and restricted chest movement, none of which can be prevented or corrected by the measuring devices. It is often not used with large children as the probe does not pick up correct readings and the belt may be too small. Infants with severe chest wall deformities will not be good candidates for this device.

▬ PULSE OXIMETRY

One of the most widely used noninvasive monitors (anesthesia, critical care, acute care, emergency room, and home care) for both infants and children is the **pulse oximeter**, which is used to measure the arterial hemoglobin saturation, referred to as the SaO_2. The SaO_2 is the percentage of arterial hemoglobin sites that are saturated. An oximeter measures the **oxygen saturation** by passing a light source thorough a perfused area over an artery to a photosensor on the other side of the perfused area.

The sensor is most often placed on the finger, toe, or ear of the infant or child, although for small infants the palm of the hand, ball of the foot, ankle, and wrist may also be used. A reusable sensor is available and used mainly for one-time spot checks, working best on fingers and toes.

Nellcor describes the workings of their sensor as follows: one side of the light sensor contains two **light-emitting diodes (LEDs)**, one of which transmits light in the red range and the other in the infrared range. The lights shine through skin, nail, tissue, venous blood, and arterial blood. A photodetector on the other side of the sensor receives the red and infrared light and measures the amount of each that has been absorbed by oxygenated and deoxygenated hemoglobin in arterial blood (Fig. 8-2). SpO_2 is the common term for oxygen saturation readings obtained from a pulse oximeter.[7]

The amount of light reflected to the sensor depends on the amount of saturated hemoglobin present in the blood at the time of the measurement. The oxygenated hemoglobin will absorb more infrared light and cause the saturation percentage to increase. The O_2/Hgb percentage is achieved by comparing the amount of infrared light to the amount of red light detected from the blood. The percentage can change with the systolic and diastolic changes in blood pressure. Most pulse oximeters also have the capacity to read and display the patient's heart rate as well as the percentage of hemoglobin saturated.

According to the American Association for Respiratory Care (AARC) Clinical Practice Guidelines, documentation of the SpO_2 measurement should be placed in the patient's chart and include (1) SpO_2; (2) patient activity level and position; (3) FiO_2 and oxygen device; (4) heart rate; (5)

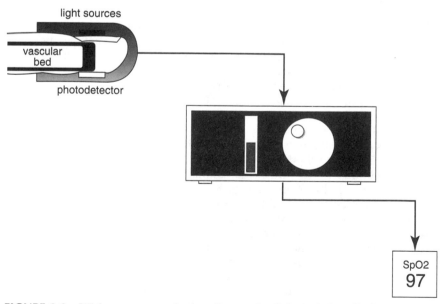

FIGURE 8-2 With sensor attached to finger, the light-emitting diodes are sending a signal through the vascular bed and transmitting it to the pulse oximeter, which displays the SpO_2 of the patient. (Redrawn from Nellcor.)

ventilator setting; (6) probe type and placement site; (7) clinical appearance of the patient; (8) alarm settings; and (9) results of any simultaneously obtained arterial and capillary blood gas measurements.[2]

The pulse oximeter has decreased the need to do frequent ABGs to monitor oxygenation in the infant and child. Additional advantages of this device include the size, lack of the need for calibration, lack of the need for site preparation, and a rapid assessment of oxygen saturation. Pulse oximeters range in size from hand-held devices to small, lightweight units that are easily portable and can be placed at the bedside. There is no calibration time required for this device as the reading is accurate from the time the blood flow is detected until it is removed from the patient. The only preparation is the attaching of the probe to the monitor and patient. Some monitors are equipped with batteries and others require an electrical source for long-term monitoring. There is no need to prepare the patient site used other than to evaluate the availability of a vascular area.

Another advantage of pulse oximetry is that numerous sites with easy access are available in both infants and children. Since the manufacturers offer the probes in a variety of sizes, there is no problem finding the correct size for the patient, making sure that the light source and the receptor site are in direct line with one another. This monitor is easily applied to both infants and children with equal effectiveness. Monitors are equipped with a default alarm system that will detect changes outside the desired range. Standard ranges are preset for pulse and saturation levels but they can be manually adjusted by the practitioner for each patient. Standard preset saturation levels are 100% (high level) and 85% (low level); for heart rate, values are preset for adults at 100 beats (high level) and 55 beats (low level). Often, as the child grows older, the adult parameters will be used.

Nellcor's pulse oximeters have been shown to be accurate to within 2% when compared to measurements made with standard laboratory instrumentation. Fetal hemoglobin does not affect the accuracy of measurement, although abnormal hemoglobin forms such as methemoglobin or carboxyhemoglobin will affect the readings.

There are some disadvantages to pulse oximetry. Since the electrodes measure only the percentage of hemoglobin that is saturated, it makes no distinction as to the source of that saturation. The value is inaccurate in the presence of methemoglobin and carboxyhemoglobin, when the saturation value detected by the oximeter will be higher than actual saturation. If the infant or child is exposed to medical dyes, the values displayed by a pulse oximeter will be less than the actual amount of oxygen saturated. Since the accuracy of the pulse oximeter is greatest between 70% and 100% saturation, hypoxic infants and children have less reliable readings.[6]

Hypothermia can also alter the reading of the device, often because of poor perfusion. Motion detections have given inaccurate readings as they lead the sensor to believe that it is detecting pulsation. Ambient light sources, such as a radiant warmer used to prevent hypothermia of the neonate, can interfere with the sensor as additional light is transmitted to the LEDs, providing abnormal readings. This problem can be corrected by covering the probe to prevent the reading of ambient light. Sensor sites need to be monitored for rubbing or pressure necrosis of the tissue. To avoid this problem, the site should be changed on a regular basis as determined by individual center protocols. The recommended time for changing a probe site of the infant or child is every 8 hours.

■ TRANSCUTANEOUS MONITORING

Transcutaneous (across the skin) monitoring is based on the principle that oxygen and carbon dioxide gases diffuse through the skin and can be measured to correlate with the ABG. A modified Clark electrode is used to measure oxygen tension and a modified Stow-Severinghaus electrode is used to measure carbon dioxide. As with other forms of noninvasive monitoring, the transcutaneous monitor is used on a continuous basis to detect trends in transcutaneous values as correlated with arterial blood gas values.

Both oxygen sensing (Fig. 8-3) and carbon dioxide sensing (Fig. 8-4) devices incorporate heating elements and thermistors to measure and control the temperature of the electrode, in addition to the gas-measuring components. The electrode is secured to the skin surface with an airtight seal to eliminate contamination by room air gases. The skin surface beneath the electrode is heated, causing increased peripheral vasodilation beneath the electrode and increased capillary blood flow to the sensor, allowing the recorded value to be similar to that of an arterialized sample. The carbon dioxide probe picks up the CO_2 beneath the skin surface because of the ease with which the CO_2 perfuses through the skin naturally. The values obtained from the transcutaneous monitor are listed as the $PtcO_2$ and $PtcCO_2$.

The transcutaneous monitor is able to obtain accurately correlated values from the infant because of the lack of adipose tissue beneath the skin surface and the ability to easily heat the skin. The infant's skin surface should be heated to between 43° to 45° C by the probe in order to obtain a correct reading. The smaller the birth weight of the infant, the easier it

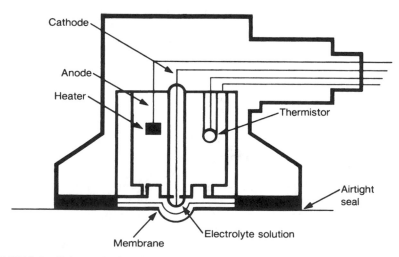

FIGURE 8-3 Schematic drawing of the electrode used to measure transcutaneous oxygen tension. (Redrawn from Novametrix Medical Systems: A User's Guide to Transcutaneous Gas Monitoring. Wallingford, CT, Novametrix Medical Systems, 1981.)

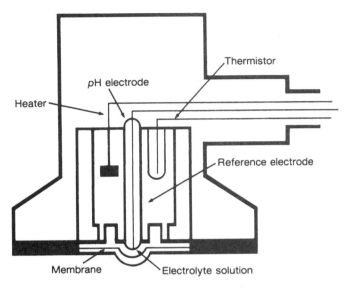

FIGURE 8-4   Schematic drawing of the electrode used to measure transcutaneous carbon dioxide tension. (Redrawn from Novametrix Medical Systems: A User's Guide to Transcutaneous Gas Monitoring. Wallingford, CT, Novametrix Medical Systems, 1981.)

is to heat the skin surface and maintain a temperature above 43° C. The pediatric patient will require higher temperatures and the skin surface will need to be checked for proper level of perfusion because of increased thickening of the skin layer as the child matures.

The electrode is normally placed on the trunk, preferably the chest, upper arm, upper thigh, shoulder, or back of the infant (Fig. 8-5). A drop of water is placed between the electrode and the patient's skin to flush out any trapped air. The probe should be changed at least every 4 hours, with more frequent changes if there are reddened areas on the skin. The site may be changed as frequently as every 2 hours. Each time the site is changed the monitor should be recalibrated.

The probe will need to be calibrated before placing it on the infant. The oxygen electrode should be accurate for a two-point calibration, using O_2 levels of zero and room air. The carbon dioxide electrode should be calibrated using a two-point calibration. Room air CO_2 cannot be used since there is such a small percentage of CO_2 in room air.

The advantages of this device are that it provides continuous noninvasive monitoring, evaluates CO_2 and O_2 at the same time, and provides information on oxygenation and ventilation when there is limited access to the blood gas sites. Since the device is used for continuous monitoring of changes in the Pa_{O_2}, it will often reflect changes by observing the trends of the patient levels. It will quickly detect a patient whose oxygenation can be improved by positioning changes, suctioning, or a slight increase in supplemental oxygen.

The disadvantages of a transcutaneous monitor are several. The device requires that continuous calibration be done on the machine itself; this causes "down" time, as the machine needs to equilibrate with the patient,

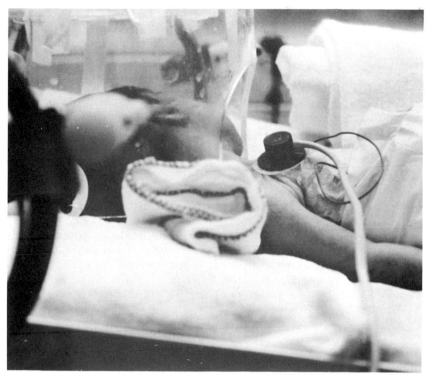

FIGURE 8-5   Transcutaneous oxygen electrode in place on the right upper chest (preductal area) of an infant receiving oxygen therapy. (Avery GB: Neonatology: Pathophysiology and Management of the Newborn, 2nd ed, p 419. Philadelphia, JB Lippincott, 1981.)

a process that requires approximately 20 minutes after the electrode is reattached. A separate machine is required for calibration of the monitor. There is no way to monitor pH values using this device, so arterial puncture may still be necessary. The amount of adipose tissue found beneath the surface of the skin can also present a problem. As the child grows, the skin changes in texture and makes perfusion of the skin more difficult.

Another complication of this monitor is that it requires heating of the element that measures transcutaneous oxygen and carbon dioxide. This often causes **erythema** (reddening of the skin) as well as blistering and burning of the skin surface, thus the site must be changed more frequently. The physical movement of the infant can cause the electrode to become loosened or detached from the skin, allowing room air to reach the sensors and provide incorrect readings by exposing the sensor to additional oxygen and reduced carbon dioxide. This causes an elevation of the $Ptco_2$ and a lowering of the $Ptcco_2$ results.

If the electrode is placed over a bony site, there is often an interruption in the reading. The skin of a premature infant is especially sensitive to the adhesive ring. The removal of this ring to change the site or calibrate the sensor can also cause removal of skin tissue itself. In some children, there can be an allergic reaction to the adhesive ring used for attachment of the electrode. The drop of water that is placed over the sensor can be lost in the placement of the electrode on the skin. Some drugs may cause inaccurate values, particularly those that affect perfusion (tolazoline, dopamine).

▬CAPNOGRAPHY

Capnography is another type of noninvasive monitor that is used to estimate the $PaCO_2$ (partial pressure of carbon dioxide) in the blood. Carbon dioxide is a product of cellular metabolism that is released into the blood in the systemic capillaries and transported to the lungs for removal. Assessing the ability to remove CO_2 from the blood is one indication of the ability of the patient to adequately ventilate the lungs. The level of CO_2 in exhaled gas is measured by the capnograph. The term for this evaluation of the exhaled gas is $PetCO_2$ (partial pressure of the end-tidal CO_2). The **capnometer** (device used to measure exhaled CO_2 tension by infrared spectrometry) provides for the CO_2 to be displayed as a number expressed in mm Hg or as a percentage of the exhaled volume. The capnometer also displays a waveform that is another indication of patterns of respiration. This monitor is often used in conjunction with the pulse oximeter to monitor the progress of the patient and determine when an arterial blood gas is appropriate.

There are two techniques utilized in the monitoring of the end-tidal CO_2. The first uses an infrared absorption spectrometer, which is based on the absorption of infrared radiation on a defined wavelength. The capnometer directs a light beam to a sample cell container and, depending on the manufacturer's specifications, this light beam will bring either a single or a double source to the sample cell. Once the collected gas is in the sample cell, a photodetector compares the amount of light from the gas to a reference cell containing a gas that is void of CO_2. The difference between the two will determine the correct CO_2 percentage.

A newer technique of infrared absorption spectroscopy utilizes a no-operator calibration that is built into the machine at the factory. When the capnometer is turned on, a 45-second calibration begins to assure reliable monitoring of the infant or child. During the warm-up period, the infrared monitor should not be placed in-line with the patient's breathing circuit. Span calibrations are performed internally by the capnograph to correct for measurements that can be affected by temperature, pressure, nitrous oxide (N_2O), and oxygen. The presence of oxygen will cause CO_2 to be falsely depressed and the presence of N_2O will cause a false elevation of the end-tidal CO_2 percentage.

There are three common methods of gathering the end-tidal CO_2 sample using a capnometer (Fig. 8-6). One is the side-stream, **distal-diverting** method, in which a continuous sample of exhaled gas is aspirated from the patient's airway and transported to the analyzer to be read. This adapter is lightweight and fits directly into the patient's breathing circuit between the endotracheal (ET) tube and the breathing circuit. A mechanism to collect water and excess humidity is placed into the circuit to prevent moisture from entering the analyzer. The water trap must be checked and emptied regularly. The lightweight adapter places little weight on the ET tube and the circuit and can be adapted to use on the nonintubated patient. This method requires a longer time to measure results but there

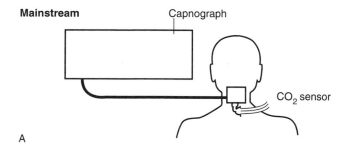

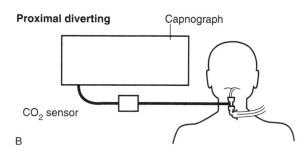

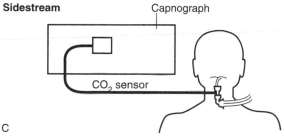

FIGURE 8-6 Mainstream, proximal diverting, and sidestream capnography. (*A*) Mainstream method involves measuring of a CO_2 sample on the exhalation side of the breathing circuit of the mouthpiece. (*B*) Proximal diverting method transports the gas partway to the capnograph and reads the CO_2 before completing transmission. (*C*) Sidestream method transports the sample to the capnograph before reading the CO_2 value. (Redrawn from Nellcor.)

is no additional dead space in the system and results are reliable unless the patient has a high respiratory rate. The high rate does not allow the sidestream method enough time to analyze one breath before the next breath arrives.

A second method is the mainstream, **nondiverting** system in which, as its name suggests, the probe is inserted directly into the exhaled gas flow so that all exhaled gas will pass directly through the analyzer. It is placed at the proximal end of the ET tube and requires a warm-up period of 5 minutes. The mainstream sensor is heated to prevent water from condensing on the in-line tube. Mainstream sample analyzers can also contribute dead space to the pediatric breathing circuit.[6] The mainstream analyzer is heavy and bulky; the weight and size of this device can cause kinking of the smaller ET tubes. The main advantage to this unit is that the results are obtained quickly. This is particularly useful for the infant or child who is breathing rapidly. This device can only be used on the patient with an artificial airway in place.

A third method is **proximal-diverting** mainstream capnography, in which CO_2 is monitored by infrared absorption of the exhaled gas sample. Monitoring begins after a warm-up period of about 45 seconds, and no operator calibration is required at start-up or during prolonged monitoring. This method offers reliable performance even when there are significant patient secretions.[5] The gas is transported a short distance to a module where the CO_2 is measured. The value is then sent to the display unit.

The proximal-diverting Nellcor 1000 (N-1000) produces waveforms and accurate changes in CO_2 airway values through the machine's response time, sample flow rate, and sample transport distance. The N-1000 provides accurate CO_2 measurements by having a response time (also termed rise time) that is able to register from 10% to 90% of a step change in airway CO_2. The significance of the response time is that it will determine the ability of the unit to accurately reflect a change in the CO_2 at the airway.[5] The sample flow rates for patients with small tidal volumes and high respiratory rates may be inaccurate if too much fresh gas is drawn in with the sample. The unit prevents this from occurring. The sample transport distance is adjusted so that the distance for the sample to be transported is less than that of the side-stream method, while avoiding the bulkiness of the mainstream method. Moisture and humidity must be removed from the exhaled gas before it reaches the measuring sensor. The TRI-GUARD system dehumidifies gas during transport and a second system clears occluding material from the airway adapter's filter.

Nellcor's N-6000 is a proximal-diverting system that consists of an airway adapter and a CO_2 sensor. This sensor weighs less than 10 g; minimizing the sensor weight is intended to decrease the risk of accidental airway displacement.[5] This device can also provide SaO_2 readings. The N-6000 provides a miniaturized, lightweight, single-beam/single-detector CO_2 sensor that has reliable performance in the presence of patient secretions and no operator calibration. The device will automatically compensate for changes in temperature, barometric pressure, and system electronics.

A capnograph can provide a graphically displayed waveform that is determined by the patient's ventilatory pattern. Figure 8-7 shows the normal waveform with five reference points identifying the steps of the exhaled breath. The waveform should start from a zero baseline (see Fig. 8-7A and B) and rise with the exhalation of CO_2 (see Fig. 8-7C). The gas will reach an alveolar plateau near the end of exhalation (see Fig. 8-7D) and return to the zero baseline with the initiation of an inspiratory breath (see Fig. 8-7E). By evaluating the waveform, the practitioner can determine whether CPR is being done effectively, ventilator settings are adequate, and work of breathing is appropriate for the infant or child.

Figure 8-8 demonstrates a waveform from an 11-year-old child with head trauma. In order to reduce intracranial pressure, it is helpful to maintain the CO_2 level between 25 and 30 mm Hg. The second waveform shows how the response to hyperventilation can be easily evaluated by the

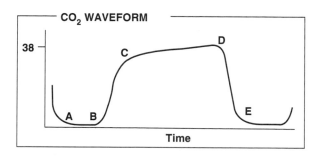

A–B: Exhalation of CO_2 free gas from dead space.

B–C: Combination of dead space and alveolar gas.

C–D: Exhalation of mostly alveolar gas (alveolar plateau).

D: "End-tidal" point—CO_2 exhalation at maximum point.

D–E: Inhalation of CO_2 free gas.

FIGURE 8-7 A normal waveform having all of the components for the $EtCO_2$ (end-tidal) to be a good estimator of $PaCO_2$. The components include: (**A**), zero baseline; (**B**), rapid, sharp uprise; (**C**), alveolar plateau; (**D**), well-defined end-tidal point; and (**E**), rapid, sharp downstroke. (Redrawn from Nellcor.)

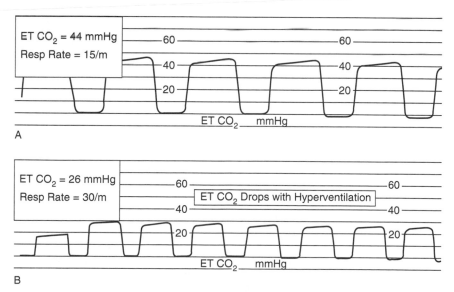

FIGURE 8-8 (**A**) Normal waveform of a mechanically ventilated 11-year-old child with head trauma by a capnograph showing a $EtCO_2$ of 44 and respiratory rate of 15 bpm. (**B**) Normal waveform of the child after adjusting the ventilator to make the patient hypercapnic. The $EtCO_2$ has been lowered to 25–30 cmH$_2$O and the respiratory rate has been increased to 30 bpm. (Redrawn from Nellcor.)

practitioner at the bedside. The common airway CO_2 graphics showing irregular patterns are demonstrated in Figure 8-9.

The advantages of a capnograph include the ability to quickly assess ventilation by monitoring the CO_2 levels and the ability to assess the breathing pattern. Another advantage is avoiding arterial puncture if the trend of the machine does not indicate abnormal levels. The monitor can also have a pulse oximeter built in to obtain SpO_2 and $PetCO_2$ along with a respiratory rate. The alarm system will indicate when CO_2 is outside of the normal range set for each individual patient. The continual reading and waveform allow the practitioner to quickly evaluate changes in the infant's or child's ventilatory pattern.

The device has some disadvantages as well. The weight of the mainstream device and the slow speed of the side-stream device can present problems. Both of these factors have been addressed with the Nellcor N-6000. The critically ill patient with a high respiratory rate may not gener-

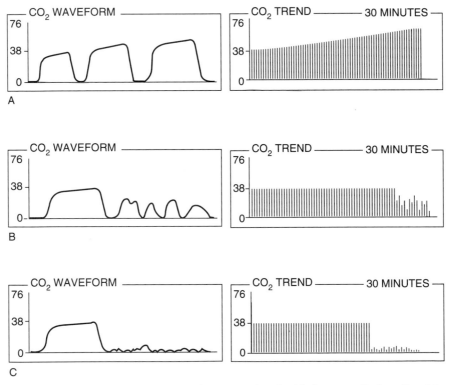

FIGURE 8-9 (**A**) Gradual rise in $EtCO_2$ associated with hypoventilation. Possible causes: (1) rising body temperature, (2) hypoventilation, (3) partial airway obstruction, such as a FBA and (4) absorption of CO_2 for an exogenous source. (**B**) Sudden drop in $EtCO_2$ to low or non-zero value with incomplete sampling of patient exhalation. Possible causes: (1) leak in the airway system, (2) partial disconnect in ventilatory circuit, (3) partial airway obstruction caused by secretions, and (4) endotracheal tube in the hypopharynx. (**C**) Sudden loss to near zero may indicate catastrophic loss of ventilation to patient. Possible causes (1) esophageal intubation, (2) complete airway disconnection from ventilation, (3) complete ventilator malfunction, and (4) total obstruction/kinked endotracheal tube. (Redrawn from Nellcor.)

ate accurate readings. The device will normally underestimate the $PaCO_2$ by 2 to 5 mm Hg and this gap will be wider if the patient is not maintaining normal ventilation-perfusion relationships.

■PULMONARY FUNCTION TESTING IN INFANTS

Pulmonary function testing of neonates is another way of noninvasively monitoring the progress of an infant or child. Testing can be done on the intubated infant, the nonintubated infant, and the child who can understand simple directions.

With the intubated neonate, it is possible to determine whether the ventilator is causing overdistention of the lungs, resulting in barotrauma, or whether there is underexpansion that may result in additional atelectasis. By directly measuring the effects of mechanical ventilation therapy through pulmonary function tests (PFTs), ventilation efficiency can, in theory, be maximized while harmful effects can be minimized. By evaluating tidal volume, **lung compliance** (change in lung volume in response to a given pressure), and **airway resistance** (pressure needed to move the gas through the airways of the lungs), the practitioner can determine the ability of the neonate's lungs to function and adjust ventilator settings to prevent further complications.

Pulmonary function testing of the neonate should cause no disturbance in the mechanical ventilation of the infant. The values obtained from this testing can be correlated with a current ABG, chest x-ray film, pulse oximetry, and clinical observations to determine or confirm the proper diagnosis or treatment of the infant. Other evaluations that can be determined from this procedure are appropriate treatment regimens, effectiveness of surfactant therapy in the premature infant, correct usage of drug therapies, and adjustments that need to be made to mechanical ventilation parameters. As lung compliance increases and airway resistance decreases, the infant will be more easily and successfully weaned from mechanical ventilation. Serial PFTs give the clinician an appropriate picture of trends in infant ventilation and guidance for therapeutic changes in treatment.

Simultaneous signals of Vt (mL/kg), airflow (V), and **transpulmonary pressure** (Ptp) are measured and integrated to determine lung mechanics and energy relationships in the system.[4] Transpulmonary pressure is the pressure that is exerted on the lungs to initiate inspiration.

There are two specific types of systems in wide use for bedside testing. One system uses a **pneumotachograph** to measure V and Vt indirectly (Fig. 8-10); the other uses a hot wire **anemometer** to quantitate V and Vt indirectly through heat loss. Both systems require placement of an esophageal balloon or a water-filled catheter in the distal esophagus to estimate Ptp.[4]

The pneumotachograph is placed in-line between the ventilator circuit and the endotracheal tube. If the infant or child is not intubated, a face mask or nasal prongs can be attached to the pneumotachograph. The measuring instrument is inside a tube and gas is able to flow through the tube, providing the results that are measured. The flow is determined by measuring the volume and integrating it with respect to time. A pneumotachograph that is larger than necessary adds excessive dead space, requiring increased amplification to pick up faint pressure gradient signals. Conversely, a device that is too small causes turbulent flows, adding resis-

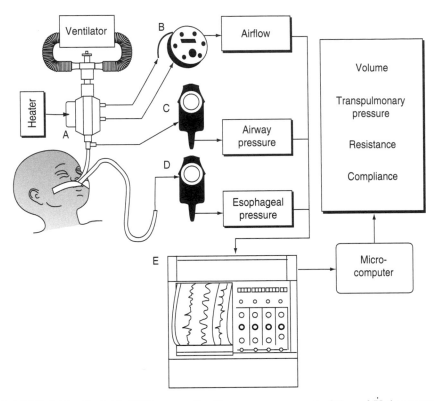

FIGURE 8-10 Bedside PFT system for direct measurement of V_1 and $\dot{V}$. A = pneumotachograph; B = differential transducer for airflow; C = transducer for airway pressure; D = transducer for esophageal pressure; E = multichannel recorder and airway monitor. (Redrawn from Cunningham MD: Monitoring pulmonary function. In Goldsmith J, Karotkin E [eds]: Assisted Ventilation of the Neonate. Philadelphia: WB Saunders, 233-244. Reprinted by permission.)

tance to the respiratory system that may influence breathing patterns.[4] In this system, water vapor can also affect the results, but this can be corrected by heating the pneumotachograph to normal body temperature or slightly higher (37°–38° C).

The second system involves the use of a hot wire anemometer that measures heat loss from the airflow to estimate gas flow across the circuit. It has been used to measure inspiratory volumes, expiratory volumes, minute ventilation, lung compliance, and airway resistance.

Humidity and temperature do not affect this device. This device will respond more quickly to flow changes, which makes it more desirable if the neonate is breathing at high respiratory rates.

The computer printout of the PFT will indicate tidal volume, lung compliance, and airway resistance on the pressure–volume loop and flow–volume loop when using bedside monitors. This is an advantage for the early detection of complications. The test is easily performed by trained personnel and is noninvasive. The PFT can be easily and quickly repeated for both the infant and the child. The tests can evaluate the need for therapies.

Disadvantages for the infant include the fact that the infant may need to be mildly sedated to perform the tests. The drug of choice for sedation is chloral hydrate. The use of a face mask may also distort the final results, making for greater accuracy in the intubated patient. The test needs to be performed by trained personnel, preferably someone with experience in both PFTs and neonatal/pediatric care.

PULMONARY FUNCTION TESTING IN CHILDREN

The child who undergoes PFTs will follow the same testing procedures as the adult as long as the child can understand the commands. The child with obstructive disease (asthma, bronchiectasis, bronchopulmonary dysplasia, and cystic fibrosis) and restrictive disease (chest deformities, atelectasis, syndromes) will be followed closely for deterioration of the lungs. The standard spirometry of slow vital capacity (to obtain volumes), forced vital capacity (to obtain flows), and MVV (minute volume ventilation) will be used for evaluation. The tests can be used in both infants and children to assess the strength of the lungs and their ability to function under anesthesia and surgery.

The lung volume measurements include the vital capacity (VC), tidal volume (Vt), expiratory reserve volume (ERV), functional residual capacity (FRC), total lung capacity (TLC), and ratio of residual volume to total lung capacity (RV/TLC). The relationship of these volumes is important for the understanding of pulmonary functions. (Fig. 8-11). Lung volumes will help to determine hyperinflation and air trapping, hypoinflation, and degree of change from a previous test. If all volumes are decreased, the child is often suffering from a restrictive problem. To evaluate an obstructive problem, the child will show a steady decrease in the size of the VC, ERV, and TLC with an increase in the RV and the RV/TLC ratio.

The flow measurements (volume/time) include the peak expiratory flow (PEF), the forced expiratory flow between the 25% and 75% volume points of a breath (FEF 25%–75%), the forced expiratory volume for a specific time period (FEVt), and forced expiratory volume as a percentage of the vital capacity (FEVt/FVC%). Table 8-1 provides a complete definition of all volumes and flows. The flow tests will reveal the amount of obstructive disease and how it responds to the use of medication to dilate the airways in the child. Tests of both volumes and flows can be conducted in a pulmonary function lab or at the patient's bedside.

The MVV is a test of the strength of the respiratory muscles. This is a difficult procedure for the child who has a restrictive deformity of the chest cavity and the child suffering from chronic obstructive disease.

The main concern with respect to the testing of children is the degree of cooperation that can be achieved with very young children of 3 to 6 years of age. Most PFTs depend on the cooperation and effort of the patient. Table 8-2 lists normal values for children from 5 to 17 years.

The peak expiratory flow is used most often with children who have hyperactive airways. There are numerous hand-held devices currently in use so that the test can be done easily, simply, and quickly in the patient's room, the emergency room, or a specific testing area. The flow is usually measured in liters per minute with an improving value as the goal. This test is also part of a flow–volume curve often done to evaluate the degree

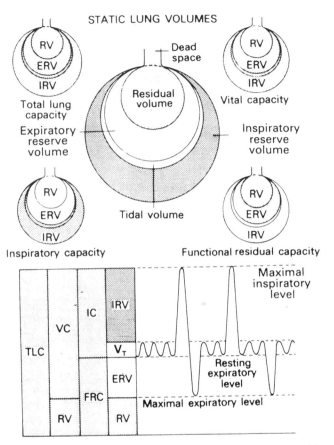

FIGURE 8-11   Division of total lung capacity into lung volumes and lung capacities. In the small diagrams surrounding the large central one, the shaded areas outline the volumes that constitute the various lung capacities. (Adapted from Comroe JH Jr et al: The Lung: Clinical Physiology and Pulmonary Function Tests, 2nd ed. Chicago, Year Book Medical Publishers, 1962.)

of obstructive disease. The values may vary according to the device used for measurement of peak flow. The hand-held devices are mainly used by children with asthma in the home setting as well as the hospital. The child can use the flow measurements to determine the need for further treatment of the airway.

Another important assessment of the child with asthma or cystic fibrosis is the pre–post bronchodilator procedure. This test involves the patient's performing the spirometry maneuver, administration of a bronchodilator with a hand-held nebulizer or metered-dose inhaler, and repetition of the spirometry maneuver. A significant test result is one where the percentage of improvement from the first to the second test is at least 15% or 100 cc.

An advantage of this form of testing is that it allows long-term assessment of pulmonary function in the child. This is a way to objectively evaluate the use of bronchodilators. The peak flow measurement is a quick

TABLE 8-1   Terms Describing Volumes and Flows

Vital capacity	Maximal amount of air that can be exhaled after a maximum inspiratory breath (VC). This capacity includes the inspiratory volume, tidal volume, and expiratory reserve volume. FVC is the term used if the exhaled vital capacity is forced.
Tidal volume	Volume of air that is either inhaled or exhaled during normal breathing (Vt). This volume is based on the size of the child.
Expiratory reserve volume	Maximal amount of air that can be exhaled beginning at the end of an exhaled tidal volume breath (ERV).
Total lung capacity	Maximum amount of air in the lung after a full inspiratory breath (TLC).
Functional residual capacity	Maximal amount of air found in the lung at the end of a normal tidal volume breath (FRC).
Peak expiratory flow/volume	Maximum amount of air flow measured from the lungs on either an inspiratory or an expiratory breath (PEF/PEV). This test is highly dependent on patient effort.
Forced expiratory flow 25%–75%	The amount of air that is forced out of the lungs during the middle 50% of the exhaled breath (FEF).
Forced expiratory volume	The amount of air that has been forcefully exhaled at either 0.5 seconds, 1.0 second, 2.0 seconds, or 3.0 seconds (FEVt). The most used of these volumes is the 1.0 second (FEV_1).
FEVt/FVC	Forced expiratory volume at a specific time compared to the forced vital capacity from a flow maneuver. This is measured as a percentage.
Maximum voluntary ventilation	Air is moved in and out of the lung as rapidly and deeply as possible. The time interval is either 10, 12, or 15 seconds. The value is extrapolated and expressed in L/min.

and fast way to evaluate acute respiratory distress in the home, hospital, or emergency room. Pulmonary function testing can also be used to evaluate the child's lung function prior to nonemergency surgery.

The main disadvantage of the pulmonary function test is that the test is effort-dependent and requires the understanding and cooperation of the child. Often, children are tired before the test is complete or fail to understand the directions and demonstrations of the pulmonary function technician. Children with cystic fibrosis often become ill while attempting the MVV maneuver. Children with asthma may have trouble with chronic coughing during the testing.

■ ECHOCARDIOGRAPHY

Echocardiography is a noninvasive diagnostic procedure that requires an understanding of cross-sectional cardiac anatomy. Components of the echocardiography study include assessing the heart and great vessels with M-mode imaging; two-dimensional imaging; and pulsed, continuous wave, and color Doppler. M-mode imaging is used to document measurements, two-dimensional imaging provides cross-sectional B-mode images of the cardiac anatomy, and Doppler imaging documents the physiologic aspect

TABLE 8-2   Normal Values for Pulmonary Function Studies in Children (All Values BTPS Unless Otherwise Noted)

TEST	FORMULA	SD	SOURCE
(Children 42–59 inches, 5–17 years old)			
FVC (L)			
Males	$0.094H - 3.04$	0.176	1
Females	$0.077H - 2.37$	0.171	1
FEV$_1$ (L)			
Males	$0.085H - 2.86$	0.159	1
Females	$0.074H - 2.48$	0.166	1
FEF$_{25\%-75\%}$ (L)			
Males	$0.094H - 2.61$	0.388	1
Females	$0.087H - 2.39$	0.347	1
PEF (L/sec)			
Males	$0.161H - 5.88$	0.451	1
Females	$0.130H - 4.51$	0.487	1
MVV (L/min)			
Males and females	$3.81H - 134$	—	1
(Children 60–78 inches, 5–17 years old)			
FVC (L)			
Males	$0.174A + 0.164H - 9.43$	0.354	1
Females	$0.102A + 0.117H - 5.87$	0.287	1
FEV$_1$ (L/sec)			
Males	$0.126A + 0.143H - 7.86$	0.303	1
Females	$0.085A + 0.100H - 4.94$	0.290	1
FEF$_{25\%-75\%}$ (L/sec)			
Males	$0.126A + 0.135H - 6.50$	0.612	1
Females	$0.83A + 0.093H - 3.50$	0.621	1
PEF (L/sec)			
Males	$0.205A + 0.181H - 9.54$	0.780	1
Females	$0.139A + 0.100H - 4.12$	0.798	1
MVV (L/min)			
Males and females	$3.81H - 134$	—	1
VC (L)			
Males	(same as FVC)		1
Females	(same as FVC)		1
FRC (L)			
Males and females	$0.067 \times e^{0.05334H}$	—	2
RV (L)			
Males and females	$0.033 \times e^{0.05334H}$	—	2

(continued)

TABLE 8-2   Normal Values for Pulmonary Function Studies in Children (All Values BTPs Unless Otherwise Noted) *(continued)*

TEST	FORMULA	SD	SOURCE
Derived lung volumes (L)			
	TLC = VC + RV		
	IC = TLC − FRC		
	ERV = VC − IC		
DLcoSB (mL CO/min/mm Hg STPD)			
Males and females	0.693H − 20.13	—	3

1. Dickman M, Schmidt CD, Gardner RM: Spirometric standards for normal children and adolescent (ages 5 years through 18 years). Am Rev Respir Dis 104:680, 1971.

2. Weng TR, Levison H: Standards of pulmonary function in children. Am Rev Respir Dis 99:879, 1969.

3. Gaensler EA, Wright GW: Evaluation of respiratory impairment. Arch Environ Health 12:146, 1966.

of the heart. High-frequency ultrasound transducers are used to transmit the ultrasound; the images are displayed on a CRT screen and can be videotaped for review and storage. The patient should be supine during the procedure with the neck extended, the head turned to one side, and the abdominal wall flaccid. Sedation may be necessary for the infant or young child so that high-quality images can be accurately obtained. If there is a suspected anomaly, the procedure is usually followed by computerized tomography (CT) scan and then magnetic resonance imaging (MRI) to make a complete diagnosis.

Scanning is done to assess both the morphology (structure and form) and the physiology (function) of the heart. The segmental approach includes identifying the position (situs) of the heart, followed by identification of the location of the vena cava and the aorta, and establishing the location of the liver and the stomach in relation to the heart. **Situs inversus**, the location of an organ in the opposite side of the chest (or thorax), can be diagnosed.

The four chambers of the heart are identified next, along with their connective membranes (septa). The transducer is manipulated on different angles and planes to visualize the entire heart. Imaging of the heart of the neonate is easily accomplished since the lungs are small and the bones of the ribs and sternum are not totally ossified at this time. The proper attachment of the tricuspid valve entering the right ventricle and the mitral valve entering the left ventricle are assessed next. The pulmonary artery and veins are assessed for abnormal size or function. The cardiac circulation is scanned for proper function, size, and position. An assessment of a patent ductus arteriosis can be done using the Doppler transducer to determine the amount of pulmonary vascular resistance. The documentation of the right and left heart blood flow velocities will indicate the presence or absence of a left-to-right shunt in the neonate or infant. The presence of common congenital cardiac complications can be determined by using ultrasound.

These tomographic views of the heart allow feedback on the ventricular function and the ejection fraction of the infant's or child's heart. The ventricular function of the heart is assessed by measuring the ability of the ventricles to pump the blood as well as by determining whether there is a ventricular septal defect (VSD), the most common congenital cardiac lesion in the neonate.[3] In the critically ill infant or child who may be septic or has severe metabolic abnormalities, echocardiography can be used to determine the presence of a reduced ventricular contraction. The ejection fraction is the portion of blood expelled from the chambers of the heart during each contraction. The ultrasound beam is produced in proportion to the velocity of the infant's blood flow. These beams can be monitored continuously for an ongoing study of the cardiac output. Pulmonary valve stenosis is the most common form of right ventricular tract obstruction.[3]

Doppler ultrasound (echocardiography) is an important means of determining congenital heart disease in the infant or child. Its main advantages are that it is noninvasive and there is no pain for the patient. It is accurate in determining the exact location and amount of disease or malformation of the organ. It is the best way to determine whether further assessment is needed. The pulsed or continuous wave Doppler provides quantitative assessment of blood flow, ventricular function, and formation of the valves of the heart. The test can be performed at the bedside. The Doppler is accurate in determining both right ventricular and pulmonary artery pressures of the infant and child.

Disadvantages of the procedure for the infant and child include the fact that the patient will usually not remain still for the procedure and most patients need mild sedation. The color Doppler is a good screening procedure for flow determinations but is limited in a functional assessment. Ventricular compliance is often difficult to determine and an inferred rather than a measured value is often used. When pulmonary hypertension is suspected, the patient should have a cardiac catheterization to accurately determine the long-term prognosis and need for surgery.

■REFERENCES

1. Ahmann E, Meny RG, Fink RJ: Use of home apnea monitors. JOGNN 21(5):394, 1992.
2. American Association for Respiratory Care: Clinical practice guidelines for pulse oximetry. Respir Care 26:1406, 1991.
3. Hagen-Ansert SL: Textbook of Diagnostic Ultrasonography, 3rd ed. Baltimore, CV Mosby, 1989.
4. Lynam LE: Pulmonary function testing: A tool for managing the mechanically ventilated patient. Neonatal Network 12:61, 1993.
5. Nellcor: Miniaturized mainstream capnography: Nellcor's ultra cap pulse oximeter and capnograph. Capnography Reference Note Number 4. Pleasanton, CA, 1992.
6. Pilchak TM: Anesthesia and monitoring equipment for pediatrics. CRNA: Clin Forum Nurse Anesth 3:64, 1992.
7. Principles of Pulse Oximetry. Pleasanton CA, Nellcor, 1991.

■BIBLIOGRAPHY

Ahrens T: Respiratory monitoring in critical care. AACN: Clinical Issues in Critical Care Nursing 4:56, 1993.
Barnhart SL, Czervinske MP: Perinatal and Pediatric Respiratory Care. Philadelphia, WB Saunders, 1995.

Burton GC, Hodgkin JE, Ward JJ: Respiratory Care: A Guide to Clinical Practice, 3rd ed. Philadelphia: JB Lippincott, 1991.

Eichenwald EC, Stark AR: Respiratory motor output: Effect of state maturation in early life. In: Haddad GG, Farber JP (eds): Developmental Neurobiology of Breathing. New York, Marcel Dekker, 1991.

Greenspan JS, Cullen JA, Zukowsky K, Antunes MJ, Spitzer AR: Pulmonary function testing in the critically ill neonate. Part I. An overview. Neonatal Network 13:9, 1994.

Healthdyne: A Parent's Guide to Infant Monitoring. Marietta GA, Healthdyne, 1993.

Higgins CB, Silverman NH, Kersting-Sommerhoff BA, Schmidt K: Congenital heart disease: Echocardiography and magnetic resonance imaging. New York, Raven, 1990.

Hess D: Monitoring in respiratory care. NBRC Horizons 19:1, 1993.

Holt WJ, Greenspan JS, Antunes MJ, Cullen JA, Spitzer AR, Wiswell TE: Pulmonary response to an inhaled bronchodilator in chronically ventilated preterm infants with suspected airway reactivity. Respiratory Care 40:145, 1995.

Koff PB, Eitzman D, Neu J: Neonatal and pediatric respiratory care, 2nd ed. St. Louis, C. V. Mosby, 1993.

Lynam LE, Algren S: Pulmonary function testing: Clinical applications. Neonatal Network 12:65, 1993.

McPherson SB: Respiratory care equipment, 5th ed. St. Louis, Mosby-Year Book, 1995.

Nellcor: Automatically Self-Calibrating Capnography in the Nellcor N-1000 Multi-function Monitor. Hayward CA, Nellcor, 1989.

Nellcor: End-Tidal CO_2 as an Aid in Monitoring CPR. Capnography Reference Note Number 1. Pleasanton CA, 1992.

Nellcor: Fetal hemoglobin. Pulse Oximetry Reference Note Number 4. Pleasanton, CA, 1987.

Nellcor: Nellcor N-1000 multi-function monitor. Capnography Reference Note Number 2. Pleasanton, CA, 1989.

Nellcor: Proximal-Diverting Capnography in the Nellcor N-1000 Multi-function Monitor. Capnography Reference Note Number 3. Pleasanton CA, 1989.

Nellcor: Technology Overview: Reflectance Sensors for Pulse oximetry. Pulse Oximetry Reference Note Number 7. Pleasanton CA, 1992.

Pulse Oximetry: An Introduction. Pleasanton CA, Nellcor, 1993.

Pulse Oximetry: Tips for Optimal Use. Pleasanton CA, Nellcor, 1993.

Pulse Oximetry: Step-by-Step Operation. Pleasanton CA, Nellcor, 1993.

Riggs J: Low flow aerosol drug delivery and pulmonary function testing. Neonatal Intensive Care 7:30, 1994.

Ruppel G: Manual of Pulmonary Function Testing, 6th ed. St. Louis, Mosby-Year Book, 1994.

Sondergeld TA: Pulmonary function testing in the NICU: Intermittent measurement versus continuous monitoring. Neonatal Intensive Care 7:20, 1994.

Whitaker K: Comprehensive perinatal and pediatric respiratory care. Albany, Delmar Publishers, 1992.

Zukowsky K, Greenspan JS, Cullen JA, Antunes MJ, Spitzer AR: Pulmonary function testing in the critically ill neonate. Part III. Case studies. Neonatal Network 13:31, 1994.

▄ SELF-ASSESSMENT QUESTIONS

1. Impedance pneumography is used to evaluate neonatal
   a. Petco$_2$
   b. respiratory rate
   c. oxygenation
   d. lung compliance

2. A disadvantage of the apnea monitor for the neonate is the
   a. restlessness during sleep
   b. alarms that are easily heard
   c. memory in the device
   d. flashing light on the monitor face

3. The most widely used noninvasive monitor is the
   a. capnometer
   b. pulse oximeter
   c. impedance pneumograph
   d. pulmonary function tests

4. An advantage to using the pulse oximeter is that it has
   a. compact size
   b. rapid assessment
   c. no required calibration
   d. all of the above

5. An infant is placed under a radiant warmer and the pulse oximeter is alarming. The reason for this could be
   a. actual amount of oxygen delivered to patient
   b. abnormal hemoglobin levels
   c. ambient light sources
   d. heating of the electrode

6. Transcutaneous monitoring can be used to evaluate
   a. oxygen diffusion
   b. carbon dioxide diffusion
   c. both oxygen and carbon dioxide diffusion

7. The most common complication of the transcutaneous monitor is
   a. erythema
   b. bruising
   c. necrosis
   d. body movement

8. When the infant is placed on capnography, the practitioner is attempting to evaluate the ability to
   a. oxygenate the tissues
   b. perfuse the tissues
   c. ventilate the lungs
   d. inhale a complete Vt breath

9. Pulmonary function tests for the infant are best performed
   a. in a PFT lab
   b. under the direct supervision of a physician
   c. with the use of a nasal cannula
   d. under mild sedation using chloral hydrate

10. An advantage to using the hot wire anemometer is
    a. ease of measurement of oxygen percentages
    b. humidity and temperature do not affect results
    c. application of the mainstream probe in-line
    d. prevention of burning and blistering of the chest

Part 3
Cardiopulmonary Disorders

Chapter 9

Pulmonary System Disorders in the Newborn

OBJECTIVES

Having completed this chapter, the reader will be able to:

1 Discuss the etiology and risk factors associated with the development of respiratory distress syndrome.

2 Describe the effects of the lack of surfactant on lung function, fluid balance in the lung, and the cardiovascular system.

3 Describe the histologic progression of respiratory distress syndrome.

4 Describe the clinical presentation of an infant with respiratory distress syndrome.

5 Describe the typical x-ray pattern of respiratory distress syndrome.

6 Discuss the treatment of the infant with respiratory distress syndrome and identify the possible complications of treatment.

7 Discuss the proposed etiologies for bronchopulmonary dysplasia.

8 List the abnormalities in physiology that result from the development of bronchopulmonary dysplasia.

9 Describe the clinical presentation of an infant with bronchopulmonary dysplasia.

10 Discuss the typical x-ray pattern of the various stages of bronchopulmonary dysplasia.

11 Describe the treatment of an infant with bronchopulmonary dysplasia.

12 Describe the type of infant who is most likely to develop meconium aspiration syndrome.

13 Explain the mechanism by which asphyxia promotes meconium aspiration syndrome.

14 Describe the two significant sequelae of meconium aspiration, and discuss the typical results of these problems in the infant.

15 Describe the various clinical presentations of infants with meconium aspiration syndrome.

16 Describe the radiologic appearance of meconium aspiration syndrome.

17 Discuss the treatment and prevention of meconium aspiration syndrome.

18 List the various types of pulmonary barotrauma and volutrauma that may occur.

19 List the factors that increase the risk of barotrauma and volutrauma.

20 Describe the usual pathology associated with the development of air leaks in the newborn.

21 Discuss the etiology or etiologies of pulmonary interstitial emphysema, pneumomediastinum, and pneumothorax.

22 Describe the pathophysiologic effects of each of the above air leaks.

23 Describe the clinical and radiologic presentation of infants with pulmonary interstitial emphysema and infants with pneumothorax.

24 Discuss the treatment and prevention of pulmonary barotrauma and volutrauma.

25 List and describe the two major types of newborn pneumonia.

26 List the risk factors associated with the development of pneumonia in the newborn.

27 List the common pathogens associated with each type of pneumonia.

28 Describe the pathophysiology of pneumonia caused by group B, β-hemolytic streptococcus.

29 Describe the features of other types of pneumonia.

30 Discuss the clinical and laboratory features of pneumonia in the newborn.

31 List the various x-ray film abnormalities that may be seen in different types of pneumonia.

32 Describe the general treatment of pneumonia.

33 Define apnea of the newborn and differentiate this disorder from periodic breathing.

34 Discuss the etiologies proposed for apnea and list the disorders with which apnea is associated.

35 Discuss the clinical manifestations, consequences, and treatment of apnea.

36 Compare the presentation of transient tachypnea of the newborn to that of respiratory distress syndrome.

37 Discuss the etiology, pathophysiology, and clinical presentation of transient tachypnea of the newborn.

38 Describe the clinical and radiologic appearance of transient tachypnea of the newborn.

39 Discuss the treatment of the infant with transient tachypnea of the newborn.

40 Describe the Wilson–Mikity syndrome, including possible etiology, pathophysiology, clinical presentation, and radiologic appearance.

41 Compare the Wilson–Mikity syndrome with bronchopulmonary dysplasia.

42 Discuss the treatment of the Wilson–Mikity syndrome.

KEY TERMS

air block
bronchopulmonary dysplasia
hyaline membrane disease
meconium
meconium aspiration syndrome

pulmonary interstitial emphysema
respiratory distress syndrome
transient tachypnea of the newborn
type II RDS

▰RESPIRATORY DISTRESS SYNDROME (HYALINE MEMBRANE DISEASE)

Respiratory distress syndrome (RDS) or hyaline membrane disease (HMD) is a syndrome associated with prematurity or stressed, high-risk infants and is the primary cause of respiratory disorders in the newborn period. RDS is caused by insufficient amounts of pulmonary surfactant or depressed surfactant activity, leading to massive atelectasis and hypoxemia. The severity of the disease increases with decreasing gestational age and is usually more severe in male infants. RDS affects approximately 20,000 to 30,000 infants each year in the United States and complicates approximately 1% of all pregnancies.[24]

Etiology

In order for an infant to have adequate respiratory function at birth, pulmonary perfusion and alveolar expansion must be adequate to support life. At 26 to 28 weeks of gestation, alveolar ducts and respiratory bronchioles are seen, but alveoli are not distinguishable. Pulmonary capillaries are present but are not in close contact with bronchioles and ducts. Alveolar development accelerates from this point, and mature alveoli lined with type I squamous epithelial cells are present by about 34 to 35 weeks of gestation. Pulmonary capillaries develop along with the alveoli.

In addition to adequate development of pulmonary capillary and alveolar tissue, mature pathways for the formation and secretion of surfactant must develop. Surfactant develops throughout gestation, with a surge in production of mature surfactant (lecithin) at about 34 weeks of gestation. Surfactants are secreted by type II cells, which also line the alveoli. Thus, the two major factors necessary for adequate lung function, development of adequate alveolar function and development of mature pulmonary surfactants, both peak at about the same time. Infants born before 35 weeks of gestation are therefore at risk for developing RDS because of pulmonary immaturity. In addition, infants of more advanced gestational age who are stressed or suffer difficulty with the neonatal transition (*e.g.*, asphyxiated infants) may have decreased production of surfactant secondary to hypoxemia and acidosis. Other high-risk factors include poorly controlled maternal diabetes, Rh incompatibility (erythroblastosis), history of RDS in siblings, and multiple gestations, in which the second and subsequent siblings are at greater risk.

The gestational age that corresponds to fetal lung maturity may vary with many conditions, some of which accelerate and some of which depress fetal lung maturation. These conditions are discussed in Chapter 1.

Pathophysiology

The primary disturbance in RDS is lack of surfactant, causing an increase in the surface tension of the alveoli. The infant must generate tremendous intrathoracic pressure gradients (25–30 mm Hg) to maintain patent alveoli. Because of a soft, pliable chest cage, the newborn infant cannot continue to generate these increased intrathoracic pressures gradients. This results in progressive atelectasis and decreased pulmonary compliance, leading to hypoxemia and metabolic acidosis. In addition, depending on the degree of prematurity, alveoli may not yet be well developed and pulmonary circulation may not be close enough to respiratory bronchioles, alveolar ducts, and alveoli to provide sufficient gas exchange, exacerbating the hypoxemia and metabolic acidosis. Overall, the atelectasis causes ventilation/perfusion imbalance and may lead to hypoventilation and hypercarbia. The resulting increase in the work of breathing also causes increased oxygen consumption, which decreases tissue oxygen delivery, and increased CO_2 production, which the infant may not be capable of eliminating. The development of the muscles of the chest wall may also be inadequate, resulting in ineffective tidal volumes and respiratory muscle fatigue.[5]

Another important property of surfactant is its role in keeping alveoli dry. The fluid balance of the lung is determined by capillary hydrostatic and oncotic pressures and by tissue hydrostatic and oncotic pressures. The net balance in a healthy lung favors a small fluid filtration out of the capillary into the interstitium, which is cleared by the lymphatic circulation. Surface tension forces are included in interstitial hydrostatic pressure. In RDS, or surfactant deficiency, surface tension forces are greater, acting to pull fluid into the alveoli. This factor, combined with damage to capillary endothelial cells by hypoxia and acidosis, causes fluid leakage into the alveoli. The fluid is rich in protein, and fibrin-clot formation occurs with the death of epithelial cells, forming the characteristic hyaline membranes.

Histologically, the progression of RDS begins as bronchial basement membrane edema and sloughing of respiratory epithelial cells. Patchy areas of atelectasis are seen. Leakage of proteinaceous fluid, caused by high surface tension forces and increased capillary permeability, occurs into air spaces, forming hyaline membranes. After about 72 hours, pulmonary macrophages appear and phagocytize the hyaline membranes. Provided that further pulmonary damage has not occurred during treatment, resolution of the disease commonly occurs in 5 to 7 days.

In addition to respiratory effects, secondary hemodynamic problems arise. With profound hypoxemia and acidosis present, pulmonary arteriolar constriction occurs, which elevates pulmonary vascular pressures. Systemic pressures may be low, resulting in initial right-to-left shunting through fetal pathways (foramen ovale and ductus arteriosus). During treatment of the infant with RDS (oxygen therapy, fluid administration, and correction of pH disturbance), the shunt may suddenly switch to left-to-right through the ductus arteriosus as pulmonary pressures are lowered and systemic pressures rise, resulting in pulmonary vascular congestion. This causes a further increase in pulmonary capillary leakage and pulmonary edema. Therefore, gradual correction of these imbalances is important, although left-to-right shunting may still occur.

The pathophysiology of RDS is summarized in Figure 9-1.

Clinical Signs and Diagnosis

The typical infant with RDS presents with signs of respiratory distress either immediately at birth or within a few hours after birth. Diagnosis includes ruling out a multitude of other conditions that can cause respiratory distress in the newborn (Table 9-1). The most difficult to distinguish is group B, β-hemolytic streptococcal or pneumococcal sepsis. The two diseases are almost identical in clinical presentation. If the maternal history is suspicious for infection, a white blood cell count with differential may be helpful. A septic infant usually demonstrates leukopenia and neutropenia with elevated bands. In addition, a gastric aspirate shake test for L/S ratio may aid in supporting the diagnosis of RDS.

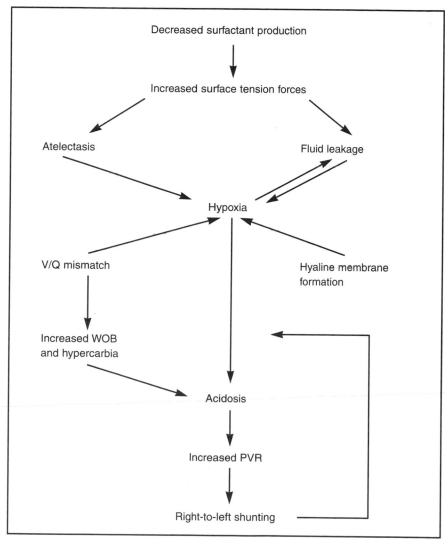

FIGURE 9-1   Pathophysiology of respiratory distress syndrome.

Symptoms worsen progressively for 2 to 3 days after onset. Breath sounds are diminished and may reveal dry, crackling sounds of air movement (rales). Clinical signs include nasal flaring (an attempt to increase airway diameter to increase airflow); intercostal, substernal, or suprasternal retractions; use of accessory muscles of breathing; tachypnea; tachycardia; and central cyanosis. Expiratory grunting, heard in the most severely afflicted infants, is a sound created by forceful exhalation through a partially closed glottis. This maneuver is an attempt to create positive end-expiratory pressure (PEEP) to aid in increasing the functional residual capacity (FRC) and maintain alveolar patency during spontaneous breathing. Paradoxical or see-saw respirations indicate the increased work

---

TABLE 9-1 Differential Diagnosis of Respiratory Distress Syndrome

Choanal atresia	Transient tachypnea of the newborn
Tracheal stenosis	Cyanotic congenital heart disease
Congenital hypoplastic lungs	Diaphragmatic hernia
Congenital pneumonias	Tracheoesophageal fistula
Neonatal sepsis	

---

of breathing, as the abdomen moves outward on inspiration and the chest cage moves inward.

As the infant becomes more hypoxic and the work of breathing increases in the first few hours after birth, peripheral vasoconstriction occurs and poor capillary refill results. The infant's color becomes pale or gray. Pitting edema may also be present, and urinary output is usually poor during the first few days.

Oxygen requirements progressively increase over the first 2 days of life. High inspired oxygen tensions are required to maintain an adequate arterial oxygen tension (50–60 mm Hg). Tissue hypoxia and poor circulatory status cause metabolic acidosis. Initially, the infant can maintain a normal to low PCO_2, but this level begins to rise as work of breathing remains high and the infant tires. As progression of the disease continues, a mixed respiratory and metabolic acidosis occurs as a result of hypoventilation and inadequate tissue oxygenation leading to anaerobic metabolism and the buildup of lactic acid.

The typical chest x-ray in RDS initially shows a diffuse, fine reticulogranular or ground-glass appearance and atelectasis. Characteristic air bronchograms may be seen in the periphery of the lung fields (Fig. 9-2). In severely affected infants, the chest x-ray may show a complete white-out, demonstrating fluid-filled and atelectatic alveoli. The lung volume is also characteristically reduced.

Management

Therapy for infants with RDS begins with careful assessment and resuscitation and includes assurance of adequate oxygenation, prevention of atelectasis, and reduction of the risk of complications.[3,24] Successful surfactant replacement therapy for infants with RDS was first described in 1980.[12] This therapy, which is discussed in detail in Chapter 23, has been helpful in reducing morbidity and mortality in infants with RDS, although it does not appear to work equally for all patients.

Initially, the primary goal of treatment is to maintain adequate oxygenation and acid–base balance. The PaO_2 should be maintained in the 50- to 80-mm Hg range,[24] with $PaCO_2$ values less than 60 mm Hg and pH greater than 7.25. If pH is allowed to fall to 7.0 or less, the risk of intraventricular hemorrhage is greatly increased.

Adequate hydration and a neutral thermal environment are also of prime importance. Frequent monitoring of arterial blood gases is important to maintain optimum PaO_2 with the lowest possible FIO_2. Pulse oximeters and transcutaneous oxygen monitors are invaluable for monitoring these infants

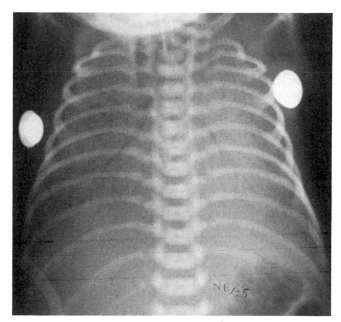

FIGURE 9-2 This premature infant presented with grunting, retractions, and cyanosis after delivery. The diffuse reticular-granular opacification, air bronchograms, and decreased lung volumes in the chest x-ray film indicate respiratory distress syndrome. (Whitsett JA, Pryhuber GS, Rice WR, Warner BB, Wert SE: Acute respiratory disorders. In Avery GB, Fletcher MA, MacDonald MG [eds]: Neonatology: Pathophysiology and Management of the Newborn, 4th ed, p. 436. Philadelphia, JB Lippincott, 1994.)

because changes in oxygenation can be detected and corrected immediately and the infant's response to routine care procedures can be observed.

Early oxygen therapy administered by oxyhood should be initiated to maintain oxygenation, but as the infant's disease progresses, oxygen therapy alone may not be sufficient. Continuous distending pressure, either by continuous positive airway pressure (CPAP) or continuous negative pressure (CNP) (see Chap. 15), in conjunction with oxygen therapy, can be used to increase FRC and prevent further atelectasis. Some studies have shown that early intervention with nasal CPAP or CNP results in better outcomes and a lower mortality rate.[13,15] General guidelines for institution of CPAP are a Pao$_2$ of 50 mm Hg or less and an FIo$_2$ of 0.60 or greater. This may vary from institution to institution, depending on experience. Nasal CPAP is usually begun at 4 to 6 cm H$_2$O and increased in increments of 2 cm H$_2$O until hypoxemia improves.[3]

Mechanical ventilation should be considered at the first signs of ventilatory failure in order to avoid severe hypoxemia and atelectasis.[24] In the infant who progresses to ventilatory failure (Paco$_2$ greater than 60 mm Hg with a pH of 7.20 or less) or if severe apneic episodes occur, mechanical ventilation is indicated. A time-cycled, pressure-limited ventilator is preferred because a wide range of I:E ratios, inspiratory times, inspiratory holds or plateaus, and lower peak airway pressures can be used to maintain adequate ventilation and oxygenation, thus avoiding some of the more serious consequences of positive pressure ventilation.

Initially, an I:E ratio of 1:1 may be beneficial to allow more inspiratory time for oxygenation. Inspiratory hold or plateau may prove beneficial in severe disease because it allows time for equilibration of pressures and improves distribution of ventilation. Inverse I:E ratios, with inspiratory time in excess of expiratory time, may be helpful in the critically ill infant for the same reasons. Inverse I:E ratios should be used judiciously and cautiously because the risk of cardiovascular effects and the incidence of air leaks are magnified by these procedures.

High-frequency ventilation (Chap. 24) may be indicated for infants who cannot be adequately oxygenated and ventilated at conventional airway pressures, respiratory rates, and FIo_2 levels. Keep in mind that the goal of ventilator therapy is to provide adequate levels of oxygenation and ventilation without inflicting unnecessary damage to the lungs.

In addition to respiratory and ventilatory support, careful attention to temperature regulation and nutrition and frequent monitoring of electrolytes, glucose, bilirubin, and urinary output are necessary. In the infant with patent ductus arteriosus (PDA), digitalis preparations or diuretics may be indicated.

Complications

Complications of the treatment of RDS must be anticipated so that each can be quickly recognized and addressed. Pulmonary air leaks (pneumothorax, pneumomediastinum, pulmonary interstitial emphysema) occur readily in premature infants and can cause rapid deterioration of the infant's clinical condition. These leaks usually occur as the infant's pulmonary status is improving, that is, as lung compliance increases. If airway pressures are not adjusted periodically, increased compliance results in increased tidal volume, which may rupture the fragile alveoli. Careful monitoring of the infant's ventilation status is extremely important so that modification of ventilatory parameters can be made to decrease the likelihood of air leaks. In addition to pulmonary air leaks, the administration of high oxygen tensions and mechanical ventilation can cause oxygen toxicity and bronchopulmonary dysplasia. Again, careful attention must be given to maintain oxygenation and ventilation using the lowest airway pressures, PEEP levels, and FIo_2 levels.

Other complications associated with treatment of the infant with RDS include intraventricular hemorrhage, infection, disseminated intravascular coagulation, and necrotizing enterocolitis.

▬ BRONCHOPULMONARY DYSPLASIA

Etiology

Bronchopulmonary dysplasia (BPD) is a chronic lung disease that develops in newborn infants treated with oxygen and positive pressure ventilation for a primary lung disorder. Approximately 7000 infants develop BPD each year, and 10% to 15% of these will die in their first year of life.[7] Specific factors that have been evaluated as causes of BPD include high oxygen concentrations, positive pressure ventilation, endotracheal intubation, duration of therapy, degree of prematurity, genetic predisposition, inflammation, and excessive fluid administration. The disease is not usually seen in infants treated with negative pressure ventilation despite the use of high oxygen concentrations. Infants treated with CPAP also show a reduced incidence of BPD.[4] Infants over 1500 g birth weight are less likely to develop BPD than are infants less than 1500 g.[19] Although the exact etiology of BPD continues to be elusive, conservative use of oxygen and positive pressure ventilation and early treatment with surfactant will probably decrease the incidence and severity of this disease.

Pathophysiology

Pathologically, BPD is characterized by several findings, which are summarized in Table 9-2. The result of these abnormalities is decreased pulmonary compliance and increased airway resistance secondary to fibrosis. In addition, ventilation/perfusion mismatching occurs, resulting in increasing oxygen requirements to maintain adequate Pao_2, at a time when the infant with uncomplicated RDS should be improving clinically. Excessive mucous secretion and air trapping occur, contributing to the development of hypercarbia. Lobar atelectasis is common in these infants, secondary to mucous plugging.

Infants with BPD also demonstrate interstitial edema and excess lung fluid. Many have left-to-right shunting through a PDA which causes pulmonary congestion. The net result is hypoxemia, pulmonary hypertension, and ultimately cor pulmonale (right heart failure secondary to lung disease).

Clinical Signs and Diagnosis

In the original description of BPD by Northway, Rosen, and Porter in 1967, the definition included radiologic, pathologic, and clinical criteria.[16] The radiologic findings were divided into four stages, which have since been utilized by practitioners worldwide. In the initial definition, much more emphasis was placed on the progression of radiologic changes than on clinical or pathologic findings. Since that time, various scoring systems have been proposed which incorporate clinical data as well as radiologic findings.[22] Table 9-3 presents a clinical scoring system which evaluates respiratory rate, dyspnea, FIo_2, $Paco_2$, and growth rate. The highest score possible is 15, with a score of 15 automatically assigned if the infant is

---

TABLE 9-2 Pathological Findings in Bronchopulmonary Dysplasia

Formation of hyaline membrane

Regeneration and repair of alveolar epithelium

Necrosis of alveolar epithelium

Bronchiolar smooth muscle metaplasia

Interstitial fibrosis

Formation of emphysematous bullae

Pulmonary hypertension

receiving mechanical ventilation. The scoring system in Table 9-4 evaluates radiographic findings. The maximum score in this system is 10 and correlates with severe cases of BPD.

Clinically, it is difficult to determine when an infant actually develops BPD because the infant is usually receiving mechanical ventilation. The normal recovery phase of RDS occurs around the 4th or 5th day after onset. If the infant demonstrates a continuing need for elevated inspired oxygen tensions and for ventilatory support at this time, the onset of BPD is likely. Chest x-ray findings at this time, however, may be difficult to differentiate from those of pneumonia, pulmonary edema, or alveolar consolidation, all of which may complicate the course of recovery from RDS. The infant with BPD requires continued high oxygen concentrations to maintain adequate Pao_2 and often exhibits persistent retractions and tachypnea. Increased $Paco_2$ requiring increased ventilatory assistance indicates the presence of air trapping and decreased compliance.

The infant usually can maintain a near-normal blood pH by compensating metabolically for respiratory acidosis. Mucous production is usually increased, and breath sounds may reveal diffuse rales and rhonchi indicative of edema and retained secretions in narrowed airways. With severe air trapping, the anteroposterior (A-P) diameter of the chest may be increased, causing a barrel-chest appearance. Pulmonary function testing may reveal decreased lung compliance and increased airway resistance. FRC may be initially reduced because of atelectasis, but it will be elevated in later stages as the result of air trapping and hyperinflation.[7] Signs of pulmonary congestion and right-sided heart failure, including peripheral edema, hepatomegaly, and jugular vein distention, may be present. Serial EKGs and echocardiography may demonstrate right ventricular hypertrophy, consistent with cor pulmonale. In addition, evaluation of the growth rate may reveal inadequate postnatal growth.

Radiologically, the initial stage of BPD is identical to severe hyaline membrane disease. In intermediate stages, diffuse haziness and opacification are seen, which may be difficult to differentiate from other causes of alveolar consolidation such as pulmonary edema or pneumonia. Areas of

TABLE 9-3 Clinical Scoring System for Bronchopulmonary Dysplasia

	SCORE			
VARIABLE	0 (normal)	1 (mild)	2 (moderate)	3 (severe)
Respiratory rate (average number/min)	<40	40–60	61–80	>80
Dyspnea (retractions)	0	Mild	Moderate	Severe
Fio_2 (Pao_2 50–70 mm Hg)	0.21	0.22–0.30	0.31–0.50	>0.50
$Paco_2$ (mm Hg)	<45	46–55	56–70	>70
Growth rate (g/d)	>25	15–24	5–15	<5

Highest score is 15. A score of 15 is assigned if the patient is receiving mechanical ventilation. (From Toce SS, Farrell PM, Leavitt PA, Samuels DP, Edwards DK: Clinical and radiographic scoring systems for assessing bronchopulmonary dysplasia. Am J Dis Child 138:581, 1984.)

TABLE 9-4 Radiographic Scoring System for Bronchopulmonary Dysplasia

	SCORE		
VARIABLE	*0*	*1*	*2*
Cardiovascular abnormalities	None	Cardiomegaly	Gross cardio-megaly or RVH or enlarged MPA
Hyperexpansion (anterior plus posterior rib count)	<14.5	14.5–16	>16 or flattened diaphragms
Emphysema	No focal areas	Scattered, small, abnormal lucencies	>1 large blebs or bullae
Fibrosis or interstitial abnormalities	None	Interstitial prominence; few abnormal, streaky densities	Dense fibrotic bands, many abnormal strands
Subjective	Mild	Moderate	Severe

RVH, right ventricular hypertrophy; MPA, main pulmonary artery. (From Toce SS, Farrell PM, Leavitt PA, Samuels DP, Edwards DK: Clinical and radiographic scoring systems for assessing bronchopulmonary dysplasia. Am J Dis Child 138:581, 1984.)

radiolucency, indicating bullae, alternate with areas of atelectasis and give a spongelike appearance to the x-ray film. In late stages, increasing size and number of emphysematous bullae and interstitial fibrosis result in a honeycomb appearance of the x-ray film. Chest x-ray films of an infant with progressively severe BPD are shown in Figure 9-3.

Management

Treatment for BPD is primarily supportive and directed toward relieving symptoms of respiratory distress and heart failure. Adequate blood gas values (Pao_2 55–70 mm Hg, $Paco_2$ 45–60 mm Hg, pH 7.25–7.40) should be maintained with the lowest possible FIo_2 and airway pressures.[1] The use of pulse oximetry and transcutaneous CO_2 measurements can be valuable in ventilator management. End-tidal CO_2 measurements may not correlate well with arterial values in infants with severe disease because of the accompanying ventilation/perfusion mismatching.[7] Weaning from mechanical ventilation is difficult and must be accomplished slowly, preferably by gradual reductions in ventilator rate to allow the infant to incrementally assume more of the work of breathing. Infants may be extubated when they have been weaned to ventilator rates of 5 to 15 breaths per minute.[7] CPAP by endotracheal tube should be avoided because of the significant airway resistance which may create increased work of breathing, fatigue, apnea, and CO_2 retention.[14]

Oxygen can be administered to spontaneously breathing infants using nasal cannula, oxyhoods, tents, or CPAP apparatus. Pulse oximetry remains invaluable in the titration of FIo_2. Arterial saturations between 90% and 95% should avoid Pao_2 values below 45 and above 100 mm Hg.[7] Increased oxygen concentrations may be required during respiratory care procedures,

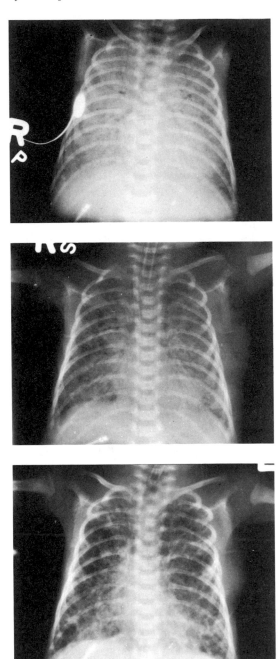

FIGURE 9-3   Stages II, III, and IV of bronchopulmonary dysplasia. Note the diffuse haziness throughout the lung fields (*top*). Cystic changes result in the spongelike appearance of Stage II (*center*). Increasing cystic formation in stage IV results in a honeycomb appearance and hyperinflation (*bottom*). (Hodgman JE: Chronic lung disorders. In Avery GB [ed]: Neonatology: Pathophysiology and Management of the Newborn, 2nd ed, p. 401. Philadelphia, JB Lippincott, 1981.)

feeding, weighing, and bathing. Some infants may require increased oxygen concentrations for a prolonged time after extubation, and an increasing number of these infants are sent home on oxygen therapy.

Adequate humidification of inspired gas is of utmost importance because of the high incidence of mucous plugging of airways and endotracheal tubes. Chest percussion and drainage and frequent suctioning are also extremely helpful.

Aerosol administration of albuterol is popular for infants with BPD. This bronchodilator may be effective in reducing airway resistance and increasing lung compliance. Cromolyn sodium has no direct bronchodilating effect but may be used to prevent bronchospasm.[7] Measurements of pulmonary mechanics in infants with BPD have shown that methylxanthines (caffeine and theophylline) can also reduce airway resistance and increase lung compliance.[6,17] Although corticosteroids have been shown to improve pulmonary mechanics, the use of systemic steroids should be reserved for ventilator-dependent infants with moderate to severe BPD because of the risks associated with prolonged administration. The use of inhaled steroids, such as beclomethasone, may be more effective and have fewer side effects when used in the treatment of infants with BPD.[7] Careful attention to fluid balance, along with digitalis preparations and diuretics, may be needed for those infants with excessive interstitial fluid, pulmonary congestion, and cor pulmonale. If PDA is a complicating factor, surgical ligation may be helpful in weaning the infant from ventilatory support. Chest x-ray improvement should not be expected because fibrotic changes do not improve rapidly. Nutritional requirements should be monitored carefully, since infants with respiratory distress may require additional energy sources to sustain weight gain and growth.

Reductions in the mortality and morbidity associated with BPD will most likely be realized by efforts to reduce its occurrence in the first place. Good prenatal care, attention to maternal health and nutrition, and prevention of premature labor can go a long way in reducing the incidence of prematurity, low birth weight, and RDS. Surfactant replacement therapy may reduce the level and duration of mechanical ventilation required and high-frequency ventilation may protect the immature lungs from barotrauma. Prophylactic supplementation of human antioxidant enzymes, such as superoxide dismutase, appears to have promise in preventing the development of BPD.[7] Respiratory care practitioners can be instrumental in the prevention and treatment of BPD by judicious use of oxygen and positive pressure ventilation and by watching the infant carefully for the signs and symptoms of complications.

Complications

The complications of BPD result from the therapy provided to the infant, primarily the risks associated with positive pressure ventilation and oxygen administration. Among the common complications are pulmonary air leaks; oxygen toxicity; intraventricular hemorrhage; and the consequences of prolonged tracheal intubation, including tracheal stenosis, tracheomalacia, and accidental extubation. Many infants with BPD have had successful weaning attempts jeopardized by airway emergencies. Infants with BPD are susceptible to infection and may become acutely ill when any bacterial or viral illness occurs. Cor pulmonale occurs as the result of hypoxemia and subsequent increases in pulmonary vascular resistance.

BPD has an overall mortality rate of approximately 30%, and most deaths occur prior to discharge from the hospital.[10] Children who are sent home frequently require oxygen therapy, diuretic therapy, bronchodilator therapy, and special formulas. Readmission to the hospital is common for these children, particularly for viral respiratory tract infections. Some studies have also reported an increased incidence of respiratory symptoms, including cough and wheezing.[10] Survival beyond 2 years, although associated with abnormalities in pulmonary function, generally allows children to function at normal capacity.[7]

▬MECONIUM ASPIRATION SYNDROME

Etiology
Meconium aspiration syndrome (MAS) is a disease seen primarily in full-term or post-term infants who have experienced some degree of asphyxia either prenatally or during the labor and delivery process. **Meconium**, a viscous green liquid, is the material contained in the fetal bowel and is composed of undigested amniotic fluid, squamous epithelial cells, and vernix. When the full-term or post-term fetus experiences in utero hypoxia, there is a redistribution of blood flow to vital organs (*i.e.*, the brain, heart, and placenta). Blood flow to the lungs, spleen, kidneys, and intestine is decreased,[4] promoting better oxygenation of the vital organs. The intestinal response to hypoxia is vasoconstriction, resulting in increased peristalsis, anal sphincter relaxation, and passage of meconium into the amniotic fluid.

The normal fetus periodically exhibits rapid, shallow respirations, moving amniotic fluid in and out of the oropharynx, with the glottis remaining closed. The asphyxiated infant, however, demonstrates deep, gasping respiratory movements, and aspiration of meconium and amniotic fluid past the glottis may occur. The post-term infant is at particular risk for MAS because of smaller amounts of amniotic fluid with which to dilute the meconium (oligohydramnios) and because of the post-term decline in placental function and consequent increase in asphyxial episodes.

The presence of meconium-stained amniotic fluid is fairly common, found in about 12% of all births, but in approximately 30% of births occurring after 42 weeks of gestation.[24] Less than half of these infants present with meconium below the vocal cords, probably because only small amounts of fluid move into the upper airways in utero. Significant amounts of meconium, however, may be inhaled as the infant takes the first few breaths at birth, carrying the meconium into the lower airways.

In addition to infants of advanced gestational age, those who are small for gestational age and those who present in the breech position are at higher risk for MAS. Infants born to toxemic, hypertensive, or obese mothers should be monitored for meconium.

Pathophysiology
There are two significant sequelae to aspiration of meconium. First is the physical presence of meconium itself, a thick, tenacious substance that obstructs airways, causing a check-valve effect in which air passes the

obstruction on inspiration but cannot exit on expiration as the airways narrow, resulting in air trapping and alveolar hyperinflation. In addition, pneumothorax or other air leaks commonly result from this type of obstruction. Ventilation/perfusion mismatching also occurs, leading to hypoxemia, alveolar hypoventilation, and hypercarbia in severely affected infants. With complete obstruction of an airway, absorption atelectasis occurs and an intrapulmonary shunt develops, compounding the hypoxemia.

The second possible result of MAS is a chemical pneumonitis, which is an acute inflammatory reaction of the bronchial and alveolar epithelium to the acidic meconium, resulting in mucosal and alveolar edema. A decrease in compliance occurs, resulting in alveolar underexpansion and impaired gas exchange. A decrease in diffusion may also occur, further interfering with oxygenation.

Because these infants are usually full-term or post-term and many have suffered intrauterine asphyxia, the pulmonary vascular bed may be hyperreactive and may exhibit vasospasm or hypoxic vasoconstriction, resulting in right-to-left shunting through a PDA or foramen ovale. This occurrence of persistent fetal circulation is a relatively common complication of MAS.

The pathophysiology of meconium aspiration syndrome is illustrated in Figure 9-4.

Clinical Signs and Diagnosis

The infant with MAS generally presents with signs of postmaturity, such as long fingernails and peeling skin. The cord and nails are stained with meconium and appear yellow. Symptoms begin at birth or shortly thereafter and include tachypnea, retractions, nasal flaring, grunting, and cyanosis. The chest may be barrel shaped, reflecting severe air trapping and alveolar hyperinflation. Apgar scores at birth are usually low, reflecting the high incidence of associated asphyxia.

The infant with mild disease will be tachypneic and able to maintain a low $PaCO_2$ in response to hypoxemia and in compensation for the metabolic acidosis characteristic of asphyxia. A moderately affected infant may gradually develop more severe distress over a 24-hour period, with the appearance of increasing hypoxemia and hypercarbia. Severely affected infants present immediately at birth with severe metabolic acidosis, hypercarbia, and hypoxemia. Coarse bronchial breath sounds with rales and rhonchi and prolonged exhalation are heard on auscultation. Cyanosis may improve with oxygen administration, depending on the presence and degree of right-to-left shunting. The definitive diagnosis of meconium aspiration is made by direct visualization of the presence of meconium below the vocal cords.

The typical chest x-ray film in severe MAS shows areas of decreased aeration, either focal or generalized. These areas alternate with areas of hyperlucency, resulting in a pattern of irregular densities throughout the lung fields (Fig. 9-5). Consolidation is common, with no increased incidence in any particular lobe. Pleural fluid accumulation and air leaks are commonly seen, especially pneumomediastinum and pneumothorax. The diaphragms may be depressed if hyperinflation is significant, although this is uncommon. The x-ray picture is clearly different from that of RDS. It is difficult, however, to differentiate from that of pneumonia, which may be important in the infant who develops a superimposed bacterial infection or the infant with intrapartum pneumonia.

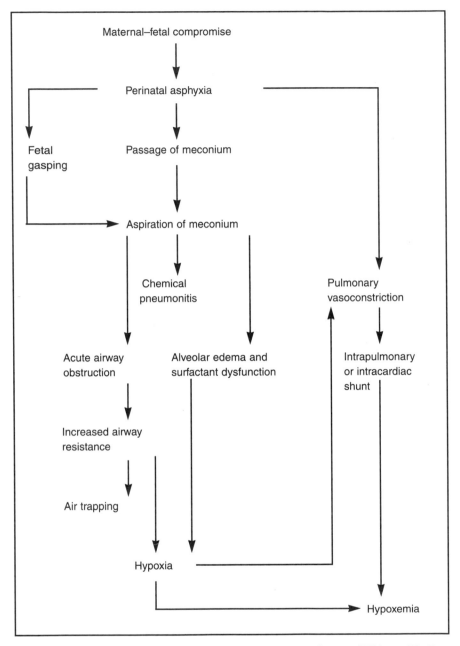

FIGURE 9-4 Pathogenesis of meconium aspiration syndrome. (Whitsett JA, Pryhuber GS, Rice WR, Warner BB, Wert SE: Acute respiratory disorders. In Avery GB, Fletcher MA, MacDonald MG [eds]: Neonatology: Pathophysiology and Management of the Newborn, 4th ed, p. 439. Philadelphia, JB Lippincott, 1994.)

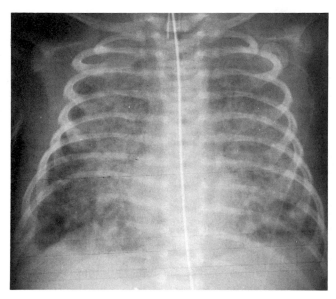

FIGURE 9-5 This full-term infant was born with fetal bradycardia and thick meconium in the amniotic fluid. Cyanosis and respiratory distress were evident within minutes of delivery. The chest x-ray film demonstrates course, irregular infiltrates, hyperinflation (left and right diaphragms at ribs 10–11), and right pleural effusion indicative of meconium aspiration syndrome. Endotracheal and nasogastic tubes are in position. (Whitsett JA, Pryhuber GS, Rice WR, Warner BB, Wert SE: Acute respiratory disorders. In Avery GB, Fletcher MA, MacDonald MG [eds]: Neonatology: Pathophysiology and Management of the Newborn, 4th ed, p. 439. Philadelphia, JB Lippincott, 1994.)

Management

Recognition of the infant at risk for meconium aspiration is of primary importance in the clinical management of the syndrome. When amniotic fluid is found to be meconium-stained or particulate, fetal heart rate monitoring for signs of distress is critical. In addition, monitoring of the high-risk infant may identify distress before membrane rupture. Prevention of meconium aspiration can be accomplished by immediate suctioning before the infant takes the first breath.

As the head is delivered, the nasopharynx and oropharynx should be suctioned thoroughly. As soon as the infant is delivered, direct visualization and intubation should be performed. Suctioning, usually with the operator's mouth supplying negative pressure through a filter mask directly to the endotracheal tube, is then performed until all meconium has been cleared. This should be done for all infants born through particulate meconium, even if meconium is not visualized in the oropharynx. The incidence of symptoms and complicating pneumothoraces is reduced when all infants with meconium staining are suctioned, compared with those who are suctioned only when meconium is seen in the oropharynx.[11] Positive pressure ventilation should not be applied until the suctioning procedure has been completed, since ventilation will move the meconium down into the lower airways.

Once the infant is initially stabilized and transported to the intensive care area, vigorous postural drainage and percussion, with frequent suctioning of the airway, should be performed. Oxygen administration may be needed and, in severe meconium aspiration, mechanical ventilation is indicated. Ventilation should be avoided if possible because of the high incidence of pneumothorax associated with MAS. If ventilation is required, an I:E ratio that allows adequate time for exhalation from partially obstructed areas of the lung should be used. Sedation and paralysis of the infant may be helpful in achieving effective ventilation.

Although meconium is sterile in utero, experimental studies have shown that meconium enhances bacterial growth, though this has not been demonstrated clinically.[4] The infant should have blood cultures drawn and be carefully monitored for possible superimposed infection. Antibiotic therapy may be indicated, and steroids may also be used against the inflammatory response in chemical pneumonitis.

High-frequency ventilation and extracorporeal membrane oxygenation have been used to treat infants who become critically ill following aspiration of meconium. These therapies are discussed in detail in Chapters 24 and 25, respectively.

Complications

The complications of meconium aspiration syndrome are primarily dependent upon the severity of the disease and the level of treatment necessary for survival. Barotrauma, especially pneumothorax and pneumomediastinum, occurs frequently in infants with check-valve airway obstructions. When increased intrathoracic pressures accompany air-trapping, the infant is also at risk of increased intracranial pressure (ICP) from reduced venous return to the heart. This increase in ICP may predispose the infant to intraventricular hemorrhage. Hyperreactivity of the pulmonary vascular bed can lead to elevations in pulmonary vascular resistance in response to hypoxia and acidosis. This can result in persistent pulmonary hypertension or persistent fetal circulation (see Chap. 11), probably the most serious complication of MAS.

▬ BAROTRAUMA AND VOLUTRAUMA: PULMONARY AIR LEAKS

Pulmonary air leak may occur as a complication of any of the life-threatening disorders of the newborn or as a result of the treatment of these disorders. Most frequently, air leaks result from the application of positive pressure mechanical ventilation. Initially, pulmonary air leaks were placed into the general category of pulmonary barotrauma, since it was presumed that these conditions were the result of excessive pressures applied to the lung. More recently, it is felt that air leaks occur as the result of excessive volume (overdistention) in portions of the lung, hence the term volutrauma has been applied.[8] Many types of air leaks can develop in the neonate, including **pulmonary interstitial emphysema** (PIE), pneumomediastinum, and pneumothorax. Less common air leaks include pneumopericardium, pneumoperitoneum, and subcutaneous emphysema. The most common risk factors for air leak include lung immaturity, RDS, aspiration syndromes, inadvertent intubation of one bronchus, mechanical ventilation, and PEEP or CPAP. Air leaks may also occur spontaneously in the newborn.

Etiology

Infants who experience air leaks pathologically present with a pattern of atelectatic alveoli adjacent to normal alveoli. When mechanical ventilation is applied, the normal alveoli may become distended and rupture. If the disease exhibits a balanced or diffuse pattern of atelectasis, air leak is less common.

PIE occurs when air is present outside the normal airways. Air dissects along peribronchial or perivascular sheaths, interlobular septa, or the visceral pleura. Preterm infants with RDS have a higher incidence of PIE than do full-term infants, which may be related to the increased distance between the alveoli and capillaries in these infants. PIE may present alone or may develop into pneumomediastinum or pneumothorax. The dissection of air into the mediastinum or pleural space actually improves the prognosis of PIE because of the relief of pressure from the interstitium and decompression of the pulmonary vessels.

Pneumomediastinum may also occur for no known reason or as a result of PIE. Air in the mediastinum is most commonly seen anterior to the heart and dissects along the diaphragm.

Pneumothorax is an accumulation of air in the pleural space, between the visceral and parietal layers of the pleura. It is the most common of all air leaks and occurs in 1% to 2% of all newborns.[23] It most likely occurs from distention and rupture of normal alveoli. When pneumothorax occurs in association with positive pressure ventilation, the pleural air may be under considerable pressure, resulting in the formation of a tension pneumothorax.

Infants with RDS usually present with pneumothorax when the initial disease is resolving and compliance is improving. The diffuse atelectasis of the initial disease process is changing to a pattern of normal alveoli next to atelectatic alveoli, and thus the incidence of pneumothorax increases at this time. Pneumothorax also occurs when airway obstruction causes peripheral distention, as in MAS.

Spontaneous pneumothorax occurs primarily in full-term infants, probably secondary to the very high negative intrathoracic pressure created with the first breath.

Pathophysiology

Pulmonary interstitial emphysema, also called **air block**, causes compression of pulmonary vessels, resulting in decreased pulmonary blood flow and increased pulmonary vascular resistance, and compression of lymphatic vessels, resulting in increased lung water. Air in the interstitium also compresses alveoli, and atelectasis follows. In addition, airways may be compressed, resulting in air trapping and distention of alveoli. If extensive enough, cor pulmonale may develop secondary to increased pulmonary vascular resistance, and right-to-left shunting (both intrapulmonary and intracardiac) will occur. Thromboembolism may occur because of sluggish or obstructed capillary flow.

In pneumomediastinum, air collection above the diaphragm, when large enough, may also compress alveoli and prevent inflation. Usually, however, mediastinal air ruptures into the pleural space and results in pneumothorax.

The effects of a pneumothorax depend primarily on its size and on the pressure of the air in the pleural space. Pneumothorax causes an increased pleural pressure, compression of the great veins, increased pulmonary vascular resistance, and decreased lung volume. A decrease in venous return occurs, causing a decrease in cardiac output. A sizable tension pneumothorax is a life-threatening condition and warrants immediate removal of the extraneous air.

Clinical Signs and Diagnosis

Infants with air leaks will generally present with tachypnea, cyanosis, and retractions caused by alveolar compression and diminished pulmonary blood flow. The onset of symptoms may be rapid or gradual, depending upon the severity of the air leak. Hypoxia results from hypoventilation and ventilation/perfusion (V/Q) mismatch. If pulmonary vascular resistance increases significantly, right-to-left shunting may occur, furthering the development of hypoxemia and resulting in decreased effectiveness of oxygen therapy. Infants with PIE may have significant air trapping, resulting in a barrel-chest appearance, or increased A-P diameter of the chest.

Pneumothorax is often associated with hypotension and severe cyanosis, resulting from the drop in cardiac output, and with a shift of the mediastinum away from the involved side, manifested by a change in the location of the apical cardiac impulse. Decreased breath sounds and reduced chest movement may be present on the involved side. Onset of symptoms may be progressive or immediate. Rapid onset usually occurs in tension pneumothorax. Severe pneumothorax results in bradypnea, bradycardia, and apnea. Arterial blood gas studies reveal acidosis, hypercarbia, and hypoxemia. Use of a high-intensity light placed against the chest wall (transillumination) may reveal increased lucency of the chest with increased pleural air. This is a valuable tool for rapid, bedside detection and evaluation of pneumothorax. Definitive diagnosis requires x-ray evidence of air leak, and stat chest films should be ordered whenever pulmonary air leak is suspected.

PIE initially presents on chest x-ray films as nodular, irregular "bubbles" originating in the hilar areas and radiating outward (Fig. 9-6). Expiratory films may be helpful in demonstrating PIE; on inspiration the bubbles may elongate and may not show very clearly on x-ray film. With time, these bubbles may converge to form large, cystic pneumatoceles. The x-ray picture will begin to clear around the 5th day in mild PIE.

Chest x-ray films for pneumothorax should be taken on expiration. A dense, dark area separating the lung from the chest wall, with absent lung markings, represents air in the pleural space (Fig. 9-7). Displacement of the mediastinal structures, including the heart, and of the trachea may occur, unless bilateral pneumothoraces are present. With the infant in the supine position, the air may layer out along the anterior chest wall, resulting in no obvious pleural air. The lung field on the involved side will, in this case, appear hyperlucent, with a sharp mediastinal border. Lateral or crosstable views may be helpful in detecting an anterior pneumothorax.

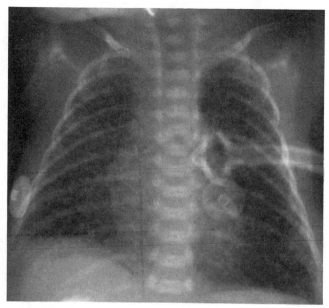

FIGURE 9-6   Chest x-ray film of pulmonary interstitial emphysema. A premature infant with severe respiratory distress syndrome requiring mechanical ventilation developed worsening respiratory acidosis and hypoxia refractory to increased ventilatory support. An anteroposterior chest x-ray film demonstrates a salt-and-pepper pattern resulting from radiolucent interstitial air surrounding compressed lung tissue. A left chest tube was placed to treat pneumothorax, a common complication of pulmonary interstitial emphysema. (Whitsett JA, Pryhuber GS, Rice WR, Warner BB, Wert SE: Acute respiratory disorders. In Avery GB, Fletcher MA, MacDonald MG [eds]: Neonatology: Pathophysiology and Management of the Newborn, 4th ed, p. 451. Philadelphia, JB Lippincott, 1994.)

Management

The best treatment for pulmonary air leaks is prevention. Ventilation should be monitored closely to avoid alveolar distention. Pressures under 30 cm H_2O are recommended to avoid PIE. In the infant who develops PIE and requires continuing ventilation, pressures should be lowered as much as possible. Administration of 100% oxygen for 10- to 15-minute intervals may facilitate reabsorption of extra-alveolar air, but the practitioner must keep in mind the hazards of high oxygen concentrations to the premature infant. Selective intubation of the uninvolved side in unilateral disease may also allow time for air to reabsorb. This technique should be reserved for the severely affected infant. Lobectomy has been performed in life-threatening PIE, although this is a drastic procedure for a potentially reversible disease. High-frequency ventilation has also been used with success.

Pneumothorax is best treated with chest tube placement and underwater seal drainage. Needle aspiration through the second or third intercostal space can be performed in an emergency to relieve pleural pressure until surgical placement of a chest tube can be accomplished. Oxygen therapy at 100% for 6 to 12 hours has been used to decrease small accu-

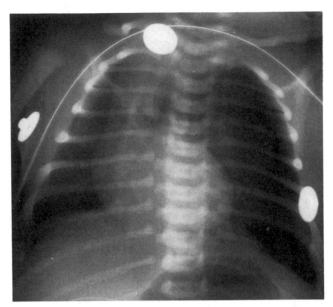

FIGURE 9-7   A full-term infant born by a difficult breech delivery presented shortly after birth with crepitus in the neck area, tachypnea, grunting, and retractions. An anteroposterior chest x-ray film demonstrates bilateral pneumothorax under tension on the left. The heart and mediastinum are compressed and shifted to the right. The left pleural air herniates across the midline. The left diaphragm is depressed and inverted. Subcutaneous emphysema is seen in the soft tissues of the neck. (Whitsett JA, Pryhuber GS, Rice WR, Warner BB, Wert SE: Acute respiratory disorders. In Avery GB, Fletcher MA, MacDonald MG [eds]: Neonatology: Pathophysiology and Management of the Newborn, 4th ed, p. 451. Philadelphia, JB Lippincott, 1994.)

mulations of air in infants who have no underlying lung disease, who are in no distress, and who have no continuous air leak. The risk of oxygen toxicity must be weighed against the benefit of this therapy; the use of 100% oxygen is controversial.[3,21]

Complications

The complications associated with pulmonary barotrauma and volutrauma are the result of either the initial development of extra-alveolar air or the subsequent treatment of the air leak. In the period following overdistention and rupture of the alveoli, decreased compliance, compression atelectasis, hypoxemia, increased pulmonary vascular resistance, and reduction in venous return may all occur. In tension pneumothorax and pneumopericardium, the excessive intrathoracic pressures can compress the vena cavae, reduce venous return, and inhibit cardiac contraction to the point where the infant becomes severely hypotensive. Intraventricular hemorrhage may occur as the result of sudden decreases in venous return to the heart and changes in cerebral blood flow.

The complications associated with the therapy for air leaks include hazards of high-concentration oxygen toxicity, namely retinopathy of prematurity and BPD. Chest tube insertion introduces the risk of hemorrhage, infection, lung puncture, and damage to the phrenic nerve.

▬PNEUMONIA

Pneumonias can be divided into two categories, depending on the route of acquisition and the age at onset of symptoms. Perinatal infections arise from transplacental infection and premature rupture of membranes. Prolonged labor and delivery and aspiration are also risk factors. Postnatal infection is usually nosocomial in nature, occurring beyond the first week of life in high-risk, low-birth-weight infants.

Etiology

The most common bacterial pathogens seen in perinatal infection are group B, β-hemolytic streptococcus (normally found in the cervical and vaginal tissue), *Escherichia coli*, *Listeria monocytogenes*, *Klebsiella pneumoniae*, and *Treponema pallidum* (causing congenital syphilis). Viral pathogens include herpes virus (HSV), cytomegalovirus (CMV), rubella, and varicella-zoster.

In postnatal infections, the most common pathogens are coagulase-positive staphylococcus, *Klebsiella pneumoniae*, and respiratory syncytial virus (RSV).

Pathophysiology

The three most common pathologic patterns associated with neonatal pneumonia are hyaline membrane formation, suppurative inflammation, and interstitial pneumonitis.[24] Group B, β-hemolytic streptococcal infection results in the development of bronchiolar and alveolar hyaline membranes, with a clinical picture virtually indistinguishable from that of RDS. The organism is spread from maternal cervical and vaginal membranes to the infant. If rupture of the membranes occurs more than 12 hours before delivery, the risk of infection is increased. Symptoms of infection may present within 1 to 2 hours or may be delayed for days, particularly if infection is secondary to aspiration of contaminated amniotic fluid. Generalized sepsis may occur in the same time period, although pneumonia is the primary finding. The preterm infant is likely to have widespread alveolar involvement, whereas full-term infants may exhibit either a localized or diffuse pattern. Infants with gram-negative infection are more likely to present with sepsis.

The viral pathogens (CMV and HSV) involve multiple body systems, sometimes including the pulmonary system. CMV does not usually present for several weeks, although acquired perinatally. The clinical picture is similar to that of BPD. HSV infection is characterized by interstitial pneumonia.

In postnatal pneumonias, staphylococcal infection is usually caused by skin or cord stump infection. Pneumonia occurs secondary to generalized sepsis and is commonly localized to one or more lobes. Accumulation of pleural fluid is common, as is the development of pneumatoceles (thin-walled, air-filled cavities). The bacteria of most concern in postnatal infection are the gram-negative enteric bacilli, especially *Klebsiella*, which causes necrotizing pneumonia, with abscess and pneumatocele formation. RSV infection usually is transmitted by infected staff members, resulting in a diffuse pneumonitis with infiltrates.

Clinical Signs and Diagnosis

In many infants, the clinical signs of pneumonia are difficult to distinguish from those of hyaline membrane disease or transient tachypnea of the newborn. Early manifestations of pneumonia and sepsis are generalized listlessness, irritability, color changes, and poor feeding. As the infection progresses, the infant becomes tachypneic, cyanotic, and hypothermic. Grunting respirations may occur, progressing to sepsis, shock, metabolic acidosis, and severe hypoxemia. Apneic episodes may also occur.

White blood cell counts in the newborn are not reliable for diagnosing infection. Leukopenia (WBC less than $5000/cm^3$) usually indicates sepsis and severe infection. A left shift (greater than 15% nonsegmented neutrophils) is also a useful diagnostic sign. Arterial blood gases will initially show only hypoxemia, progressing to metabolic acidosis as sepsis develops. Blood cultures are useful in identifying the etiologic pathogen.

Chest x-ray films may be helpful in the differential diagnosis of some of these pathogens from other respiratory diseases in the newborn, but are not particularly helpful in others. The clinical and x-ray presentation of group B, β-hemolytic streptococcus infection is nearly identical to that of RDS. Staphylococcal pneumonias generally demonstrate lobar consolidation and pneumatoceles. *Klebsiella* infection is associated with lobar infiltrates and bulging fissures. General patterns of lung infection include atelectasis, which may result in a "smudged" or "dirty lung" appearance on x-ray films; pleural effusions; and relative overexpansion of noninvolved areas.

Management

After cultures of blood and other sources (such as sputum and gastric aspirate) have been obtained, broad-spectrum antibiotic therapy, such as a combination of ampicillin and kanamycin, may be administered. More specific antibiotic therapy may be needed for nosocomial infection because these organisms are likely to be resistant to commonly used broad-spectrum drugs. Results of blood and other cultures will be helpful in adjusting antibiotic therapy. Oxygenation, adequate humidification, and good bronchial hygiene are important to maintain adequate pulmonary status. Mechanical ventilation should be initiated if indicated on the basis of clinical assessment and arterial blood gas monitoring.

Complications

The prognosis of neonatal pneumonia in full-term infants is good, while premature and low-birth-weight infants have a higher mortality rate.[10] Common complications include hypoxemia, ventilatory failure, necrotizing enterocolitis, and sepsis. Infants who require mechanical ventilation face the additional hazards of retinopathy of prematurity, air leaks, intraventricular hemorrhage, and BPD.

▰APNEA OF PREMATURITY

Apnea is defined as the absence of breathing for more than 20 seconds or cessation of breathing for a shorter duration which is accompanied by bradycardia or cyanosis. This should not be confused with periodic breathing, which is an irregular breathing pattern associated with shorter apneic periods of 5 to 10 seconds. Periodic breathing is usually benign. Heart rate usually decreases with apnea, and color changes may be noted, along with hypoxemia. None of these clinical signs are present in periodic breathing.

Etiology

The exact cause of apnea is not known, although many theories have been proposed. Virtually all very low-birth-weight infants have periodic breathing, and many will also have apneic episodes. The number and severity of apneic periods decreases with increasing gestational age and should resolve between 34 and 36 postconceptional weeks.[18] Periods of apnea are rare in full-term infants (38–42 weeks' gestation) and are usually associated with other causes, such as birth asphyxia, intracranial disease, or respiratory depression caused by medications.[9]

It has been shown that preterm infants have a higher resting $PaCO_2$ and a decreased ventilatory response to CO_2, perhaps due to an immature central nervous system. Hypoxia associated with apnea also decreases the ventilatory response to CO_2. The incidence of apnea during active (REM) sleep is much higher than during quiet (non-REM) sleep.[9] Since premature infants can spend up to 80% of their sleep time in REM sleep,[3] we would expect higher frequencies of apnea than in full-term infants who spend approximately 50% of their sleep time in REM sleep. Decreases in skeletal muscle tone also occur during active sleep, which further increases the compliance of the newborn chest. The increased compliance results in paradoxical breathing patterns in which a larger amount of diaphragmatic energy becomes wasted.[9] It is currently believed that respiratory muscles fatigue more easily in these infants, resulting in periodic breathing or apnea.

Infants respond to many illnesses with apnea. These illnesses include infections, seizures, hypoglycemia, hypocalcemia, hyponatremia, serious intracranial bleeding, and anemia.[18] In addition, apnea may occur in association with hyperthermia, PDA, and maternal narcotic use.

Pathophysiology

Apnea is commonly associated with bradycardia, cyanosis, and, if it progresses to periods of 45 seconds or longer, hypotonia and unresponsiveness. Frequent apneic episodes may lead to cerebral hypoxia and ischemia, resulting in hypoxic–ischemic brain injury.

Clinical Signs and Diagnosis

Apnea presents as absence of breathing in excess of 20 seconds, associated with cyanosis, bradycardia (heart rate less than 80/min), and hypoxemia. Snoring, choking, mouth breathing, decreased muscle tone, and changes in the respiratory pattern may also occur.[3] Other clinical manifestations are associated with the underlying disorders that may predispose the infant to apnea.

Management and Complications

All infants less than 34 weeks' gestational age should be monitored for apneic spells for at least the first week of life. Chest movement may persist during episodes of apnea caused by obstruction of the upper airway.

Impedance apnea monitors, which respond to chest movement, may not detect these types of apneic periods. Monitoring of heart rate should always accompany monitoring of respiration. When a monitor sounds, the practitioner must respond to the infant, and not to the monitor. Look at the infant carefully, noting respiratory efforts, cyanosis, and heart rate.

Most apneic spells in premature infants respond to tactile stimulation, such as gently shaking the hand or foot or rubbing the abdomen or back. If the infant does not respond to tactile stimulation, positive pressure ventilation should be initiated at FIo_2 of 0.40 or equal to the FIo_2 received by the infant prior to the episode.[20] Chest compressions should be performed if the heart rate falls below 80 beats per minute or if the infant is hypotensive. Once stabilized, the infant should be carefully evaluated in order to identify the underlying cause of the apnea. Evaluation includes physical examination, arterial blood gases, complete blood count, serum glucose, calcium, and electrolytes. If infection is suspected, appropriate cultures should be taken.

If an underlying disorder is identified, it is treated appropriately. If hypoxemia is documented by blood gas measurement, pulse oximetry, or transcutaneous monitoring, oxygen therapy should be initiated. Frequently, FIo_2 of 0.23 to 0.25 is effective in decreasing apneic episodes.[3] If no cause can be identified, theophylline, a methylxanthine that stimulates the central nervous system and increases ventilation, may be administered. Serum theophylline levels should be maintained at 7 to 12 mg/dL, although lower levels may also be effective.[20] CPAP (2–5 cm H_2O) has also been used to treat apneic episodes, and concurrent oxygen administration is recommended to relieve hypoxemia as both a cause and an effect of apnea. Additional measures include avoidance of elevated body temperature, use of some form of stimulation such as a rocking bed, and tactile or auditory stimulation when an apneic episode occurs.

Once therapy has been initiated, the infant should be carefully monitored for the occurrence of continued episodes. If apnea persists despite therapy, mechanical ventilation may be needed.

Most premature infants should outgrow apnea of prematurity by the time they reach 40 weeks postconceptional age. Apnea that persists beyond this period should be examined closely for the underlying cause. Polysomnography (recording of chest motion and heart rate over a period of time) can be helpful in determining the need for continued monitoring. Since there may be a higher incidence of sudden infant death syndrome (SIDS) in infants with apnea of prematurity, these infants may be sent home with an apnea monitor.[3]

■TRANSIENT TACHYPNEA OF THE NEWBORN

Transient tachypnea of the newborn (TTN) was first described in 1966 by Avery and colleagues[2] and is now also called **type II RDS** or "wet lung" syndrome. This condition presents initially with clinical symptoms similar to those of mild RDS in the first 24 to 48 hours after birth, and is a relatively mild, self-limited condition. As the name implies, the major manifestation of this disorder is tachypnea, with respiratory rates as high as 150 breaths per minute.

Etiology

Newborns affected with TTN are usually near-term or full-term infants of appropriate size for their gestational age. History may include maternal analgesia or anesthesia during labor or an episode of intrauterine asphyxia. Maternal bleeding, maternal diabetes, cesarean section, and prolapsed umbilical cord have all been related to an increased incidence of TTN.

It was initially proposed that the syndrome was the result of delayed absorption of the fetal lung liquid. Since that time, others have supported this hypothesis, although the exact cause of TTN remains unknown. An alternate theory is that TTN is caused by immaturity of the pulmonary surfactant system.[24]

Pathophysiology

The infant may be somewhat depressed at birth, resulting in an accumulation of mucus and secretions. The swallowing and cough mechanisms may also be diminished. Lack of adequate inspiratory effort or a cesarean delivery may lead to delayed circulatory changeover and shunt closure, as well as to decreased absorption of fetal pulmonary liquid. The increased amount of fluid remaining in the lung leads to reduced lung compliance, decreased tidal volume, and increased dead space. Pulmonary capillary congestion with interstitial or pulmonary edema may occur.

Clinical Signs and Diagnosis

The typical infant with TTN has good Apgar scores at birth. Several hours later however, nasal flaring, grunting, and retractions may be noted. Cyanosis may be present but responds well to simple oxygen therapy. Tachypnea occurs, with respiratory rates as high as 100 to 150 breaths per minute. Arterial blood gas studies reveal mild hypoxemia, with possible respiratory and metabolic acidosis. Breath sounds are usually clear unless significant pulmonary edema is present.

Chest x-ray findings initially appear normal. At about 12 hours of age, signs of pulmonary congestion appear, resulting in heavy central markings (Fig. 9-8). Distention may occur, manifested by peripheral hyperlucency, flattened diaphragms, and bulging of intercostal spaces. Patchy pulmonary infiltrates may be seen in some infants.

The diagnosis of TTN is made by exclusion of other causes of respiratory distress and with the aid of the chest x-ray. Within about 24 to 48 hours, signs of respiratory distress disappear. Absorption of lung fluid occurs because of lymphatic clearance. Oxygen requirements usually decrease to room air by 48 hours of age.

Management and Complications

Treatment of the infant with TTN is generally supportive and directed at relieving the signs of respiratory distress. Adequate oxygenation is usually achieved by administration of oxygen by hood. Hypoxemia generally responds well to FIo_2 of 0.40 or lower. CPAP may be indicated in infants who require higher FIo_2 levels or who have persistent chest retractions. Mechanical ventilation is rarely needed. The infant's position should be changed frequently and oral feedings withheld until the tachypnea

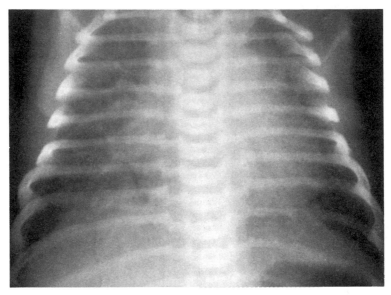

FIGURE 9-8   This full-term infant was born by cesarean section and developed tachypnea and grunting that resolved 48 hours after birth. Perihilar vascular densities, streaky opacities of interstitial edema, fluid in the interlobar fissures, small pleural effusions, and cardiomegaly are observed on the radiograph. These features are indicative of transient tachypnea of the newborn. (Whitsett JA, Pryhuber GS, Rice WR, Warner BB, Wert SE: Acute respiratory disorders. In Avery GB, Fletcher MA, MacDonald MG [eds]: Neonatology: Pathophysiology and Management of the Newborn, 4th ed, p. 449. Philadelphia, JB Lippincott, 1994.)

resolves. Since the symptoms of TTN can mimic those of neonatal pneumonia, broad-spectrum antibiotics may be started.

Complications occur rarely in infants with TTN and are primarily related to the risks of therapy, including the hazards of oxygen therapy. Newborns treated with CPAP are at minimal risk for pulmonary air leaks.

▬WILSON–MIKITY SYNDROME

Wilson–Mikity syndrome (also known as Mikity–Wilson syndrome or pulmonary dysmaturity) is a chronic lung disease seen exclusively in preterm infants. Clinically, it is difficult to differentiate from BPD, although the infant's history is usually quite different.

Etiology

There is no known etiology for Wilson–Mikity syndrome. Because it is a disease of premature infants, there is speculation that compensatory emphysematous changes occur as a result of lung immaturity. Maternal bleeding and asphyxia may be associated with its occurrence.

Pathophysiology

Pulmonary changes are similar to those of BPD, except that fibrosis is not present. Alternating areas of distention and atelectasis occur. On autopsy,

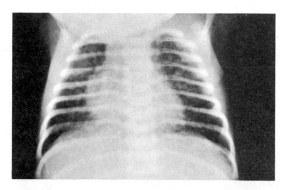

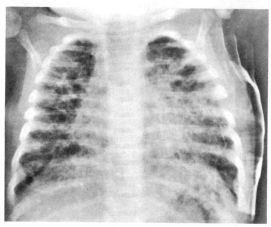

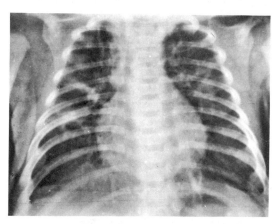

FIGURE 9-9 Radiologic appearance and progression of Wilson–Mikity syndrome. Early development of streaky densities, particularly in the upper lobes (*top*). Cystic densities throughout the lung fields, similar to bronchopulmonary dysplasia (*center*). Streaky infiltrates persist in upper lobes during recovery, with overdistention of lower lobes (*bottom*). (Hodgman JE: Chronic lung disorders. In Avery GB [ed]: Neonatology: Pathophysiology and Management of the Newborn, 2nd ed, p 407. Philadelphia, JB Lippincott, 1981.)

alveolar septa have been seen to be underdeveloped, but there is no evidence of epithelial damage or fibrosis. Alveolar distention and subsequent ventilation/perfusion mismatch is the reason for clinical symptoms.

Clinical Signs and Diagnosis

Onset of symptoms occurs during the first week of life. Tachypnea, cyanosis, and retractions are early symptoms and often progress to apnea. Ventilatory assistance may be required by the second week of life, as hypercarbia and ventilatory failure follow. Arterial blood gas studies initially show hypoxemia, progressing to respiratory acidosis.

Initially, chest x-ray findings are essentially normal. By the end of the first week, there may be bilateral streaky upper lobe infiltrates (Fig. 9-9). Small cystic areas are seen in all lobes. In later stages, the cystic areas at the bases enlarge and the lower lung fields become hyperlucent because of distention. Streaky infiltrates persist in upper lobes. It is difficult to differentiate Wilson–Mikity syndrome from middle- to late-stage BPD on the basis of x-ray examination, but infants with BPD have a very different history, including treatment with oxygen and positive pressure ventilation.

Management and Complications

Treatment of these infants is primarily supportive. Supplemental oxygen is administered to maintain PaO_2 and may be needed for long-term therapy, including home oxygen therapy. Ventilatory support may be needed for apnea or CO_2 retention. Careful attention should be given to maintenance of the lowest airway pressures and FIO_2 possible to maintain adequate ventilation and oxygenation. These factors may superimpose oxygen toxicity changes on an already chronic disease.

Two thirds of infants with Wilson–Mikity syndrome survive the acute phase and begin a gradual recovery. The disease is generally resolved by the time the infant reaches 2 years of age.[23]

■REFERENCES

1. Abman SH, Wolfe RR, Accurso FJ, Koops BL, Bowman M, Wiggins JW Jr: Pulmonary vascular response to oxygen in infants with bronchopulmonary dysplasia. Pediatrics 75:80, 1985.
2. Avery ME, Gatewood OB, Brumley G: Transient tachypnea of the newborn. Am J Dis Child 111:380, 1966.
3. Boyle KM, Baker VL, Cassaday CJ: Neonatal pulmonary disorders. In Barnhart SL, Czervinske MP (eds): Perinatal and Pediatric Respiratory Care. Philadelphia, WB Saunders, 1995.
4. Brady J: Management of meconium aspiration syndrome. In Thibeault D, Gregory G (eds): Neonatal Pulmonary Care. Menlo Park, CA, Addison-Wesley, 1979.
5. Burchfield D, Neu J: Neonatal parenchymal disease. In Koff PB, Eitzman D, Neu J (eds): Neonatal and Pediatric Respiratory Care, 2nd ed. St. Louis, Mosby-Year Book, 1993.
6. Davis JM, Bhutani VK, Stefano JL, Fox WW, Spitzer AR: Changes in pulmonary mechanics after caffeine administration in infants with bronchopulmonary dysplasia. Pediatr Pulmonol 6:49, 1989.
7. Davis JM, Rosenfeld WN: Chronic lung disease. In Avery GB, Fletcher MA, MacDonald MG (eds): Neonatology: Pathophysiology and Management of the Newborn, 4th ed. Philadelphia, JB Lippincott, 1994.
8. Dreyfuss D, Saumon G: Barotrauma is volutrauma, but which volume is the one responsible? Intensive Care Med 18:139, 1992.

9. Eichenwald EC, Stark AR: Apnea of prematurity. In Koff PB, Eitzman D, Neu J (eds): Neonatal and Pediatric Respiratory Care, 2nd ed. St. Louis, Mosby-Year Book, 1993.
10. Fiascone JM, Vreeland PN, Frantz ID III: Neonatal lung disease and respiratory care. In Burton GG, Hodgkin JE, Ward JJ (eds): Respiratory Care: A Guide to Clinical Practice, 3rd ed. Philadelphia, JB Lippincott, 1991.
11. Fletcher M: Respiratory distress syndrome and other respiratory diseases in neonates. In Burton GG, Hodgkin J (eds): Respiratory Care: A Guide to Clinical Practice, 2nd ed. Philadelphia, JB Lippincott, 1984.
12. Fujiwara T, Maeta H, Chida S, Morita T, Watabe Y, Abe T: Artificial surfactant therapy in hyaline membrane disease. Lancet 1:55, 1980.
13. Gerard P, Fox WW, Outerbridge EW: Early versus late introduction of continuous negative pressure in the management of idiopathic respiratory distress syndrome. J Pediatr 87:591, 1975.
14. Kim EH: Successful extubation of newborn infants without pre-extubation trial of continuous positive airway pressure. J Perinatol 9:72, 1989.
15. Krouskop RW, Brown EG, Sweet AY: The early use of continuous positive airway pressure in the treatment of IRDS. J Pediatr 87:263, 1975.
16. Northway WH Jr, Rosen C, Porter DY: Pulmonary disease following respirator therapy of hyaline membrane disease. N Engl J Med 76:357, 1967.
17. Rooklin AR, Moomjian AS, Shutack JG, Schwartz JG: Theophylline therapy in bronchopulmonary dysplasia. J Pediatr 95:882, 1979.
18. Scanlon JW: The very-low-birth-weight infant. In Avery GB, Fletcher MA, MacDonald MG (eds): Neonatology: Pathophysiology and Management of the Newborn, 4th ed. Philadelphia, JB Lippincott, 1994.
19. Shannon D: Chronic complications of respiratory therapy in the newborn. In Thibeault D, Gregory G (eds): Neonatal Pulmonary Care. Menlo Park, CA, Addison-Wesley, 1979.
20. Stark AR: Apnea. In Cloherty JP, Stark AR (eds): Manual of Neonatal Care, 2nd ed. Boston, Little, Brown, 1985.
21. Stiles AD: Air leak: Pneumothorax, pneumomediastinum, pulmonary interstitial emphysema, pneumopericardium. In Cloherty JP, Stark AR (eds): Manual of Neonatal Care, 2nd ed. Boston, Little, Brown, 1985.
22. Toce SS, Farrell PM, Leavitt PA, Samuels DP, Edwards DK: Clinical and radiographic scoring systems for assessing bronchopulmonary dysplasia. Am J Dis Child 138:581, 1984.
23. Whitaker KB: Comprehensive Perinatal and Pediatric Respiratory Care. Albany, NY, Delmar Publishers, 1992.
24. Whitsett JA, Pryhuber GS, Rice WR, Warner BB, Wert SE: Acute respiratory disorders. In Avery GB, Fletcher MA, MacDonald MG (eds): Neonatology: Pathophysiology and Management of the Newborn, 4th ed. Philadelphia, JB Lippincott, 1994.

■ SELF-ASSESSMENT QUESTIONS

1. Which of the following conditions is the primary cause of respiratory disorders in the newborn period?
   a. meconium aspiration
   b. hyaline membrane disease
   c. transient tachypnea of the newborn
   d. apnea of prematurity

2. What is the primary cause of respiratory distress syndrome in the newborn?
   a. low birth weight
   b. aspiration of amniotic fluid
   c. delayed absorption of fetal lung fluid
   d. insufficient amount of pulmonary surfactant

3. The chronic lung disease that develops in newborn infants treated with oxygen and mechanical ventilation is
   a. bronchopulmonary dysplasia
   b. Wilson–Mikity syndrome

c. hyaline membrane disease
d. persistent pulmonary hypertension

4. Radiologically, the initial stage of BPD is identical to
   a. viral pneumonia
   b. transient tachypnea of the newborn
   c. hyaline membrane disease
   d. pneumothorax

5. The post-term infant is at greater risk for meconium aspiration syndrome because of
   I. smaller amount of amniotic fluid
   II. higher birth weight
   III. decline in placental function
   a. I only
   b. III only
   c. I and III
   d. I, II, and III

6. The first step in the management of an infant who may have aspirated meconium is to
   a. begin positive pressure ventilation
   b. immediately dry the infant
   c. place the infant in a 40% oxyhood
   d. suction the airway

7. Risk factors for pulmonary barotrauma include
   a. mechanical ventilation
   b. prematurity
   c. respiratory distress syndrome
   d. all of the above

8. Which of the following pathogens commonly causes pneumonia in the postnatal period?
   a. coagulase-positive staphylococcus
   b. cytomegalovirus
   c. rubella
   d. *Escherichia coli*

9. Which of the following is *not* used in treating infants with apnea of prematurity?
   a. theophylline
   b. CPAP
   c. tolazoline
   d. oxygen

10. What is the primary cause of transient tachypnea of the newborn?
    a. low birth weight
    b. aspiration of amniotic fluid
    c. delayed absorption of fetal lung fluid
    d. insufficient amount of pulmonary surfactant

Chapter 10

Pulmonary Disorders in Children

EARL FULCHER, JR.

OBJECTIVES

Having completed this chapter, the reader will be able to:

1 Identify differences in clinical signs, symptoms, and medical history that may assist one in distinguishing between causes of lower airway obstruction.

2 Identify factors that have increased the life expectancy of children born with cystic fibrosis.

3 Describe how pneumonia may cause an exacerbation of underlying cardiopulmonary disease in children.

4 Identify differences in clinical signs, symptoms, and medical history that may help one in distinguishing between croup, epiglottitis, and foreign body aspiration.

5 Discuss appropriate management techniques for the child suspected of having epiglottitis.

6 Identify indications for providing nonconventional methods of supporting gas exchange in the child with respiratory failure. Describe advantages of these nonconventional techniques.

KEY TERMS

acute lung injury	methacholine challenge
acute respiratory distress syndrome	pneumonia
autosomal recessive	spasmodic croup
bronchiolitis	status asthmaticus
epiglottitis	tracheomalacia
laryngotracheobronchitis	

Pulmonary disorders constitute the most frequent cause of illness in the young child and infant.[182] The purpose of this chapter is not to provide a comprehensive review of all pulmonary conditions that affect the pediatric patient, but to provide instead a concise analysis of the etiology, pathophysiology, clinical signs, diagnosis, and management of 10 common pediatric pulmonary disorders. The pulmonary disorders that will be addressed include asthma, cystic fibrosis, bronchiolitis, pneumonia, croup, epiglottitis, foreign body aspiration, tracheomalacia, near drowning, and respiratory failure.

ASTHMA

Etiology
Asthma is a condition caused by hyperreactive airways. The patient with asthma can have an "attack" triggered by various allergic and nonallergic stimuli. Pediatric asthma affects 5% to 10% of all children in the United States[167] and is a common cause of absenteeism in school-aged children.[137] Hospitalization rates and mortality rates in pediatric asthma have increased in the last several years.[35,90,92] The reasons for this increase are severalfold and will be discussed in the management section below.

Pathophysiology
The lower airways of the patient with asthma are hyperresponsive to various allergic and nonallergic stimuli.[92,117,133] Examples of common allergic and nonallergic stimuli that may lead to airway hyperreactivity in the pediatric patient are listed in Table 10-1. The classic pathological condition that occurs during an asthma "attack" is spasm of the bronchial smooth muscle. Bronchospasm usually occurs within the first hour after exposure to airway stimuli. This reactivity of the bronchial smooth muscle is often termed the *early phase* of an asthma attack.[116,133] However, bronchospasm is only part of the pathology that exists during an asthma exacerbation. Recent research has proved that airway inflammation plays a significant role in the pathophysiology of asthma. The airways release a host of inflammatory mediators that lead to hypersecretion of mucus, goblet-cell hyperplasia, smooth muscle hypertrophy, and an influx of other inflammatory cells into the airways. The increased volume of mucus mixes with the inflammatory cells to form thick, tenacious plugs that occlude small airways. This inflammatory process may occur hours after exposure to the stimuli and the initial bronchospasm. Therefore, the resultant inflammatory process is often referred to as the *late phase* of an asthma attack.[90,117,133]

TABLE 10-1   Common Allergic and Nonallergic Stimuli in Asthma

ALLERGIC STIMULI	NONALLERGIC STIMULI
Cigarette smoke	Cold air
Pollen	Heightened emotional response
Grass clippings	Exercise
Dust mites	
Animal dander	
Viruses	
Exhaust fumes	

This combination of bronchospasm and an inflammatory process causes a significant degree of airway obstruction. Small airway obstruction leads to air trapping and a potential auto-PEEP effect that produces ventilation/perfusion abnormalities with hypoxic vasoconstriction. Recent clinical research has shown that inflammation and airway obstruction exist even in clinically stable patients.[10,175]

Clinical Signs and Diagnosis

The child who is experiencing an asthma exacerbation may first present with a cough and dyspnea. The presence of a cough is often the first sign of small airway obstruction in the child. Children may also complain of chest tightness along with dyspnea. Wheezing with decreased air entry will usually be heard upon auscultation. The child who is experiencing a moderate or severe attack may be heard wheezing without the use of a stethoscope.

An asthma attack should not be ruled out if a child does not present with noticeable wheezing. As stated in Chapter 6, the airway obstruction may be so severe that there is not enough air movement for a wheeze to be heard. Children who are experiencing a severe asthma attack may also be diaphoretic and cyanotic. As always, cyanosis is a late, grave sign of respiratory insufficiency and must be treated immediately.

A child experiencing an asthma attack will usually be tachypneic and tachycardic and may display use of accessory muscles. Pulsus paradoxus may also be present in the child with a moderate or severe exacerbation.[172,182] The initial chest x-ray film typically reveals hyperinflated lungs with flattened diaphragms and relatively clear lung fields. Subsequent chest x-ray film may show increased opacity with consolidated lung tissue if the inflammatory process is allowed to continue without intervention.

Blood gas results will vary depending on the degree of airway obstruction.[32,90,182] Initially, a child may have normal blood gas values or a respiratory alkalosis secondary to increased alveolar ventilation. As the inflammatory process continues and mucus plugging leads to increased airway obstruction, the $PaCO_2$ will begin to rise with worsening hypoxemia. The presence of hypercarbia with a moderate to severe hypoxemia is the definitive sign that a child has progressed to a **status asthmaticus** condition (acute, severe, prolonged episode of asthma) and requires immediate and aggressive therapy in order to prevent respiratory failure. Even the presence of a $PaCO_2$ in the range of 40 to 45 mm Hg should warn the clinician of a deteriorating condition.[90] Another sign of severe pulmonary insufficiency in the older child is the inability to speak in complete sentences owing to shortness of breath.

The diagnosis of asthma in the child is made primarily on a history of recurrent episodes of reversible airway obstruction triggered by certain allergic or nonallergic stimuli.[92,117,137] Table 10-1 lists common allergic and nonallergic stimuli. A family history of asthma or atopy may predispose a child to the development of asthma. Children who have a history of repeated episodes of viral bronchiolitis, pneumonia, and gastroesophageal reflux or a history of bronchopulmonary dysplasia are also at increased risk to develop reactive airways.[114,117] The differential diagnosis for children suspected of having asthma includes the aforementioned conditions as well as cystic fibrosis, foreign body aspiration, congenital airway malformations, pulmonary edema, and obliterative bronchiolitis.[117,137]

A definitive diagnosis of asthma is often difficult to obtain in the young child. Pulmonary function tests measuring expiratory flowrates and lung volumes may prove useful in the older child in detecting small airway obstruction. The reversibility of the child's airway obstruction can be assessed with prebronchodilator and postbronchodilator spirometry. The degree of airway responsiveness may also be assessed through the use of a **methacholine challenge**. For this test, the child inhales a small amount of aerosolized methacholine, a respiratory irritant, and then performs a forced vital capacity maneuver. The more responsive the child's airways, the smaller the amount of methacholine required to produce a significant decrease in pulmonary function. Pulmonary function examinations and the methacholine challenge are usually limited to children 5 years of age or older.[92,141] A final measurement that may prove helpful in the diagnosis of childhood asthma is a test for the presence of specific IgE antibodies. Many children with asthma and atopy have elevated levels of IgE present in their serum.[92,114]

Management and Complications

The management of a child with an attack of asthma is based on the need to relieve the airway obstruction caused by bronchospasm and then prevent "late-phase" inflammatory reactions through the use of certain anti-inflammatory agents. Therefore, the primary medications used in the treatment of asthma in children are inhaled beta-adrenergic bronchodilators and corticosteroids.

Inhaled beta-2 specific bronchodilators are first-line therapy for the treatment of an asthma attack. The administration of inhaled bronchodilator agents is described in detail here because this is the area in which most respiratory care practitioners will actively participate in patient management. Inhaled albuterol, as well as the agent terbutaline, has proved to be safe and effective in the treatment of childhood asthma.[35,117] The guidelines published by the National Institutes of Health recommend the use of 0.15 mg/kg/dose of albuterol for the treatment of pediatric asthma. The recommended frequency is every 4 to 6 hours with a maximum dosage of 5 mg.[117] However, albuterol aerosols may be given every 20 minutes to the unstable patient in the emergency department. There also have been reports comparing the recommended dosage of albuterol with protocols utilizing 0.3 mg/kg/dose. The higher albuterol dosage was found to be as safe as the lower dosage and was associated with an increase in effectiveness.[150] In my experience, administering up to 5 mg of nebulized albuterol every 2 hours to pediatric patients has no significant side effects. The clinician should titrate the dosage of inhaled bronchodilators to the individual requirements of the patient and not by specific guidelines based on body weight.[131]

The child suffering from a severe exacerbation who does not respond initially to frequent beta-adrenergic aerosols may be given a trial of continuous nebulization. The administration of 10 to 15 mg of albuterol per hour has been shown to improve pulmonary function in those children who were at risk of requiring mechanical ventilation.[11,23,124] Continuous nebulization of terbutaline has also proved to be safe and effective.[112] The child who receives continuous bronchodilator nebulization should be monitored closely via ECG and pulse oximetry for side effects of this therapy such as arrhythmias, hypokalemia, and increased ventilation/perfusion mismatch.[35]

Inhaled bronchodilators are commonly administered to children via a small volume nebulizer (SVN) or metered dose inhaler (MDI). The MDI requires coordination skills that may be difficult for children younger than the age of 7 to master. However, the addition of a spacer device may allow the child as young as 3 to be treated adequately with an MDI.[62,131] Recently, the use of an MDI and spacer proved to be as effective as an SVN in the treatment of asthmatics older than 2 years of age.[26] An SVN is typically employed when treating the younger child incapable of using an MDI correctly or the child who is in severe distress. An SVN employs higher doses than an MDI and may be more effective than an MDI in the treatment of severely ill asthmatics.[16,62] An inhaled bronchodilator delivered via SVN to a young child or infant is usually given with a mask or "blown to the face."

The pediatric clinician must remember that only 10% to 12% of an aerosolized drug is delivered to the patient using a mouthpiece and proper technique.[62,131] Therefore, much less of the drug will be deposited in the small airways of the child when the mask or "blow-by" methods are employed. Less than 1% of the drug cromolyn sodium (Intal) was absorbed by infants who received the drug via SVN and mask.[143] The dosage of aerosolized bronchodilator should, therefore, be regulated according to patient response. An improved patient response is usually determined by an increase in the forced expiratory volume in one second (FEV_1) or peak expiratory flow rate (PEFR) of 12% to 15% above baseline.[117,141] Usual signs of improvement after a bronchodilator aerosol administration include decreased wheezing in the asthmatic patient, suggesting a positive response. However, the patient with severe airway obstruction may present with minimal air movement on the initial examination and display wheezing *after* bronchodilator therapy. It is in this scenario that wheezing may actually be a sign of improvement.

The use of anti-inflammatory agents is the other primary method of managing the pediatric asthma patient. These agents decrease airway hyperresponsiveness to various allergic stimuli and irritants and prevent late-phase reactions during acute asthma exacerbations. The agents cromolyn sodium (Intal) and nedocromil sodium (Tilade) are now considered to be first-line therapy in the treatment of mild to moderate asthma. Intal may be given via MDI or small-volume nebulizer, whereas Tilade is only offered in MDI form. It may take several weeks of consistent therapy with these agents before a decrease in airway responsiveness is noted. The onset time is approximately 2 to 4 weeks for Intal and 1 to 2 weeks for Tilade.

Corticosteroids, such as prednisone and methylprednisolone, are the other group of anti-inflammatory agents that are frequently employed in the management of asthma. Steroid therapy should be administered after all acute asthma exacerbations to prevent late-phase reactions and for all moderate to severe asthmatics who are unresponsive to Intal or Tilade.[42,92,117] Corticosteroids should initially be administered via inhalation in order to decrease systemic side effects.[43,133] Of concern with the use of steroid therapy for pediatric asthma patients are the risks of adrenal suppression, growth retardation, and cataracts.[43,92] However, recent research has shown that the risks of cataracts and growth retardation are minimized when inhaled dosages are kept at less than 800 µg per day.[43] Children with moderate to severe asthma may require oral steroid therapy in addition to or in place of Intal or Tilade. Corticosteroids should be administered orally or intravenously to all children who require hospitalization or admission to an emergency department.[35,92,117]

Theophylline is now considered a second-line drug in the management of pediatric asthma.[35,92,159] It may be useful in the treatment of nocturnal or steroid-dependent asthma, especially in its time-release forms.[37,92,117] The recommended serum level for theophylline therapy is now 5 to 15 µg/mL instead of 10 to 20 µg/mL. Research has shown that the degree of bronchodilation at a level of 20 µg/mL is not significantly greater than that achieved at 15 µg/mL. Side effects of theophylline therapy, such as irritability and behavior and learning difficulties, are often present in children at serum levels greater than 15 µg/mL.[92,117]

Oxygen therapy should be employed in the management of the child with asthma who displays clinical signs of hypoxemia or who has hypoxemia documented by pulse oximetry or blood gas analysis. Supplemental oxygen should be titrated to keep SpO_2 values greater than 92% and the PaO_2 greater than 80 mm Hg.[35] Small volume nebulizers used for bronchodilator administration should be powered by oxygen instead of compressed air so that the risk of hypoxemia is minimized during the treatment.

Mechanical ventilation should be reserved for those children who experience a severe asthma attack and are not responsive to a combination of continuous bronchodilator nebulization and intravenous steroids.[35,90] The combination of bronchospasm and mucus plugging during a severe asthma exacerbation causes air trapping, alveolar overdistention, and the presence of auto-PEEP in the lungs even before mechanical ventilation is initiated.[35,90] Therefore, the risk of pulmonary air leaks and hemodynamic compromise is greatly increased during positive pressure ventilation.

The goal for mechanically ventilating the pediatric asthma patient must be to employ a strategy that will minimize these risks. This strategy should include the use of tidal volumes of 10 mL/kg or less and an I:E ratio of 1:3 or less. The application of PEEP must be approached cautiously since these patients will already have some degree of intrinsic PEEP with areas of alveolar overdistention.

During positive pressure ventilation of the patient with severe asthma, peak airway pressures may often rise to very high levels (40 to 80 cm H_2O). It must be understood that the elevated pressures occur because of the extremely high airway resistance present in these patients.[25,64,104] The high peak airway pressures are generated in the endotracheal tube and airways and *not* at the alveolar level. In a study by Leatherman and colleagues, no incidents of barotrauma occurred in 42 severe asthmatics who were mechanically ventilated, despite an average peak airway pressure of 68 cm H_2O.[93] Therefore, the practitioner should focus on keeping the end-inspiratory plateau pressure (peak alveolar pressure) below 35 to 40 cm H_2O and not be as concerned with elevated *peak* airway pressures. The pediatric clinician should also be hesitant to decrease inspiratory flowrates in order to decrease peak airway pressures. When the peak flow rate is decreased during volume-cycled ventilation, the I:E ratio may increase to the point that air trapping and auto-PEEP increase.[64,93] By employing these general guidelines for mechanical ventilation, the likelihood of iatrogenic lung injury can be decreased.

A final issue that must be discussed in the management of pediatric asthma is patient education. Proper patient education may play a significant role in decreasing the morbidity and mortality of pediatric asthma.[91,92] A predominant risk factor for asthma mortality is a patient's lack of understanding of the severity of the disease, how to recognize an impending attack, and how to utilize medications properly.[91,92] This lack of knowledge and misconception about the severity of asthma is demonstrated by children as well as by their parents.

Asthma education includes the identification of common allergic stimuli, proper use of medications including MDI instructions, and proper use of a peak flowmeter to predict and treat an asthma attack.[37,117] Excellent asthma education materials are available from the National Asthma Education Program as well as several pharmaceutical companies. Recent research has proved that appropriate asthma education can decrease the morbidity and hospitalization rates in children with asthma.[111] However, there are few institutions where respiratory care practitioners are directly involved in the development and management of pediatric asthma education programs. The pediatric respiratory care practitioner should seek to become involved in asthma education and *not* leave this task to other professionals who are not as well trained in pulmonary therapeutics.[73] At a minimum, the pediatric respiratory care practitioner should be familiar with the *Executive Summary: Guidelines for the Diagnosis and Management of Asthma* published by the National Institutes of Health and have the ability to properly instruct a child in the use of an MDI and home peak flow monitoring.

The prevalence of severe asthma and the mortality rates of asthma in children have increased in recent years. Reasons for this increase as listed in the literature are as follows:[35,91,92]

1. Low socioeconomic class
2. Lack of proper parental support and medical facilities
3. Lack of knowledge and understanding of severity of asthma and its proper management by patients, parents, and clinicians
4. Severe attacks triggered by foods
5. Misdiagnosis (especially in young children)
6. Psychosocial problems (drug abuse, depression, and manipulative use of asthma)

Despite these sobering facts, our knowledge and understanding of asthma and its treatment have also increased significantly over the last several years. As pediatric clinicians, we must acquire this knowledge first for ourselves and then teach our young patients and their parents how best to manage this disease. Only through education and prevention will we decrease the number of young asthmatics who cross our emergency department doorways.

CYSTIC FIBROSIS

Etiology

Cystic fibrosis is an autosomal recessive disorder that is prompted by mutations of a single gene pinpointed on the seventh chromosome. The term **autosomal recessive** means that the cystic fibrosis (CF) gene can occur in either males or females and that the CF gene will not be dominant if paired with a normal gene. A child who receives one CF gene and one normal gene from his or her parents would be a carrier of the CF trait but would *not* have CF. Parents who are both carriers of the CF gene have a 25% chance of producing a child with cystic fibrosis.

This disease affects nearly every organ system in the body that contains epithelial surfaces.[81] In the Caucasian American population, CF has the highest mortality for genetic diseases, with an incidence of approximately one in every 2500 live births. It occurs in approximately one in every 17,000 African Americans and is very rare in the Asian population.[87]

Pathophysiology

CF causes a change in the transport of chloride and sodium ions across the epithelial surfaces of the lungs, pancreas, intestinal mucous glands, and sweat glands. This alteration in ion flow manifests itself as dehydration of secretions in the ducts and airways, which then leads to blockages of pancreatic ducts and the small airways of the lung. The viscous secretions block the pancreatic ducts and disallow the flow of enzymes necessary for food digestion. The altered ion transport may also lead to small bowel obstruction and will cause an increase in chloride loss from the sweat glands.

The presence of thick, tenacious secretions in the airways of the patient with CF creates a perfect growth medium for bacteria. The respiratory tract of a patient with CF is typically colonized very early in life by the *Staphylococcus aureus* organism, and then later by *Haemophilus influenza* and *Pseudomonas aeruginosa* bacteria. After colonization occurs, there usually begins a recurring cycle of infection, inflammation, and airway obstruction that leads to pulmonary dysfunction.[162]

Pseudomonas aeruginosa is the organism most often implicated in these cycles of infection and inflammation.[139] Airway inflammation may trigger bronchospasm in some individuals with CF.[121] The inflammatory process causes an increase in airway resistance, which leads to air trapping with a typical obstructive component noted on pulmonary function tests. The combination of airway inflammation and mucus plugging may cause the development of a cascade of pulmonary events that includes bronchiolitis, atelectasis, cyst formation, and bronchiectasis. As the lung disease progresses in the latter years of a CF patient's life, increased ventilation/perfusion mismatch leads to hypoxemia, pulmonary hypertension, and eventually cor pulmonale.[121]

Clinical Signs and Diagnosis

Children with CF may present with signs and symptoms of the disease as a newborn or later during childhood, depending upon the particular genetic mutation present. However, the initial symptoms and severity of CF may vary even among children in the same family with identical genotypes.[172]

The presence of meconium ileus within the first 2 days of life is highly indicative of cystic fibrosis. Meconium ileus occurs in 10% to 15% of CF cases.[30] Other common indications of CF in early childhood include a salty taste to the child's skin when kissed; failure to thrive; recurrent respiratory tract infections; a family history of CF; prolonged neonatal jaundice; rectal prolapse; and frequent, greasy, foul-smelling stools. However, atypical cases of CF may display little pancreatic involvement or clinically significant pulmonary insufficiency. Therefore, the pediatric clinician must maintain a high index of suspicion when working with children who display one or a combination of the conditions listed above.[121,179]

A sweat chloride test is performed to help confirm the diagnosis of CF in children who present with clinical signs and symptoms of the disease (Fig. 10-1). The chloride ion is unable to be reabsorbed into epithelial cells in individuals with CF; therefore, an abnormally high salt content is present in their sweat. A positive sweat chloride test consists of chloride values of greater than 60 mEq/L in each of two sweat samples obtained on different days. Chloride measurements of 40 to 60 mEq/L are inconclusive and require repeated testing and further review of clinical indicators.[121,179] The sweat chloride test should only be performed in the laboratories of established CF centers in order to decrease false positive and negative results.[140] A positive sweat chloride test is now often followed by genetic testing, which can identify the presence of the more common CF gene mutations.[172,179]

Management and Complications

The management of CF basically involves the treatment and prevention of pancreatic insufficiency and respiratory tract infections. Pancreatic insufficiency combines with the thick mucus found in the small bowel to cause maldigestion of foods and malabsorption of fats. Dietitians work with the child's physician to treat this process through the use of pancreatic enzymes and vitamin supplements. The pancreatic enzymes come in a capsule or powder form and are taken orally prior to meals or heavy snacks.[30] Pancreatic enzyme therapy and vitamin supplementation are adequate for proper weight gain in many CF patients. Occasionally, some CF patients require high-calorie, high-fat diets to maintain their ideal body weight.[30,121]

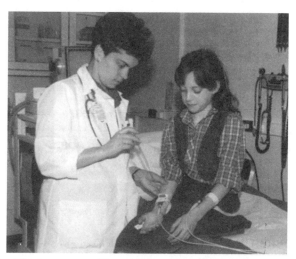

FIGURE 10-1   The sweat test. (Cunningham JC, Taussig LM: An Introduction to Cystic Fibrosis for Patients and Families. Bethesda, MD, Cystic Fibrosis Foundation, 1991.)

The pediatric respiratory care practitioner must realize that most children with CF have increased workloads placed on their respiratory muscles because of the obstructive nature of their lung disease. The respiratory musculature consumes many calories during the breathing process, especially during a respiratory tract infection. Therefore, adequate nutrition and, perhaps, an increased calorie intake are required by these individuals to maintain proper respiratory muscle function.

Bronchopulmonary dysfunction secondary to infection is the cause of more than 90% of CF deaths.[33,162] Therefore, antibiotic therapy has proved to be a mainstay in the treatment of CF and is used to control, and at times attempt to prevent, infectious exacerbation of the disease.[121,179] The antibiotic tobramycin, a member of the aminoglycoside group, has proved to be particularly effective in combatting gram-negative organisms such as *Pseudomonas aeruginosa*. Other antibiotics commonly used include third-generation cephalosporins such as ceftazidime and quinolones such as ciprofloxacin and ofloxacin. During an acute infectious exacerbation, the CF patient is typically admitted to the hospital for 10 to 14 days of intravenous antibiotic therapy and aggressive pulmonary hygiene. However, recent advances in home antibiotic therapy may provide therapeutic and financial benefits.[57,179]

Antibiotics may also be aerosolized for the treatment or prevention of a pulmonary infection.[57,109] Aerosolized antibiotics may offer several advantages, as listed in Table 10-2. They are typically delivered by either a small volume nebulizer using a low dose strategy or a large-volume ultrasonic nebulizer using a high dose strategy. The aminoglycosides, tobramycin and gentamicin, are the most common antibiotics delivered via aerosol.[75]

Most CF patients will display some degree of small airway obstruction secondary to the presence of thick, dried mucus. These thick, tenacious secretions are present in the airways with or without a pulmonary infection.[179] Therefore, the other mainstay in the management of CF is chest physical therapy (CPT) (see Chap. 18). CPT is typically thought of as the use of postural drainage and therapeutic chest percussion to mobilize secretions and improve pulmonary function.[6,40] This conventional form of CPT is still provided as the primary method of airway clearance in most CF centers located in the United States. Conventional postural drainage and percussion has been used for over 30 years in the CF patient and is recommended by some authorities for treatment of small airway obstruc-

---

TABLE 10-2   Advantages of Aerosolized Antibiotics

1. Slow decline in pulmonary function when used in conjunction with other therapy

2. Systemic side effects minimized when compared with intravenous (IV) therapy

3. Antibiotic administered directly to the source of infection

4. Inhibitory concentrations of antibiotic in sputum much greater than IV therapy

5. Increase effectiveness of antibiotic when used in conjunction with IV therapy

6. Decrease frequency of hospitalizations when used regularly in home

7. Maintain antibiotic efficacy after IV therapy discontinued

tion beginning at the time of diagnosis.[40,179,180] Although some studies show little or no change in certain pulmonary function values after a single CPT session,[6] long-term evaluations demonstrate a decline in pulmonary function when conventional CPT is *not* administered.[36,135] Percussion of the chest may be applied either with one's hands or with various mechanical percussors or vibrators.

There is evidence in the literature that percussion may cause hypoxemia and worsening of pulmonary function in the CF patient.[126] Therefore, chest percussion must be performed judiciously in these patients, with appropriate monitoring for hypoxemia and increased work of breathing. CF patients usually require at least 2 to 3 minutes of chest percussion in 10 different postural drainage positions to ensure adequate clearance of all lung segments.[58,107] The CPT sessions are usually administered three to four times a day during a hospital admission and once or twice a day at home.

Other forms of CPT have recently been made available in the United States and offer alternative techniques for airway clearance. Positive expiratory pressure (PEP) therapy has been widely used in Europe for many years and has now gained acceptance in the United States as a method to recruit atelectatic airways and improve mucus mobilization.[58] The patient exhales via mask or mouthpiece through a flow resistor, which creates PEP and allows collateral ventilation of partially obstructed airways through the pores of Kohn. The improved collateral ventilation places gas distal to the partial obstruction, which enhances the mobilization of the mucus during a huff cough or forced expiratory technique.[6,58,102] The primary advantage of PEP therapy is that it can be performed independently by most patients 3 years of age and older, whereas conventional CPT typically requires the assistance of another person.[58,102] PEP has been compared with traditional CPT in several studies, with the results demonstrating a trend toward a greater improvement in pulmonary function with PEP therapy.[58,115,120]

Other airway clearance techniques currently used in the CF population include high-frequency chest wall oscillation devices, a flutter valve device, and exercise. The chest wall devices provide high-frequency oscillations to the chest wall via an inflatable, air-filled vest or a cuirass shell. The device offers another airway clearance technique that can be delivered independently, but it is expensive and has not yet proved to be superior to conventional CPT.[1,177] The flutter valve device combines the use of PEP therapy with high-frequency airway oscillations. This device incorporates the use of a flow resistor with a loosely supported steel ball (see Chap. 18). As the patient exhales through the device, PEP is created and the vibrations of the steel ball produce high-frequency oscillations at about 15 Hz, which are transmitted to the airways.[57,58] The flutter valve device is compact, cost-effective, can be used independently, and has shown improved sputum clearance when compared with conventional CPT.[18]

A final, simple method of improving mucus clearance in the CF patient is exercise. Exercise offers the advantage of improving or maintaining cardiovascular health while providing the child with an additional therapy that is understood and accepted by peers.[30,58]

Medicated aerosol therapy is commonly used in the management of CF. The use of aerosolized bronchodilators in the treatment of CF is based on the presence of reversible bronchospasm. Bronchodilator therapy is effective in about 30% of CF patients.[179] Recent advances in CF research have made available two other medications that are delivered to the airways via aerosol. Recombinant human DNase (Pulmozyme) and amiloride enhance the mobilization of thick, dried secretions by different methods (see Chap. 17). Amiloride is a sodium channel blocker that is commonly used as a diuretic. When delivered by aerosol to the CF patient, amiloride prevents the reabsorption of sodium into airway epithelial cells, allowing water to accumulate on the airway surface and thin existing mucus.[133,179]

Recombinant human DNase is a mucolytic agent that is capable of decreasing the viscosity of mucus when a pulmonary infection is present. During a pulmonary infection, neutrophils converge on the area and release DNA, which is a viscous polyanion. RhDNase breaks down the DNA and thins the mucus. RhDNase does *not* decrease the viscosity of mucus in those individuals without a pulmonary infection.[57,179] Research has demonstrated that both medications offer some improvement in mucociliary clearance and pulmonary function.[69,88,129]

Supplemental oxygen therapy may be required for the management of CF as the disease progresses and evidence of cor pulmonale appears.[179] Individuals with CF should be offered oxygen conservation devices, such as liquid pulsed oxygen, to allow more time for travel and social activities. Novel therapies for the CF patient include gene therapy and lung transplantation. The affected gene that causes CF was located in 1989; since then, intense research has been underway to find a way to replace the recessive CF gene in the airways with a normal gene. This potential therapy offers the first chance at actually treating the cause of this disease instead of its symptoms.[57,179] However, gene therapy remains in phase I FDA trials as researchers have yet to find a safe, effective way to transfer the gene to airway epithelial cells (personal communication, Cystic Fibrosis Foundation, 1996). Lung transplantation has recently been used in the treatment of CF patients who have severe pulmonary dysfunction and meet the other requirements for receiving an organ transplant. The 2-year survival rate is 50% to 60%.[57,179] Unfortunately, a major drawback to this approach in the United States is the lack of suitable organs.[74,179]

Cystic fibrosis is a serious genetic disorder that may, at times, be very difficult to manage. Complications that may occur in the management of CF include pneumothorax, hemoptysis, rectal prolapse, intestinal obstruction, cirrhosis, and pancreatitis.[57,121] Despite the potential for serious complications, individuals today have a median survival age of 29 years, whereas the survival age for CF was only 10.6 years in 1966 and 20 years in 1981. There are currently many individuals with CF who are living well into their 40s and 50s.[31] Improvements in antibiotic therapy, nutritional supplementation, and airway clearance techniques have significantly enhanced the life expectancy and quality of life in individuals with CF.

BRONCHIOLITIS

Etiology
Bronchiolitis is the most common cause of lower respiratory tract obstruction in the young child. It commonly occurs in children younger than 2 years of age and is typically viral in origin. The usual pathogens are respiratory syncytial virus (RSV) and the parainfluenza viruses. Viral

bronchiolitis occurs more frequently during the fall and winter months.[68,137,174] The viruses are transmitted via contact with infected secretions, such as an infected child wiping his or her nose or eyes and then touching an uninfected child. The causative virus is also commonly transmitted to an infant by an older family member who presents with symptoms of a common cold.[55,154] Therefore, infection control measures should include cohorting patients and the use of gowns and gloves by health care workers.[55,174]

Pathophysiology

Viral bronchiolitis is characterized by an inflammatory process that occurs in the small bronchi and bronchioles of the infected child. The caliber of the airways in the lower respiratory tract of the young child or infant is extremely small, which places the child at increased risk for bronchiolar occlusion. The small airways become obstructed during the inflammatory process by an influx of inflammatory cells, increased amounts of viscous pulmonary secretions, mucosal edema, and possible smooth muscle contraction. This obstructive process leads to patchy areas of atelectasis and hyperinflation.[55,174]

Infants younger than 6 weeks of age or those with underlying cardiopulmonary, immunodeficiency, or neuromuscular disorders are at increased risk to develop a severe pulmonary infection. These infants may develop an acute viral interstitial pneumonia instead of the typical bronchiolitis pattern. The viral pneumonia produces alveolar and mucosal edema, with the possibility of formation of alveolar hyaline membranes.[174]

Clinical Signs and Diagnosis

Diagnosis of bronchiolitis is usually made by analysis of nasopharyngeal cultures, past medical history, and clinical signs and symptoms. A nasopharyngeal specimen may be obtained via a sterile swab or suction catheter and analyzed with immunofluorescent staining techniques for the presence of the RSV antigen.[80] A positive RSV culture with evidence of a lower respiratory tract infection virtually assures the clinician that the child has viral bronchiolitis.

A child with viral bronchiolitis presents with a history of a viral upper respiratory tract infection (common cold) that precedes the signs of the lower respiratory tract illness. Common signs and symptoms of lower respiratory tract involvement include a congested cough, wheezing, tachypnea, and low-grade fever. Auscultation of the chest may also reveal wet rales in conjunction with expiratory wheezing. A chest x-ray film reveals the presence of hyperinflation, peribronchiolar thickening, and possible patchy consolidation. The signs and symptoms of viral bronchiolitis will typically resolve in 7 to 10 days, which coincides with a decrease in the viral shedding.

Management and Complications

Despite the prevalence of bronchiolitis in children, most infants acquire only a mild form of the condition and do *not* require hospitalization for treatment.[55,154] Until recently, the treatment of viral bronchiolitis in the hospitalized child has been primarily supportive. The child is treated with a combination of pulmonary and nutritional therapeutics to maintain adequate hydration, ventilation, and perfusion.[137,174,182]

In early 1996, an RSV-specific immunoglobulin was released for the treatment and prevention of bronchiolitis caused by RSV (personal communication, Med Immune, Inc., 1996). The immunoglobulin has been extensively studied in patients at increased risk for acquiring a severe RSV infection. The RSV-specific immunoglobulin boosts the child's own immune response when infected with the respiratory syncytial virus. Given in monthly intervals during the fall and winter months, the immune globulin has proved to reduce both the incidence and severity of RSV-associated bronchiolitis and pneumonia.[52,59] This preventive therapy may change the way in which all children at risk for acquiring a severe RSV infection are treated.

Common pulmonary therapeutics used for the treatment of viral bronchiolitis include supplemental oxygen, chest physical therapy, aerosolized bronchodilators, theophylline, antiviral agents, and mechanical ventilation. Supplemental oxygen should be provided to any infected child who displays clinical signs of hypoxemia or has an SpO_2 less than 92% or PaO_2 less than 70 torr (see Chap. 14). Mechanical ventilation should be instituted in any child who displays poor ventilation and oxygenation despite optimal use of other pulmonary therapeutics or in any child who displays impending respiratory failure. Excellent reviews for the use of mechanical ventilation in infants with a severe viral bronchiolitis or pneumonitis have been published (see also Chap. 16 of this text).

The use of beta-adrenergic and anticholinergic bronchodilators in the treatment of viral bronchiolitis has remained controversial despite many years of clinical research and review.[131,152,174] Many studies have shown a significant improvement in pulmonary function and clinical score after administration of aerosolized beta-adrenergic drugs such as albuterol.[86,103,169] Other researchers have shown either little change in pulmonary function and clinical scores or a *decrease* in pulmonary function and oxygenation after bronchodilator administration. Potential reasons for these discrepancies include the following:

- Imprecise, nonstandard pulmonary function testing techniques in infants
- Varying drug dosages and aerosol delivery techniques
- Measurement of pulmonary function soon after a single treatment versus measuring outcomes after a series of treatments over a period of hours or days
- Evaluation of infants at differing stages of their disease, which may influence aerosol deposition
- Evaluation of infants with and without laboratory evidence of a viral or bacterial pulmonary infection

When this array of compounding factors is considered along with the results of current studies, it can be concluded that there is a subgroup of children who will show improvement with use of aerosolized bronchodilators.[131,174] Earlier thoughts that infants had few airway beta-receptors or underdeveloped bronchial smooth muscle[97,105] have essentially been proved untrue. Many recent clinical studies have proved that bronchial smooth muscle constriction does indeed occur in the young infant and the smooth muscle constriction can be reversed with the use of an aerosolized bronchodilator.[116,168]

A trial regimen of bronchodilator therapy is, therefore, recommended for all infants who present with clinical signs and symptoms of viral bronchiolitis.[131,174] This recommendation can also be made given the likelihood that the clinician may not be able to differentiate between the infant who presents with viral bronchiolitis and the child who presents with his or her *first* asthma attack induced by a viral infection. The bronchodilator therapy should be administered using standard drug dosages, such as albuterol at 0.15 to 0.30 mg/kg or metaproterenol at 0.01 to 0.025 mL/kg.[131,169] The nebulizer should be powered with oxygen and vital signs and pulse oximetry monitoring should be performed before and after each treatment.[174]

Other bronchoactive drugs have been studied in the treatment of viral bronchiolitis. Racemic epinephrine has recently been shown to be more effective than albuterol in the treatment of hospitalized infants admitted for viral bronchiolitis. The children showed a quicker improvement with racemic epinephrine as compared with albuterol, with no difference in adverse side effects.[134,144] Reasons for this difference may be the vasoconstrictor effects of racemic epinephrine, as well as the increased effect of a greater equipotent dosage of racemic epinephrine (0.1 mL/kg of racemic epinephrine versus 0.03 mL/kg of albuterol). The anticholinergic drug ipratropium bromide has also been studied for treatment of viral bronchiolitis. When combined with albuterol, infants showed no additional improvement with the ipratropium bromide as compared with aerosolized therapy with albuterol alone.[149]

Perhaps the most controversial medicated aerosol currently approved for the treatment of viral bronchiolitis is the antiviral agent ribavirin. Ribavirin is a nucleoside analogue that interrupts viral shedding in both DNA and RNA viruses, including the respiratory syncytial virus (RSV).[133] It is administered via a small particle aerosol generator (SPAG) that produces a large volume of aerosol particles in the respirable range. It has been shown to decrease viral shedding and improve clinical symptoms in children who have bronchiolitis or pneumonia caused by RSV.[12,164] However, much of the research demonstrating improved outcomes with ribavirin therapy as compared with a control group was performed on infants who had only mild to moderate disease.[12,55,164]

As stated previously, infants with an underlying cardiopulmonary disorder, such as bronchopulmonary dysplasia, are thought to have a more severe disease course when infected with RSV.[2,56] Therefore, ribavirin is recommended for those infants with an underlying cardiopulmonary disorder as well as very young infants and those who require mechanical ventilation (Table 10-3). Despite these recommendations by the American Academy of Pediatrics, the clinical efficacy and cost effectiveness of ribavirin continues to be called into question.[55,174,183] Recent research by Meert and colleagues has shown that the antiviral agent does not significantly decrease the number of mechanical ventilator days, use of supplemental oxygen, or length of hospitalization in those infants who require assisted ventilation.[108] Previous research did demonstrate a decrease in these factors, but this group used a placebo of sterile water in their control group as compared with the placebo of normal saline used by Meert and colleagues.[156]

The use of ribavirin in those children with underlying congenital heart disease who acquire an RSV pneumonia has also been questioned. Retrospective data have shown the mortality rate in this group to be signifi-

TABLE 10-3   American Academy of Pediatrics Recommendations for the Use of Ribavirin in RSV Pneumonia

1. Underlying congenital heart disease
2. Underlying chronic lung conditions (bronchopulmonary dysplasia)
3. Immunosuppressed children (HIV, organ transplants)
4. Infants <6 weeks of age
5. Severe pneumonitis caused by RSV with PaO_2 <65 mm Hg and increasing $PaCO_2$
6. Children requiring mechanical ventilation

cantly less than previously thought, thanks to improvements in medical intensive care and surgical correction.[113] A recent survey of pediatric critical care physicians also raises concerns for the increased likelihood of bronchospasm and ventilator malfunctions in children treated with aerosolized ribavirin.[9]

A critical cost–benefit analysis must, therefore, be performed whenever the use of aerosolized ribavirin is questioned. The drug itself costs approximately $1500 for a 3-day course of therapy, not including the additional charges for personnel and the many precautions that must be followed to limit occupational exposure.[9] Ribavirin has been reported to be carcinogenic and teratogenic in animals and to cause conjunctivitis and skin rashes in some health care providers.[76] An alternative method for the nonintubated patient is shown in Figure 10-2. This system should enhance the delivery of ribavirin to the child while decreasing the likelihood of occupational exposure.[24]

Chest physical therapy (CPT) is another modality that is traditionally employed in the treatment of children with bronchiolitis. As mentioned earlier, these children will often have increased mucus production, which may lead to atelectasis and infection if the child is not kept well hydrated and the secretions mobilized. CPT has not been proved to improve pulmonary function or clinical symptoms in children with bronchiolitis, although limited research has been performed in this area.

Theophylline therapy is another modality that may be employed in the treatment of bronchiolitis. It is often used for its bronchodilator effects, although there is some evidence that theophylline may improve pulmonary function in critically ill infants by enhancing diaphragmatic contractility.[174] Schena and colleagues reported a decrease in total system resistance with a concomitant decrease in arterial CO_2 when intravenous aminophylline was used in four mechanically ventilated infants.[148] Other research in children with only a mild to moderate infection showed no improvement in the clinical course.[22] Since other bronchoactive medications have greater beta-adrenergic activity, there seems to be little need for the routine use of theophylline in the treatment of bronchiolitis except in those children who are critically ill. However, as with CPT, more research is needed before absolute recommendations can be made.

Complications of bronchiolitis include apnea in young infants and a residual decrease in pulmonary function, although this decline may not be

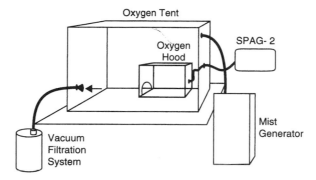

FIGURE 10-2 Oxygen hood within an oxygen tent canopy for ribavirin administration. (Cefaratt JL, Steinberg EA: An alternative method for delivery of ribavirin to nonventilated pediatric patients. Respir Care 37 [8]:877,1992.)

clinically apparent in school-aged children.[55,78] There also seems to be an increased likelihood that young children who suffer a moderate to severe course of bronchiolitis may develop asthma or reactive airway disease when they are older.[114,127] Despite these complications, the mortality rate for those children hospitalized with RSV-associated bronchiolitis is less than 1%.[55]

■ PNEUMONIA

Etiology
Pneumonia is a rather loose term that encompasses a wide range of disease states. Pneumonia is typically thought of as an infectious process of the pulmonary system that causes an inflammatory reaction near the acinus region of the lung. The pathogen or insult that results in a pneumonia may be transmitted to the lungs by inhalation or via the bloodstream.[50,51] Pediatric pneumonia is most often caused by either the RSV or parainfluenza viruses.[50,52] Other causative viral agents include the adenoviruses and varicella (chickenpox), whereas the mycoplasma organisms are a typical cause of pneumonia in children over 5 years of age.[50,53] Pediatric cases of pneumonia are *not* frequently caused by bacteria. The most common bacterial pathogens that lead to pneumonia are the *Streptococcus pneumoniae* (pneumococcus), *Staphylococcus,* and *Haemophilus influenzae* type B organisms.[50,51,53]

Pathophysiology
The degree and area of pathological involvement during pediatric pneumonia will vary with the causative agent, age of the patient, and presence of underlying cardiopulmonary and immunosuppressive disorders. Children with an underlying disorder, such as bronchopulmonary dysplasia, may develop a severe pneumonia and require hospitalization, whereas previously healthy children may require only supportive therapy in the home.[52,54,55] Younger children and infants may display a more severe disease course when compared with older children because their airways are

much smaller and more likely to be occluded. The small functional residual capacity of a young child is also easily lost when pathogens invade the lung parenchyma.

The *Pneumococcus* and *H. influenzae* bacteria will cause lobar consolidation, whereas *Staphylococcus* and many viral organisms produce a more diffuse involvement of the lung parenchyma. Regardless of whether the pneumonia is isolated in one lobe or disseminated throughout the lung, there will be an influx of plasma cells and lymphocytes into the involved area. This inflammatory reaction in the parenchyma and small airways of the lung will result in alveolar and interstitial edema, which will lead to areas of atelectasis and lung consolidation. As the infection progresses, an empyema or pleural effusion may form during bacterial pneumonias. The child's mucus will become thickened because of the presence of the pathogen and the accumulation of inflammatory cells. In children with underlying hyperreactive airways, such as those with asthma and CF, the release of inflammatory mediators may cause smooth muscle constriction throughout the small airways.[50-52,56]

Clinical Signs and Diagnosis

Signs and symptoms of pediatric pneumonia, as with the pathophysiology, will vary with the causative agent, age of the patient, and presence of any underlying disorders. Common clinical findings during pediatric pneumonia are listed in Table 10-4.

It may be especially difficult to distinguish between viral and bacterial pneumonias when looking only at clinical signs and symptoms. However, bacterial infections often present with a sudden onset accompanied by a high fever, whereas a viral pneumonia is often preceded by a common cold and a low-grade fever. Bacterial pathogens are also more likely to produce lobar consolidation and pleural effusions than are viral pathogens.[50,53,54]

The diagnosis of pediatric pneumonia is often based on assessment of the child's signs and symptoms, along with the findings on chest x-ray films, blood cultures, and a complete blood count (CBC). A white blood cell count (WBC) of greater than 15,000 mm^3 is indicative of a bacterial pathogen, whereas a WBC of less than 11,000 mm^3 may be present during a viral infection. Blood cultures are seldom positive in children with pneumonia, since viruses are the most common pathogens and only 15% to

---

TABLE 10-4   Common Clinical Signs and Symptoms in Pneumonia

Fever—low-grade if viral pneumonia

Cough—productive with purulent sputum if bacterial pneumonia

Tachypnea

Retractions—intercostal and substernal

Adventitious breath sounds—wheezing, rales, or decreased over affected segments

Dull percussion note over affected segments

Malaise

Vomiting—caused by thickened sputum

25% of patients with community-acquired pneumonia have blood-borne pathogens.[50,57] Children who present with viral upper respiratory symptoms during the fall and winter months may undergo nasal washing or aspirate to determine the presence of RSV.

To better determine the exact cause of a pneumonia, a sample of expectorated sputum should be sent for culture and gram stain.[50] Unfortunately, most infants and young children will be unable to produce a sputum sample upon demand that is not contaminated with the normal flora of the upper airway. If the child is critically ill or immunocompromised, a sample may be obtained via tracheal aspirate, needle biopsy, or bronchoalveolar lavage (BAL).[50,51,57]

Management and Complications

The successful treatment of pneumonia is based on making an accurate determination of the cause of the condition. Children who display positive cultures from respiratory or blood specimens should begin a course of antibiotic therapy based on the organism's sensitivity. Initially, broad-spectrum antibiotics are administered unless specific, highly resistant organisms are present on the culture.[50,51,53,57] Aerosolized antibiotics have proved successful in the treatment of certain gram-negative pneumonias, such as those caused by a *Pseudomonas aeruginosa* infection in the CF patient.[58,59,60] The antiviral agent ribavirin may be employed in the treatment of RSV-associated pneumonia, although its use remains controversial.[61] A pneumonia caused by the influenza virus may be effectively treated with the antiviral agent amantadine.[52,57]

Once appropriate antibiotic or antiviral medications are instituted, all other care remains supportive. Children who present with signs or documented evidence of hypoxemia should be treated with supplemental oxygen therapy. Those who display signs of respiratory failure may require positive pressure ventilation or continuous positive airway pressure (CPAP) via endotracheal tube or noninvasive interfaces such as a nasal mask. Antipyretics should be employed for the child's comfort and to decrease tissue oxygen consumption. The child should also be kept well hydrated to decrease the risks of thick, dried pulmonary secretions.[50]

Chest physical therapy is frequently ordered by physicians for children diagnosed with pneumonia.[62] However, research into the use of traditional chest physical therapy (postural drainage, percussion, vibration) has proved that CPT offers little improvement in pneumonia and perhaps may increase atelectasis and lower the PaO_2 in some patients.[63-65] Therefore, CPT should be ordered only in those patients with an underlying disorder, such as CF or bronchiectasis, who produce sputum in excess of 25 mL/day, and in those children who show evidence of atelectasis secondary to mucus plugging.[57,72]

Most previously healthy children who acquire a mild pneumonia recover completely with no cardiopulmonary impairments. Children with underlying cardiopulmonary disorders or those who suffer a severe pneumonia may develop a number of complications, which may include empyema, pleural effusion, pneumothorax, pulmonary hemorrhage, and respiratory failure requiring endotracheal intubation and mechanical ventilation.[50,51,66,67] There is evidence that some children who endure a severe bout of pneumonia may have a residual decrease in pulmonary function that may not be clinically apparent.[54,68]

CROUP

Etiology

The upper airway disorder referred to as croup is more accurately termed *viral laryngotracheobronchitis* (LTB). LTB is the most common cause of upper airway obstruction in children aged 6 months to 3 years. It is most often caused by parainfluenza viruses types I and II, RSV, or the influenza virus.[51,69,70] There is also evidence of *Mycoplasma pneumoniae* leading to LTB in older children.[71] LTB occurs most often during the late fall and winter months, as do most viral-associated disorders.[70]

Pathophysiology

The pathology of LTB that causes its classic symptoms is a swelling of the subglottic region of the upper airway. This section of the upper airway is anatomically the smallest portion in young children because of the stricture placed around it by the cricoid cartilage. As the term **laryngotracheobronchitis** suggests, there may also be inflammation of the trachea and mainstem bronchi. The inflammatory process produces mucosal edema, which can significantly reduce the cross-sectional area of the airway and greatly increase airway resistance.

Clinical Signs and Diagnosis

Children and infants with LTB typically present with a history of a common cold that precedes the croup-like symptoms by 1 to 3 days. Common clinical signs of LTB include a low-grade fever, barking cough, stridor, hoarseness, suprasternal retractions, and tachypnea (see Table 10-5 for a comparison with epiglottitis and foreign body aspiration). Children who have recurrent episodes of croup-like symptoms without the presence of a viral infection are said to have **spasmodic croup**. Spasmodic croup is thought to be allergic in nature, and children will recover fully within 3 to 6 hours. Viral LTB has a recovery period of 2 to 6 days.[69,70,73,74]

The diagnosis of viral LTB is usually made clinically, based on the classic signs and symptoms listed above. Radiographic confirmation of the diagnosis may be made with lateral or anteroposterior views of the neck that demonstrate subglottic narrowing and a normal epiglottis. The classic "steeple sign" will be present on an anteroposterior view of the neck (Fig. 10-3).[69,70,73] Differential diagnosis of viral LTB includes epiglottitis, bacterial tracheitis, foreign body aspiration, diphtheria, retropharyngeal abscess, and laryngeal thermal injury.[50,69]

Management and Complications

Many children who acquire viral LTB may only need supportive care in the home. Parents or guardians who treat their child at home after consultation with a physician are encouraged to keep their child calm and content to lessen the increased respiratory efforts that crying and agitation will produce. Caregivers may also attempt to soothe the swollen airway by having the child breathe humidified air from a cool-mist vaporizer or holding the child in a steam-filled bathroom or outside in the cool night air. If these actions do not produce noticeable improvement within an hour or if the child continues to have audible stridor while sleeping, the physician should again be consulted.[74,75]

TABLE 10-5 Comparison of Viral Croup, Epiglottitis, and Foreign Body Aspiration (FBA)

	VIRAL CROUP	EPIGLOTTITIS	FBA
Age range	6 months–3 years	2 years–adult	7 months–4 years
Etiology	Viral (seasonal)	Bacterial	Foodstuffs or toys
Onset of symptoms	Gradual	Acute	Acute
Clinical Signs			
Stridor	Yes	Rare	Yes
Cough	Yes—barking	Rare	Yes
Hoarseness	Yes	Yes	May occur
Wheezing	Rare	No	May occur
Dysphagia	No	Yes	May occur
Temperature	<101°F	>101°F	Normal
Cyanosis	Rare	<20%	May occur
X-ray findings	Subglottic narrowing (steeple sign)	Enlarged epiglottis (thumb sign)	Object may or may not be seen
Treatment			
Intubation	Only 3%–6%	Yes—all cases	Rarely required
R. epinephrine	Useful	Not effective	Not effective
Steroids	Useful	Rarely used	Not effective
Antibiotics	Not effective	Yes—all cases	If secondary bacterial infection occurs
Bronchoscopy	Seldom used	Occasionally used	Yes—most cases

Viral LTB is usually treated in the hospital with a combination of cool aerosol therapy, inhaled racemic epinephrine, and steroids. An intramuscular injection of dexamethasone at 0.6 mg/kg or an equipotent dose of oral prednisone is now recommended for any child who requires inhaled racemic epinephrine upon admission to the hospital emergency department. These potent anti-inflammatory agents have been shown to decrease the severity of LTB and the need for repeated racemic epinephrine treatments.[70,73] An intramuscular injection of dexamethasone may be preferred over oral prednisone in the young infant because of the very bitter taste of prednisone. Recently, the use of aerosolized steroids have been shown to improve the clinical outcomes of children treated for LTB in the emergency department.[80–82] However, there is currently no corticosteroid approved in the United States for use in an aerosol solution.

The onset of action for parenteral steroid therapy is probably between 3 and 6 hours.[70,73] Therefore, aerosolized racemic epinephrine is given to relieve the upper airway obstruction until the steroids begin to take effect. Racemic epinephrine should be administered at a dosage of 0.05 mL/kg or a dosage of 0.25 mL for infants and 0.5 mL for older children.[70,76] Racemic epinephrine is a potent alpha-adrenergic compound that will

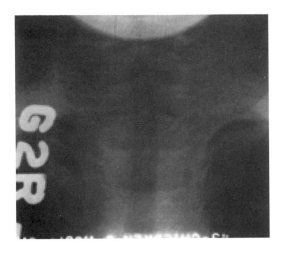

FIGURE 10-3 Typical antero-posterior neck radiograph in viral laryngotracheobronchitis demonstrating subglottic narrowing. (Cressman WR, Myer CM III: Diagnosis and management of croup and epiglottitis. Pediatr Clin North Am 41 [2]:265, 1994.)

decrease mucosal swelling and thereby reduce airway resistance and work of breathing. Maximum benefit will occur within 1 to 2 hours.[77]

Many hospitals and physicians used to require that any child who received a racemic epinephrine aerosol in the emergency department be admitted to the hospital for fear of a rebound effect that could lead to worsened airway obstruction.[69] However, recent research has proved this complication of racemic epinephrine therapy to be rare. Many children may be safely discharged after 2 to 4 hours of observation following racemic epinephrine and corticosteroid therapy.[76,78,79,101] Pediatric practitioners should also remember to allow the child's parent or guardian to administer the racemic epinephrine aerosol. The airway obstruction in a young child, who is already anxious because of an increased work of breathing, may be worsened when a stranger attempts to blow a cold mist into his or her face.

The other mainstay in the treatment of viral LTB is the use of a cool aerosol to soothe the child's inflamed airways.[69,70,83] This therapy is commonly administered to the child in the emergency department or hospital via an aerosol "croup" tent or an all-purpose nebulizer. As mentioned earlier, parents or guardians are often counseled to attempt the same therapy at home with the use of vaporizers or the steam produced by a running bathroom shower.[74] Despite its common use, research has proved cool aerosol therapy to offer no additional benefit when the child is kept well hydrated. In fact, it has been postulated that the relief a child receives from cool aerosol therapy may come not from the increased humidity but from the comfort provided by a parent holding them in the croup tent or steam-filled bathroom.[70] Most experienced pediatric practitioners will testify that the young toddler with croup will not remain enclosed in the croup tent without a parent or guardian getting in the tent with him or her.

The most feared complication of LTB is the need for an artificial airway. Although this complication should always be anticipated and respected, the incidence of endotracheal intubation for the treatment of LTB is only 3% to 6%.[50,69] Endotracheal intubation should be performed on the child with worsening airway obstruction who displays hypercarbia and moderate to severe hypoxemia despite repeated racemic epinephrine treatments and corticosteroid therapy. These children can usually be successfully extubated in 2 to 5 days when the airway inflammation has decreased and pulmonary secretions are minimal.[50,69]

▬EPIGLOTTITIS

Etiology
Epiglottitis is a true airway emergency that is caused by the acute inflammation and swelling of supraglottic structures. This gross swelling of the epiglottis and arytenoids may lead to partial or complete upper airway obstruction. The causative agent in over 80% of cases is *Haemophilus influenzae* type B bacteria. Children who acquire epiglottitis are generally older than those affected by croup and typically range from 2 to 6 years of age.[50,70] Although this emergency airway disorder still occurs occasionally in children and adults, its incidence has dramatically decreased since the introduction of conjugate vaccines for the *H. influenzae* organism that may be given during infancy.[84]

Pathophysiology
As described previously, the swelling of the epiglottis and other supraglottic structures will produce partial to complete airway obstruction. The inflamed and enlarged epiglottis and arytenoids may actually prolapse through the vocal cords as inspiratory effort increases (Fig. 10-4). The enlarged epiglottis, which usually covers the glottis during swallowing, may partially cover the esophageal opening as well and lead to dysphagia. If the child becomes agitated and inspiratory effort greatly increases, or if the gag reflex is stimulated by use of a tongue blade or other instrument, *complete* airway obstruction may occur.[50,69,70]

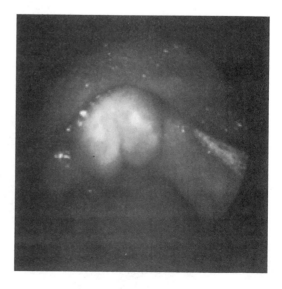

FIGURE 10-4 Swollen, distorted epiglottis seen in a case of epiglottis by direct laryngoscopy. (Cressman WR, Myer CM III: Diagnosis and management of croup and epiglottitis. Pediatr Clin North Am 41 [2]:265, 1994.)

Clinical Signs and Diagnosis

The child with epiglottitis typically presents with an acute onset of upper airway obstruction and fever occurring in the last 4 to 8 hours (see Table 10-5). The child will appear either lethargic or irritated, depending on his or her age and the severity of the condition. The child will usually sit upright in a "tripod" position, with the neck elevated to better maintain the airway. The older child will complain of hoarseness and pain when vocal efforts are made. Stridor or other adventitious breath sounds are uncommon. The child may be drooling secondary to the inability to swallow. The child often has a "toxic" appearance, with a temperature greater than 38°C. Suprasternal retractions and nasal flaring may also be present, but cyanosis may not appear until complete airway obstruction is impending.[50,69,70,75]

The pediatric clinician should immediately suspect epiglottitis if a child presents with signs of bacterial septicemia and an acute onset of upper airway obstruction. If epiglottitis is suspected, diagnosis should be made by a physician only during direct laryngoscopy or flexible fiberoptic bronchoscopy. The definitive treatment for epiglottitis is the placement of an artificial airway in the operating room. This procedure should not be delayed in order to obtain radiographs for confirmation of supraglottic swelling.[70]

The differential diagnosis includes viral croup, foreign body aspiration, bacterial tracheitis, upper airway burns, retropharyngeal abscess, and epiglottic hemangioma.[69,70] If the child's history and clinical symptoms do not strongly suggest epiglottitis, then lateral neck x-rays may be obtained. If epiglottitis is present, the lateral neck film would reveal the classic "thumb sign" of a swollen epiglottis, as well as enlarged aryepiglottic folds (Fig. 10-5).[69,70,75]

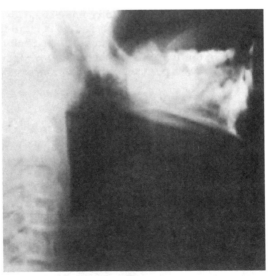

FIGURE 10-5 Lateral neck radiograph showing a positive "thumb" sign and ballooning of the hypopharynx. (Oski FA et al [eds]: Principles and Practice of Pediatrics, 2nd ed. Philadelphia, JB Lippincott, 1994.)

Management and Complications

The primary complication of epiglottitis is the occurrence of complete airway obstruction and respiratory arrest prior to the placement of an artificial airway. This complication can be avoided and mortality and morbidity minimized if a high index of suspicion and caution is maintained during the assessment and diagnosis of the child.

When epiglottitis is suspected, the child should be kept as calm as possible by allowing him or her to sit in the parent's lap and avoiding any unnecessary tests or procedures. Most importantly, the child's mouth or tonsils should *not* be examined until all personnel and equipment have been gathered for the placement of an artificial airway. A tympanic temperature device should be utilized instead of an oral thermometer, and arterial or venipunctures should *not* be performed until the artificial airway is in place. If the child appears cyanotic, supplemental oxygen may be delivered via "blow-by" method with the parent holding the oxygen tubing near the child's face. An oxygen mask should not be placed on the child if he or she becomes even slightly upset upon seeing the mask. The parent or guardian should be allowed to continue to hold the child if a lateral neck x-ray film is ordered and during the trip to the operating room.[50,70,85]

Once the decision is made to assess the child's airway via laryngoscopy or bronchoscopy, the most skilled pediatric anesthesiologist, pediatric surgeon, ENT surgeon, or pediatrician should be notified and the child taken to the operating room. The inspection and subsequent intubation of the trachea should be performed by the most skilled physician available after the child has received gaseous anesthesia and continues to breathe spontaneously. An endotracheal tube one size smaller than normal is typically placed nasally. If the trachea cannot be intubated, a tracheostomy must be performed, although this is a rare occurrence.

Once the artificial airway is in place, intravenous sedation should be administered and blood as well as laryngeal cultures obtained. The child should then be transferred to the ICU, where mechanical ventilation is instituted along with appropriate monitoring. Intravenous antibiotic therapy is then started with a combination of ampicillin and chloramphenicol. If the blood or laryngeal cultures reveal a bacteria other than *H. influenzae* type B, then antibiotic therapy is adjusted accordingly. The child typically requires intubation for 24 to 48 hours. Extubation is based on the absence of supraglottic swelling during periodic laryngoscopy or bronchoscopy by a skilled physician. The child's ability to swallow and the presence of an audible airleak around the endotracheal tube are also indications that successful extubation is possible. Once successfully extubated, the child may be transferred to a general floor care area to continue a 10-day course of antibiotics. The child may be discharged home to complete antibiotic therapy once all signs of infection and upper airway obstruction have disappeared.

■ FOREIGN BODY ASPIRATION

Etiology

Children aged 7 months to 4 years of age are at risk for aspirating a foreign body into the larynx, trachea, or bronchi. Children of this age group often explore their environment through touch and taste, thereby increasing their risk for foreign body aspiration. Common objects that may be aspirated by young children include small toys, balloons, hot dogs, beans, peanuts, coins, and buttons.[50,53,75]

Pathophysiology

The severity of respiratory compromise caused by the presence of a foreign body in the airway will depend on the size of the object, degree of obstruction, and location of the object.[50] A large object that completely occludes the trachea or larynx will lead to respiratory arrest and death if the object cannot be removed quickly with the Heimlich maneuver or by other means available to health care personnel.[53]

Foreign bodies that create only a partial obstruction in the upper or lower airways may produce inflammation and swelling around the object, which could worsen the obstruction. Small objects that deposit distal to the mainstem bronchi may produce a "ball-valve" effect, resulting in air-trapping and the potential for a pneumothorax. Objects aspirated into the lower airways, especially organic objects, can produce a local pneumonia or areas of atelectasis.[53]

Clinical Signs and Diagnosis

Aspiration of a foreign body should be considered in any child who presents with a sudden onset of airway obstruction.[69] The diagnosis of foreign body aspiration is highly probable in the child who displays signs of acute airway obstruction without signs and symptoms of a bacterial or viral infection.

The first evidence that should lead the pediatric practitioner to suspect foreign body aspiration is a history of coughing and gagging followed by stridor and/or wheezing while the child was eating or playing with small objects (see Table 10-5). Objects that lodge in the laryngeal area are more likely to produce stridor, coughing, and gagging, whereas objects lodged in the lower airways will likely produce wheezing, signs of air trapping, and symptoms of a possible secondary bacterial infection.[50,53]

Lateral and anteroposterior chest radiographs or video fluoroscopy may be used to assist in the diagnosis of foreign body aspiration; however, certain plastics and foodstuffs may be radiolucent on x-ray.[50,53] Flexible fiberoptic bronchoscopy may be used to assist in the diagnosis if the child presents with little physical evidence of aspiration and radiographs prove negative. However, the object should not be manipulated during fiberoptic bronchoscopy, as most pediatric-sized flexible bronchoscopes lack the forceps or brushes necessary for removal.[86]

Management and Complications

Children who aspirate foreign bodies seldom cough up the object spontaneously. Objects that are deposited in the laryngeal area may be removed via direct laryngoscopy by a skilled physician.[53] As mentioned previously, the presence of a foreign body in the trachea or bronchi can be confirmed with the use of a flexible fiberoptic bronchoscope.[108] The object should not be removed with the flexible bronchoscope unless a small-sized adult bronchoscope that contains the necessary accessories for foreign body removal can be utilized.[87] The definitive treatment for the removal of a foreign body located distal to the larynx is the use of *rigid* bronchoscopy while the child is under general anesthesia.[86,88,89]

Potential complications of foreign body aspiration include the potential for pulmonary airleak if the object is lodged distal to the trachea. Cardiopulmonary arrest and death may occur if the foreign body is dislodged from a lower airway during a cough and then occludes the opposite mainstem bronchus.[108] The possibility for bronchiectasis also exists if the object remains in the airway for some period of time and produces mucus accumulation and infection. A pneumonia may develop if certain organic materials are aspirated or if incomplete removal occurs during bronchoscopy. Any bronchial or parenchymal infection may require repeat bronchoscopy, antibiotic therapy, and bronchial hygiene therapy.[50]

▬TRACHEOMALACIA

Etiology

Tracheomalacia is a softening of the cartilage in the tracheal rings that leads to various degrees of airway obstruction. It is the most common congenital anomaly involving the trachea.[90] Other common causes of tracheomalacia include prolonged endotracheal intubation, elevated peak airway pressures during positive pressure ventilation, esophageal atresia, and tracheoesophageal fistula. This deformity of the tracheal cartilage may also be caused by extrinsic compression of the trachea by vascular rings, innominate arteries, tumors, or cysts. Tracheomalacia typically presents during the newborn period but may also manifest during childhood if one of the above conditions occurs.[86,90-92]

Pathophysiology

Tracheomalacia usually involves only the lower half of the trachea, but the entire trachea can be affected. This deformity of the tracheal rings causes the trachea to lose its stability during exhalation and, occasionally, during inspiration. As the child forcefully exhales or coughs, the trachea collapses on itself, which produces air trapping. The trachea may also collapse during a deep breath or gasp as the intraluminal pressure in the trachea becomes negative.[90,91]

Clinical Signs and Diagnosis

The characteristic symptom of tracheomalacia is a barking cough similar to the sound made by a seal. A coarse wheeze may also be heard during exhalation. The child could present with stridor and a barking cough if the malacia affects the upper portion of the trachea. The wheezing and/or stridor will be unresponsive to aerosolized beta-adrenergic therapy. Tracheomalacia is differentiated from croup because of the absence of a viral prodrome and the presence of any of the various causes listed above. Symptoms of tracheomalacia may also present when an endotracheal or tracheostomy tube is removed. The endotracheal tube will provide artificial support to the airway and cause signs of malacia to manifest once the tube is removed.[90,91]

The diagnosis of tracheomalacia is confirmed either by the use of a rigid bronchoscope or during flexible fiberoptic bronchoscopy.[93,94] Regardless of whether flexible or rigid bronchoscopy is utilized, the child must be allowed to breathe spontaneously during the procedure. The bronchoscopist will then be able to visualize the collapse of the trachea during a forced exhalation and confirm the diagnosis.[86,91]

Management and Complications

The treatment for tracheomalacia is, most often, time. As the child grows and develops, the trachea will become more rigid and the symptoms should disappear. Most children outgrow this disorder by 2 to 3 years of age.[90-92] A tracheostomy may be necessary on the rare occasion that the malacia does not improve with age or the disorder leads to life-threatening airway obstruction.[92]

▬ NEAR-DROWNING

Etiology

Near-drowning is defined as the survival of a victim of submersion for *greater* than 24 hours. Drowning is defined as the death of a submersion victim within 24 hours of the incident.[95,96]

Accidents are the leading cause of death in childhood, and drowning is second only to motor vehicle accidents as the most common cause of accidental death in children.[97,98] Drowning or near-drowning accidents most often occur in toddlers 1 to 4 years of age and in teenage males. Nonsupervision of young children is the most common cause of near-drowning accidents in the toddler age group. Alcohol, horseplay, and daredevil activities are the common factors associated with most drowning deaths in teenage males.[96,98]

Near-drownings occur most frequently in waters that are familiar to the victim. Toddlers and infants have drowned in bathtubs, toilets, buckets of water, and swimming pools or hot tubs of their parents or neighbors. Teenagers most often drown in diving accidents, falls, or boating accidents.[50,96,98] Teenage males also increase their risk of drowning when they attempt to swim further than they are physically capable.[95]

Pathophysiology

A child's body undergoes a rapid chain of events once he or she becomes submerged under water. The end result for nearly all near-drowning victims is a state of hypoxia and acidosis.[96] The sequence of pathological events that occurs during a near-drowning or drowning event is outlined in Figure 10-6.

A child may or may not aspirate water once submerged. Approximately 10% of near-drowning victims have reflex laryngospasm, which minimizes the amount of liquid aspirated into the lungs. This reflex causes the so-called "dry drowning."[96] Another reflex that may improve survival in near-drowning victims is the "diving reflex." This reflex occurs as the child's face hits the cold water and the CNS is stimulated by the trigeminal nerve, which causes bradycardia, a transient increase in arterial blood pressure, and peripheral vasoconstriction. The peripheral vasoconstriction shunts blood to the heart and brain, which increases the chance of survival with normal neurological function.[98]

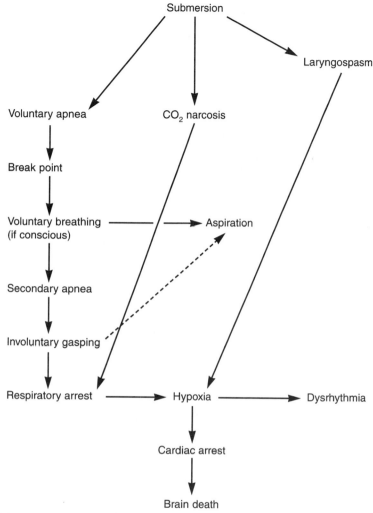

FIGURE 10-6　Sequence of respiratory reflexes occurring in drowning. (Levin DL et al: Drowning and near-drowning. Pediatr Clin North Am 40 [2]: 321,1993.)

Whether a child aspirates fresh water or salt water is of little consequence. Electrolyte changes and alterations in intravascular volume will be minimal in both instances.[50,96] Salt water is hypertonic and, when aspirated, causes an influx of water and plasma proteins into the alveoli and interstitial space. This influx of water into the alveolar region washes out the endogenous surfactant. Fresh water is typically hypotonic, and when aspirated it moves readily into the pulmonary vasculature. The movement of fresh water across the alveolar–capillary membrane causes surfactant inactivation or dysfunction.[95] Regardless of the tonicity of the water aspirated, the end result is the formation of pulmonary edema, atelectasis, bronchospasm, and hypoxic vasoconstriction that manifests clinically as hypoxia and acidosis. The presence of noxious substances in the aspirated water, such as gram-negative bacteria, fungi, algae, and sewage, may cause a severe pneumonitis and further alveolar damage.[96] Children who experience a near-drowning incident are also at *high risk* to develop acute respiratory distress syndrome (ARDS) because of the presence of increased pulmonary capillary permeability and alveolar inflammation.[50,99]

The neurologic outcome of near-drowning accidents is determined by the temperature of the water, length of submersion, age of the child, time before CPR efforts are initiated, and length of time without a pulse. The longer a child is submerged or left in a hypoxic state, the sooner cerebral hypoxia and edema will begin, which may lead to brain death.[50,95,96,98] Most drownings and near-drownings in the United States occur in warm water, so the time in which a child can survive without oxygen is usually 4 to 6 minutes.[96,100] Children who are submerged in cold water (0° to 15°C) from 40 to 60 minutes have survived with their neurological function intact, although these outcomes are *not* typical. It is thought that children can survive longer submersion times in cold water because of the diving reflex and a slowing of the cerebral metabolic rate.[96,98]

Clinical Signs and Diagnosis

The diagnosis of near-drowning is obviously made at the scene of the accident as the child is pulled from the water. As stated previously, morbidity and mortality are determined by the temperature of the water, length of submersion, age of the child, time before CPR efforts were initiated, and length of time without a pulse. Therefore, bystanders and emergency personnel must gather and clarify as much of this information as possible. In addition, a sample of the water may be obtained, which could help predict and treat certain pulmonary sequelae.[96]

The clinical signs and symptoms found in the near-drowning victim will vary greatly with the length of submersion, temperature of the water, and presence of any traumatic injury associated with the submersion accident. Clinical signs may range from a child who is alert and hypothermic with normal respiratory efforts to a child who is apneic and pulseless with no reflexes intact.[50,95] Two clinical signs that occur in nearly every near-drowning victim are hypoxemia and some degree of hypothermia.[96]

Arterial blood gases typically reveal severe hypoxemia with a large alveolar-to-arterial O_2 gradient and a mixed acidosis with initial pH values of 7.00 to 7.10.[50,96,98] As mentioned previously, electrolyte disturbances and the effects of hemoconcentration or hemodilution because of fluid shifts are minimal. Chest x-ray films taken within the first few hours of the incident may reveal only mild congestion of the pulmonary vasculature. If a significant amount of water was aspirated, the x-ray will begin to demonstrate areas of atelectasis with diffuse pulmonary edema 24 to 48 hours after the initial insult.[50,98] Signs and symptoms of ARDS may not be clinically present until 2 to 3 days after the submersion accident.

The child who aspirates water or other foreign material during a near-drowning incident may display wheezing secondary to bronchospasm. As pulmonary edema forms, rales or crackles may also be heard upon auscultation. Rescuers may note moderate to large amounts of frothy, white, blood-tinged secretions as the victim coughs or the airways are suctioned.

The child who is submerged for several minutes or who aspirated a generous amount of water will display signs of respiratory distress once spontaneous respirations begin.[50,96,98] These signs include tachypnea or bradypnea, intercostal and sternal retractions, and evidence of hypoxemia. Many near-drowning victims will appear cyanotic because of the combination of hypothermia and hypoxemia.

Neurologic impairment may be assessed by determining states of consciousness and checking reflexes.[95] This assessment should be done using the Glasgow Coma Scale (Table 10-6). The child should also be observed closely for the presence of seizures.[98] Pupil reactivity in a near-drowning victim is *not* an adequate predictor of neurologic impairment.[96,102]

Management and Complications

Perhaps the most important treatment for a near-drowning victim is the rapid recognition of apnea and/or pulselessness with an appropriate response by bystanders or emergency personnel. It has been observed that timely initiation of cardiopulmonary resuscitation (CPR) improves the outcome for many children who suffer a near-drowning accident.[96,98,102]

TABLE 10-6   Modified Glasgow Coma Scale for Infants and Children

	CHILD	INFANT	SCORE
Eye opening	Spontaneous	Spontaneous	4
	To verbal stimuli	To verbal stimuli	3
	To pain only	To pain only	2
	No response	No response	1
Verbal response	Oriented, appropriate	Coos and babbles	5
	Confused	Irritable cries	4
	Inappropriate words	Cries to pain	3
	Incomprehensible words or nonspecific sounds	Moans to pain	2
	No response	No response	1
Motor response	Obeys commands	Moves spontaneously and purposefully	6
	Localizes painful stimulus	Withdraws to touch	5
	Withdraws in response to pain	Withdraws in response to pain	4
	Flexion in response to pain	Decorticate posturing (abnormal flexion) in response to pain	3
	Extension in response to pain	Decerebrate posturing (abnormal extension) in response to pain	2
	No response	No response	1

(Used with permission from Hazinski MF: Neurologic disorders. In Hazinski MF [ed]: Nursing Care of the Critically Ill Child, 2nd ed. St. Louis, Mosby–Year Book, 1992: 549.)

Emergency personnel should attempt resuscitation on any child who has been submerged for less than 1 hour in water with a temperature less than 70°F. There is little evidence of children surviving submersions of greater than 1 hour with intact neurologic function.[96,98] The child's wet clothing should be removed and replaced with warm, dry clothing or linen. Supplemental oxygen should be delivered as soon as possible to all victims. The use of the Heimlich maneuver in near-drowning victims is controversial. Its use should probably be limited to the child with evidence of upper airway obstruction.[96,100]

If the child is pulseless and apneic, basic CPR should continue and then advanced cardiac life support procedures (ACLS) provided as soon as possible. Intravenous lines should be established if possible for the administration of fluids and cardiotonic medications such as epinephrine and atropine.[98,103] However, it has been noted that children who require cardiotonic drugs to establish a perfusing cardiac rhythm have a high incidence of death or survival with severe neurologic impairment.[102] In addition, children who enter the emergency department pulseless, apneic, and normothermic have a high probability of death or survival in a vegetative state.[50,98]

The child who is apneic, obtunded, or in severe respiratory distress at the accident scene should receive positive pressure ventilation via a bag-valve-mask unit. The child may be intubated in the field if an experienced, ACLS-trained individual is available at the accident scene. Whether endotracheal intubation is performed in the field or emergency department, personnel must be aware of the possibility of aspiration of gastric contents. The near-drowning victim may swallow a significant amount of water, so suction equipment must be readily available. A nasogastric tube should also be inserted to decrease the risk of aspiration.[95,98] A child who requires intubation and mechanical ventilation for severe hypoxemia or hypercapnia will typically develop ARDS. These patients should be treated with conventional or nonconventional forms of ventilatory support to optimize alveolar recruitment, minimize pulmonary vasoconstriction, and avoid lung overdistention (see the section below on respiratory failure).

The other mainstay in treating the near-drowning patient is rewarming techniques. Resuscitation should continue on a near-drowning victim until the core temperature reaches 92°F. If the child does not have a perfusing cardiac rhythm with a core temperature of 92°F, then the likelihood of survival is extremely poor.[96] Warming techniques vary but usually include warming blankets, heated IV solutions, and heated humidified O_2 therapy. The humidified oxygen should be delivered to the patient's airway at a temperature of 105° to 108°F.[96] Although the use of heated humidified oxygen is a standard rewarming technique,[95,96] its ability to significantly increase the core body temperature has recently been called into question.[104,105]

Other techniques used to manage the near-drowning victim include intracranial pressure (ICP) monitoring and hyperventilation in any child who requires mechanical ventilation and who displays neurologic depression. The ICP should be maintained at less than 20 torr, if possible, while keeping cerebral perfusion pressure greater than 50 torr.[96,98] If the ICP cannot be controlled with hyperventilation and diuretic therapy, the use of a barbiturate-induced coma may be indicated.[106,107] The technique of maintaining a near-drowning victim in a relative hypothermic state to reduce cerebral edema and cerebral metabolism is no longer considered therapeutic, as the risks of an altered white-blood cell count outweigh the potential benefit.[98,106,107]

Potential complications of near-drowning in the pediatric victim are many. The most devastating is severely impaired neurologic function. Other complications include renal failure, hepatic failure, sepsis, pneumonia, and diffuse intravascular coagulation (DIC).[50,96]

▬ RESPIRATORY FAILURE

Etiology

The term *respiratory failure* encompasses a wide range of potential meanings. Respiratory failure is defined here as being synonymous with **acute lung injury** (ALI) or **acute respiratory distress syndrome** (ARDS). At a recent American–European Conference on ARDS, the "A" in ARDS was changed from *adult* to *acute* to include the many pediatric patients that are affected by this syndrome.[109,112,113] ALI has been defined as an inflammatory syndrome with an acute onset that results in an increased permeability of the pulmonary vasculature. This results in refractory hypoxemia caused by an increased intrapulmonary shunt. ARDS is now defined as a more severe form of ALI. Therefore, only those patients with a severe form of ALI should be labeled as having ARDS, whereas those with a milder form of ALI should not receive the ARDS classification. Those children who develop pulmonary edema and refractory hypoxemia secondary to left heart failure (cardiogenic pulmonary edema) or hypervolumia should not be classified as having ALI or ARDS.[109,110]

There are many different causes of ALI and ARDS. These varied conditions may be identified as either direct or indirect pulmonary injury (Table 10-7). The most common conditions associated with ALI include sepsis, aspiration pneumonitis, primary pneumonia, and multiple trauma.[99,109,110]

Pathophysiology

ALI or ARDS can occur when a child's lungs are subjected either directly or indirectly to an inflammatory reaction at the alveolar–capillary interface. This inflammatory process occurs because of an influx of neutrophils, macrophages, and lymphocytes into the acinus of the lung. These inflammatory cells release inflammatory mediators such as proteolytic

---

TABLE 10-7   Common Conditions Associated With ALI and ARDS

DIRECT LUNG INJURY	INDIRECT LUNG INJURY
Aspiration pneumonitis	Sepsis
Near-drowning	Nonthoracic trauma
Primary pneumonia	Shock
Smoke inhalation	Burns
Thoracic trauma	Pulmonary embolism
	Multiple transfusions

enzymes, which damage the pulmonary endothelium and basement membrane. This damage to the basement membrane results in an increased permeability, with the result being pulmonary edema. The combination of pulmonary edema and the presence of inflammatory mediators then leads to surfactant inactivation or dysfunction.[99,109]

High permeability pulmonary edema and surfactant dysfunction manifests as decreased lung compliance and refractory hypoxemia. The decreased lung compliance occurs because of a decreased functional residual capacity (FRC) secondary to atelectasis and fluid-filled alveoli. Although this process was once believed to be homogenous, it is now recognized that the ARDS-affected lung is actually a mixture of aerated sections and collapsed, fluid-filled alveoli. Therefore, tidal ventilations in the ARDS patient will likely result in most of the tidal volume being preferentially distributed to the aerated portions of lung.[110,111]

This cascade of pathological events occurs in three distinct stages. The *acute* or *exudative phase* occurs within 12 to 48 hours of the initial lung injury and involves the influx of monocytes and neutrophils. The classic formation of hyaline membranes occurs during this stage. The *subacute* or *proliferative stage* occurs at 4 to 10 days and is characterized by a decrease in hyaline membrane formation and pulmonary edema, with some regeneration of type I cells. The lungs seem to undergo a repair and healing phase during the subacute stage. Eight to 10 days following the initial insult, varying degrees of interstitial and alveolar fibrosis form during the *chronic* or *fibrotic stage*.[99] It should be the goal of the pediatric clinician to minimize the degree of lung injury that occurs during the acute and subacute stages, thereby reducing or eliminating the effects of the fibrotic stage.

Hypoxemia and the influx of inflammatory mediators also cause pulmonary hypertension with a concomitant increase in right ventricular work. The increased myocardial work and increased work of breathing caused by this cascade of events results in an increased oxygen consumption, which places an even greater burden on the cardiopulmonary system.

Clinical Signs and Diagnosis

The diagnosis of ALI is made when an acute onset of hypoxemic respiratory failure is associated with one of the various conditions listed in Table 10-7. ALI is further characterized by diffuse, bilateral, alveolar infiltrates on the chest x-ray film and a PaO_2/FIO_2 of less than 300 torr (regardless of PEEP level) with no evidence of left heart dysfunction. ARDS is diagnosed by the presence of all the characteristics of ALI with the distinction of a PaO_2/FIO_2 of less than 200 torr.[109,110]

There are four clinical phases of ARDS. During the first phase, the child displays signs of respiratory distress such as tachypnea and dyspnea after the initial lung injury. However, the child will usually have a normal chest x-ray film with little change in PaO_2. The second phase is described as latent, since the child will display some clinical signs of decreased respiratory distress. This apparent improvement occurs despite the beginning of the acute or exudative pathologic stage of lung injury.[99,110]

The latent clinical phase is short-lived as the clinical signs of acute, severe lung injury begin to appear during the third clinical phase. It is during the third phase that the patient displays signs of severe respiratory distress such as tachypnea, grunting, and retractions. The child's hypoxemia will be refractory to an FIO_2 of greater than 50%, while the $PaCO_2$ may remain normal or begin to increase. The diffuse, bilateral, alveolar infiltrates are now evident on a chest x-ray film. It is at this point that the child will typically require endotracheal intubation and mechanical ventilation.

If the lung injury is worsened by mechanical ventilation and FIO_2 levels greater than 50% during this acute, clinical phase, the child will likely progress to the fourth clinical phase of ARDS. This phase is characterized by the formation of pulmonary fibrosis and the appearance of multiple system organ failure. Pediatric patients who progress to this fourth clinical phase of ARDS experience a high mortality rate. The mortality rate for pediatric ARDS victims is estimated to be approximately 60%.[99,110,113]

Management and Complications
Most children who acquire ARDS or ALI will require endotracheal intubation and mechanical ventilation. Adjustment and titration of mechanical ventilation in these patients can be very precarious because of the increased risk of iatrogenic lung injury. Young children are especially at risk to develop ventilator-induced lung injury because their high chest wall compliance offers little resistance to lung overdistention.[110] Therefore, mechanical ventilation of the pediatric ARDS patient must be performed in a manner that will be least harmful to the child's lungs while maintaining adequate oxygenation and ventilation. At times a "normal" $PaCO_2$ may be sacrificed in order to minimize the potential for overdistention of the compliant portions of the lung and thereby reduce the risk of lung injury. This is the concept of "permissive hypercapnia."[110,114,115] It is interesting that the concept of permissive hypercapnia has been championed in recent years as a method of reducing ventilator-induced lung injury during ARDS, although most neonatal clinicians have ventilated neonates with infant RDS in this fashion for many years. Fortunately, the technique of allowing the $PaCO_2$ to rise to moderately high levels (50 to 80 torr) by using physiologic tidal volumes is now being advocated for use in pediatric ARDS.[110]

The issue of whether ventilator-induced lung injury is caused by excessive pressure (barotrauma) or excessive volume (volutrauma) has been extensively reviewed by other authors and researchers.[110,114,116,117] It is evident in both human and animal studies that it is supraphysiologic tidal volumes (12 to 15 mL/kg) that lead to iatrogenic lung injury and *not* increased peak airway pressures.[115,118–122] Using the scientific evidence now available, guidelines for performing conventional mechanical ventilation in the pediatric ARDS patient can be formed. These guidelines are listed in Table 10-8.

Since the pathology of ALI and ARDS involves surfactant dysfunction or inactivation, the potential for use of surfactant replacement therapy would seem promising. Exogenous surfactant therapy has proved to be extremely successful in the treatment of infant RDS; however, these infants suffer from surfactant deficiency and not surfactant dysfunction. Little research has been done in the treatment of pediatric ARDS with surfactant replacement therapy. Initial studies in both adult and pediatric patients have shown transient improvements in oxygenation indices and lung compliance, but few patients have been enrolled in these projects.[123–125] The difficulty in administering surfactant therapy to pediatric and adult ARDS patients will be determining whether the solution should

TABLE 10-8   Guidelines for Use of Conventional Mechanical Ventilation in Pediatric ARDS

1. Restrict exhaled Vt to 5–7 mL/kg (physiologic range)

2. Maintain PEEP *above* inflection point on inspiratory limb of pressure–volume curve (range of 5–15 cm H_2O)

3. Avoid rates >40 breaths/min to reduce risks of auto-PEEP

4. Increase inspiratory time after maximum PEEP reached (avoid I:E ratios ≥1.5:1 to reduce risk of auto-PEEP)

5. Accept PaO_2 of 50–60 torr

6. Maintain some degree of hypercapnia ($PaCO_2$ >50 torr)

(Modified from Kacmarek RM, Hickling KG: Permissive hypercapnia. Respir Care 38[4]:373, 1993, Table 3; and Heulitt MJ, Anders M, Benham D: Acute respiratory distress syndrome in pediatric patients. Redirecting therapy to reduce iatrogenic lung injury. Respir Care 40[1]:74, 1995.)

be given via intratracheal bolus or aerosol. Initial research has shown that aerosolized exogenous surfactant will typically deposit in the compliant and aerated portions of the lung instead of in the atelectatic or partially collapsed areas.[124,127] In addition, a multicenter, randomized study on the use of aerosolized, artificial surfactant in sepsis-induced, adult ARDS patients showed *no* significant effect on oxygenation indices, duration of mechanical ventilation, or mortality.[126]

Infants and toddlers who develop ARDS could potentially be given intratracheal boluses of exogenous surfactant, just as neonates are.[125] However, larger, older children would require extremely high amounts of the currently available surfactant preparations since the dosing is 4 or 5 mL/kg via intratracheal bolus. This amount of liquid bolused into the trachea of the older child could be both physiologically detrimental and very expensive. Multicenter, randomized, controlled clinical trials are needed to decide whether surfactant replacement therapy in pediatric ARDS will significantly reduce mortality and morbidity.

Some children who are mechanically ventilated for ARDS using the guidelines listed in Table 10-8 may continue to display poor oxygenation and ventilation, with evidence of iatrogenic lung injury. These patients may be offered one of several unconventional approaches for support of gas exchange. The four unconventional techniques discussed here include extracorporeal membrane oxygenation, high-frequency oscillatory ventilation, nitric oxide therapy, and partial liquid ventilation. All of these techniques offer the possibility of improved gas exchange while minimizing the use of high FIO_2 levels and reducing the risks associated with volumetric overdistention of the lungs.[140] These techniques may one day become standard therapy for the treatment of the pediatric ARDS patient.

Extracorporeal membrane oxygenation (ECMO) is an invasive technique that supports gas exchange via partial cardiopulmonary bypass while allowing the lung time to "rest" or heal (see Chap. 25). ECMO has proved to be an extremely successful therapy for the treatment of respiratory failure in newborns[128] and has the potential to decrease the mortality of pediatric ARDS patients in whom other strategies have failed.[110,129] However, it is important that ECMO be employed *before* lung injury becomes irreversible and severe pulmonary fibrosis begins.[130] ECMO and the other unconventional techniques discussed here may be beneficial if used in a timely manner during the ARDS pathological process, but must *not* be used to prolong death.

High-frequency oscillatory ventilation (HFOV) is an exciting form of mechanical ventilation that typically uses respiratory rates of 300 to 900 breaths/min with tidal volumes less than anatomic deadspace (see Chap. 24). The mechanical breaths fluctuate around a mean airway pressure that can be set on the ventilator independent of other adjustments. When used in diffuse, noncompliant lung disease, the mean airway pressure is initially increased 2 to 5 cm H_2O above the mean pressure used during conventional mechanical ventilation in order to optimize lung volume.[133,141] This "high volume" strategy has the advantage of keeping the lung volume relatively constant since the high frequency breaths are delivered at volumes less than deadspace. When used judiciously, this strategy virtually eliminates the alveolar stretch injury and shear stress of small airways that can occur during conventional ventilation as alveoli collapse upon expiration and then are forcefully reopened during inspiration.[129,134,141] This HFOV high volume technique has proved successful, when compared with conventional mechanical ventilation, in the treatment of pediatric respiratory failure.[131,132]

Nitric oxide (NO) therapy and partial liquid ventilation are relatively new clinical techniques still undergoing FDA trials at the time of this writing. NO is a gas that produces vasodilation in the pulmonary vasculature when inhaled and has little effect on systemic vascular resistance. NO can be combined with conventional mechanical ventilation or HFOV to help alleviate the pulmonary hypertension present in ARDS and thereby improve oxygenation. Initial clinical reports are encouraging, but much research is required before NO therapy can be recommended as treatment for pediatric ARDS.[110,135,136]

Partial liquid ventilation (PLV) is perhaps the most promising new therapy for the treatment of ARDS in the pediatric patient. PLV uses liquid perfluorocarbons to support the functional residual capacity (FRC) of the lung (i.e., "liquid PEEP") instead of the conventional air/oxygen gas mixture. The patient's FRC is actually filled with the liquid perfluorocarbon via tracheal instillation (approximately 30 mL/kg) while gas ventilation continues with a conventional ventilator. The liquid perfluorocarbons are biologically inert, colorless, and odorless; possess low surface tension; and will not wash away endogenous surfactant. Oxygen is 20 times more soluble in perfluorocarbons than in water. These properties allow the liquid chemical to readily support gas exchange and distribute throughout the lung in a uniform fashion, in contrast to gas ventilation, in which the delivered tidal volume preferentially inflates and overdistends the normal alveolar units. PLV produces homogenous recruitment and expansion of the lung, thereby improving ventilation-to-perfusion ratios with a concomitant improvement in oxygenation (Fig. 10-7). PLV has proved to be safe and effective in the treatment of ARDS.[137-139] Multicenter trials are ongoing to decide whether PLV will be approved for general use in the ARDS patient.

As stated previously, the mortality rate for pediatric ARDS is approximately 60%. The most common cause of death in the ARDS patient is multiple system organ failure. However, respiratory failure and iatrogenic

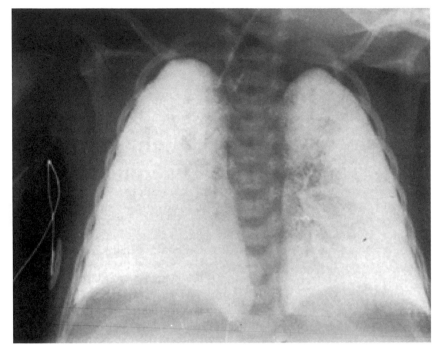

FIGURE 10-7   Lung filled with perfluorochemical. Note image enhancement capability of liquid, and homogenous expansion of lung fields. (Greenspan JS: Physiology and clinical role of liquid ventilation therapy. J Perinatol 16 [2]:S47,1996.)

lung injury definitely contribute to the mortality of these patients.[110,115] Complications in survivors of ARDS or ALI vary with the severity of the initial insult, age of the patient, and type of therapy employed. Most children who survive do so with little neurological or pulmonary impairment. The most common pulmonary function abnormality is a decrease in diffusing capacity.[99,110]

Perhaps the only way to significantly decrease mortality and morbidity from ARDS is to be able to accurately predict when ARDS or ALI may develop and then treat it quickly and efficiently without causing further lung damage. Until this can be done, the techniques discussed above should be employed while we continue to learn more about ARDS and how our interventions contribute to its pathology.[140]

■ REFERENCES

1. Arens R, Gozal D, Omlin KJ, et al: Comparison of high-frequency chest compression and conventional chest physiotherapy in hospitalized patients with cystic fibrosis. Am J Respir Crit Care Med 150(4):1154, 1994.
2. American Academy of Pediatrics, Committee on Infectious Diseases: Use of ribavirin in the treatment of respiratory syncytial virus infection. Pediatrics 92:502, 1993.
3. American Association for Respiratory Care: Clinical practice guideline: Postural drainage therapy. Respir Care 36(12):1418, 1991.
4. American Heart Association: Textbook of Advanced Cardiac Life Support. Dallas TX, American Heart Association, 1994.

5. American Heart Association: Textbook of Basic Life Support. Dallas TX, American Heart Association, 1994.
6. Anderson JB, Falk M: Chest physiotherapy in the pediatric age group. Respir Care 36(6):545, 1991.
7. Anzueto A, Baughman RP, Guntupalli KK, Weg JG, Wiedeman HP, Raventos AA: Aerosolized surfactant in adults with sepsis-induced acute respiratory distress syndrome. N Engl J Med 334(22):1417, 1996.
8. Arnold JH, Hanson JH, Toro-Figuero LO, Gutierrez J, Berens RJ, Anglin DL: Prospective, randomized comparison of high-frequency oscillatory ventilation and conventional mechanical ventilation in pediatric respiratory failure. Crit Care Med 22(10):1530, 1994.
9. Arnold JH, Truog RD, Thompson JE, Fackler JC: High frequency oscillatory ventilation in pediatric respiratory failure. Crit Care Med 21(2):272, 1993.
10. Azzawi M, Bradley B, Jeffery PK, et al: Identification of activated T lymphocytes and eosinophils in bronchial biopsies in stable atopic asthma. Am Rev Respir Dis 142:1407, 1990.
11. Ba M, Thiverge RL, Lapierre JG, et al: Effects of continuous inhalation of ralbuterol in acute asthma. Am Rev Respir Dis 135:A326, 1987.
12. Barry W, Cockburn F, Cornal R, Price JF, Sutherland G, Vasdag A: Ribavirin aerosol for acute bronchiolitis. Arch Disabled Child 61:593, 1986.
13. Bartlett RH, Gazzaniga AB, Toomasian J, Corwin AG, Roloff D, Rucker R: Extracorporeal membrane oxygenation (ECMO) in neonatal respiratory failure. Ann Surg 204(3):236, 1986.
14. Behera D, Jindal SK, Malik SK: Removal of foreign bodies in children [letter]. Chest 93(5):1116, 1988.
15. Bernard GR, Artigus A, Brigham KL, Carlet J, Falke K, Hudson L, Lamy M, et al, and the Concensus Committee: The American-European Consensus Conference on ARDS: Definitions, mechanisms, relevant outcomes, and clinical trial coordination. Am J Repir Crit Care Med 149:818,1994.
16. Blake KV, Hoppe M, Harmon E, et al: Relative amount of albuterol delivered to lung receptors from a metered-dose inhaler and sebulizer solution: Bioassay by histamine bronchoprovocation. Chest 101:309, 1992.
17. Bohn DJ, Biggar WD, Smith CR, Conn AW, Barker GA: Influence of hypothermia, barbiturate therapy, and intracranial pressure monitoring on morbidity and mortality after near-drowning. Crit Care Med 14(6):529, 1986.
18. Bolek JE: Variations of positive expiratory pressure [abstract]. Pediatr Pulmonol Suppl 9:93, 1993.
19. Bower LK, Betit P: Extracorporeal life support and high-frequency oscillatory ventilation: Alternatives for the neonate in severe respiratory failure. Respir Care 40(1):61, 1995.
20. Bowton DL, Kong DL: High tidal volume ventilation produces increased lung water in oleic acid-injured rabbit lungs. Crit Care Med 17(9):908, 1989.
21. Branson RD, Chatburn RL: Humidification of inspired gases during mechanical ventilation. Respir Care 38(5):461, 1993.
22. Brooks LJ, Cropp GJ: Theophylline therapy in bronchiolitis. Am J Disabled Child 135:934, 1981.
23. Calcone A, Wolkove N, Stern E, et al: Continuous nebulization of albuterol in acute asthma. Chest 97:693, 1990.
24. Cefaratt JL, Steinberg EA: An alternative method for delivery of ribavirin to nonventilated pediatric patients. Respir Care 37(8):877, 1992.
25. Chatburn RL: Principles and practice of neonatal and pediatric mechanical ventilation. Respir Care 36(6):569, 1991.
26. Chou KJ, Cunningham SJ, Crain EF: Metered dose inhalers with spacers versus nebulizers for pediatric asthma. Arch Pediatr Adolesc Med 149(2):201, 1995.
27. Clark RH, Null DM: High-frequncy oscillatory ventilation. In Pomerance JJ, Richardson CJ (eds): Neonatology for the Clinician. East Norwalk, CT, Appleton and Lange, 1993.
28. Connors AF, Hommon WE, Martin RJ, Rogers RM: Chest physical therapy: The immediate effect on oxygenation in acutely ill patients. Chest 78:559, 1980.
29. Cressman WR, Myer CM: Diagnosis and management of croup and epiglottitis. Pediatr Clin North Am 41(2):265, 1994.
30. Cunningham JC, Taussig LM: What is cystic fibrosis? In An Introduction to Cystic Fibrosis for Patients and Families. Bethesda, MD, Cystic Fibrosis Foundation, 1991.

31. Cystic Fibrosis Foundation Data Registry Report for 1989. Bethesda, MD, Cystic Fibrosis Foundation, 1990.
32. Dantzker DR: Obstructive lung disease. In Dantzker DR, MacIntyre NR, Bakow ED (eds): Comprehensive Respiratory Care. Philadelphia, WB Saunders, 1995.
33. Davis PB (ed): Cystic Fibrosis. New York, Marcel Dekker, 1993.
34. DeBruin W, Notterman DA, Magid M, Godwin T, Johnston S: Acute hypoxemic respiratory failure in infants and children: Clinical and pathologic characteristics. Crit Care Med 20(9):1223, 1992.
35. DeNicola LK, Monem GF, Gale MO, Kissroon N: Treatment of critical status asthmaticus in children. Pediatr Clin North Am 41(6):1293, 1994.
36. Desmond K, Schwerk F, Thomas E, Beaudry P, Coates A: Immediate and long-term effects of chest physiotherapy in patients with cystic fibrosis. J Pediatr 103:538, 1983.
37. Donohue T: Ambulatory care of the adult asthma patient. In Kussin PS, MacIntyre N (eds): Adult asthma. Respir Clin North Am 1(2):193, 1995.
38. Dreyfuss D, Basset G, Soler P, Saumon G: Intermittent positive pressure hyperventilation with high inflation pressures produces pulmonary microvascular injury in rats. Am Rev Respir Dis 132(4):880, 1985.
39. Dreyfuss D, Soler P, Basset G, Saumon G: High inflation pressure pulmonary edema: Respective effects of high airway pressure, high tidal volume, and positive end-expiratory pressure. Am Rev Respir Dis 137(5):1159, 1988.
40. Eid N, Buchheit J, Neuling M, Phelps H: Chest physiotherapy in review. Respir Care 36(4):270, 1991.
41. Faix RG, Viscardi RM, DiPietro MA, Nicks JJ: Adult respiratory distress syndrome in full-term newborns. Pediatrics 83(6):97, 1989.
42. Fan LL, Sparks LM, Fix EJ: Flexible fiberoptic endoscopy for airway problems in a pediatric intensive care unit. Chest 93(3):556, 1988.
43. Fawcett DD: Inhaled anti-inflammatory agents in childhood asthma: Theory and practice. Respir Care 40(1):108, 1995.
44. Fitzgerald D, Mellis C, Johnson M, Allen H, Cooper P, Van Asperen P: Nebulized budesonide is as effective as nebulized adrenaline in moderately severe croup. Pediatrics 97(5):722, 1996.
45. Foy HM: Infections caused by Mycoplasma pneumonia and possible carrier state in different populations of patients. Clin Infect Dis 17(Suppl 1):537, 1993.
46. Gattinoni L, Pesenti A, Avalli L, Rossi F, Bambino M: Pressure-volume curve of total respiratory system in acute respiratory failure: Computed tomographic scan study. Am Rev Respir Dis 136(3):730, 1987.
47. Green CG: Assessment of the pediatric airway by flexible bronchoscopy. Respir Care 36(6):555, 1991.
48. Green CG, Eisenberg J, Leong AM, Nathanson I, Schnapf BM, Wood RE: Flexible endoscopy of the pediatric airway. Am Rev Respir Dis 145(1):233, 1992.
49. Green J: Recognizing epiglottitis: How to identify and respond to this pediatric crisis. Nursing 8:33, 1992.
50. Greenspan JS: Physiology and clinical role of liquid ventilation therapy. J Perinatol 16(2) (Part 2):547, 1996.
51. Groothuis JR, Gutierrez KM, Lauer BA: Respiratory syncytial virus infection in children with dysplasia. Pediatrics 82:199, 1988.
52. Groothius JR, Simoes EA, Levin MJ, et al: Prophylactic administration of respiratory syncytial virus immune globulin to high-risk infants and young children. N Engl J Med 329:1524, 1993.
53. Guzzetta PC, Anderson KD, Eichelberger MR, et al: General surgery. In Avery GB, Fletcher MA, MacDonald MG (eds): Neonatology: Pathophysiology and Management of the Newborn, 4th ed. Philadelphia, JB Lippincott, 1994.
54. Haas CF, Weg JG: Exogenous surfactant therapy: An update. Respir Care 41(5):397, 1996.
55. Hall CB: Respiratory syncytial virus: What we know now. Contemp Pediatr Nov:1, 1993.
56. Hall CB, McBride JT, Gala CL, Hildreth SW, Schnabel KC: Ribavirin treatment of respiratory syncytial viral infection in infants with underlying cardiopulmonary disease. JAMA 254(21):3047, 1985.
57. Hardy KA: Advances in our understanding and care for patients with cystic fibrosis. Respir Care 38(3):282, 1993.
58. Hardy KA: A review of airway clearance: New techniques, indications, and recommendations. Respir Care 39(5):440, 1994.

59. Hemming VG, Prince GA, Groothuis JR, Siber GR: Hyperimmune globulins in prevention and treatment of respiratory syncytial virus infections. Clin Microbiol Rev 8(1):22, 1995.
60. Hen J: Current management of upper airway obstruction. Pediatr Annual 15(4):276, 1986.
61. Herridge MS, Slutsky AS: High-frequency ventilation: A ventilatory technique that merits revisiting. Respir Care 41(5):385, 1996.
62. Hess D: Aerosol therapy. In Kussin PS, MacIntyre N (eds): Adult asthma. Respir Clin North Am 1(2):235, 1995.
63. Hess D, Bigatello L, Kacmarek RM, Ritz R, Head CA, Hurford WE: Use of inhaled nitric oxide in patients with acute respiratory distress syndrome. Respir Care 41(5):424, 1996.
64. Hess DR, Kacmarek RM: Asthma. In Essentials of Mechanical Ventilation. New York, McGraw-Hill, 1996.
65. Heulitt MJ, Anders M, Benham O: Acute respiratory distress syndrome in pediatric patients: Redirecting therapy to reduce iatrogenic lung injury. Respir Care 40(1):74, 1995.
66. Hickling KG, Walsh J, Henderson S, Jackson R: Low mortality rate in adult respiratory distress syndrome using low-volume, pressure-limited ventilation with permissive hypercapnia: A prospective study. Crit Care Med 22(10):1568, 1994.
67. Hirschl RB: Laboratory and clinical experience with liquid ventilation in respiratory failure. Respir Care 41(6):529, 1996.
68. Hoffman JI: Lung disease in children. In Rudolph AM, Hoffman JI, Axelrod S (eds): Pediatrics. Norwalk, CT, Appleton and Lange, 1987.
69. Hubbarb RC, McElvaney NG, Birrer P, et al: A preliminary study of aerosolized recombinant human deoxyribonuclease I in the treatment of cystic fibrosis. N Engl J Med 326(12):812, 1992.
70. Hughes DM, Lesouef PN, Landau LI: Effect of salbutamol on respiratory mechanics in bronchiolitis. Pediatr Research 22(1):83, 1987.
71. Hurst JM, Branson RD: Liquid breathing—partial liquid ventilation. Respir Care 41(5):416, 1996.
72. Husby S, Agertoft L, Mortensen S, Pedersen S: Treatment of croup with nebulized steroid (budesonide): A double blind, placebo-controlled study. Arch Disabled Child 68(3):352, 1993.
73. Interiano B, Guntupalli KK: Metered-dose inhalers: Do health care providers know what to teach? Arch Intern Med 153:81, 1993.
74. Jenkinson SG: Lung transplantation: An update. Respir Care 38(3):278, 1993.
75. Jew LL, Hart L: Inhaled aminoglycosides in cystic fibrosis. DICP, Annals Pharmacother 24:711, 1990.
76. Kacmarek RM: Ribavirin and pentamidine aerosols: Caregiver beware! (Editorial). Respir Care 35:1034, 1990.
77. Kacmarek RM, Hickling KG: Permissive hypercapnia. Respir Care 38(4):373, 1993.
78. Kattan M, Keens TG, Lapierre JG, Levison H, Bryan AC, Reilly BJ: Pulmonary function abnormalities in sympton-free children after bronchiolitis. Pediatrics 59(5):638, 1977.
79. Kelley PB, Simon JE: Racemic epinephrine use in croup and disposition. Am J Emerg Med 10(3):181, 1992.
80. Brooks J: Acute bronchiolitis. In Kempe H, Silver H, O'Brien D, Fulginiti V (eds): Current Pediatric Diagnosis and Treatment. Norwalk, CT, Appleton and Lange, 1987.
81. Kerem B, Rommers JM, Buchanan et al: Identification of cystic fibrosis gene: Genetic analysis. Science 245:1073, 1989.
82. Kiiski R, Rakala J, Kari A, Emili J: Effect of tidal volume on gas exchange and oxygen transport in the adult respiratory distress syndrome. Am Rev Respir Dis 146:1131, 1992.
83. Kinsella JP, Abman SH: Clinical approaches to the use of high-frequency oscillatory ventilation in neonatal respiratory failure. J Perinatol 16(2) (Part 2):552, 1996.
84. Kinsella JP, Abman SH: Clinical pathophysiology of persistent pulmonary hypertension of the newborn and the role of inhaled nitric oxide therapy. J Perinatol 16(2) (Part 2):524, 1996.
85. Klassen TP, Feldman ME, Watters LK, Sutcliffe T, Rowe PC: Nebulized budesonide for children with mild-to-moderate croup. New Engl J Med 331(5):285, 1994.
86. Klassen TP, Rowe PC, Sutcliffe T, Ropp LJ, McDowell IW, Li MM: Randomized trial of salbutamol in acute bronchiolitis. J Pediatr 1188(5):807, 1991.

87. Klinger KW: Genetics of cystic fibrosis. Semin Respir Med 6:233, 1985.
88. Knowels MR, Church NL, Waltner WE, et al: A pilot study of aerosolized amiloride for the treatment of lung disease in cystic fibrosis. N Engl J Med 322:1189, 1990.
89. Kunkel NC, Baker MD: Use of racemic epinephrine, dexumethasone, and mist in outpatient management of croup. Pediatr Emerg Care 12(3):156, 1996.
90. Kussin PS: Pathophysiology and management of life-threatening asthma. In Kussin PS, MacIntyre N (eds): Adult asthma. Respir Clin North Am 1(2):177, 1995.
91. Kussin PS, Fulkerson WJ: The rising tide of asthma. In Kussin PS, MacIntyre N (eds): Adult asthma. Respir Clin North Am 1(2):163, 1995.
92. Larsen GL: Asthma in children. New Engl J Med 326(23):1540, 1992.
93. Leatherman J, Ravenscraft SA, Iber C, Clemenson S, Davies S: High peak inflation pressures do not predict basotrauma during mechanical ventilation of status asthma [abstract]. Am Rev Respir Dis 139:A154, 1989.
94. Ledwith CA, Shea LM, Mauro RD. Safety and efficacy of nebulized racemic epinephrine in conjunction with oral dexamethasone and mist in the outpatient treatment of croup. Ann Emerg Med 25(3):331, 1995.
95. Lee PC, Helsmoortel CM, Cohn SM, Firk MP: Are low tidal volumes safe? Chest 97(27):430, 1990.
96. Lenney W, Milner AD: Alpha and beta adrenergic stimulants in bronchiolitis and wheezy bronchitis in children under 18 months of age. Arch Dis Child 53:532, 1978.
97. Lenney W, Milner AD: At what age do bronchodilator drugs work? Arch Dis Child 53:532, 1978.
98. Lewis J, Ikegami M, Tabor B, Jobe A, Absolom D: Aerosolized surfactant is preferentially deposited in normal versus injured regions of lung in a heterogenous lung injury model [abstract]. Am Rev Respir Dis 145(4, Part 2): A184, 1992.
99. Lewis RM: Chest physical therapy: Time for a redefinition and a renaming [editorial]. Respir Care 37(5):419, 1992.
100. Levin DL, Morriss FC, Roro LO, Brink LW, Turner GR: Drowning and near-drowning. Pediatr Clin North Am 40(2):321, 1993.
101. Littlewood JM, Smye SW, Cunliffe H: Aerosol antibiotic treatment in cystic fibrosis. Arch Dis Child 68:788, 1993.
102. Mahlmeister MJ, Fink JB, Hoffman GL, Fifer LF: Positive-expiratory-pressure mask therapy: Theoretical and practical considerations and a review of the literature. Respir Care 36(11):1218, 1991.
103. Mallol J, Burrueto L, Girardi G, et al: Use of nebulized bronchodilators in infants under 1 year of age: Analysis of four forms of therapy. Pediatr Pulmonol 3:298, 1987.
104. Manning HL: Peak airway pressure: Why the fuss? Chest 105:242, 1994.
105. Matsuba K, Thurlbeck WM: A morphometric study of bronchial and bronchiolar walls in children. Am Rev Respir Dis 105:908, 1972.
106. McDonald NE, Hall CB, Suffin SC, et al: Respiratory syncytial viral infection in infants with congenital heart disease. N Engl J Med 307:397, 1982.
107. McDougal J: Chest physiotherapy how-to booklet. Birmingham AL, Children's Hospital of Alabama, 1991.
108. Meert KL, Sarnaik AP, Gelmini MJ, et al: Aerosolized ribavirin in mechanically ventilated infants with respiratory syncytial virus lower respiratory tract disease. Crit Care Med 22:566, 1994.
109. Michael BC: Antibacterial therapy in cystic fibrosis. Chest 94(Suppl. 2):129s, 1994.
110. Modell JH: Treatment of near-drowning: Is there a role for HYPER therapy (editorial). Crit Care Med 14(6):593, 1986.
111. Moe EL, Eisenber JO, Vallmer WM, Wall MA, Steners FJ, Hollis JF: Implementation of "Open Airways" as an educational intervention for children with asthma in an HMO. J Pediatr Health Care 6(5):251, 1992.
112. Moler FW, Hurwitz ME, Custer JR: Improvement in clinical asthma score and $PaCO_2$ in children with severe asthma treated with continuously nebulized terbutaline. J Allergy Clin Immunol 81(6):1101, 1988.
113. Moler FW, Khan AS, Meliones JN, et al: Respiratory syncytial virus morbidity and mortality estimates in congenital heart disease patients: A recent experience. Crit Care Med 20:1406, 1992.
114. Morgan WJ, Martinez FD: Risk factors for developing wheezing and asthma in childhood. Pediatr Clin North Am 39(6):1185, 1992.
115. Mortensen J, Falk M, Groth S, Jensen C: The effects of postural drainage and positive expiratory pressure physiotherapy on tracheobronchial clearance in cystic fibrosis. Chest 100(5):1350, 1991.

116. Motoyama EK, Fort MD, Kelsh KW, Mutich RL, Guthrie RD: Early onset of airway reactivity in premature infants with bronchopulmonary dysplasia. Am Rev Respir Dis 136:50, 1987.

117. National Institutes of Health: Executive summary: Guidelines for the diagnosis and management of asthma. Publication No. 91-3042A; June 1991.

118. Nemiroff MJ: Near-drowning. Respir Care 37(6):600, 1992.

119. Nichter MA, Everett PB: Childhood near drowning: Is cardiopulmonary resuscitation always indicated? Crit Care Med 17(10):993, 1989.

120. Oberwaldner B, Evans JC, Zach MS: Forced expirations against a variable resistance: A new chest physiotherapy method in cystic fibrosis. Pediatr Pulmonol 2(6):358, 1986.

121. Orenstein DM: Cystic fibrosis. Respir Care 36(7):746, 1991.

122. O'Rourke PP: ECMO: Where have we been? Where are we going? Respir Care 36(7):683, 1991.

123. Outwater KM, Crone RK: Management of respiratory failure in infants with acute viral bronchiolitis. Am J Dis Child 138:1071, 1984.

124. Papo MC, Frank J, Thompson AE: A prospective, randomized study of continuous versus intermittent nebulized albuterol for severe status asthmaticus in children. Crit Care Med 21:1479, 1993.

125. Predergast M, Jones JS, Hartman D: Racemic epinephrine in the treatment of laryngotracheitis: Can we identify children for outpatient therapy? Am J Emerg Med 12(6):613, 1994.

126. Pryor JA, Webber BA, Hodson ME: Effect of chest physiotherapy on oxygen saturation with cystic fibrosis. Thorax 45(1):77, 1990.

127. Pulland CR, Hey EN: Wheezing, asthma, and pulmonary dysfunction 10 years after infection with respiratory syncytial virus in infancy. Br Med J 284:1665, 1982.

128. Radford M: Effect of salbutamol in infants with wheezy bronchitis. Arch Dis Child 50:535, 1975.

129. Ramsey BW: The Pulmozyme (rnDNase) Study Group. A summary of the results of phase III multicenter clinical trial. Aerosol administration of recombinant human DNase reduces the risk of respiratory tract infections and improves pulmonary function in patients with cystic fibrosis. Pediatr Pulmonol 9:152, 1993.

130. Ramsey BW, Darkin HL, Eisenberg JD, et al: Efficacy of aerosolized tobramycin in patients with cystic fibrosis. N Engl J Med 328(24):1740, 1993.

131. Rau JL: Delivery of aerosolized drugs to neonatal and pediatric patients. Respir Care 36(6):514, 1991.

132. Rau JL: Humidity and aerosol therapy. In Barnes TA (ed): Core Textbook of Respiratory Care Practice, 2nd ed. St. Louis, Mosby–Year Book, 1994.

133. Rau JL: Respiratory Care Pharmacology, 4th ed. St. Louis, Mosby–Year Book, 1994.

134. Reijonen T, Korppi M, Pitkakangas S, Tenhola S, Remes K: The clinical efficacy of nebulized racemic epinephrine and albuterol in acute bronchiolitis. Arch Pediatr Adolesc Med 149(6):686, 1995.

135. Reisman J, Rivington-Law B, Corey M, et al: Role of conventional therapy in cystic fibrosis. J Pediatr 103:538, 1983.

136. Ring JC, Stidham GL: Novel therapies for acute respiratory failure. Pediatr Clin North Am 41(6):1325, 1994.

137. Roberts KB: Respiratory disorders. In Roberts KB (ed): Manual of Clinical Problems in Pediatrics, 2nd ed. Boston, Little, Brown, 1985.

138. Roberts KB: Upper airway obstruction accidents. In Roberts KB (ed): Manual of Clinical Problems in Pediatrics, 2nd ed. Boston, Little, Brown, 1985.

139. Rosenberg M, Ramsey B: Evolution of airway microbiology in infants with cystic fibrosis: Role of nonpseudomonal and pseudomonal pathogens. Semin Respir Infect 7(3):158, 1992.

140. Rosenstein BJ, Lanbaum TS, Gordes D, Brusilow SW: Cystic fibrosis: Problems encountered with sweat testing. JAMA 240:1987, 1978.

141. Ruppel G: Manual of Pulmonary Function Testing. St. Louis, CV Mosby, 1986.

142. Rutter N, Milner AD, Hiller EJ: Effect of bronchodilators on respiratory resistance in infants and young children with bronchiolitis and wheezing bronchitis. Arch Dis Child 50:719, 1975.

143. Salmon B, Wilson NM, Silverman M: How much aerosol reaches the lungs of wheezy infants and toddlers? Arch Dis Child 65:401, 1990.

144. Sanchez I, De Koster J, Powell RE, Wolstein R, Chernick V: Effect of racemic epinephrine and salbutamol on clinical score and pulmonary mechanics in infants with bronchiolitis. J Pediatr 122(1):145, 1993.

145. Sarnaik AP, Lieh-Lai M: Adult respiratory distress syndrome in children. Pediatr Clin North Am 41(2):337, 1994.
146. Schellhose DE, Graham LM, Fix EJ, Spark LM, Fan LL: Diagnosis of tracheal injury in mechanically ventilated premature infants by flexible bronchoscopy. Chest 98(5):1219, 1990.
147. Schellhose DE, Leland LF: Flexible endoscopy in the diagnosis and management of neonatal and pediatric airway and pulmonary disorders. Respir Care 40(1):48, 1995.
148. Schena JA, Crone RK, Thompson JE: The use of aminophylline in severe bronchiolitis. Crit Care Med 12:225, 1984.
149. Schuh S, Johnson D, Canny G, et al: Efficacy of adding nebulized ipratropium bromide to nebulized albuterol therapy in acute bronchiolitis. Pediatrics 90(6):920, 1992.
150. Schuh S, Reider MJ, Canny G, et al: Nebulized albuterol in acute childhood asthma: Comparison of two doses. Pediatrics 86(4):509, 1990.
151. Sessler DI: Objections to humidification editorial (letter). Respir Care 38(10):1113, 1993.
152. Silverman M: Bronchodilators for wheezy infants? Arch Dis Child 59:84, 1984.
153. Skolnik N: Croup. J Fam Pract 37(2):165, 1993.
154. Skoner D, Caliguiri L: The wheezing infant. Pediatr Clin North Am 35:1011, 1988.
155. Smith AL, Ramsey BW, Hedges DL, et al: Safety of aerosol tobramycin administration for 3 months to patients with cystic fibrosis. Pediatr Pulmonol 7:265, 1989.
156. Smith DW, Frankel LR, Mathers LH, et al: A controlled trial of aerosolized ribavirin in infants receiving mechanical ventilation for severe respiratory syncytial virus infection. New Engl J Med 325:24, 1991.
157. Stapleton T: Chest physiotherapy in primary pneumonia [letter]. Br Med J 291:143, 1985.
158. Stokes GM, Milner AD, Hodges GC, Henry RL, Elpinick MC: Nebulized therapy in acute severe bronchiolitis in infancy. Arch Dis Child 58:279, 1983.
159. Stoloff SW: The changing role of theophylline in pediatric asthma. Am Fam Physician 49(4):839, 1994.
160. Stone CS: Respiratory disorders. In Pediatric Nurse Practitioner Certification Review Guide. Potomac, MD, Health Leadership Associates, 1994.
161. Stretton M, Newth CJ: Patient education guide: What to do when your child has croup. J Respir Dis 16(2):217, 1995.
162. Stutman HR, Marks MI: Pulmonary infections in children with cystic fibrosis. Review. Semin Respir Infect 2(3):166, 1987.
163. Sullivan LM, Kacmarek RM: Arrest following a prolonged course of periodic coughing and fever in a child. Respir Care 38(10):1103, 1993.
164. Taber LH, Knight V, Gilbert BE, et al: Ribavirin aerosol treatment of bronchiolitis associated with respiratory syncytial virus infection in infants. Pediatrics 72(5):613, 1983.
165. Tabers Medical Dictionary, 17th ed. Philadelphia, FA Davis, 1993.
166. Tapson VF, Kussin PS: Respiratory tract infections. In Dantzker DR, MacIntyre NR, Bakow ED (eds): Comprehensive Respiratory Care. Philadelphia, WB Saunders, 1995.
167. Taylor WR, Newacheck PW: Impact of childhood asthma on health. Pediatrics 90:657, 1992.
168. Tepper RS: Airway reactivity in infants: A positive response to methacholine and metaproterenol. J Appl Physiology 62:1155, 1987.
169. Tepper RS, Rosenberg D, Eigen H, and Reister T: Bronchodilators responsiveness in infants with bronchiolitis. Pediatr Pulmonol 17:81, 1994.
170. Thomas DO: Near-drowning. In Quick Reference to Pediatric Emergency Nursing. Gaithersburg, MD, Aspen, 1991.
171. Thomas NJ, Webb SA, Smith J, Tecklenburg FW, Habib AM: The use of exogenous surfactant in three pediatric patients following gastric aspiration. Respir Care 39(9):912, 1994.
172. Tizzano EF, Buchwald M: Recent advances in cystic fibrosis research. J Pediatr 122(6):985, 1993.
173. Valdepena HG, Wald ER, Rose E, Ungkanont K, Casselbrant MC: Epiglottitis and Haemophilus influenzae immunization: The Pittsburgh experience—a five-year review. Pediatrics 96(3):424, 1995.
174. Walker TA, Khurana S, Tilden SJ. Viral respiratory infections. Pediatr Clin North Am 41(6):1365, 1994.
175. Wardlaw AJ, Dunnette S, Gleich GJ, Collins JV, Kay AB: Eosinophils and mast cells in bronchoalveolar lavage in subjects with mild asthma: Relationship to bronchial hyperreactivity. Am Rev Respir Dis 137:162, 1988.

176. West KW, Grosfeld JL: Surgical disorders. In Pomerance JJ, Richerdson CJ (eds): Neonatology for the Clinician. East Norwalk, CT, Appleton and Lange, 1993.
177. Whitman J, Van Beusekon R, Olson S, Worm M, Indihar F: Preliminary evaluation of high-frequency chest compression for secretion clearance in mechanically ventilated patients. Respir Care 38(9):1081, 1993.
178. Wiedemann H, Gaughman R, deBoisblanc B, Schuster D, Caldwell E, Weg J, et al: A multi-center trial in human sepsis-induced ARDS of an aerosolized synthetic surfactant (Exosurf) [abstract]. Am Rev Respir Dis 145(4, Part 2):A184, 1992.
179. Wilmott RW, Fiedler MA: Recent advances in the treatment of cystic fibrosis. Pediatr Clin North Am 41(3):431, 1994.
180. Wood RE: Treatment of cystic fibrosis lung disease in the first two years. Pediatr Pulmonol 68s, 1989.
181. Wood RE, Sherman JM: The airways. In Carlo WA, Chatburn RL (eds): Neonatal Respiratory Care, 2nd ed. Chicago, Mosby–Year Book, 1988.
182. Zander J, Hazinski MF: Pulmonary disorders. In Hazinski MF (ed): Nursing Care of the Critically Ill Child, 2nd ed. Chicago, Mosby–Year Book, 1992.
183. Zucker AR, Meadow ML: Pediatric critical care physicians' attitudes about guidelines for the use of ribavirin in critically ill children with respiratory syncytial virus pneumonia. Crit Care Med 23(4):767, 1995.

■SELF-ASSESSMENT QUESTIONS

1. Identify which medications are necessary for the treatment of the early phase of an asthma attack and which are necessary for treatment or prevention of the late phase. Why are these medications used in this manner?

2. Identify at least three ways in which the respiratory care practitioner can educate the pediatric asthma patient on how to better manage the disorder.

3. Identify at least three therapies that have helped to increase the life expectancy of the cystic fibrosis patient.

4. What techniques may be employed to prevent the child who is status asthmaticus from requiring mechanical ventilation?

5. Is a trial of inhaled bronchodilator therapy warranted in the infant who is wheezing and has a positive RSV culture? Why?

6. Identify clinical signs and symptoms that may help in distinguishing between foreign body aspiration and croup.

7. Identify three possible causes of tracheomalacia and describe the most common therapy for this disorder.

8. What factors are predictive of mortality in the near-drowning victim?

9. Describe the difference between acute lung injury (ALI) and acute respiratory distress syndrome (ARDS).

10. State specific techniques that should be employed when providing conventional mechanical ventilation to the pediatric ARDS patient. Why should such a strategy be used?

Chapter 11

Congenital Cardiovascular Disorders

ROBERT R. FLUCK, JR.

OBJECTIVES

Having completed this chapter, the reader will be able to:

1 Describe the etiology, pathophysiology (including hemodynamic derangements), clinical presentation (including methods of diagnosis), management, and complications of the following congenital cardiovascular disorders:

persistent pulmonary hypertension

patent ductus arteriosus

ventricular septal defect

atrial septal defect

tetralogy of Fallot

transposition of the great vessels

total anomalous pulmonary venous return

coarctation of the aorta

hypoplastic left heart syndrome

truncus arteriosus

tricuspid atresia

aortic stenosis

Eisenmenger syndrome

KEY TERMS

acyanotic heart disease
cyanotic heart disease
patent ductus arteriosus
ostium secundum defect
tetralogy of Fallot

Blalock-Taussig shunt
Rashkind procedure
coarctation of the aorta
Norwood procedure
truncus arteriosus

▬ PERSISTENT PULMONARY HYPERTENSION

Persistent pulmonary hypertension (PPHN), formerly called persistent fetal circulation (PFC), is a syndrome characterized by severe hypoxemia and cyanosis. It occurs in about 1 in 1000 live births. Because of the failure of the pulmonary vascular resistance to fall normally at birth, pulmonary artery pressure remains high and right-to-left shunting through the ductus arteriosus and foramen ovale occurs.

Etiology

The smooth muscle cells in the pulmonary circulation of the full-term neonate are very reactive to hypoxia and hypercarbia. At birth, the physical effect of ventilation of the lung combines with the decreased partial pressure of carbon dioxide and increased partial pressure of oxygen to decrease pulmonary vascular resistance (PVR) below that of systemic vascular resistance. This process allows the transition to extrauterine circulation. PPHN develops when the drop in PVR does not occur. The elevated pressure in the pulmonary circulation is then maintained because the neonate has a greater potential than the adult in response to stress both to cause proliferation of smooth muscle cells in the tunica media and also to manufacture more protein, forming the matrix in the vessel walls. Additionally, return to the more normal vascular structure occurs much more slowly and perhaps incompletely in the neonate compared to the adult once the stress has been removed. Some investigators feel that this condition leaves some abnormality in the pulmonary vascular wall which makes the individual more susceptible to the development of pulmonary hypertension later in life.[1-5]

Those infants who develop PPHN frequently have Apgar scores of less than or equal to 5 at 1 and 5 minutes. About half have a history of perinatal asphyxia. Chronic intrauterine hypoxia may result in PPHN secondary to hypertrophy of the tunica media of pulmonary arteries combined with polycythemia. Increased hematocrit has been shown to increase PVR and thus decrease cardiac output.

Common precursors for PPHN include meconium aspiration syndrome; respiratory distress syndrome (RDS); pneumonia, especially that caused by group B streptococci; abnormalities of the pulmonary vascular bed such that pulmonary hypertension persists despite the correction of acidosis, hypoxia, hypercapnia, or lung inflammation (the group best described as having persistent fetal circulation); maternal receipt of prostaglandin synthesis inhibitors such as aspirin or indomethacin; and hypoplastic lungs, as in the case of congenital diaphragmatic hernia (CDH), in which both lungs are smaller than normal, yielding a decreased cross-sectional area of the pulmonary vascular bed. Anything else that results in hypoxia and hypoventilation, such as central nervous system disease, may also contribute to the development of PPHN.

Pathophysiology

The primary abnormality of PPHN is pulmonary hypertension such that pulmonary artery pressures exceed systemic arterial pressures, resulting in a right-to-left extracardiac shunt through the ductus arteriosus. Owing to the decrease in pulmonary circulation, there is a reversal of the normal atrial pressure gradient and, thus, intracardiac right-to-left shunting through the foramen ovale. The result is severe hypoxemia with cyanosis; there is normocapnia as long as alveolar ventilation can be maintained. Because of the right-to-left shunts, the hypoxemia is refractory to oxygen administration. Resolution occurs in days to weeks.

Clinical Manifestations

In a neonate presenting with refractory hypoxemia, the differential diagnosis includes pulmonary disease, congenital cardiac disease, and PPHN. The diagnosis is arrived at by eliminating possibilities in an orderly fashion (Table 11-1). The infant is first placed in an oxyhood with an FIO_2 of 1.0 for 10 minutes. If there is parenchymal lung disease causing ventilation/perfusion (V/Q) mismatch, the PaO_2 will be greater than 100 mm Hg. If the PaO_2 is *less than* 50 mm Hg, there most likely is a fixed right-to-left shunt, due either to PPHN or cyanotic congenital cardiac disease. In this case, the presence of ductal shunting should be confirmed by obtaining preductal (right radial or temporal artery) and postductal (umbilical artery) samples with the infant breathing 100% oxygen. A differential of *greater than* 15 mm Hg is considered indicative of ductal shunting. Of course, since the majority of infants with PPHN have ductal shunting, this does not confirm or deny PPHN.

Next in the differential diagnosis of PPHN is the hyperoxia–hyperventilation test. The infant is hyperventilated with a manual resuscitator with 100% oxygen. The therapist monitors the effectiveness of the ventilation via a pressure manometer, breath sounds, color, and the presence of good chest excursion. The $PaCO_2$ is maintained between 20 and 25 mm Hg (by use of arterial blood gases), a range which has been shown to yield maximal pulmonary vasodilation. If PPHN is the problem, the PaO_2 will generally rise to greater than 100 mm Hg. Transcutaneous oxygen and carbon dioxide monitoring is extremely useful in this circumstance, as sudden

---

TABLE 11-1 Differential Diagnosis of Persistent Pulmonary Hypertension (PPHN)

1. Perform hyperoxia test (place infant in 100% hood).

   a. PaO_2 > 100 mm Hg: parenchymal lung disease

   b. PaO_2 = 50 to 100 mm Hg: either parenchymal disease or cardiovascular disease

   c. PaO_2 < 50 mm Hg: fixed right to left shunt

2. If fixed right-to-left shunt is present or suspected, obtain preductal and postductal arterial samples.

   a. >15 mm Hg difference in PaO_2 values: ductal shunting

   b. <15 mm Hg difference in PaO_2 values: no ductal shunting

3. Perform hyperoxia–hyperventilation test: mechanically hyperventilate infant with 100% oxygen until $PaCO_2$ of 20 to 25 mm Hg is reached.

   a. PaO_2 100 mm Hg with hyperventilation: PPHN

   b. PaO_2 < 100 mm Hg with hyperventilation: R/O congenital heart disease with echocardiography or other diagnostic technique

      (1) Abnormal echo: congenital heart disease

      (2) Normal echo: probably PPHN

changes in the infant's condition can be detected immediately and the effectiveness of ventilation can be assessed constantly. In certain cases of congenital cardiac disease, particularly hypoplastic left heart syndrome, the infant's condition may rapidly worsen as blood flow, which comes almost exclusively from the right ventricle, is preferentially directed to the pulmonary circulation.

The typical infant with PPHN is full-term or post-term and presents, usually within the first 24 hours of life, with tachypnea, mild to moderate respiratory distress, and hypoxemia, with or without cyanosis, which is refractory to oxygen therapy. The chest x-ray film will usually be relatively normal, with perhaps decreased pulmonary vascular markings, thus ruling out active pulmonary disease. Signs of heart failure are infrequently present. Breath sounds will be normal. Heart sounds will be characterized by a holosystolic murmur. A right ventricular heave or systolic sternal lift may be present because of the increased right ventricular workload. Echocardiography will enable the team to rule out the existence of congenital cardiac disease.

Treatment

The primary goal in treatment of PPHN is reduction of PVR. Initially, the infant should remain in an oxyhood with 100% oxygen, as high FIO_2 will aid in pulmonary vasodilation. As with any neonate, maintenance of a neutral thermal environment will minimize oxygen consumption.

If RDS is the precipitating factor in PPHN, there are several means of treating the problem. Exogenous surfactant can be administered to reverse atelectasis and attendant alveolar hypoxia (see Chap. 23). Should assisted ventilation be necessary, several approaches are possible. Liquid ventilation eliminates surface tension by eliminating the air–liquid interface. That feature, combined with the relative incompressibility of liquid, provides very uniform ventilation. Partial liquid ventilation also is beneficial and simpler technically than liquid ventilation. The most recent development in partial liquid ventilation is perfluorocarbon-assisted gas exchange. High-frequency jet ventilation and high-frequency oscillation have been effective in increasing ventilation, lowering $PaCO_2$, and causing pulmonary vasodilation. Tracheal gas insufflation, the process of flushing the dead space in the large airways with the inspiratory gas mixture during exhalation to allow a reduction in the tidal volume and thus peak pressure, has recently shown promise.

Still somewhat experimental for support of the neonate with insufficient gas exchange is extracorporeal membrane oxygenation (ECMO), as discussed in Chapter 25. As it is very expensive and labor intensive, it is available at a limited number of centers. Considering the time for transport to a center offering ECMO, the decision to transfer care needs to be made in a timely fashion. ECMO offers better results than conventional therapy (mechanical ventilation), especially in cases of CDH or group B streptococcus sepsis. The ongoing concern with ECMO is that, in one series, 22% of the infants developed some sort of intracranial vascular abnormality.[6]

For conventional ventilation, the gold standard used to be the critical PCO_2, maintaining the $PaCO_2$ between 25 and 30 mm Hg and the pH at about 7.50. However, hyperventilation has never undergone controlled clinical trials. It may contribute to lung injury. Finally, there is an association between the requirement for prolonged hyperventilation and both sensorineural hearing loss and worsened developmental outcome.

The latest and most promising treatment for PPHN is nitric oxide (NO). While it is a selective pulmonary vasodilator, it is not effective in all cases, such as CDH. An improvement in oxygenation, however, does not necessarily predict recovery. There are several other considerations or concerns regarding administration of NO. The optimum dose has not yet been determined. NO by itself in sufficient concentration is toxic, requiring a system to scavenge the gas before it escapes into the air in the patient's room. In the presence of oxygen, NO oxidizes to nitrogen dioxide (NO_2). Thus, NO is shipped in nitrogen. NO_2 is a component of smog and is a pulmonary irritant. Since oxidation begins as soon as NO is exposed to oxygen, long transit times in ventilator circuits need to be avoided. Finally, NO oxidizes normal hemoglobin into methemoglobin. Consequently, the patient's methemoglobin levels must be monitored during treatment with NO.

General vasodilators have been tried in the past, most notably tolazoline (Priscoline). The major disadvantage of these nonselective vasodilators is that they also dilate the systemic vascular system, resulting in two problems: systemic hypotension and inability to facilitate the transition of the circulation to extrauterine existence. Thus, these drugs are seldom used.

CONGENITAL HEART DISEASE

Embryologically, the heart is structurally developed by 8 weeks of gestation. Congenital heart disease results from inadequate formation of specialized tissues during this time period. The etiology of these defects is not always clear and is probably multifactorial. Some defects may be familial in incidence, and some defects are more prominent in one gender than the other. Males, for example, are more likely to have coarctation of the aorta, aortic stenosis, and transposition of the great vessels; females are more prone to atrial septal defects and patent ductus arteriosus. Maternal diabetes and maternal rubella are associated with an increase in defects. Congenital cardiac disease may be part of the constellation of defects associated with a given chromosomal abnormality. For example, between 67% and 100% of patients with Marfan syndrome have associated cardiac anomalies (Abraham Lincoln had Marfan syndrome); nearly 50% of those with Trisomy 21 (Down syndrome) have congenital cardiac disease.

Certain signs and symptoms may lead to the suspicion of congenital cardiac disease. Cyanosis may be due to right-to-left shunting or secondary to left heart failure resulting in pulmonary edema. There may be a murmur, clubbing, and frequent respiratory infections. The infant may exhibit fatigue and exercise intolerance, which is manifest by feeding and sucking difficulties accompanied by cyanotic episodes. Failure to thrive or gain weight appropriate for age and gender may be a sign of left-to-right shunting.

Congenital cardiac diseases are generally categorized in one of two ways: (1) those resulting in left-to-right shunting (**acyanotic** diseases), in which blood is shunted from the left side to the right side of the heart, resulting in pulmonary congestion and increased left ventricular volume work; and (2) those resulting in right-to-left shunting, in which deoxygenated blood is shunted from the right side of the heart to the left side, resulting in severe hypoxemia and possibly cyanosis. Either of these types of shunts results in hemodynamic disturbances.

Four consequences of congenital heart disease affect the overall circulation. The first is volume overload, which occurs when more than the normal amount of blood enters the ventricle. The result is increased ventricular work, ventricular hypertrophy, and, if the overload is severe enough, ventricular failure. The second is pressure overload. When an obstruction to outflow of blood from a ventricle is present, there is also increased ventricular work, hypertrophy, and failure. The third possible consequence is desaturation secondary to a right-to-left shunt; this leads to insufficient tissue oxygenation and acidosis, both of which decrease the effectiveness of cardiac pumping. Last is decreased net cardiac output. While this may be the final result of any of the above three problems, it can also be a primary problem, as in hypoplastic left heart syndrome. Some defects may cause only one of these disturbances but others may lead to any combination.

■PATENT DUCTUS ARTERIOSUS

Etiology

The ductus arteriosus connects the pulmonary artery to the dorsal aorta, generally at the aortic isthmus, just distal to the left subclavian artery (Fig. 11-1). The ductus normally closes functionally by the end of the first day of life as a result of a combination of increased arterial oxygen tension and decreased prostaglandin levels; the effectiveness of these stimuli is modified by the amount of ductal muscle mass, which tends to be less in premature infants. If the ductus does not constrict when pulmonary artery pressure falls and systemic pressures increase, there will be a left-to-right shunt. Depending on the relationship between these two pressures, there may also be a small right-to-left or bidirectional shunt.

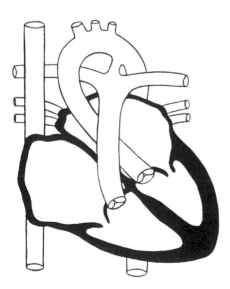

FIGURE 11-1 Patent ductus arteriosus. Note the persistence of the fetal channel connecting the descending aorta and the pulmonary artery.

Patent ductus arteriosus (PDA) may be present as an isolated defect or in combination with other congenital cardiac defects. As an isolated defect, it is found in 60% to 70% of infants born with congenital rubella. It is seen in just under 4% of all neonates with symptomatic cardiac disease, with a greater prevalence in females. PDA is also seen in hyaline membrane disease, prematurity, and infants born at high altitude; there is no gender difference among these groups.

Pathophysiology

The ductus arteriosus normally closes as a result of decreased prostaglandin levels and increased arterial oxygen tension; prostaglandin E_1 may be used in those situations in which patency is necessary to support systemic or pulmonary blood flow. Spontaneous closure may not be so effective in the premature infant with decreased muscle development in the ductus arteriosus; indomethacin, a prostaglandin inhibitor, may be effective in closing the ductus in this situation. A PDA in a term infant is generally not responsive to pharmacologic closure.

The magnitude of the shunt across the ductus depends on the size of the ductus. If the ductus is small, the shunt will have insignificant hemodynamic consequences. However, if the ductus is of moderate size, the volume of blood being shunted into the pulmonary circulation will be large enough to cause left ventricular volume overload, elevated left atrial pressure, pulmonary edema, and congestive heart failure (CHF).

The premature infant with the same magnitude of shunt may develop CHF sooner than the term infant. This is due to two problems: (1) incomplete development of the medial muscles in the pulmonary arteries, resulting in a lower PVR and, thus, more pulmonary blood flow; and (2) incomplete development of the myocardium which is, thus, less functional.

An infant with a large PDA will develop pulmonary hypertension because of the large volume of blood shunted into the pulmonary circulation as well as the direct transmission of systemic pressure into the pulmonary circulation through this large defect. The right ventricle will also fail as a result of the increased pulmonary artery pressure. Pulmonary vascular obstructive disease may develop subsequently in those infants with moderate to large PDAs.

Clinical Manifestations

A continuous murmur is usually not heard except in some small premature infants. There is, more commonly, a crescendo systolic murmur, often with clicks. S_2 may be difficult to hear. The infant with a large defect will have bounding pulses, a wide pulse pressure, and a hyperactive apex.

Additional signs and symptoms can include those of CHF, recurrent pulmonary infections, and failure to thrive. CHF may not develop in the term infant until weeks after birth, but may be manifest much sooner in the premature infant.

The chest x-ray film will show cardiac enlargement, left atrial enlargement, prominent pulmonary vessels, and a prominent main pulmonary artery. The electrocardiogram (EKG) will show left ventricular hypertrophy, sometimes left atrial hypertrophy, and ST and T wave changes if the failure is severe.

Echocardiography will show the ductus arteriosus and its size; color Doppler echocardiography will show the direction of flow across it and also disturbed pulmonary artery flow. In the presence of large defects, there will be left ventricular enlargement, left atrial enlargement, and right ventricular hypertension with resultant flattening of the interventricular septum.

Treatment

Medical treatment, where appropriate, may be the method of choice. There are two types of medical treatment available. Use of indomethacin in larger, less premature infants has been successful in about 85% of those cases. Failure of closure with indomethacin does not adversely affect subsequent surgical closure. Indomethacin would seem to be contraindicated in very small premature neonates as they have a much higher failure rate and also a much higher rate of complications, including intestinal perforation, renal failure, and bleeding. Percutaneous transcatheter ductal closure (PTDC) devices (Rashkind devices) are also gaining popularity. They seem to be most effective in vessels less than 5 mm in diameter. The use of PTDC devices results in more frequent recurrence of ductal patency than does surgical closure.

What some would consider the gold standard in treatment is surgical closure. This can take several forms. An open procedure, involving a left thoracotomy, can be performed either by simple ligation (at both ends and the middle) or division and ligation. The performance of the surgery without insertion of a chest tube represents an important improvement in open procedures. When the ductus is clamped, the normal hemodynamic changes are increased systemic pressure and decreased pulmonary artery pressure. If pulmonary artery pressure increases and systemic pressure decreases, this indicates that the shunt was right-to-left and surgical closure is contraindicated at this time. Video-assisted thoracoscopy, in which fiberoptic bundles and tools are passed through two 5-mm holes, is under development. Traditional ligation with or without division is associated with very low morbidity and mortality rates.

■ VENTRICULAR SEPTAL DEFECT

Ventricular septal defect (VSD) is the most common congenital cardiac defect (Fig. 11-2). It may be small or large, single or multiple, and occur as an isolated defect or in combination with other defects. It is most commonly found in the membranous portion of the interventricular septum. Although only 10% of VSDs cause symptoms, they are the most common cause of CHF after the second week of life.

Pathophysiology

The infant with a small VSD will be asymptomatic. With a larger defect, as PVR decreases after birth, a left-to-right shunt will develop which will cause both volume and pressure overload of the right ventricle. Most infants have sufficient decrease in PVR to become symptomatic by the second week of life, although others, possibly with delayed decrease of PVR, may not become symptomatic until 3 months of age. Premature infants will exhibit the clinical picture of CHF sooner than full-term infants

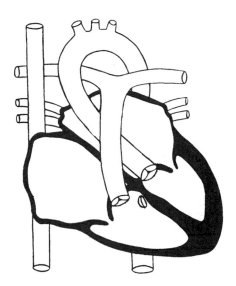

FIGURE 11-2 Ventricular septal defect. Note the opening in the wall between the right and left ventricles.

because the premature infant has less fully developed musculature in the pulmonary vascular bed.

The increased pulmonary blood flow causes an increase in the size of the pulmonary arteries and left atrium. The increased size of these structures predisposes the infant to mechanical obstruction of an airway and atelectasis. The infant has lower lung compliance and is, therefore, more susceptible to respiratory infections and respiratory distress. Because of the increased pressure load on the right ventricle, it will ultimately fail. If the symptomatic VSD is not corrected, the child may develop pulmonary vascular obstructive disease. It is possible for a VSD to become smaller or even close spontaneously, especially with small defects, thus alleviating symptoms.

Clinical Manifestations
The clinical picture of a VSD depends upon its size. A small defect will be associated with a harsh systolic murmur heard best at the lower left sternal border. The infant with the large defect will present with tachypnea (with a rate consistently >60/min), tachycardia, diaphoresis, decreased oral intake, fatigue with feeding, and perhaps a pulmonary infection.

The chest x-ray film will show cardiac enlargement, increased pulmonary blood flow, and possibly pulmonary edema. The EKG will show left and, in the picture of pulmonary hypertension, right ventricular hypertrophy. Echocardiography will confirm the diagnosis, showing not only size, location, and number of defects but associated and unsuspected defects such as PDA, coarctation of the aorta, left and right ventricular outflow tract obstruction, and atrial septal defect.

Treatment
The asymptomatic infant with a VSD usually requires no treatment but should be followed closely. Some infants with progressively increasing pulmonary vascular resistance will begin to show the picture of **tetralogy of**

Fallot as right ventricular hypertrophy develops. Any infant with EKG changes indicating right ventricular hypertrophy should be reevaluated. In infants who develop CHF, digoxin and diuretics are indicated; those who fail to do well on this regimen may respond to afterload reduction with angiotensin converting enzyme (ACE) inhibitors. Pulmonary infections should be treated appropriately with antibiotics, bronchodilators, and perhaps chest physical therapy and postural drainage. Repair or palliation should be effected in the infant who is refractory to maximal medical therapy as evidenced by failure to grow, repeated hospitalizations for pulmonary infection, or significantly elevated pulmonary artery pressure after 6 months of age.

Once it has been decided that the infant has failed conventional medical therapy, there are several possible surgical options. The most common, and most successful, for the single isolated VSD (not accompanied by another cardiac defect) is patching. Some authors would recommend patching for most of these types of VSDs as the mortality and morbidity are nearly zero for these uncomplicated cases. Morbidity and mortality increase when there are multiple septal defects; the surgeon needs to use a ventricular approach rather than the transatrial approach; or the VSD occurs with another cardiac defect, even an atrial septal defect, which is relatively benign by itself. Besides the traditional patching with Dacron patches, other approaches under investigation include umbrella closure, both transcutaneously as well as during surgery, and patching using biological glue instead of sutures.

■ ATRIAL SEPTAL DEFECT

There are several types of atrial septal defects (ASDs), depending on the source one uses. Virtually all neonates have a persistent foramen ovale (PFO), which closes functionally when the atrial pressure gradient reverses from the pressure on the right greater than on the left before birth to pressure on the left greater than on the right after birth. The foramen ovale is still able to be traversed by a catheter in a small percentage of adults (Fig. 11-3).

The **ostium secundum defect**, the most common form of ASD, is located high in the interatrial septum, in the vicinity of the FO. It rarely causes symptoms and is usually discovered during a workup for another defect or failure to thrive. It usually does not cause failure and can, thus, simply be observed until the child is older.

Defects of the endocardial cushion account for 4% of congenital cardiac defects; they can be partial, resulting in an ostium primum defect, or complete, causing a complete atrioventricular (AV) canal. The ostium primum defect is located low in the interatrial septum and is associated with a cleft medial (septal) mitral leaflet and consequent mitral regurgitation. The complete AV canal causes a connection among all four cardiac chambers with resultant chaotic mixing of the blood as it travels through the central circulation.

The sinus venosus defect is located high in the interatrial septum near the junction of the superior vena cava and is often associated with anomalous pulmonary venous drainage.

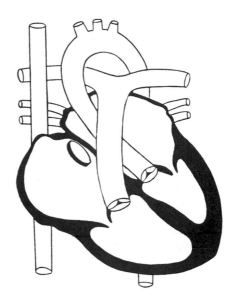

FIGURE 11-3 Atrial septal defect. Note the opening in the wall between the right and left atria.

Pathophysiology

The hemodynamics of an ASD depend on the type of defect, its size, and the presence of any associated defects. The PFO usually closes functionally shortly after birth and, therefore, is of no consequence. Many ostium secundum defects also close spontaneously within the first year of life, leading to a suspicion that they may simply have been misdiagnosed PFOs. The most serious hemodynamic consequences accompany endocardial cushion defects. In the ostium primum, there will usually be mitral regurgitation with its resultant increased left atrial pressure and subsequent pulmonary congestion. There can also be volume overload on the right heart due to a left-to-right shunt across the atrial septum or regurgitation from the left ventricle into the right atrium through the cleft mitral valve. The result can be severe CHF. In addition, streaming of blood from the inferior vena cava across the large, low defect can lead to arterial desaturation. The complete AV canal causes additional right ventricular and pulmonary hypertension due to left-to-right shunting through ventricular septal defects. Children with complete AV canals are prone to develop pulmonary vascular obstructive disease.

Clinical Manifestations

The symptomatic infant with an ostium primum defect frequently has significant mitral regurgitation. There may be failure to thrive and a history of multiple pulmonary infections. There may be mild cyanosis with complete AV canal. Auscultatory findings may include an S_1 obscured by a pansystolic murmur, an accentuated S_2, and a loud S_3. Infants with Down syndrome, paradoxically, may exhibit no auscultatory abnormalities. The chest x-ray film shows cardiac enlargement and prominent pulmonary vasculature, especially the main pulmonary artery. The EKG shows left-axis deviation. Echocardiography will show the anatomic features of the defects. Patients with complete AV canals may require cardiac catheterization to clearly delineate any associated lesions and determine the presence of elevated pulmonary vascular resistance.

Treatment
In patients who exhibit refractory CHF or pulmonary hypertension, surgical repair is the preferred treatment. In infants who are less than 2.5 to 3 kg or have other serious illness, pulmonary artery banding may provide sufficient palliation to allow repair to be postponed to a later time. With complete repair of an isolated primum defect, there is usually excellent prognosis. Without surgery, the prognosis is grim, with a 50% mortality rate of symptomatic infants by 1 year of age.

■TETRALOGY OF FALLOT
Tetralogy of Fallot (TOF) was the first cyanotic congenital cardiac defect described. It is characterized by a large VSD, pulmonary stenosis (either valvar, right ventricular infundibular, or both), right ventricular hypertrophy, and overriding or dextroposition of the aorta (Fig. 11-4). The result is a reduction in pulmonary blood flow with accompanying cyanosis. This defect comprises approximately 6% to 7% of all congenital cardiac defects and is the most common cyanotic congenital cardiac malformation. As with other defects, it may be present as an isolated defect or in combination with others including PDA, endocardial cushion defect, dextrocardia, and ASD. If it is combined with an ASD it is termed pentalogy of Fallot. The severity can range from an isolated, sometimes asymptomatic TOF in an otherwise healthy infant to multiple cardiac abnormalities combined with lethal noncardiac defects.

Pathophysiology
Pulmonary blood flow is determined by the severity of the right ventricular outflow tract obstruction, systemic vascular resistance, presence of

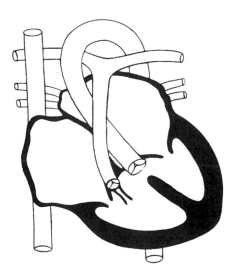

FIGURE 11-4 Tetralogy of Fallot. Note the large opening in the ventricular septum, the narrowing of the entrance to the pulmonary artery as it leaves the right ventricle, and the position of the aorta as it overrides the opening in the ventricular septal wall.

PDA, and possible presence of other collateral supply for the pulmonary circulation. Systemic and pulmonary pressures can be the same depending on the size of the VSD. The amount of right-to-left shunt depends directly on the severity of the pulmonary stenosis and inversely on the systemic vascular resistance.

The lesion of TOF is progressive; one fourth of individuals who have this condition are cyanotic at birth, three fourths are cyanotic by 1 year of age, and nearly all are cyanotic by age 20. Hypoxemia can be exacerbated by a hyperpneic spell (as during a temper tantrum), infundibular spasm, or closure of the ductus arteriosus. This results in decreased pulmonary blood flow and worsening metabolic acidosis for which the body cannot compensate owing to the insufficient pulmonary blood flow.

Clinical Manifestations

The usual presentation of the patient with TOF is with cyanosis and exertional dyspnea. Those infants with relatively mild pulmonary stenosis or extensive collateral circulation may develop CHF due to a left-to-right shunt. The chest x-ray film shows the apex of the heart tilted upward because of the hypertrophied right ventricle, yielding a "boot-shaped" heart. The EKG will nearly always show both right axis deviation and right ventricular hypertrophy. If both of these are not present, the clinician should consider major associated defects or alternative diagnoses. Echocardiography will show hypertrophy of the free wall of the right ventricle and the overriding aorta. Catheterization may show equal right and left ventricular pressures with normal pulmonary artery pressures. Angiography is helpful to determine the anatomy of the pulmonary vascular bed, including the site of stenosis, and to detect any systemic-to-pulmonary collaterals.

Treatment

There is some controversy over when to perform corrective surgery on infants with TOF. The momentum has been toward earlier operative intervention, driven by the need in some congenital defects to perform correction shortly after birth. In looking at the long-term picture, one must evaluate attrition rate while awaiting surgery, mortality after palliation, operative mortality, late hemodynamic result, and late mortality.

Some feel that the classic **Blalock-Taussig shunt**, an end-to-side anastomosis of the subclavian artery (usually on the right) to the pulmonary artery, or a 4- or 5-mm polytetrafluoroethylene (PTFE) graft, remains an appropriate procedure when pulmonary blood flow must be augmented, as in the case of critical pulmonic stenosis or atresia.[7] Others support two-stage repair (palliation initially followed by complete correction) in children who weigh less than 8 kg or are less than 12 months old.[8] The Waterston–Cooley shunt (between the ascending aorta and right pulmonary artery) and the Potts shunt (between the descending aorta and left pulmonary artery) have fallen into disuse, the Potts because it is difficult to "take down" (reverse) when total correction is performed.

Uva and colleagues feel that early repair is the preferred technique (defining early as less than 6 months).[9] That view is supported by Murphy et al., who list older age at time of surgery, previous heart failure, and a postoperative right ventricle to left ventricle systolic pressure ratio greater than 0.5 as significantly associated with higher rates of long-term mortality.[10] Starnes et al. feel that palliation has become controversial; they perform a complete repair for TOF at the time of presentation, regardless of the patient's age.[11] They cite Sullivan's data implicating increased time of uncorrected physiology as the cause of ventricular ectopy, both in the short term as well as the long term.[12] This ectopy is accepted as the primary cause of late deaths following repair of TOF.

Another controversy surrounds the location of the incision for repair of the VSD. Previously, a transventricular approach was used. However, Karl and colleagues support the transatrial approach, citing several studies which note a strong correlation between the occurrence of ventricular dysrhythmias and the size of the right ventricular incision.[13] Repair involves closing the VSD with a Dacron patch; extra tissue in the right ventricular outflow tract is excised and the pulmonary artery is enlarged with a pericardial patch as necessary.

Prior to surgical intervention, medical treatment addresses many factors. Oxygen can palliate hypoxia; morphine will reduce preload and thus myocardial oxygen demands; its sedation during a " spell" will further reduce myocardial work. Intravenous sodium bicarbonate will help treat metabolic acidosis. Prostaglandin E_1 may reopen the ductus arteriosus or maintain it in an open state and, thus, improve pulmonary blood flow. Phenylephrine may also be needed to increase systemic vascular resistance in order to improve pulmonary blood flow.

▀ TRANSPOSITION OF THE GREAT VESSELS

In transposition of the great vessels (TGV), the aorta arises from the right ventricle and the pulmonary artery from the left ventricle, yielding two parallel circulations instead of the normal series circulations (Fig. 11-5). The most common form of TGV is D-transposition, in which the aorta is anterior to the pulmonary artery instead of posterior to it. It is one of the

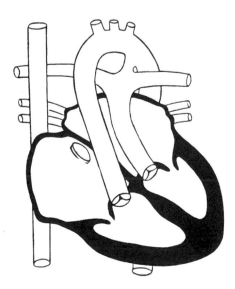

FIGURE 11-5 Transposition of the great vessels. Note the origin of the aorta in the right ventricle and the main pulmonary artery in the left ventricle, which is the reverse of normal. Also present are an atrial septal defect and a patent ductus arteriosus, which allow the pulmonary and systemic circulations to mix.

most common congenital cardiac defects and also a major cause of death in the newborn who does not undergo surgery. Prior to the development of balloon atrial septostomy and procedures for palliation and correction, 90% of infants with TGV died within the first year of life; mortality now stands around 10% with aggressive medical and surgical treatment.[14,15]

Pathophysiology

Oxygenated blood from the pulmonary veins makes a continuous circuit through the left atrium, left ventricle, pulmonary circulation, and back again, while deoxygenated blood circulates through the right atrium, right ventricle, aorta, systemic circulation, and back again to the right atrium. Without some form of communication between the two circulations (such as PDA, ASD, or VSD), there is no mixing of the blood and extrauterine existence is difficult and brief. The infant may initially present in little distress until the ductus arteriosus and foramen ovale close; then, cyanosis may become severe. The presence of a VSD may initially mask the problem until some time later when the VSD becomes smaller and causes cyanosis. The VSD will also cause both volume and pressure overload on the left ventricle, leading to CHF. It can also lead to pulmonary vascular obstructive disease with time.

Clinical Manifestations

In infants without a VSD, cyanosis with mild tachypnea will develop shortly after birth. Although cyanotic and tachypneic, the infant does not have other signs of respiratory distress, a condition sometimes called peaceful cyanosis. The EKG shows both right axis deviation and right ventricular hypertrophy. Since these two patterns are so consistently seen in this defect, their absence should cause one to search for associated anomalies or alternative diagnoses, such as single ventricle or straddling tricuspid valve. Echocardiography may be useful in demonstrating the switch in vessels. Cardiac catheterization is important for measuring pressures in both the vessels and chambers and also for clarifying the coronary artery anatomy; the presence of anomalous coronary arteries may preclude or at least decrease the chances of success of an arterial switch procedure. Catheterization will show right ventricular pressure at systemic levels. The pressure in the left ventricle will depend upon two factors—the size of the VSD and the presence of pulmonary stenosis. Left atrial pressure may be elevated, especially in the absence of an ASD.

One of the most important diagnostic tests is inhalation of 100% oxygen for a brief period of time. Failure of the arterial PO_2 to rise more than about 30 mm Hg is strong presumptive evidence of complete transposition; it highlights the inadequate mixing between the pulmonary and systemic circulations.

The chest x-ray film may initially be normal. In older children, it will show prominent pulmonary vascular markings and an enlarged "egg-shaped" heart. Other than cyanosis, the physical examination may be unremarkable, with murmurs variable and perhaps a loud second heart sound.

Treatment

A newborn diagnosed with TGV may need rapid treatment. Initial infusion of prostaglandin E_1 may help maintain an open ductus arteriosus until surgical intervention can be accomplished. The primary temporizing procedure is the Rashkind procedure, or balloon atrial septostomy (BAS), which is most useful in infants less than 3 months of age. A balloon-tipped catheter is passed through the inferior vena cava, right atrium, and foramen ovale into the left atrium. It is inflated with 3 to 5 mL of contrast medium and pulled forcibly back into the right atrium, rupturing the foramen ovale and allowing blood to flow from left to right atrium. In older children, a blade septostomy may be performed. A catheter with a retractable blade in its tip is passed through the foramen ovale. The blade is exposed and drawn back through the atrial septum, creating a linear incision which is then enlarged by BAS.

In those in whom the BAS is insufficient, the first level of surgery is the Blalock-Hanlon atrial septectomy. This improves mixing of the left and right sides, lowers left atrial pressure, and relieves pulmonary congestion. It is rarely used.

Total correction can be accomplished by three mechanisms, none of which is without complications. The first method of total correction involves an atrial switch procedure. In the Mustard procedure, a conduit is constructed of pericardium which ducts flow from the cavae and coronary sinus to the mitral valve and left ventricle and from there to the pulmonary artery. The blood from the pulmonary veins drains over this patch through the tricuspid valve into the right ventricle and is pumped into the systemic circulation. The Senning procedure accomplishes the same end using the remaining atrial septum to form the baffle. Long-term hazards of both of these procedures include caval obstruction and atrial dysrhythmias.

The second method of correction is the Rastelli procedure. In this operation, the main pulmonary artery is divided and the proximal end is oversewn; a Dacron graft is then sewn around the aortic valve. The other end of the graft is sewn to the VSD, making an internal channel to the aorta from the left ventricle. A right ventriculotomy is made and a Dacron tube is used to connect the right ventricle to the distal main pulmonary artery. Right ventricular performance may suffer, however, as a consequence of a lack of pulmonic valve.

The third method is a true correction, as it switches the output of the ventricles to the appropriate side. This is termed the arterial switch or Jatene procedure; its use is limited to those situations in which coronary artery anatomy is relatively normal.[16] The aorta and pulmonary artery are divided. The aorta is rotated forward and the proximal pulmonary artery (which is arising from the left ventricle) is sewn to the distal aorta. The coronary arteries are reimplanted in the pulmonary artery; the "holes" left in the aorta are repaired. The proximal aorta (arising from the right ventricle) is anastomosed to the distal pulmonary artery. This procedure normalizes ventricular function, returning the high-pressure pumping to the left ventricle and avoiding problems of right ventricular failure seen with the atrial switch surgeries. It should be performed relatively soon after birth, as the left ventricle loses its ability to generate systemic pressures quickly as the pulmonary vascular resistance and pulmonary artery pressure fall. However, pulmonary artery stenosis may develop later, especially in those who had an accompanying VSD which needed to be patched.[15] The incidence of this problem is being reduced as the procedure is refined.

▬TOTAL ANOMALOUS PULMONARY VENOUS RETURN

Total anomalous pulmonary venous return (TAPVR) is also termed total anomalous pulmonary veins and total anomalous pulmonary venous connection. In this defect, all of the pulmonary venous drainage returns to the right side of the heart, either directly or via systemic venous channels. There are four types of TAPVR:

1. Supracardiac, in which all four pulmonary veins drain into a common pulmonary venous trunk posterior to the heart and then usually into the left innominate vein via a "vertical anomalous pulmonary vein" (Fig. 11-6)
2. Cardiac, in which the pulmonary veins connect directly with the right atrium or drain into the coronary sinus
3. Infracardiac, in which blood from a common pulmonary venous trunk drains into a vein which passes through the diaphragm at the esophageal hiatus and from there into the inferior vena cava, portal vein, or ductus venosus
4. Mixed type, in which drainage from each lung is different.

Even though TAPVR accounts for only a small percent of congenital cardiac defects, it is important for two reasons: (1) it is a truly surgical disease which often needs prompt treatment but has a good prognosis after surgery, and (2) it is frequently misdiagnosed as pulmonary disease, delaying appropriate surgical treatment.

Pathophysiology

There are two major subclassifications of infants with TAPVR: those with obstructed pulmonary veins and those with unobstructed pulmonary veins. Unobstructed pulmonary veins cause a large left-to-right shunt with

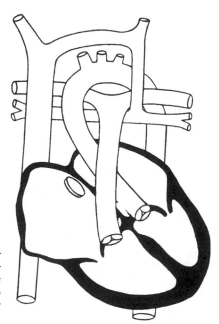

FIGURE 11-6 Total anomalous pulmonary venous return. Note the connection of the pulmonary veins to the venous drainage system and thus into the right atrium of the heart, rather than to the left atrium.

CHF and pulmonary artery hypertension. The maintenance of systemic flow depends on the presence of a PDA or a PFO, which allows right-to-left shunting. Because of the mixing of oxygenated blood with systemic venous blood in the right atrium, cyanosis is usually not marked. In fact, the oxygen content in this type of defect tends to be the same in all four chambers of the heart. Unobstructed TAPVR is, with TGV, the only congenital defect in which the oxygen content in the pulmonary artery is equal to or greater than that in the aorta. In the case of obstructed pulmonary veins, there is pulmonary venous hypertension, pulmonary edema, pulmonary arterial hypertension, and marked cyanosis. The cyanosis is worse in the obstructed form of TAPVR because the interatrial shunt, although present, is less effective.

Clinical Manifestations
The infant with the unobstructed variety of TAPVR usually does not present until after the immediate neonatal period. As the PVR drops, there is an increase in pulmonary blood flow with resulting pulmonary edema, CHF, and mild cyanosis. The infant with obstructed TAPVR typically presents as critically ill, cyanotic, and tachypneic within 1 week of birth. The chest x-ray film in unobstructed TAPVR, especially of the supracardiac type, shows a "snowman" appearance due to the tremendous vascular engorgement in the superior mediastinum. The chest radiograph may be unremarkable regarding the heart in obstructed TAPVR until the terminal stage; the lungs, however, will show a reticular appearance similar to that seen in interstitial pneumonia as a consequence of the pulmonary venous obstruction. The EKG reveals right atrial enlargement as evidenced by tall, peaked P waves, right ventricular hypertrophy, and a right axis deviation; there is also a Q wave in the right chest leads. Echocardiography may show lack of pulmonary venous connections to the left atrium, leftward bulge of the interatrial septum, and the presence of the pulmonary venous channel posterior to the heart. Although the diagnosis may be missed with echocardiography alone, use of color Doppler imaging to determine flow aids in arriving at the correct diagnosis. Cardiac catheterization combined with angiocardiography was formerly considered the best way to establish a definitive diagnosis and determine the anatomy of the blood vessels. Echocardiography has become the preferred means of diagnosis of TAPVR with the latest advances in technology and techniques.

Treatment
Those infants with obstructed TAPVR often present as critically ill and require rapid, if not immediate, surgical intervention. Initial oxygen therapy or mechanical ventilation may be necessary. When surgery is necessary within the first 24 hours of life, without an intervening period for stabilization, mortality is generally high. In one series, every infant requiring emergency intubation and ventilation died.[17] Anatomic type, however, is not a determinant of surgical results. Regardless of the anatomic type, correction is accomplished by redirecting pulmonary venous flow to the left atrium, either by direct connection (in the supracardiac or infracardiac types) or by an intracardiac baffle (in the types draining directly to the right atrium or the coronary sinus). The cornerstones of optimal treat-

ment are early diagnosis and early surgical intervention without a prolonged attempt at medical management. Long-term survival depends on unobstructed connection between the pulmonary venous system and the left atrium.

▬COARCTATION OF THE AORTA

Coarctation of the aorta affects approximately 6% of those infants with congenital cardiac disease, appearing more frequently in those weighing less than 2.5 kg. It is best separated into simple and complex categories for consideration of presentation and treatment. Simple coarctation involves a constriction at the aortic isthmus, usually at or just below a PDA. The complex defect includes hypoplasia of the entire aortic arch, with or without a specific site of narrowing; a PDA; and one or more of the following: VSD, endocardial cushion defect, aortic stenosis, mitral stenosis or regurgitation, subaortic stenosis, hypoplastic left ventricle and ascending aorta, and endocardial fibroelastosis (a condition that results in gross cardiomegaly, pulmonary edema, and, often, left lower lobe atelectasis secondary to bronchial obstruction due to the enlarged heart).

Pathophysiology

Because only about one quarter of the ventricular output passes through the aortic isthmus in utero, compared with about 60% through the ductus arteriosus, the isthmus is the smallest part of the aorta. Following transition to extrauterine life, the isthmus normally grows; in simple coarctation, a constricting band develops at the point of connection of the ductus arteriosus to the aorta. The constriction may worsen in the immediate postnatal period as the ductus itself constricts. There may be hypertrophy and endothelial thickening at the site of coarctation as the infant grows. The effect is an increased pressure load on the left ventricle to which may be added an increased volume load if a large PDA exists. Once the left ventricle is unable to sustain its output in the face of the added volume or pressure load, failure ensues with elevated left ventricular end-diastolic pressure and pulmonary edema.

In complex coarctation, one finds pulmonary artery hypertension, blood flow to the descending aorta supplied by the ductus arteriosus, usually a large intracardiac shunt, and elevated pulmonary blood flow. The right side of the heart is dilated and hypertrophied. There is volume and pressure overload on both ventricles with resultant biventricular failure. The pressures in the right ventricle, pulmonary artery, and ascending and descending aorta are the same. Peripheral pulse pressure is normal and pulses are equal. Should the ductus constrict or close, femoral pulses diminish and a picture of shock with renal and mesenteric hypoperfusion and metabolic acidosis develops.

Clinical Manifestations

Infants with simple coarctation may be asymptomatic initially. Lower extremity pulses are absent or diminished and delayed compared to brachial pulses. Pulse pressure in the lower extremities may be as narrow as 10 mm Hg. While systolic pressure is higher in the upper extremities than in the lower, marked hypertension is uncommon. The chest radiograph shows cardiac enlargement with pulmonary venous congestion. The EKG shows early right ventricular hypertrophy with left ventricular hypertrophy in the older infant. Echocardiography will demonstrate the location and severity of the constriction along with the presence of any associated defects.

The infant with complex coarctation will usually present in failure early in the neonatal period. Pulses in the lower extremities are diminished or may wax and wane with changes in ductal patency. The chest radiograph shows cardiac enlargement and pulmonary edema. The EKG shows right axis deviation, and right atrial and ventricular hypertrophy. The EKG will allow elucidation of the complete picture.

Treatment

Medical treatment is aimed at improving congestive failure; there may be considerable success with medical treatment alone initially. However, the infant who is refractory to medical management or who presents with severe signs and symptoms will require surgery. There are several possible techniques, depending on the location, extent, and severity of the coarctation itself and the type and presence of associated defects. Simplest is resection of the constricted area with an end-to-end anastomosis; this may sometimes result in recurrent coarctation. If there is not enough vessel to reanastomose the ends, a Dacron or PTFE graft may be inserted. If the area of coarctation is more extensive, a side patch aortoplasty may be used. The subclavian flap angioplasty is useful in the neonate. Formerly, a left thoracotomy was the preferred approach. However, some authors have suggested that a median sternotomy is preferable in that it facilitates side patch aortoplasty and also cardiopulmonary bypass when it is necessary to repair associated defects simultaneously.[18]

▬ HYPOPLASTIC LEFT HEART SYNDROME

Hypoplastic left heart syndrome (HLHS) encompasses a constellation of defects including aortic valve atresia, mitral valve atresia, severe left ventricular and proximal aortic hypoplasia, and, frequently, coarctation of the aorta and left ventricular endocardial fibroelastosis. According to the New England Regional Infant Cardiac Program, HLHS comprises 7% to 8% of congenital heart disease seen in the first year of life and is the most common cause of death due to cardiac disease in neonates.[19] It is universally fatal if left untreated.

Pathophysiology

With the combination of a hypoplastic (and thus ineffective) left ventricle and aortic and mitral hypoplasia, flow through the left side of the heart is virtually nonexistent. Systemic flow is provided by the right ventricle through the ductus arteriosus, with blood flowing retrograde to the aortic arch and coronary arteries. Pulmonary venous return must pass through an ASD or PFO to the right atrium. Oxygen saturation is the same in the right ventricle, pulmonary artery, and aorta. Maintenance of adequate systemic perfusion is dependent upon the maintenance of (1) adequate intravascular volume, (2) a PDA, and (3) a balance between pulmonary and systemic vascular resistances.

Clinical Manifestations

Signs and symptoms present nearly immediately upon constriction of the ductus arteriosus. A clinical picture of shock will develop and the infant will become gray, with weak peripheral pulses. These episodes may be intermittent as the ductus arteriosus alternately opens and constricts. The chest radiograph shows cardiac enlargement and pulmonary vascular engorgement. The EKG demonstrates right atrial hypertrophy, right ventricular hypertrophy, and right axis deviation. Echocardiography allows the diagnosis to be made by demonstrating a small or nonfunctional left ventricle.

Treatment

As recently as 1986, HLHS was not considered a surgical disease; the only treatment offered was "comfort care," allowing the infant to die with the support of its family. There are now two surgical options available for HLHS: transplantation and the **Norwood procedure**. The technical aspects of transplantation are well developed, as is the immunosuppressive regime. The major stumbling block remains the lack of hearts for transplantation into neonates. As heart failure or an infection secondary to failure can result in the death of the infant prior to transplantation, after 1 month without location of a suitable donor, one must consider other surgical options.[20]

The Norwood procedure occurs in two (or three) stages. The first stage is based upon three principles:

1. Attachment of the right ventricle directly to the aorta
2. Regulation of pulmonary blood flow for proper growth of the pulmonary vascular bed to avoid development of both pulmonary vascular obstructive disease and volume overload on the right ventricle; this is accomplished by insertion of a systemic arterial–pulmonary arterial shunt
3. Establishment of a large connection between the atria[21]

The second stage is a Fontan procedure, in which the systemic arterial–pulmonary arterial shunt is removed and a systemic venous–pulmonary arterial connection is made. As experience with the Norwood procedure increased, it became clear that a two-stage Fontan procedure worked better for many infants. Initially, the superior vena cava is connected to the pulmonary arteries in what is termed a hemi-Fontan procedure; in 6 months, the inferior vena cava is then channelled to the pulmonary arteries. The staged Fontan was instituted because removal of the systemic arterial-pulmonary arterial shunt caused a rapid decrease in the end-diastolic volume of the right ventricle. Since the wall thickness increased under these circumstances, the diastolic compliance of the ventricle fell, reducing filling and thus cardiac output. The success of the Norwood procedure is limited by the ability of the right ventricle to assume the pressure load of systemic perfusion.

Regardless of the procedure chosen, preoperative management is similar. Prostaglandin E_1 is infused to insure patency of the ductus arteriosus. Pulmonary and systemic vascular resistances are adjusted to maintain systemic blood flow. Minimal oxygen administration and even hypoventilation on mechanical ventilation will prevent a decrease in

PVR, whereas an infusion of sodium nitroprusside may be needed to decrease systemic vascular resistance. Postoperative management concentrates on minimizing PVR by using the lowest possible mean airway pressure consistent with maintenance of $PaCO_2$ in the range of 20 to 30 mm Hg.

▬TRUNCUS ARTERIOSUS

In this defect, the **truncus arteriosus** fails to divide into the aorta and the pulmonary artery. This single vessel supplies both the pulmonary and systemic circulations and is accompanied by a high ventricular septal defect. The single semilunar valve may have extra leaflets; it also may be incompetent. Additionally, this defect is frequently accompanied by extracardiac congenital defects, such as the DiGeorge anomaly, a congenital immunologic deficiency.

Pathophysiology

Owing to the presence of the large VSD and common ventricular outflow, the systemic and pulmonary flows mix with resulting cyanosis. The degree of cyanosis is determined by the amount of pulmonary blood flow, which is affected by obstruction in the proximal pulmonary arteries. Relatively little obstruction will result in a large left-to-right shunt and CHF. Thus, CHF and cyanosis are at opposite poles, with low pulmonary vascular resistance favoring gas exchange but contributing to CHF. Pulmonary vascular obstructive disease will develop rapidly under these circumstances, as early as 1 year of age.

Clinical Manifestations

Truncus arteriosus resembles VSD more than other cyanotic lesions. Except for the cyanosis (as discussed earlier), signs and symptoms usually do not develop until PVR has fallen sufficiently to allow a large left-to-right shunt. There is tachypnea in addition to the cyanosis. There is a murmur resembling that of a VSD and bounding peripheral pulses. The chest radiograph shows an enlarged heart and pulmonary vascular engorgement. The EKG may not be helpful, showing left, right, or biventricular hypertrophy.

Treatment

Medical treatment is rarely successful for this defect. While banding of the pulmonary arteries was once done, the technical difficulties in creating equal obstructions limited its effectiveness; additionally, the procedure was just palliative. Correction is now usually undertaken by 6 weeks of age. The VSD is repaired through a ventriculotomy. A new right ventricular outflow tract is created and connected to the pulmonary arteries, which are disconnected from the truncus. Previously, a Dacron graft with a heterograft valve was used for this conduit. A human homograft, because it is available in many sizes, is now preferred.[22] Early risk factors for death include severe truncal valve regurgitation, interrupted aortic arch, coronary artery anomalies, and repair at greater than 100 days of age.[23] Long-term outcome may be influenced by competence of the trunk valve and also by stenosis of the pulmonary arteries.

▄TRICUSPID ATRESIA

In this relatively rare disease, there is no tricuspid valve and thus no connection between the right atrium and right ventricle. All of the systemic venous return proceeds through the foramen ovale to the left atrium and then to the left ventricle. In addition, the right ventricle is usually hypoplastic and the pulmonic valve stenotic.

Pathophysiology

The major problem in tricuspid atresia without associated anomalies is the decreased pulmonary blood flow. Blood flow to the lungs occurs through a PDA and via a ventricular septal defect through a small right ventricle and some degree of pulmonary stenosis. Cyanosis will reflect the degree of obstruction of flow to the lungs.

Clinical Manifestations

The infants are found to be cyanotic. The chest radiograph shows a heart of normal size or slightly enlarged, with decreased pulmonary vascular markings. The EKG shows a left-axis deviation. The definitive diagnosis is made with echocardiography.

Treatment

It is ideal to wait until the infant is at least 1 year old; waiting 3 years or more is preferable before performing the Fontan procedure. In the immediate postnatal period, infusion of prostaglandin E_1 will maintain a PDA. Subsequently, a Blalock-Taussig shunt (subclavian artery to pulmonary artery) can be inserted to allow the infant to grow. Once the child has grown sufficiently, the Fontan procedure, in which the right atrium is connected to the pulmonary artery, can be performed. The good surgical candidate will have low pulmonary pressures and resistance.

▄AORTIC STENOSIS

Obstruction to outflow from the left ventricle can occur below the aortic valve, at the valve itself, distal to the valve, or in some combination. Subaortic stenosis may be discrete (composed of a membrane), tunnel (characterized by tubular narrowing of the left ventricular outflow tract), or functional (a condition known variously as hypertrophic cardiomyopathy, hypertrophic obstructive cardiomyopathy, or idiopathic hypertrophic subaortic stenosis). Stenosis of the aortic valve itself can be due to a smaller annulus than normal, fusion of commissures, fewer cusps than normal (both bicuspid and unicuspid valves are found), or some combination of the above. Supravalvular stenosis, like subaortic stenosis, comes in three varieties: (1) membranous, caused by the presence of a membrane with a single perforation; (2) hourglass, in which the media and intima of the ascending aorta are severely thickened, giving the characteristic shape; and (3) hypoplasia of the ascending aorta and (in 1 out of 5 cases) some of the vessels of the aortic arch.

Pathophysiology

As long as the left ventricle is capable of handling the additional pressure workload imposed upon it, cardiac output will be maintained. However, there will be hypertrophy of the ventricle; this will ultimately lead to angina, as the muscle develops faster than its blood supply. Once the ventricle fails, CHF, pulmonary edema, and peripheral vascular collapse (in the worst case) will develop. Exertional syncope also ensues, as the ventricle fails suddenly when asked to increase its output in the face of high resistance in the outflow tract.

Clinical Manifestations
The infant presenting early usually has aortic valve disease rather than subvalvular or supravalvular obstruction. The baby will be tachypneic and perhaps pale or cyanotic. The chest radiograph will show cardiac enlargement and increased pulmonary venous markings. The EKG will show biventricular enlargement. The echocardiogram will provide the details of the lesion.

Treatment
While even mild stenosis may progress, those presenting with mild disease fare better than those with moderate disease.[24] Initial palliation previously was by valvulotomy. More recently, percutaneous transluminal balloon aortic valvuloplasty has been gaining greater acceptance. Ultimately, many will require valve replacement, a procedure delayed as long as possible to allow the patient and aortic annulus to approach adult size.[25] These patients will continue to require observation throughout their lives for complications following surgery. Supravalvular obstruction is usually treated surgically with patch aortoplasty, which consists of a lateral incision, relief of the obstruction, and placement of a Dacron patch over the opening. Subaortic stenosis of the discrete type lends itself readily to surgical resection, although with a somewhat high rate of recurrence.[26]

Treatment for hypertrophic obstructive cardiomyopathy remains to be clearly elucidated. Many different drugs have potential benefit, but also potential serious side effects. Surgery, either removal of the excess tissue or simple incision into the stenotic area, also shows promise.

▀ EISENMENGER SYNDROME
This syndrome is based on the existence of a large systemic-to-pulmonary connection at the aortopulmonary, ventricular, or atrial level with pulmonary artery pressures at or near systemic level and a reversed or bidirectional shunt between the two circulations. The condition was first described by Victor Eisenmenger in 1897 in a case report of a 32-year-old man who had died; autopsy findings included a large VSD with aortic overriding, right ventricular hypertrophy, and pulmonary artery atheromatous changes. This was subsequently named Eisenmenger's complex by Wood, who termed any other anatomical condition resulting in the same physiology Eisenmenger syndrome (and listed at least 12 of these possible conditions).[27]

Pathophysiology
Under normal circumstances, a connection between the systemic and pulmonary circulations results in a left-to-right shunt, since systemic vascular resistance, and therefore pressure, are usually greater than the corresponding values for the pulmonary circulation. When pulmonary vascular resis-

tance increases, often as a result of increased flow leading to changes in the pulmonary vascular bed, the shunt becomes either bidirectional (as pressures equalize) or reversed (as pulmonary artery pressure exceeds systemic arterial pressure). The pulmonary vascular changes include extension of muscle into normally nonmuscular peripheral arteries, medial hypertrophy of more proximal muscular arteries, and a reduced number of peripheral vessels.[28]

Clinical Manifestations

In one series of over 200 patients, the most common causative lesions were VSD (33%), ASD of secundum variety (30%), and PDA (14%).[29] The presentation commonly included dyspnea on exertion, palpitations, edema, hemoptysis, and syncope. Physical findings include clubbing of digits, central cyanosis, and a prominent jugular venous "a" wave, beyond those of the specific etiologic lesion. The chest radiograph shows cardiomegaly, almost invariably a prominent main pulmonary artery segment, and diminished peripheral vascular markings. The EKG will show deviation of the right axis along with right atrial and ventricular hypertrophy. Echocardiography will allow determination of the anatomy of the lesion and Doppler echocardiography will identify direction and magnitude of the shunt, along with valvular dysfunction.

Treatment

Nonsurgical therapy aims to avoid or reduce complications resulting from hypoxia, CHF, infection, and hematologic abnormalities. Regardless of the specific drugs used, the prognosis is grim once permanent changes in the pulmonary vascular bed occur. Surgical treatment involves either heart–lung transplantation or single-lung transplantation with repair of intracardiac defects. While transplantation may seem to be the definitive answer, the potential complications of immunosuppressive therapy and rejection are considerable; they may be preferable to those of chronic hypoxia, however.

■REFERENCES

1. Tucker A, Anderson K, Babyak S, White W: Pulmonary hypertension and increased pulmonary vascular reactivity in rats exposed at 10,000 ft since birth. Chest 93:185S, 1988.
2. Caslin A, Heath D, Smith P: Influence of hypobaric hypoxia in infancy on the subsequent development of vasoconstrictive pulmonary vascular disease in the Wistar albino rat. J Pathol 163:133, 1991.
3. Hakim T, Mortola J: Pulmonary vascular resistance in adult rats exposed to hypoxia in the neonatal period. Can J Physiol Pharmacol 68:419, 1989.
4. Hampl V, Jerge J: Perinatal hypoxia increases hypoxic pulmonary vasoconstriction in adult rats recovering from chronic exposure to hypoxia. Am Rev Respir Dis 142:619, 1990.
5. Kolar F, Osiadal B, Prochazka J, Pelouch V, Widimsky J: Comparison of cardiopulmonary response to intermittent high-altitude hypoxia in young and adult rats. Respiration 56:57, 1989.
6. Taylor G, Short B, Fitz C: Imaging of cerebrovascular injury in infants treated with extracorporeal membrane oxygenation. J Pediatr 114:635, 1989.
7. Gold JP, Violaris K, Engle MA, Klein AA, Ehlers KH, Lang SJ, Levin AR, Moran F, O'Loughlin JE, Snyder MS, Fatica N, Notterman DS, Isom OW: A five-year clinical experience with 112 Blalock-Taussig shunts. J Card Surg 8:9, 1993.
8. John S, John C, Bashi VV, Ravikumar E, Kaul P, Choudhury SP, Prasad KMS, Kanhere VM, Jha A, Krishnaswami S: Tetralogy of Fallot: Intracardiac repair in 840 infants. Cardiovasc Surg 1(3):285, 1993.

9. Uva MS, Lacour-Gayet F, Komiya T, Serraf A, Bruniaux J, Touchot A, Roux D, Petit J, Panché C: Surgery for tetralogy of Fallot at less than six months. J Thorac Cardiovasc Surg 107:1291, 1994.

10. Murphy JG, Gersh BJ, Mair DD, Fuster V, McGoon MD, Ilstrup DM, McGoon DC, Kirklin JW, Danielson GK: Long-term outcome in patients undergoing surgical repair of tetralogy of Fallot. N Engl J Med 329:593, 1993.

11. Starnes VA, Luciani GB, Latter DA, Griffin ML: Current surgical management of tetralogy of Fallot. Ann Thoracic Surg 58:211, 1994.

12. Sullivan ID, Prebiterio P, Gooch VM: Is ventricular arrhythmia in repaired tetralogy of Fallot an effect of operation or a consequence of the course of the disease? Br Heart J 58:40, 1987.

13. Karl TR, Sano S, Pornviliwan S, Mee RBB: Tetralogy of Fallot: Favorable outcomes of nonneonatal transatrial transpulmonary repair. Ann Thorac Surg 54:903, 1992.

14. Hallman GL, Cooley DA, Gutgesell HP: Surgical Treatment of Congenital Heart Disease, 3rd ed. Philadelphia, Lea and Febiger, 1987.

15. Flanagan MF, Fyler DC: Cardiac disease. In Avery GB, Fletcher MA, MacDonald MG (eds): Neonatology: Pathophysiology and Management of the Newborn, 4th ed. Philadelphia, JB Lippincott, 1994.

16. Alexander JA, Knauf DG, Greene MA, van Mierop LHS, O'Brien DJ: The changing strategies in operation for transposition of the great vessels. Ann Thorac Surg 58:1278, 1994.

17. Cobanoglu A, Menashe VD: Total anomalous pulmonary venous connection in neonates and young infants: Repair in the current era. Ann Thorac Surg 55:43, 1993.

18. DeLeon SY, Downey FX, Baumgartner NE, Ow EP, Quinones JA, Torres L, Ilbawi MN, Pifarré R: Transsternal repair of coarctation and associated cardiac defects. Ann Thorac Surg 58:179, 1994.

19. Fyler DC: Report of the New England Regional Infant Cardiac Program. Pediatrics 65(Suppl):463, 1980.

20. Zahka KG, Spector M, Hanisch D: Hypoplastic left heart syndrome: Norwood operation, transplantation, or compassionate care. Clin in Perinatol 20:145, 1993.

21. Norwood WI: Hypoplastic left heart syndrome. Ann Thorac Surg 52:688, 1991.

22. Turley K: Current method of repair of truncus arteriosus. J Cardiac Surg 7:1, 1992.

23. Hanley FL, Heinemann MK, Jonas RA, Mayer JE, Cook NR, Wessel DL, Castaneda AR: Repair of truncus arteriosus in the neonate. J Thorac Cardiovasc Surg 105:1047, 1993.

24. Kitchiner DJ, Jackson M, Walsh K, Peart I, Arnold R: Incidence and prognosis of congenital aortic valve stenosis in Liverpool (1960—1990). Br Heart J 69:71, 1993.

25. Bashore TM, Lieberman EB: Aortic/mitral obstruction and coarctation of the aorta. Cardiol Clin 11:617, 1993.

26. Jacobs JP, Palatrianos GM, Cintron JR, Kaiser GA: Transaortic resection of the subaortic membrane: Treatment for subvalvular aortic stenosis. Chest 106:46, 1994.

27. Wood P: The Eisenmenger syndrome or pulmonary hypertension with reversed central shunt. Br Med J 2:701, 1958.

28. Collins-Nakai RL, Rabinovitch M: Pulmonary vascular obstructive disease. Cardiol Clin 11:675, 1993.

29. Saha A, Balakrishnan KG, Jaiswal PK, Venkitachalam CG, Tharakan J, Titus T, Kutty R: Prognosis for patients with Eisenmenger syndrome of various aetiology. Int J Cardiol 45:199, 1994.

▪SELF-ASSESSMENT QUESTIONS

1. What are three common precursors for PPHN?

2. What are possible treatments for PPHN and drawbacks of each?

3. What are the four possible consequences of congenital cardiac disease related to the circulatory system?

4. Traditional treatment of PDA involves either administration of indomethacin or open surgical ligation. What are two newer techniques?

5. What is the pathophysiology that predisposes the infant with a large VSD to pulmonary complications?

6. List and describe the anatomy of four types of ASDs.

7. What is the common major hemodynamic consequence of both tetralogy of Fallot and tricuspid atresia?

8. Early and accurate diagnosis of TAPVR is important, even though this defect accounts for only a small percentage of congenital cardiac defects. What are the two reasons for this?

9. What defects are potentially present in the constellation of complex coarctation of the aorta?

10. What are the three treatment options presently available for HLHS and what are the considerations for each?

Chapter 12

Congenital Anomalies

OBJECTIVES

Having completed this chapter, the reader will be able to:

1 List the causes of choanal atresia.

2 Discuss the pathophysiologic effects, clinical presentation, diagnosis, and treatment of both unilateral and bilateral choanal atresia.

3 Describe the pathophysiology of Pierre-Robin syndrome, and state the most common other congenital defect associated with this disorder.

4 Discuss the clinical manifestations and treatment of Pierre-Robin syndrome.

5 State the causes of congenital diaphragmatic hernia and the most common location of this defect.

6 Discuss the effects of congenital diaphragmatic hernia on the cardiac and pulmonary systems.

7 Describe the clinical and radiographic presentation of congenital diaphragmatic hernia.

8 Discuss the use of bag-mask ventilation in infants born with congenital diaphragmatic hernia.

9 Discuss the problems associated with mechanical ventilation of infants with congenital diaphragmatic hernia, both preoperatively and postoperatively.

10 Describe the surgical treatment for congenital diaphragmatic hernia.

11 State three major features of the history of infants born with tracheoesophageal fistula.

12 List and describe the five types of tracheoesophageal fistula.

13 Discuss the general problems, clinical and radiograph presentation, and treatment of tracheoesophageal fistula.

14 Describe the pathophysiology, clinical presentation, and management of infants with omphaloceles and gastroschisis.

KEY TERMS

choanae
choanal atresia
contralateral
dextrocardia

gastroschisis
glossoptosis
micrognathia
omphalocele

CHOANAL ATRESIA

The **choanae** are the two openings in the posterior portion of the nasal cavity, directing airflow into the nasopharynx. The choanae are separated by the posterior nasal septum. **Choanal atresia** results from choanal stenosis, a bony choanal septum, or a complete membrane obstructing the nasal passage. The primary result is occlusion or blockage of the airway between the posterior nasal passage and the nasopharynx. This anomaly occurs in approximately 1 in 7000 births.[6]

Choanal atresia may be bilateral or unilateral; unilateral atresia is more common. Twenty percent to 50% of infants with choanal atresia have associated defects. These have been described as CHARGE association defects, with the acronym representing *c*olobomata of the eyes, *h*eart defects, *r*enal anomaly, *g*rowth and mental retardation, gastroesophageal reflux, and *e*ar deficits.[1] If choanal atresia is identified in a newborn, a thorough examination is indicated to search for associated defects.

Pathophysiology

Newborn infants are obligate nose breathers for the first 6 to 8 weeks of life. If an obstruction prevents air passage through the nose, the infant will demonstrate signs of respiratory distress. In bilateral choanal atresia, the respiratory distress will become apparent soon after birth, accompanied by severe cyanosis and inability to ventilate. The infant will become asphyxiated unless an airway is established. A characteristic feature of bilateral atresia is that the respiratory distress disappears when the infant cries and then worsens when the infant starts nursing or sucking.

In unilateral choanal atresia, the infant has less severe symptoms, and the diagnosis of choanal atresia may actually be delayed for several years.

Clinical Signs and Diagnosis

The infant with bilateral choanal atresia presents immediately after birth with cyanosis and retractions. In unilateral or partial obstruction, labored nasal breathing or inspiratory stridor may be heard. A high inspiratory resistance causes the soft, pliable extrathoracic airways to collapse, resulting in stridor on inspiration. If the obstruction is not relieved, pulmonary hypertension secondary to hypoxia and acidosis leads to right heart failure. In complete bilateral obstruction, the infant may become severely cyanotic and is at risk for asphyxiation unless the obstruction is relieved by insertion of an oral airway.

Cyanosis and inability to ventilate properly occur during sucking or feeding, leading to the suspicion of partial or unilateral choanal atresia. Diagnosis should actually begin in the delivery room when a catheter (6 Fr.) is passed through the nares into the nasopharynx as part of the routine newborn examination.[6] A thin, flexible nasopharyngoscope may also be used to attempt visualization of the region. The most accurate method of documenting the exact location and extent of the atresia is a high-resolution computed tomography (CT) scan.[6] Because nasal edema may mimic choanal atresia, a topical nasal decongestant can be administered before the procedure to decrease edema and to rule out this possibility.

Management and Complications

Immediate treatment for choanal atresia involves provision of a patent airway. Tracheotomy was performed in the past, but management is now more conservative. Insertion of an oral airway to position the tongue anteriorly will allow the infant to breathe through the oropharynx and relieve the symptoms of respiratory distress. A McGovern nipple (large rubber nipple with an enlarged hole) or a nipple with the end cut off will also relieve distress.

Early surgical repair is indicated. A transnasal or transpalatal approach may be used and the obstruction is enlarged or perforated. Some surgeons prefer to perform an initial transnasal repair in the newborn, followed by a transpalatal procedure when the child is larger.[6] Large-bore plastic tubes (stents) are inserted and kept in place for several weeks or months following surgical repair. It is important to keep the tubes clear of secretions in order to prevent obstruction. Feeding can begin as soon as one naris is patent and the infant can be discharged once the parents have been trained in suctioning and maintaining the airway.

Immediate complications of bilateral choanal atresia include airway obstruction and the risk of hypoxia and asphyxiation if the defect is not identified and treated promptly. Long-term postoperative complications include scarring and closure of the choanae so that further dilation and reinsertion of the stents may be necessary.

▆ PIERRE-ROBIN SYNDROME

Pierre-Robin syndrome is characterized by **glossoptosis** (downward displacement of the tongue) and **micrognathia** (underdevelopment of the jaw). The tongue is large in comparison to mandible size, predisposing the infant to airway obstruction. This defect is frequently associated with cleft palate.

Pathophysiology

Micrognathia, or hypoplasia of the mandible, causes the tongue position to be more posterior than normal. Airway obstruction occurs as a result of the tongue falling back into the hypopharynx. During sucking and swallowing, the negative pressure that is created pulls the tongue upward into the cleft palate and obstructs the nasopharynx. The airway obstruction causes respiratory distress and insufficiency.

Clinical Signs and Diagnosis

The symptoms of Pierre-Robin syndrome vary from minor respiratory distress to severe airway obstruction depending on the extent of the anomaly and the presence of other anomalies. In severe obstruction, sternal, intercostal, substernal, and suprasternal retractions are seen. The infant has choking and gagging episodes during feeding and may hyperextend the neck in an attempt to relieve the obstruction. Cyanotic episodes occur and may be severe enough to cause brain damage and death. The diagnosis is made on the basis of physical examination and a history of airway obstruction.

As the infant grows, the glossoptosis and feeding problems may diminish in severity by the age of 6 months.

Management and Complications

To alleviate the airway obstruction, the infant should be placed in the prone position with the face down. Towel rolls are placed under the shoulders and forehead to maintain this position; this keeps the tongue more anterior and prevents obstruction of the airway. A nasotracheal tube may be inserted to maintain a patent airway and also prevent the pulling upward of the tongue during sucking. The tube can be kept in position until the infant has grown or can have surgical correction. For mild cases, carefully supervised oral feedings may be possible. If more severe symptoms of respiratory distress are present, the infant is fed by means of a nasogastric or gastrostomy tube. Particular attention must be given to positioning the infant during any type of feeding because the risk of aspiration is high.

Various surgical procedures can be performed to relieve airway obstruction. A heavy suture may be sewn through the base of the tongue out to traction or tied around a button attached to the skin of the chin. This procedure, or the insertion of a nasotracheal tube, will maintain the child until the mandible has grown sufficiently. Tracheostomy may be indicated for very severe problems and life-threatening episodes of obstruction. The airway problems are self-limiting, and treatment will provide relief of obstruction until the child grows.

Complications of Pierre-Robin syndrome include failure to thrive, malnutrition, chronic hypoxia, and pneumonia.[11]

■ CONGENITAL DIAPHRAGMATIC HERNIA

Congenital diaphragmatic hernia is caused by a failure of the posterolateral portion (foramen of Bochdalek) of the diaphragm to close properly or by failure of the pleural peritoneal membrane to develop. The incidence of congenital diaphragmatic hernia varies from 1 in 2200 births to 1 in 3000 births.[6,10]

Pathophysiology

The pathologic changes that accompany the failure of the diaphragm to form include herniation of the intestines into the thorax, hypoplasia of the lung on the affected (ipsilateral) side, and underdevelopment of the abdomen. The lung on the opposite (**contralateral**) side may also be compressed by the shift of the heart and great vessels.

Eighty-five percent to 90% of congenital diaphragmatic hernias occur on the left side. It is thought that right-sided defects occur more rarely because the liver partially occludes the diaphragmatic defect and prevents herniation of the intestines into the thoracic cavity. Symptoms of right-sided hernias are less severe and the mortality rate is lower.

The intestinal contents enter through the hernia at about the 8th week of gestational development. The lung on that side, therefore, has less than the normal number of alveoli, retarded pulmonary capillary development, and cuboidal cells lining the endothelial tissue. After birth, the presence of the intestines in the thoracic cavity prevent expansion of the lung, causing respiratory insufficiency and decreased cardiac performance. A mediastinal shift to the unaffected side impinges on inflation of the developed lung. **Dextrocardia** is seen in the most common form of diaphragmatic hernia, secondary to the mediastinal shift.

Secondary to the underdeveloped pulmonary capillary bed and intestinal impingement on the capillaries, a high pulmonary vascular resistance is maintained after birth. Persistent fetal circulation and right-to-left shunting may result and further complicate the respiratory insufficiency. Severe hypoxia and acidosis may persist until the intestines are surgically removed from the thoracic cavity.

Clinical Signs and Diagnosis

The infant born with congenital diaphragmatic hernia presents immediately after birth with respiratory distress and cyanosis. A barrel-shaped chest and scaphoid abdomen may be present, since the intestines are in the thoracic cavity rather than in the abdominal cavity. Right-sided heart sounds indicate dextrocardia, confirmed by chest x-ray. The cardiac impulse may also be displaced. Breath sounds will be decreased or absent, and bowel sounds may be heard over the chest. After birth, gas enters and dilates the bowel, compromising ventilation and cardiac status.

The severity of the respiratory distress will prompt the practitioner to obtain a chest x-ray, which will confirm the diagnosis (Fig. 12-1). The gas-filled bowel will be visualized in the thoracic cavity and the abdominal cavity will be airless. Dextrocardia will be seen if the intestines are on the left side of the chest. Contrast media are not needed to confirm the diagnosis.

Arterial blood gas studies reveal a respiratory and metabolic acidosis from hypoventilation and severe hypoxia.

Diagnosis of congenital diaphragmatic hernia may be made prenatally by ultrasound examination of the fetus. If a prenatal diagnosis is made,

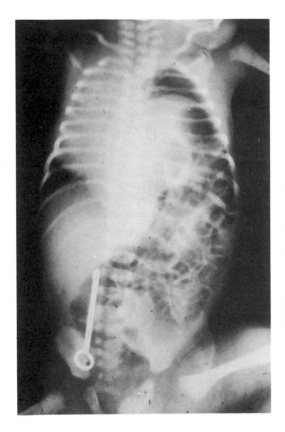

FIGURE 12-1 X-ray film of left diaphragmatic hernia with loops of bowel well up into the chest. Although most diaphragmatic hernias do not have a sac, the smooth curve of the sac in this instance is visible. Notice the heart is displaced to the border of the right chest. (Guzzeta PC, Anderson KD, Eichelberger MR, Newman KD, Rouse TM, Schnitzer JJ, Boyajian M, Tomaski SM: General surgery. In Avery GB, Fletcher MA, MacDonald MG [eds]: Neonatology: Pathophysiology and Treatment of the Newborn, 4th ed, p. 922. Philadelphia, JB Lippincott, 1994.)

delivery of the infant should take place in a center that is equipped to handle the potential problems. Lung maturity should be assessed by lecithin/sphingomyelin (L/S) ratio, and prenatal steroids can be given if there is doubt about pulmonary maturity.[10]

Management and Complications

Congenital diaphragmatic hernia is no longer considered a surgical emergency and stabilization of the infant prior to surgery may improve the eventual outcome.[6] The immediate goal is to reverse the hypoxia, hypercarbia, and acidosis present at birth in order to minimize persistent fetal circulation with its right-to-left shunting across the ductus arteriosus. This may be accomplished with mechanical ventilation with 100% oxygen, sedation with narcotics, muscle paralysis, controlled alkalosis with hyperventilation, intravenous bicarbonate, and vasopressors.[6,11] A nasogastric tube is inserted to decrease gas distention of the intestines and allow some expansion of the lung. Bag-mask ventilation should not be used because this is likely to increase the amount of air in the intestines and further compromise ventilation. Once an artificial airway has been established, low ventilating pressures must be used because of severe bilateral restriction of lung expansion; the incidences of pneumothorax and barotrauma are high. High-frequency ventilation may be valuable because of the ability to adequately ventilate the infant at lower airway pressures. Some centers may use extracorporeal membrane oxygenation (ECMO) to stabilize the infant before surgery (see Chap. 25).

Surgery is performed using either an abdominal or thoracic approach. The intestines are carefully withdrawn into the abdominal cavity, and the diaphragmatic defect is sutured closed. The use of prosthetic material to create a "patch" may be necessary if the defect is large and adequate diaphragmatic tissue is not available. Because the abdomen has not accommodated the intestines throughout gestational development, a pouch may have to be created to hold the intestines. If the intestines are replaced into the small abdominal cavity, the increased pressure on the diaphragm will prevent adequate ventilation postoperatively. The pouch can be repaired after the infant grows and stabilizes.

Cautious postoperative use of the ventilator is important. Mechanical ventilation may be required for a period of hours to days.[11] The lung on the affected side is underdeveloped and the temptation to reexpand it after repair of the hernia must be resisted. Pneumothorax may occur easily and is an unwanted complication in an already severely compromised infant. Ventilation should be accomplished using the lowest possible airway pressure to maintain an adequate $PaCO_2$. A high FIO_2 may be required. Positive end-expiratory pressure is usually not indicated for these infants, but, if it becomes necessary, low levels should be used. High-frequency ventilation and ECMO may also be helpful during the postoperative period.

It has been proposed that following surgical repair, infants may be classified into three groups.[4] In the first group are newborns who have an uncomplicated postoperative course and do very well. The second group consists of infants with pulmonary hypoplasia that is so severe that it is incompatible with life, and they generally do not survive despite aggressive treatment. Infants in the third group do well for 8 to 24 hours following repair, the so-called "honeymoon period," and then develop increasing hypoxia and acidosis.[11] Persistent pulmonary hypertension and right-to-left shunting complicate the postoperative course of these infants (see Chap. 11). Tolazoline (Priscoline) may be used to vasodilate and decrease pulmonary vascular resistance. The usual treatment for persistent right-to-left shunting includes hyperventilation, which may be difficult to accomplish in these infants because of pulmonary hypoplasia and the high incidence of pneumothorax.

Future modalities for the treatment of infants with congenital diaphragmatic hernia include surfactant replacement therapy, intratracheal pulmonary ventilation, and pulmonary lobar transplantation.[2,12] Prenatal surgical correction of the diaphragmatic defect has also been proposed, but there are many ethical issues that must be addressed before in utero repair becomes an accepted form of treatment.

▀TRACHEOESOPHAGEAL FISTULA

The exact cause of esophageal atresia and tracheoesophageal fistula (TEF) is unknown. During embryonic development, the trachea and esophagus develop from the same diverticulum of the foregut and are recognizable as early as 22 to 23 days after fertilization.[7] By 34 to 36 days of gestation, the trachea and esophagus should divide into separate channels. Esophageal atresia and TEF result when this separation and development is interrupted or incomplete.

TEF and esophageal atresia occur in about 1 of 3000 to 4500 births.[6] About one third of the infants are born prematurely and a maternal history of hydramnios is often associated with these infants, since the infant is unable to swallow amniotic fluid. In many of the infants born with TEF defects, other anomalies are present, and have been described as the VACTERL syndrome (vertebral, anal, cardiac, tracheal, esophageal, renal, and limb anomalies).[9] In a study of 84 infants, Grosfeld and Ballantine reported that 31 (37%) had cardiac anomalies, 18 (21.4%) had gastrointestinal malformations, and 6 (7%) had the VACTERL association.[5] The most common cardiac lesion is ventricular septal defect, followed by patent ductus arteriosus and tetralogy of Fallot.[6]

Pathophysiology

TEF presents in one of five different forms (Fig. 12-2). The most common is a blind esophageal pouch with the lower esophagus attached to the trachea. Eight-six percent of infants will have this form of TEF.[6] The rarest form is the double fistula. Signs and symptoms are very similar in all types of TEF and will be presented here generally.

The central clinical problem in TEF is aspiration of saliva and reflux of gastric contents into the trachea and lungs. A chemical aspiration pneumonitis results. When crying, the infant closes the glottis, which forces air into the fistula, dilates the stomach, and causes respiratory insufficiency that results from elevation of the diaphragm. Immediate management of these infants is directed primarily at stabilization and prevention of aspiration.

Clinical Signs and Diagnosis

The infant presents with symptoms early after birth. Excess salivation and drooling are seen first. Episodes of choking, gagging, and dyspnea occur,

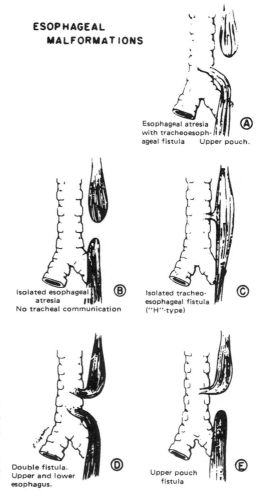

ESOPHAGEAL
MALFORMATIONS

Esophageal atresia
with tracheoesoph-
ageal fistula   Upper pouch.   Ⓐ

Isolated esophageal   Ⓑ
atresia
No tracheal communication

Isolated tracheo-   Ⓒ
esophageal fistula
("H"-type)

Double fistula.   Ⓓ
Upper and lower
esophagus.

Upper pouch   Ⓔ
fistula

FIGURE 12-2 Representations of the various forms of esophageal malformations associated with tracheoesophageal fistula. (Nardid GL, Zuidema GD: Surgery, 3rd ed. Boston, Little Brown, 1972.)

especially with feeding. When crying or coughing, the infant has a distended abdomen which is the result of forcing air through the fistula and into the stomach.

Chest x-ray film may reveal pneumonia, atelectasis, and an elevated diaphragm. Chest and abdominal x-ray films show a dilated esophageal pouch and either the presence or absence of air in the abdomen, depending on the type of fistula. Chemical pneumonitis may be present on chest x-ray film if the infant has aspirated. Contrast media may be used to outline the blind pouch but must be suctioned out immediately to prevent aspiration (Fig. 12-3).

Diagnosis can also be determined by the inability to pass a large catheter slowly into the esophagus. A fairly large, inflexible catheter must be used to prevent coiling within the pouch, leading the clinician to believe it has passed into the stomach.

Ultrasound examination of the heart and great vessels is valuable in identifying any cardiac anomalies that may be present. Bronchoscopy may

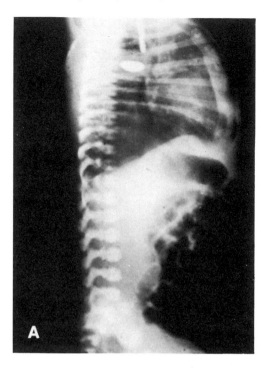

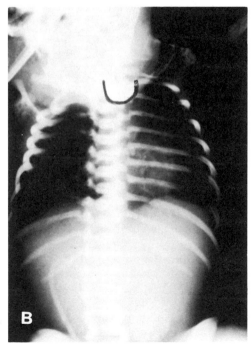

FIGURE 12-3 (*A*) Lateral radiograph of a baby with esophageal atresia and tracheoesophageal fistula reveals a small meniscus of barium in the upper pouch. Gas is present in the stomach and intestinal tract because of the fistulous connection to the trachea. In this radiograph, some air in the lower esophageal segment can be seen in the posterior mediastinum. (*B*) In a radiograph of a patient with isolated esophageal atresia, the upper pouch is outlined with barium. There is no air below the diaphragm. (*C*) In a barium swallow in a patient with H-type isolated esophageal atresia, a normal-sized lumen of the esophagus is seen. Dye has spilled into the trachea, outlining the upper trachea and larynx. The fistula is at the level of the clavicle. (Guzzeta PC, Anderson KD, Eichelberger MR, et al: General surgery. In Avery GB, Fletcher MA, MacDonald MG [eds]: Neonatology: Pathophysiology and Treatment of the Newborn, 4th ed, p. 925. Philadelphia, JB Lippincott, 1994.) (*Continues*)

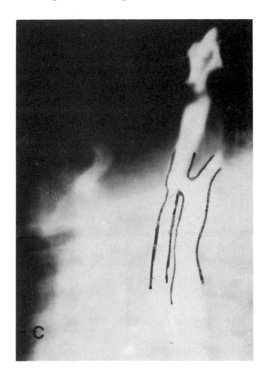

FIGURE 12-3 (Continued.)

also be useful in locating the exact location of the fistula.[6] Prenatal ultrasound examinations can identify TEF in some fetuses.

Management and Complications
Stabilization of the infant is the most immediate concern. Surgery for the infant with TEF may be delayed if the infant poses a high surgical risk because of prematurity, associated anomalies, or aspiration pneumonia. The infant should be kept on a radiant warmer in a 30-degree, upright position to decrease the chance of gastric reflux. A nasogastric tube is inserted into the upper esophageal pouch and suction applied to remove excess secretions. Adequate humidification, chest physiotherapy, oxygen administration, and broad-spectrum antibiotics are indicated for the treatment of aspiration pneumonitis. The infant is fed by means of a gastrostomy tube if surgical correction will be delayed.

Once the infant has been stabilized, surgery is performed through a right thoracotomy. The lower segment of the esophagus is detached from the trachea and the fistula is sutured closed. The blind pouch is then opened and anastomosed to the lower segment of the esophagus. Infants are maintained on intravenous nutrition postoperatively and oral feedings can be started on the 5th or 6th day if there is no evidence of complications.[6] Care must be taken not to disrupt the tracheal or esophageal sutures if suctioning or reintubation are required.

The major complication in the preoperative stage is aspiration pneumonia. Following surgical repair, complications include esophageal strictures, gastroesophageal reflux, recurrent fistula, and tracheomalacia. Respiratory complications have been noted in up to 50% of patients postoperatively and include apnea, bradycardia, aspiration, recurrent pneumonia, and respiratory arrest.[3] The survival rate for infants with esophageal atresia has improved steadily and is as high as 100% in infants from one center who were stable prior to surgery and had a primary repair.[6] Infants who were unstable and required multiple surgeries had lower survival rates, and deaths were often due to associated anomalies, such as cardiac defects and congenital diaphragmatic hernia.

▀ ABDOMINAL WALL DEFECTS

Omphalocele and gastroschisis are defects of the abdominal wall in which a portion of the abdominal contents are outside the cavity. They result from abnormal or incomplete development of the layers of the abdominal wall during gestation. An **omphalocele** is a condition in which the protruding intestines are contained within a translucent membrane or sac and the umbilical cord originates from within this membrane (Fig. 12-4). The sac is usually intact, but it may be ruptured during the delivery of the infant. In **gastroschisis**, the defect is usually lateral to the umbilical stump and the protruding intestines are not contained within a membrane (Fig. 12-5). Infants with omphaloceles may also have associated defects, such as congenital heart disease, intestinal atresia, or an imperforate anus.

Pathophysiology

During gestation, the pressure of the abdominal contents against the abdominal wall provides a stimulus for continued growth of the layers of the wall. If a large portion of the intestines develop outside of the abdomen, the cavity may be underdeveloped, making surgical repair more difficult. The development of the intestines and abdominal organs is usually not affected by the presence of an omphalocele or gastroschisis,

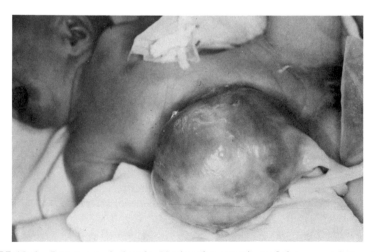

FIGURE 12-4   Large omphalocele. Notice the covering of the sac and its relation to the umbilicus, which protrudes from the lower portion. (Guzzeta PC, Anderson KD, Eichelberger MR, et al: General surgery. In Avery GB, Fletcher MA, MacDonald MG [eds]: Neonatology: Pathophysiology and Treatment of the Newborn, 4th ed, p. 945. Philadelphia, JB Lippincott, 1994.)

although malrotation may occur since the intestine is not fixed inside the cavity. The greatest risk to the infant is from trauma during the delivery process and from infection in the immediate postnatal period.

The respiratory status of the infant may be compromised following surgery if there is not sufficient room in the abdominal cavity to accommodate the structures that developed outside the abdomen. When the intestines are returned to the abdomen, they apply pressure against the diaphragm and limit its movement, a situation which may cause respiratory failure.

Clinical Signs and Diagnosis

The diagnosis of these abnormalities is made entirely by physical examination at the time of delivery. The defects may also be identified prenatally by ultrasound examination. Prenatal diagnosis allows time to arrange transport of the mother to a perinatal center that can provide the resources needed to care for these infants. Because of the frequency of associated anomalies, careful examination of all other systems should follow identification of these problems.

Management and Complications

Immediately after delivery, the intestines and other protruding structures should be carefully covered with sterile, saline-soaked gauze to prevent drying and infection. This covering is also important in maintaining the temperature of the infant. No pressure should be placed on the intestines, since this can reduce blood flow to the structures and may also apply upward pressure against the diaphragm, impeding respiratory efforts.[6] A nasogastric tube may be inserted to remove gastric secretions and prevent aspiration.[8] Intravenous fluids are administered

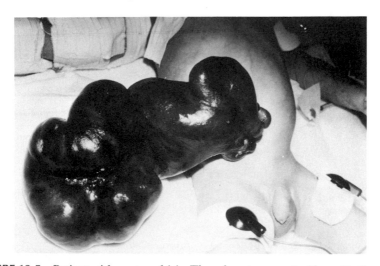

FIGURE 12-5 Patient with gastroschisis. The edematous, matted bowel is the result of the intestines floating freely in the amniotic fluid. Remarkably, these distorted viscera ultimately fit back into the abdominal cavity and assume a normal appearance and function. (Guzzeta PC, Anderson KD, Eichelberger MR, et al: General surgery. In Avery GB, Fletcher MA, MacDonald MG [eds]: Neonatology: Pathophysiology and Treatment of the Newborn, 4th ed, p. 946. Philadelphia, JB Lippincott, 1994.)

to provide hydration and glucose, and prophylactic antibiotics may also be given.

Surgical repair should be performed as soon as the infant is stabilized. If the abdominal cavity is large enough to accommodate the intestines and other structures, complete repair may be accomplished in a single procedure in which the viscera are returned to the abdomen and the defect sutured closed. If this is not possible, an extra-abdominal prosthetic compartment is fashioned out of a Silastic material and sutured to the edges of the defect to protect the protruding viscera. Over the next 7 to 10 days, the pressure of the extra-abdominal contents against the internal contents will expand the abdominal cavity to the point where total closure is possible. During this time, the infant should be supported with intravenous feeding and careful observation for signs of respiratory distress.

Respiratory complications are not generally seen in infants who undergo a primary surgical repair. Infants who require multiple corrective procedures are at higher risk for complications.[11] Mortality and complications are more often the result of associated anomalies, rather than the primary abdominal wall defects or their surgical repair. The most common complications in the postoperative period are infection, increased intra-abdominal pressure, and respiratory distress.[8]

▰REFERENCES

1. Coniglio J, Manzione J, Hengerer A: Anatomic findings and management of choanal atresia and the CHARGE association. Ann Otol Rhinol Laryngol 97:448, 1988.
2. Cromblehome TM, Adzick NS, Hardy K, Longaker MT, Bradley SM, Duncan BW, Verrier ED, Harrison ME: Pulmonary lobar transplantation in neonatal swine: A model for treatment of congenital diaphragmatic hernia. J Pediatr Surg 25:11, 1990.
3. Delius RE, Wheatly MJ, Coram AG: Etiology and management of respiratory complications after repair of esophageal atresia with tracheoesophageal fistula. Surgery 112:527, 1992.
4. Fiascone JM, Vreeland PN, Frantz ID: Neonatal lung disease and respiratory care. In Burton GG, Hodgkin JE, Ward JJ (eds): Respiratory Care: A Guide to Clinical Practice, 3rd ed. Philadelphia, JB Lippincott, 1991.
5. Grosfeld JL. Ballantine TDN: Esophageal atresia and tracheoesophageal fistula: Effect of delayed thoracotomy on survival. Surgery 84:394, 1978.
6. Guzzeta PC, Anderson KD, Eichelberger MR, Newman KD, Rouse TM, Schnitzer JJ, Boyajian M, Tomaski SM: General surgery. In Avery GB, Fletcher MA, MacDonald MG (eds): Neonatology: Pathophysiology and Treatment of the Newborn, 4th ed. Philadelphia, JB Lippincott, 1994.
7. Hopkins WA: The esophagus. In Gray SW, Skandalakis JE (eds): Embryology for Surgeons. Philadelphia, WB Saunders, 1972.
8. Powers L, Burrington J, Gardner SL, Merenstein GB: Pediatric surgery. In Merenstein GB, Gardner SL (eds): Handbook of Neonatal Intensive Care, 2nd ed. St. Louis, CV Mosby, 1989.
9. Quan L, Smith DW: The VATER association: Vertebral defects, anal atresia, T-E fistula with esophageal atresia, radial and renal dysplasia: A spectrum of associated defects. J Pediatr 104:7, 1973.
10. Tapper D: Surgical emergencies in the newborn. In Cloherty JP, Stark AR (eds): Manual of Neonatal Care, 2nd ed. Boston, Little, Brown, 1985.
11. Tracy T, Silen ML, Weber TR, Czervinske MP: Neonatal disorders that affect respiratory care. In Barnhart SL, Czervinske MP (eds): Perinatal and Pediatric Respiratory Care. Philadelphia, WB Saunders, 1995.
12. Wilson JM, Thompson JR, Schnitzer JJ, Bower LK, Lillehei CW, Perlman ND, Kolobow T: Intratracheal pulmonary ventilation and congenital diaphragmatic hernia: A report of two cases. J Pediatr Surg 25:1048, 1990.

▬SELF-ASSESSMENT QUESTIONS

1. Occlusion or blockage of the airway between the posterior nasal passage and the nasopharynx is known as
   a. omphalocele
   b. choanal atresia
   c. glossoptosis
   d. meningomyelocele

2. Immediate treatment for an infant with choanal atresia consists of
   a. insertion of an oral airway
   b. nasotracheal intubation
   c. tracheotomy
   d. positioning the infant in a prone position

3. Diagnosis of Pierre-Robin syndrome is made on the basis of
   a. lateral cervical neck x-ray
   b. serum protein analysis
   c. physical examination
   d. bronchoscopy

4. Initial treatment of the infant with micrognathia and glossoptosis consists of
   a. insertion of an oral airway
   b. nasotracheal intubation
   c. tracheotomy
   d. positioning the infant in a prone position

5. Congenital diaphragmatic hernia occurs most often on the _____ side.
   a. right
   b. left

6. Clinical signs of diaphragmatic hernia include
   I. scaphoid abdomen
   II. cyanosis
   III. excessive drooling
   IV. decreased breath sounds
   a. II and III   c. I, II, and III
   b. I and IV   d. I, II, and IV

7. Persistent pulmonary hypertension and right-to-left shunting often complicate the treatment of
   a. gastroschisis
   b. congenital diaphragmatic hernia
   c. tracheoesophageal fistula
   d. Pierre-Robin syndrome

8. The central problem for infants with tracheoesophageal fistula is
   a. incomplete closure of the foramen of Bochdalek
   b. aspiration of saliva and gastroesophageal reflux
   c. blockage of the nasal airway
   d. hypoplasia of the mandible

9. The major complication following corrective surgery for tracheoesophageal fistula is
   a. persistent pulmonary hypertension
   b. infection
   c. pneumothorax
   d. aspiration pneumonia

10. A condition in which the intestines protrude through the abdominal wall and are contained within a translucent membrane is known as
    a. gastroschisis
    b. omphalocele
    c. glossoptosis
    d. diaphragmatic hernia

Chapter **13**

Neurologic Disorders

JAMES LAWSON

OBJECTIVES

Having completed this chapter, the reader will be able to:

1 Identify the most common form of muscular dystrophy.

2 Identify the age at which muscular dystrophy is thought to be most common.

3 Describe methods used to diagnose the patient with muscular dystrophy.

4 Describe changes in pulmonary function seen in patients with muscular dystrophy.

5 Describe the treatment of a patient with muscular dystrophy.

6 Describe the clinical presentation of Reye's syndrome.

7 Explain the clinical features of Reye's syndrome.

8 Explain the five stages of Reye's syndrome.

9 Describe the treatment of the patient with Reye's syndrome.

10 Explain the purpose of intubation and why mechanical ventilation is used in the treatment of Reye's syndrome.

11 State the definition of cerebral palsy.

12 Describe the type of infant afflicted with cerebral palsy.

13 Identify the diagnostic tools used to determine the onset of cerebral palsy.

14 Describe the use of electroencephalograms in verifying neurologic activity in patients with cerebral palsy.

15 Describe the treatment of a patient with cerebral palsy.

16 Identify the causes of epilepsy.

17 Describe the different types of seizures.

KEY TERMS

athetosis
cerebral palsy
Duchenne's dystrophy
electroencephalogram
electromyogram

encephalopathy
epilepsy
Reye's syndrome
Scott cannula

■MUSCULAR DYSTROPHY

Muscular dystrophies are hereditary conditions characterized by progressive muscle weakness. The most common form is **Duchenne's dystrophy**. This disease is inherited as a sex-linked recessive trait and occurs in early childhood. Muscle weakness is usually present at 2 to 4 years of age. This disease has a rapid progression, with patients being confined to a wheelchair by 10 to 12 years of age.[13]

Etiology

Inheritance of muscular dystrophies can be both genetic and autosomal. Duchenne's muscular dystrophy is a multisystem disease that affects the skeletal muscles, heart, and brain.[6] Skeletal muscles are weakened with fixed scoliosis and tendon contractures. In the heart, cardiomyopathy associated with cardiac arrhythmias is frequently seen.

Pathophysiology

These genetically transmitted diseases cause progressive atrophy in skeletal muscle or degeneration of neural tissue. The cause is unknown but appears to be an inborn error of metabolism. Serum creatinine phosphokinase is increased in affected patients.[6]

Clinical Signs and Diagnosis

Because of muscle weakness, once the child starts to walk certain abnormalities can be detected. Simple movements like standing from a sitting position and climbing steps become difficult. As a result of a decrease in ambulation, the patient's pulmonary function tests (PFTs) are altered. Abnormalities in PFTs include a decreased maximal expiratory pressure, decreased total lung capacity, decreased residual volume, and decreased vital capacity (VC).[6,13]

An increase in serum creatinine phosphokinase acts as a diagnostic aid, especially when dealing with a symptomatic child with a family history of muscular dystrophy. Confirmation can also be made by performing a muscle biopsy and an **electromyogram** (EMG), a test used to trace the contraction of a muscle as a result of electrical stimulation.[5,13]

Management and Complications

Physical and orthopedic therapy should be implemented for supportive measures. Preventive measures should also be taken to reduce the incidence of infection. When infection occurs, good pulmonary cleansing with the aid of assisted coughing and deep breathing should be implemented. PFTs should be performed on a routine basis throughout the year to monitor the patient's pulmonary reserve. Intermittent positive pressure breathing therapy should be instituted for volume expansion when a patient's VC drops below 80% of the predicted level.[13] Due to respiratory muscle impairment, mechanical ventilation may be necessary. Respiratory care practitioners may come into contact with patients with muscular dystrophy in hospitals, extended care facilities, and patients' homes.

Respiratory muscle weakness may occur in some patients, with ventilation becoming impaired at night. Mechanical ventilation then becomes necessary either at night or continuously. Because of a decrease in lung volumes, these patients are prone to frequent respiratory tract infections. Most of these patients die from respiratory failure by 30 years of age.[13]

■REYE'S SYNDROME

Reye's syndrome is a life-threatening, noncontagious illness that initially causes a deterioration of liver function and encephalopathy of the brain. **Encephalopathy** is defined as any dysfunction of the brain. To a lesser degree, other organs of the body may be affected.

Etiology

Reye's syndrome appears to be associated with typical childhood illnesses such as influenza type B and varicella. Some studies have found an increased risk of Reye's syndrome after use of aspirin during a viral illness.[10,11] Reye's syndrome is one of the most common causes of encephalopathy in children; without proper treatment, massive cerebral edema may result. An epidemic of influenza or chicken pox is commonly followed by an increase in the number of cases of Reye's syndrome.[11] The primary months are January, February, and March but cases have been reported in every month.[10] This disease usually affects children from infancy to approximately 19 years of age.[5]

Pathophysiology

As liver function deteriorates as a result of the abnormal accumulation of fat in the liver and other organs, the ammonia processing capability of the liver is damaged. Ammonia (NH_3) is accumulated in the liver and is eventually released into the bloodstream and the brain. This increase in ammonia will cause renal impairment since the kidneys now have to buffer excessive amounts of ammonia.[7] Liver deterioration also causes an accumulation of fat in the liver cells and eventually leads to a loss of normal liver function. Following liver and kidney malfunction, fluid imbalance results. This causes the accumulation of fluid in the brain cells resulting in an increased intracranial pressure (ICP).[7] The increased ICP can cause respiratory arrest and irreversible cortical damage.

Clinical Signs and Diagnosis

Typically, a child with Reye's syndrome has been healthy until developing persistent nausea and vomiting, usually beginning 3 to 7 days after an ordinary viral infection such as influenza or chicken pox.[11,12] The patients are unlikely to have a fever. Other early signs of Reye's syndrome are listlessness, loss of energy, drowsiness, irritability, aggressiveness, confusion, and irrational behavior.[7] Table 13-1 describes the stages of Reye's syndrome.

Diagnosis of the early stages of Reye's syndrome can be achieved by obtaining serum enzyme levels including aspartate aminotransferase (AST [SGOT]) and alanine aminotransferase (ALT [SGPT]).[7] Any deviation from normal values strongly suggests Reye's syndrome. In making this diagnosis, every possible pathology that would cause a biochemical abnormality should be ruled out, such as meningitis, encephalitis, exogenous toxins, and drug overdose or abuse. If blood tests show an increased ammonia level, Reye's syndrome should be suspected. An **electroen-**

TABLE 13-1   **Five Classic Stages of Reye's Syndrome**

STAGE	CONDITION	DESCRIPTION
I	Mild	Quiet, lethargic, normal respirations, normal skeletal muscle tone, normal heart rate, normal pupillary response
II	Moderate	Stuporous, slurred speech, ataxia, hyperpnea, normal pupillary response
III	Severe	Agitated delirium, seizure activity, hyperpnea, tachycardia, pupils dilated
IV	Critical	Comatose, decerebrate posturing, no response to painful stimuli, brainstem respirations (Cheyne-Stokes and apneustic), and doll's eyes
V	Brain death	Coma, flaccid paralysis, apnea, variable heart rate, pupils fixed and dilated

cephalogram (EEG) may be performed to detect any unusual brain wave activity that may indicate encephalopathy.[13]

Management and Complications

Management of patients with Reye's syndrome may vary somewhat based on severity. In stage I, patients may need correction of any electrolyte imbalance and management of serum glucose levels. Stage II requires monitoring in an intensive care unit, and more aggressive treatment should be considered at this point. Elective intubation should be initiated for protection of the patient's airway and mechanical ventilation initiated to maintain Pa_{O_2} levels between 100 and 150 mm Hg and Pa_{CO_2} levels between 20 and 28 mm Hg. Radial arterial line insertion should be considered for frequent arterial blood gas readings and a pulmonary artery (Swan Ganz) catheter placed for frequent hemodynamic monitoring. These patients may rapidly progress to a comatose state. Stage III involves a comatose patient. Continuation of the supportive care given in stages I and II is needed. Paralyzing agents such as pancuronium bromide (Pavulon) or curare should be used to control ventilation and reduce oxygen consumption. Capnography can be implemented to monitor patient end tidal CO_2 (ET_{CO_2}). ET_{CO_2} should correlate well with the patient's Pa_{CO_2} and changes in ICP.

Surgical intervention may be necessary to insert a catheter in order to monitor ICP. The **Scott cannula** is commonly used for this purpose. The cannula is placed in the lateral ventricle of the brain to closely monitor the ICP. Normal ICP is 10 to 15 mm Hg; ICP should be kept at or below this normal level. Cerebral perfusion pressure should be kept greater than 50 mm Hg by reducing ICP while maintaining arterial blood pressure.[13] Management of the cerebral edema associated with Reye's syndrome is the major factor affecting the outcome of the patient. By using osmotic diuretics such as mannitol, mild diuresis can be performed without affecting electrolyte and acid–base balance. With the aid of mechanical ventilation, the patient can be hyperventilated, thus causing cerebral vasoconstriction.

Because of the multiple organ involvement seen in Reye's syndrome, many body processes may be affected. This may cause hypoglycemia, increased fluid levels in the brain resulting in increased ICP, and hypoxemia.[7] ICP may become elevated enough to cause irreversible brain damage.

CEREBRAL PALSY

Cerebral palsy (CP) can be defined as a motor function disorder resulting from damage to a child's brain. This damage may be associated with low-birth-weight infants or with critically ill neonates with respiratory problems. CP is associated with a group of conditions caused by a permanent, non-progressive brain defect or lesion present at birth or shortly after.

Etiology

If the diagnosis of CP is to be made, the damage must be nonprogressive and have occurred prenatally, during birth, or in childhood.[10] This disorder is usually associated with premature or abnormal births and intra-partum asphyxia, resulting in damage to the nervous system.[4,9]

A major cause of CP is prematurity. Other prenatal causes include a lack of oxygen to the fetal brain caused by pinching and/or kinking of the umbilical cord.[4] Shock caused by any condition relating to maternal blood loss is also a factor. Any damage to the brain at birth may cause CP. During infancy and early childhood, any type of head trauma or cerebral infection such as meningitis or encephalitis may cause CP.[4,9]

Pathophysiology

Abnormal development of the placenta or any kinking or knotting of the umbilical cord greatly contributes to the risk of the infant developing CP by interfering with the supply of oxygen to the fetal brain, resulting in fetal asphyxia. Following an anoxic episode, the brain swells, causing blood vessels to rupture. Swelling of the brain may lead to increased ICP and impairment of neurologic function.

Clinical Signs and Diagnosis

Clinical signs are often not evident at birth. After 6 months of age, the primitive exaggerated tendon reflexes persist, interfering with normal movement and causing a delay in motor development. The child has difficulty sitting, rolling over, crawling, walking, smiling, and making speech sounds.[3] Spasticity, **athetosis** (involuntary twisting movements in the hands and fingers), and mixed muscle reaction are the most common types of muscle and movement disorders. A child with spastic CP has difficulty initiating movement, while a child with antheoid CP has difficulty controlling both movement and posture.[3,5] Because of the high prevalence of brain damage, children with mixed muscle reaction have a higher incidence of mental retardation.

CP is often diagnosed from a child's medical history. Examination of the child's nervous system is most important. To confirm or assess the extent and possible location of brain damage, a computerized tomography scan may be performed. Seizures can occur in patients with CP; EEGs are used to measure the electrical activity of the brain. With the aid of EEGs, seizure spikes or any other asymmetries can be noted.[6,13]

Management

Primary treatment for CP consists of supporting patients to enable them to live with their disability. Certain considerations also need to be addressed, such as the age of the child and the severity of the involvement. Orthopedic treatment, such as the use of braces, splints, and casts, has been beneficial in helping to stabilize arm and leg positions to prevent contractions and deformities of the bones.[3] Physical therapy methods include exercise and walking, if possible, along with range-of-motion exercises, which may aid in reducing the level of disability.[3] The respiratory care practitioner should consider volume expansion exercises if the patient is immobile or confined to a wheelchair. By using incentive spirometry and coughing and deep breathing exercises, the occurrence of atelectasis and pneumonia may be reduced.

▬ EPILEPSY AND SEIZURES

Epilepsy, sometimes called seizure disorder, is a medical condition in which people are susceptible to recurring seizures of various types. Epilepsy is not a disease; it is a sign or symptom of an underlying neurological disorder.

Etiology

A seizure is a brief episode of sudden, excessive electrical activity in the brain that affects its normal functions and produces changes in a person's movements, behavior, or consciousness. The kind of seizure a person has depends on how much of the brain is affected. This interference with normal brain activity is variable and can range from life threatening to barely noticeable.[2]

There is no single cause of epilepsy, since many factors can injure the nerve cells in the brain. The common causes of seizures in children are listed in Table 13-2.

Clinical Signs and Types of Seizures

In some cases, the child experiences a sensation or warning called an aura. These auras are changes in body sensations that vary from person to person. Young children may not be aware of these feelings. In children the signs and symptoms are reflected in the type of seizure involved and are categorized as either generalized or partial. Different types of seizures are described in detail in Table 13-3.

TABLE 13-2 Causes of Seizures

Idiopathic—no known cause

Birth injury

Congenital defects

Fever

Infection

Toxic substances

Trauma

TABLE 13-3 Types of Seizures

Generalized Seizures: These happen when all or most of the brain is affected. So much of the brain is involved that the child may lose consciousness.

Generalized tonic clonic seizure is the type of seizure that used to be called grand mal. The child loses consciousness, falls, stiffens, then shakes uncontrollably for a minute or two. Although dramatic, this type of seizure is rarely a medical emergency.

Myoclonic seizure lasts a shorter time. It causes a massive muscle jerk that may throw the child to the ground.

Atonic seizure causes sudden falls. It lasts only a few moments but can happen frequently.

Absence seizure is very brief, lasts only a few seconds, and resembles a blank stare or daydreaming. While it is occurring, the child is completely unaware of his or her surroundings. It begins and ends suddenly.

Infantile spasms occur in infants. They are clusters of brief jerking or jackknife movements.

Partial Seizures. These happen when only part of the brain is affected, although they can spread to the whole brain and cause generalized tonic clonic seizures. When seizure activity remains in one area, the following types of seizures may occur:

Simple partial affects the senses, feelings, emotions, and movement. Objects may look bigger or smaller; there may be hallucinations of sight or sound. The child can feel unexplained pain, fear, or anger. A hand or leg may shake. The child does not lose consciousness.

Complex partial may start like a simple partial seizure but progress to cause loss of awareness and automatic movements that resemble a trance-like stage. Automatic movements can take almost any form but are not under conscious control. A complex partial seizure lasts only a minute or two, but confusion afterwards may last much longer.

Diagnosis and Management

The diagnosis of most seizure disorders can be made on the basis of their obvious clinical manifestations. However, psychomotor and petit mal seizures can sometimes have atypical clinical signs that make diagnosis more difficult. The electroencephalogram (EEG) is the most useful test in the evaluation of seizures and should be given to any child suspected of having a seizure. Electrodes placed on different areas of the scalp record the electrical impulses caused by brain activity. The testing session should include a period of wakefulness with hyperventilation and intermittent photic stimulation, and a period of light sleep.

Further testing is dictated by the clinical situation. A computed tomography (CT) scan can be helpful in determining the location and extent of the cerebral lesion. A lumbar puncture (spinal tap) is indicated if there is any possibility of central nervous system infection.[8] Some children may have metabolic disorders that require additional testing.

Treatment

Treatment of epilepsy has made enormous advances through the use of anticonvulsant medications. The increased knowledge of the metabolism of these drugs and their interactions has aided physicians in treating this disorder. One of the most significant factors is the ability to measure serum levels. Some of the more commonly used drugs are phenobarbital, phenytoin (Dilantin), valproic acid (Depakene), and carbamazepine (Tegretol).[1] The choice of drug is determined by the type of seizure, a drug's side effects, and the needs of the particular child.

▄ REFERENCES

1. Blackman JA: Medical Aspects of Developmental Disabilities in Children from Birth to Three, rev. Rockville MD, Aspen, 1984.
2. Epilepsy Foundation of America: Epilepsy and Seizures. Washington DC, Epilepsy Foundation of America, 1990.
3. Fetters L: Measurement and treatment in cerebral palsy: An argument for a new approach. Physical Therapy 6:244, 1991.
4. Gaffney G, Sellers S, Flavel V, Squire M, Johnson A: Case control study of intrapartum care, cerebral palsy and perinatal death. British Med J Mar 19:743, 1994.
5. Green M, Haggerty RJ: Ambulatory Pediatrics. Philadelphia, WB Saunders, 1990.
6. Hughes JG, John GF: Synopsis of Pediatrics. St. Louis, CV Mosby, 1984.
7. Kelly KJ: Respiratory care of the neurologically injured and neuromuscular impaired child. In Koff PB, Eitzman D, Neu J (eds): Neonatal and Pediatric Respiratory Care, 2nd ed. St. Louis, Mosby-Year Book, 1993.
8. Levine MD: Developmental Behavioral Pediatrics. Philadelphia, WB Saunders, 1983.
9. Miller G. Cerebral palsy and minor congenital anomalies. Clin Ped 30:97, 1991.
10. Miller HC, Stephen M: Hemorrhagic varicella: A case report and review of the complications of varicella in children. Am J of Emerg Med 11:633, 1993.
11. National Reye's Syndrome Foundation: Reye's Syndrome Annual 7:1, 1992.
12. Quam DA: Recognizing a case of Reye's syndrome. American Family Physician 50:1491, 1994.
13. Schidlow DV, Smith DS: A Practical Guide to Pediatric Respiratory Diseases. Philadelphia, Hanley and Belfus, 1994.

▄ SELF-ASSESSMENT QUESTIONS

1. At what age does muscle weakness present in infants with muscular dystrophy?
   a. 6 months   c. 2 years
   b. 1 year   d. 6 years

2. Signs and symptoms of muscular dystrophy include
       I. decreased residual volume
       II. increased tidal volume
       III. decreased vital capacity
          a. I only   c. I and II
          b. II only   d. I and III

3. _____ is defined as any dysfunction of the brain.
   a. encephalopathy   c. neuritis
   b. encephalitis   d. polyneuritis

4. Clinical signs of Reye's syndrome include
   a. persistent nausea and vomiting
   b. afebrile
   c. irrational behavior
   d. all of the above

5. Diagnosis of Reye's syndrome is based upon the finding of
   a. serum enzyme levels
   b. alanine aminotransferase
   c. increased serum ammonia levels
   d. all of the above

6. A child exhibiting slurred speech, ataxia, and hyperpnea is in which stage of Reye's syndrome?
   a. stage I
   b. stage II
   c. stage III
   d. stage IV

7. In the child with Reye's syndrome, PaO$_2$ levels should be maintained at
   a. 50 to 80 mm Hg
   b. 70 to 90 mm Hg
   c. 100 to 150 mm Hg
   d. 150 to 200 mm Hg

8. _____ is a disorder resulting from damage to an infant's brain associated with prematurity.
   a. muscular dystrophy
   b. Reye's syndrome
   c. Duchenne's dystrophy
   d. cerebral palsy

Part 4
Respiratory Therapeutics

Chapter **14**

Oxygen Therapy

KIM V. HILL

OBJECTIVES

Having completed this chapter, the reader will be able to:

1 List the indications for oxygen therapy.

2 List and describe the types of hypoxia and give examples of each.

3 Discuss the signs and symptoms associated with each type of hypoxia.

4 Discuss the principles of oxygen administration in the newborn and child.

5 Identify and describe the oxygen administration devices used with infants and pediatric patients.

6 Discuss the advantages and disadvantages of each type of oxygen administration device.

7 Describe the hazards associated with the use of oxygen therapy.

8 Describe the etiology, pathophysiology, prevention, and treatment of retinopathy of prematurity.

9 List the factors that contribute to the development of bronchopulmonary dysplasia and absorption atelectasis.

10 Discuss the clinical application of helium–oxygen therapy.

KEY TERMS

absorption atelectasis
central cyanosis
dysoxia
high-flow system
hypoxemia

hypoxia
low-flow system
oxyhood
peripheral cyanosis
retinopathy of prematurity

Oxygen is a colorless, odorless, and tasteless gas required for the life of all organ systems in the human body. It has been the most widely used therapeutic agent in respiratory care for decades, not only in the adult, but in the infant and child as well. The practitioner must remember that oxygen is a drug and should be administered with care. It is common knowledge that prolonged exposure to elevated concentrations of oxygen may cause toxic side effects. Cautious administration of oxygen is especially important in premature infants because of their susceptibility to the hazards of this drug. This chapter will discuss the importance of oxygen delivery, potential hazards or side effects, and equipment utilized in providing oxygen to the newborn and child.

▰ INDICATIONS

The primary indication for oxygen therapy is to supply an adequate amount of oxygen to the tissues.[11] An adequate level of oxygen is defined as that amount which allows the tissues to perform their normal metabolic functions. In most cases, the PaO_2 is used as an indicator to determine the need for additional oxygen delivery to the tissues, but other factors also play an important role.

The specific indications for oxygen therapy as determined by the American Association for Respiratory Care Clinical Practice Guidelines for Oxygen Therapy in the Acute Care Hospital are as follows:

1. Documented hypoxemia, in which arterial oxygen tensions (PaO_2) of less than 60 mm Hg or arterial saturations (SaO_2) of less than 90% on room air are obtained; or when PaO_2 and/or SaO_2 levels are below desirable ranges for specific clinical situations in children and infants more than 28 days old.
2. In neonates, PaO_2 levels of less than 50 mm Hg and/or SaO_2 levels of less than 88% or capillary oxygen tension (PcO_2) levels of less than 40 mm Hg are indication for oxygen therapy.[1]

Types of Hypoxia

Hypoxia is defined as inadequate oxygen at the tissue level, whereas **hypoxemia** is a reduction of the oxygen content in the arterial blood and can be caused by low PaO_2 values, low hemoglobin levels, or abnormal hemoglobin saturations. Any or all of these factors may reduce the amount of oxygen carried to the tissues.[13] There are three basic categories of hypoxia: hypoxemia, reduced blood flow, and **dysoxia**, an abnormal metabolic state in which the tissues are unable to properly utilize the oxygen available to them. Table 14-1 summarizes the causes and primary indications of hypoxia.

A variety of signs and symptoms may result from hypoxia, depending upon its severity and duration. Clinical findings associated with hypoxia include tachypnea, dyspnea, cyanosis, tachycardia, restlessness, and confusion.[13] In severe cases of hypoxia, bradycardia and arrhythmias may develop. These signs and symptoms will vary from patient to patient.

One of the most commonly reported signs of severe hypoxia is cyanosis. Cyanosis is a bluish discoloration of the skin, mucous membranes, and nail beds, and is caused by an abnormally high amount of reduced hemoglobin (Hb-) in the capillaries, or when at least 5 g % of reduced hemoglobin is present.[13]

There are two types of cyanosis, peripheral and central, and it is important to differentiate between the two types when evaluating the oxygen status of the patient. **Peripheral cyanosis** exists when there is excessive Hb- in the venous blood and occurs when the tissues are extracting more

TABLE 14-1 Types of Hypoxia

CAUSE	PRIMARY INDICATOR	MECHANISM	EXAMPLE
Hypoxemia			
Low PIO_2	Low PaO_2	Reduced P_B	High altitude
Hypoventilation	Low PaO_2, High $PaCO_2$	Decreased VA	Drug overdose
Diffusion defect	Low PaO_2, High $PaCO_2$ on air, resolves with O_2	Barrier at A-C membrane	Pulmonary edema, HMD
Anatomic shunt	Low PaO_2, High P(A-a) on air, does not resolve with O_2	Blood flow between right and left side of circulation	Congenital heart disease
Physiologic shunt	Low PaO_2, High P(A-a) on air, does not respond with O_2	Perfusion without ventilation	Atelectasis
Hb Deficiency			
Absolute	Low Hb content	Loss of Hb	Hemorrhage
Relative	Abnormal SaO_2 Reduced CaO_2	Abnormal Hb	Methemoglobin
Reduced Blood Flow			
Reduced blood flow	Increased $C(a-v)O_2$	Decreased perfusion	Shock, ischemia
Dysoxia			
Dysoxia	Normal CaO_2, Increased CvO_2	Disruption of cellular enzymes	Cyanide poisoning, septic shock

(Scanlan CL: Patterns of cardiopulmonary dysfunction. In Scanlan CL, Spearman C, Sheldon RL [eds]: Egan's Fundamentals of Respiratory Care, 6th ed. St. Louis, Mosby-Year Book, 1995.)

oxygen from the blood than under normal circumstances. This extraction can be a result of poor perfusion. **Central cyanosis** occurs when saturation of arterial hemoglobin is reduced and can be detected in the capillary beds of the lips and the lining of the cheeks. In normally oxygenated capillary blood, about 2.5 g of reduced Hb- exists and results in a saturation level of approximately 75% and a PaO_2 of about 40 mm Hg.[13] Therefore, central cyanosis would be expected with PaO_2 levels below 40 mm Hg.

Cyanosis may be a poor indicator of hypoxia since not all hypoxic states produce cyanosis. High carboxyhemoglobin levels and cyanide poisoning are two examples in which death can result from hypoxia without cyanosis.[13] Increases in oxygen content also add to the degree of cyanosis. Patients who have polycythemia (high Hb levels) can be cyanotic and still have a normal PaO_2 level, whereas patients with anemia (low Hb levels) can be hypoxic long before cyanosis appears.[13] Other factors that can affect the degree of cyanosis include the perception of the examiners, ambient light, color of the skin, and presence of abnormal hemoglobin such as high fetal hemoglobin levels or methemoglobin. One final factor that may hide the signs of cyanosis is hyperbilirubinemia, which causes a jaundiced appearance of the skin.[13,16] All of these factors must be considered and contribute to the unreliability of cyanosis as an indicator of hypoxia.

▬ PRINCIPLES OF OXYGEN ADMINISTRATION

Arterial blood gas values for the normal full-term infant at birth (Table 14-2) tend to show mild metabolic acidosis with hypoxemia. The differences from normal adult values are primarily due to the stressful events of delivery and the lower buffering capacity of the newborn's blood. The mild hypoxemia and acidosis do not require treatment since, during the first week of life, blood gas values gradually approach normal adult ranges, except for a slightly lower PaO_2.[16] It would be unnecessary to try to maintain normal adult blood gas values in premature or otherwise compromised newborns because they simply do not require treatment.

The PaO_2 of an infant receiving oxygen therapy should be maintained between 50 and 80 mm Hg.[5] Adequate tissue oxygenation can be maintained at this level while reducing the risks from toxic levels of oxygen. The only exception to this PaO_2 range is for the infant being treated for persistent fetal circulation, where high levels of oxygen are administered to reduce pulmonary vasoconstriction.[5]

Oxygen therapy for the newborn and child should be tailored to the individual patient. Infants have remarkable mechanisms for compensating for hypoxia, including polycythemia, increased cardiac output, decreased affinity of hemoglobin for oxygen, and preferential shunting of blood to vital organs. The patient's ability to compensate should be considered when providing oxygen therapy.[5]

▬ METHODS OF OXYGEN ADMINISTRATION

Oxygen from a cylinder or wall source is cold and dry and must be warmed and humidified before therapeutic application. Many devices

TABLE 14-2 Blood Gas Values for Normal-Term Infants (5 Hours of Age)

PARAMETER	VALUE
pH	7.34
$PaCO_2$	35 mm Hg
PaO_2	74 mm Hg
HCO_3^-	19 mEq/L
Base excess	−5

(Scanlan CL: Patterns of cardiopulmonary dysfunction. In Scanlan CL, Spearman C, Sheldon RL [eds]: Egan's Fundamentals of Respiratory Care, 6th ed. St. Louis, Mosby-Year Book, 1995.)

used to deliver oxygen to newborn infants and children are very similar to those used for adult patients. These devices are classified as either low-flow or high-flow devices. A **low-flow system** is one in which only a portion of the patient's total inspired minute volume is provided by the device, and the patient must entrain the remainder of their minute volume from the room air. The amount of entrained air will affect the FIO_2 delivered. A **high-flow system**, on the other hand, is one in which the patient's total inspired minute volume is delivered by the device itself. These devices provide 100% of the patient's requirements and give precise oxygen concentrations.

Low-Flow Devices

Examples of low-flow devices commonly used in the newborn and child include nasal cannulas, simple oxygen masks, and partial and nonrebreathing masks.[8] Nasal cannulas (Fig. 14-1) are ideal for use in long-term oxygen therapy in stable patients who require low FIO_2 ranges such as in the treatment of the infant with bronchopulmonary dysplasia (BPD). Cannulas with short nasal prongs are available for use in premature infants and newborns. Flowmeters for infants using nasal cannulas should be calibrated in small increments such as quarters or tenths of a liter per minute. Excessive flow through nasal cannulas may yield extremely high oxygen percentages and may also cause drying of the nasal mucosa and

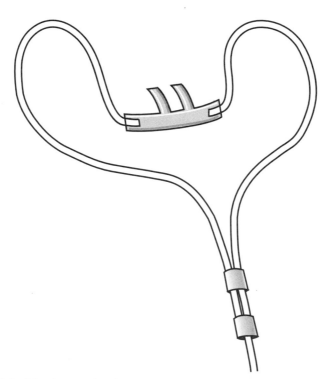

FIGURE 14-1 Nasal cannula. (Respiratory Therapy Review Entry Level Study Guide. Kettering, OH, RTS Publishing Company, 1996. Used with permission.)

sinus drainage. Flowrates used in infants and children with nasal cannulas range from 0.10 to 4.0 L/min.[12] Simple masks (Fig. 14-2) supply a slightly higher FIO_2 than the nasal cannula and may be poorly tolerated by the infant and child. Partial and nonrebreathing masks are suitable for short-term use in an emergency situation.[4] Caution should be taken with the administration of high oxygen concentrations from nonrebreathing masks in order to prevent any adverse effects from high levels of oxygen.

While exact oxygen concentrations with low-flow devices are uncertain in the infant and child, more attention should be paid to the oxygen saturation level as monitored by pulse oximetry as a guide for adequate oxygenation. Table 14-3 lists infant and pediatric oxygen administration devices and their respective flowrates and delivered oxygen concentrations.

High-Flow Devices

Venturi masks or air entrainment masks are examples of high-flow systems which will provide the patient's total inspired minute volume. These devices differ in design from manufacturer to manufacturer but usually incorporate air entrainment ports and a jet orifice to deliver specific oxygen concentrations with relatively high total flow ranges. The FIO_2 delivered depends upon the size of the entrainment ports and jet orifice and the oxygen flow through the jet orifice.[4] Large-volume nebulizers can also be used to deliver oxygen to children. These devices incorporate an air entrainment system similar to that of the Venturi mask. Nebulizers can be used in conjunction with aerosol masks, tracheostomy masks (Fig. 14-3), and face tents to provide specific concentrations of oxygen to the pediatric patient.[8] These devices are not recommended for use in newborns because the sound level intensities they produce can be damaging to the infant's organ of Corti and may cause hearing loss.[10]

Oxygen hoods or **oxyhoods** (Fig. 14-4) are probably the most common form of short-term oxygen delivery for the newborn.[8] Oxygen hoods are clear plastic boxes or cylinders that usually surround the infant's head and have an opening for the infant's neck. Located on the rear of the oxyhood is a port for the connection of large-bore tubing for oxygen delivery and humidification. Some types of oxyhoods incorporate soft plastic panels

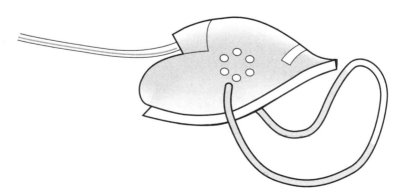

FIGURE 14-2 Simple oxygen mask. (Respiratory Therapy Review Entry Level Study Guide. Kettering, OH, RTS Publishing Company, 1996. Used with permission.)

TABLE 14-3 Oxygen Administration Devices

DEVICE	FLOWRATE	FIO$_2$	ADVANTAGES	DISADVANTAGES
Nasal cannula	.10–4 L/min	Variable	Good for long-term care in chronic disease, usually well tolerated, easy to apply, lightweight	Active infants may not tolerate, inaccurate FIO$_2$, insufficient humidity
Masks: simple, partial rebreather, nonrebreather	Minimum 6 L/min	Variable	Higher concentrations of FIO$_2$ over cannula, good for transport	CO$_2$ buildup with insufficient flowrates, inaccurate FIO$_2$, not tolerated well by infants and small children, pressure necrosis
Oxyhood	Minimum 7 L/min	21%–100%	Stable FIO$_2$, not interrupted by routine care of infant, warmed and humidified gas at any FIO$_2$ when used with a blender	Noise levels may cause hearing loss, overheating may cause apnea and dehydration, underheating will cause increased oxygen consumption, inadequate flow will cause CO$_2$ buildup, high flows may cause "layering" of O$_2$
Tents	Minimum 10 L/min	21%–50%	Cool aerosol	Varying FIO$_2$, hard to stabilize, fog or mist with higher outputs from nebulizer, danger of asphyxiation, fire hazard with use of electric or battery-operated toys/equipment
Isolette/incubator		21%–70%	Warmed humidified gas, stable FIO$_2$ when used in conjunction with hoods	Varying FIO$_2$ without hoods, long stabilization time, risk of bacterial contamination

similar to those of an oxygen tent. An oxygen blender should be used in conjunction with the oxyhood to deliver precise oxygen concentrations. Flow from the blender is warmed and humidified by using a heated humidifier, such as a wick-type or passover humidifier.

Nebulizers can be used in conjunction with oxyhoods but should only be used with blenders to reduce the noise levels produced by these devices. As mentioned earlier, noise levels caused by equipment used in the neonatal intensive care unit can be hazardous to the infant's hearing and may lead to hearing loss. Mishoe and colleagues conducted a study on sound levels produced by respiratory care equipment in the neonatal intensive care unit and reported that hearing loss from noise exposure is related to the intensity, frequency, and duration of exposure to the sound.[10] They studied the noise levels produced from nebulizers and humidifiers at different flowrates and FIO$_2$s in conjunction with two different types of oxyhoods. Results revealed that sound levels were significantly higher from nebulizers than humidifiers, and that sound levels were

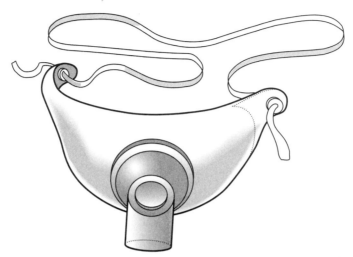

FIGURE 14-3   Tracheostomy collar. (Respiratory Therapy Review Entry Level Study Guide. Kettering, OH, RTS Publishing Company, 1996. Used with permission.)

also much higher when using the soft plastic hoods than when using the harder plastic hoods. These results suggest that nebulizers should not be used in the neonatal intensive care unit because of the noise levels produced. Also, heated humidifiers are recommended because they produce much less noise. The study also suggests that the lowest possible flowrate should be used to reduce noise levels.

Oxygen percentage is monitored inside the hood using an oxygen analyzer. Many oxygen analyzing devices incorporate alarms to warn of changing inspired oxygen concentrations. However, a layering effect of oxygen may occur when using high oxygen levels. This layering produces higher oxygen levels at the bottom of the hood; thus, analyzation should be carried out as close to the infant's face as possible, particularly in the unstable infant.[8] In addition, the temperature in the hood should be monitored to avoid overheating or underheating of the infant.

The oxyhood maintains a stable FIO_2 at any concentration around the infant's head, while leaving the body accessible for care. Oxyhoods can also be used inside incubators so that the infant may be maintained in a neutral thermal environment without the disadvantage of changing oxygen concentrations whenever the incubator is opened.

The use of an oxyhood is not without possible hazards. Overheating of the gas may cause apnea and dehydration, whereas underheating may cause increased oxygen consumption in the infant. If an oxyhood is used inside an isolette, care should be taken to maintain the hood temperature and the isolette temperature at the same level so that a neutral thermal environment for the infant can be sustained. In addition, flow must be maintained at an adequate level to flush exhaled gas, with its elevated carbon dioxide content, from the hood. A flow of 7 L/min is usually adequate for this purpose.[8] Care must also be taken to avoid pressure necrosis around the infant's neck from a hood that is not properly sized.

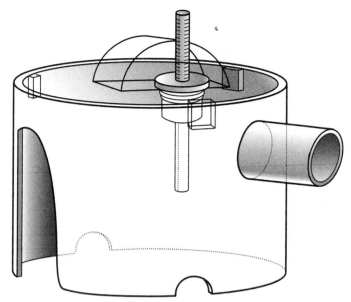

FIGURE 14-4   Oxyhood. (Respiratory Therapy Review Entry Level Study Guide. Kettering, OH, RTS Publishing Company, 1996. Used with permission.)

Mist Tents

Mist tents (Fig. 14-5) have been used in the past to deliver oxygen to adults and children. Today, they are almost exclusively used to deliver oxygen and humidity to infants and children, especially in the treatment of croup.[8]

Tents are designed for use with a metal frame that attaches to the bed or as a self-contained unit on which a large plastic enclosure is attached to cover the entire patient. Mist tents usually incorporate some type of device for providing a cool, humidified environment. This may be accomplished by using a high-powered aerosol generator powered by compressed air or oxygen that is cooled and circulated, such as in the case of most modern refrigeration units, or by using atomizers or nebulizers in conjunction with ice, thus providing an aerosol and cool environment with oxygen concentrations titrated inline. Oxygen concentrations in any kind of tent are variable, at best, because of the problems associated with leaks that can occur with improperly sealed canopies. Concentrations over 50% are difficult to achieve.[8] For best results, canopies should be tucked in around the patient's bed and side openings kept zipped to prevent fluctuations in FIO_2. Also, as with oxyhoods, frequent analyzation of oxygen near the patient's face is suggested so that accurate FIO_2s are delivered. Flowrates from atomizers or nebulizers should be adequate to flush out any excess CO_2.

Hazards associated with the use of tents include fog or thick mist from high output nebulizers, overhydration from high levels of moisture, and, most importantly, asphyxiation from collapse of the tent or by accidental lodging of the infant's head between the mattress and tent itself. Danger of fire from an oxygen-enriched environment is also a major hazard asso-

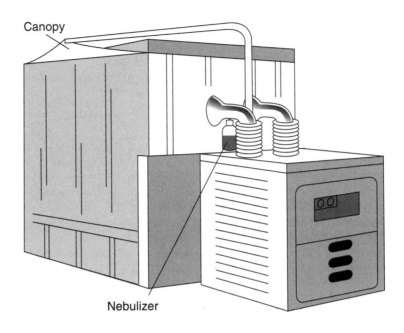

FIGURE 14-5   Mist tent. (Respiratory Therapy Review Entry Level Study Guide. Kettering, OH, RTS Publishing Company, 1996. Used with permission.)

ciated with the use of tents. Sparks can be produced from electric or battery-operated toys, nurse call buttons, electric percussors, and static electricity. These devices should be prohibited when tents are in use. As with any device, hazards can be avoided by proper instruction and observation by parents and health care team members.

Isolettes and Incubators
Incubators were initially designed to maintain a warm, humidified environment for the newborn. Modern isolettes or incubators may be used with varying degrees of success to deliver low concentrations of oxygen. Some isolettes incorporate an inlet nipple adapter which allows oxygen to be supplied from a flowmeter and small-bore tubing. Oxygen concentrations of about 40% can be provided, depending on the oxygen flowrate. These devices also incorporate a "red flag" which, when raised, covers the air entrainment ports and raises the FIO_2 to about 60% to 70%. Typically, these devices are not used to deliver oxygen, but rather are used to maintain humidity and temperature levels for infants. The more common method of oxygen delivery to an infant in an isolette is the use of a hood inside the isolette. Hoods are able to maintain stable oxygen concentrations for the infant while nursing care is being performed.

There are several disadvantages associated with the use of isolettes or incubators for oxygen delivery. The oxygen concentration delivered is not precise and therefore not appropriate for care of the unstable or critically ill infant. Each time the isolette is opened for nursing care or other procedures, the air within is diluted with room air, causing frequent fluctuations in FIO_2. High oxygen tensions are difficult to achieve and maintain, and stabilization of oxygen percentage requires several minutes. In addition, there is increased risk of bacterial growth within the isolette because the oxygen is humidified, thus providing a warm, moist atmosphere for microorganisms in the interior of the isolette.

▬HAZARDS OF OXYGEN THERAPY

Several studies published in the 1940s noted that oxygen therapy reduced apnea, cyanosis, and brain injury in preterm infants.[6,7,15] This finding led to indiscriminate use of oxygen therapy in the 1940s and 1950s and a subsequent increase in the incidence of retrolental fibroplasia (now referred to as retinopathy of prematurity), consequent loss of vision, and the development of BPD.[2] Since then, our understanding of the pathophysiology of the toxic effects of oxygen has improved, and technological advances have improved our ability to monitor infants receiving oxygen therapy. The knowledge base is still incomplete, however, and the design of controlled human studies is difficult at best.

When initiating oxygen therapy, it is better to give too much than too little. The dangers of hypoxia far outweigh the dangers of temporary hyperoxia. Excessive PaO_2 levels revealed by arterial blood analysis following establishment of oxygen therapy may be decreased by the use of non-invasive monitoring or serial blood gas sampling.

Retinopathy of Prematurity

Retinopathy was first described by Terry in 1942 and was called retrolental fibroplasia.[17] In 1984, the term retrolental fibroplasia was replaced with **retinopathy of prematurity** (ROP) to designate this occurrence primarily affecting preterm infants.[8] ROP is most commonly associated with preterm infants weighing less than 1500 g who have received some form of supplemental oxygen. ROP can occur around the time of delivery or at any subsequent point from the injury of immature retinal vessels.

ROP is identified in five stages. Stage I is indicated by a thin white line (demarcation line) which separates the vascularized retina from the unvascularized retina.[3] This stage is characterized by constriction of immature retinal vessels in response to excessive oxygen tensions (PaO_2). The second proliferative phase, stage II, is characterized by an elevated ridge that is wider and may extend into the vitreous and retina. These vessels will remain constricted and become permanently occluded. By stage III, there is formation of new vessels in an attempt to oxygenate the retina. All of these factors combine with earlier stages to cause retinal detachment in stage IV. Stage V is total retinal detachment and blindness. ROP may result in varying degrees of sight loss. The American Academy of Pediatrics recommends screening the eyes of infants of less than 36 weeks gestational age or weighing less than 2000 g who have received supplemental oxygen, or infants weighing less than 1000 g who have not received supplemental oxygen. Screening should preferably be performed between 4 and 8 weeks postnatally, with regular follow-up visits every 2 to 3 weeks if there is any sign of abnormality.[9]

The three major factors that contribute to the development of ROP include arterial oxygen tension, maturity of retinal vessels, and duration of hyperoxia. Other factors may also be associated with the development of ROP including gestational age, intraventricular hemorrhage, sepsis, and low birth weight. However, the most important factor contributing to ROP is prematurity itself.[8]

Cryotherapy is done using a small, freezing cataract probe to treat stage III and early stage IV ROP. If done in time, cryotherapy has been known to reduce the chance of poor outcomes; however 25% of patients receiving this therapy still proceed to retinal detachment. Complications from this type of therapy include apnea, bradycardia, and decreased oxygen saturation. Vitrectomy and lensectomy procedures have been performed in severe cases of ROP in both eyes. Laser therapy is not performed in cases of ROP due to the lack of sufficient experience.[3]

Complications that occur with ROP include nearsightedness, misalignment of the eyes, rhythmic oscillation of the eye ball, lazy eye, secondary cataracts, glaucoma, retinal pigment changes, signs of inflammation, one-sided vision, and corneal degeneration. Late retinal detachment may also occur at any point.[3]

Prevention of ROP should be directed toward keeping PaO_2 levels as low as possible while maintaining adequate oxygenation to the tissues and decreasing the duration of exposure to oxygen.[3] Blood samples should be obtained frequently from an arterial site that represents blood supply to the head to determine the oxygen tension in the retinal vessels. A peripheral artery or umbilical artery should be used in the absence of a ductal shunt; the right radial, brachial, or temporal artery should be used if ductal shunting exists. Additionally, transcutaneous oxygen monitoring or pulse oximetry should be utilized for critically ill premature infants. Infants often demonstrate frequent swings in PaO_2 levels that may not be detected by isolated blood gas measurements. Although noninvasive monitoring of oxygenation using transcutaneous electrode or oximetry has limitations, it remains an effective method for guiding oxygen therapy in most cases.

Bronchopulmonary Dysplasia

BPD is a chronic lung disease that occurs primarily in premature infants who have had prolonged treatment with oxygen and positive pressure ventilation for hyaline membrane disease. One theory that is widely accepted is that the pulmonary destruction seen with this disorder is caused by oxygen free radicals produced in the reduction of molecular oxygen. This theory states that the generation of partially reduced oxygen products is increased and is responsible for the cytotoxicity of oxygen. Biochemical products such as hydrogen peroxide interact with components and cause metabolic and structural changes in the cells themselves, especially the cells of the lungs. BPD is characterized by fibroblastic and granular epithelial cell development, increased collagen synthesis, and decreased surfactant production. These changes result in pulmonary fibrosis and emphysema.[8] The etiology, pathophysiology, diagnosis, and treatment of BPD are discussed in detail in Chapter 9.

Absorption Atelectasis

Absorption atelectasis generally occurs when FIo$_2$ levels of greater than 50% are used.[14] In the alveoli and blood, nitrogen is the primary gas that maintains the residual volume. When a patient is subjected to high levels of oxygen, the nitrogen content in the blood and alveoli is usually reduced within several minutes by replacement of oxygen and may cause alveolar collapse. When this occurs, oxygen is rapidly absorbed into the blood. This phenomenon occurs most often with ventilation/perfusion mismatches, where perfusion is in excess of ventilation. Therefore, absorption atelectasis reduces vital capacity and increases shunting of blood through the lung.[11]

■HELIUM–OXYGEN THERAPY

Helium has a very low density and reduces the pressure needed to move air in and out of areas where turbulent flow is present, such as in the large airways of the lungs. With less pressure required to move air, the patient's work of breathing can be substantially reduced, especially in cases of large airway obstruction. For over 60 years, helium has been used in the management of large airway obstruction and has been shown to be effective in the treatment of certain patients with chronic obstructive pulmonary disease, various types of upper airway obstruction, postextubation stridor in pediatric patients, and refractory viral croup.[14]

Administration of helium must be combined with oxygen because helium is an inert gas that will not sustain life. The usual combination of helium and oxygen is at least 20% oxygen and 80% helium, with helium replacing the normal amount of nitrogen present in room air. Helium–oxygen is also available in a mixture of 30% oxygen and 70% helium. The additional oxygen can be helpful in treating patients with hypoxemia in conjunction with large airway obstruction. Both mixtures are commercially available in convenient, premixed cylinders which are much safer and easier for the practitioner to use. It is generally recommended that this gas mixture be administered with a closed-system administration device, such as a nonrebreathing mask. Nasal cannulas or other low-flow devices are not recommended because the patient may entrain room air which could dilute the gas mixture and affect the outcome of the therapy. The use of oxygen hoods is also discouraged because the helium will tend to concentrate at the top of the hood, which decreases the helium concentration delivered to the infant. Helium–oxygen mixtures can also be given to ventilated patients with cuffed endotracheal tubes.

When gas mixtures are administered, the practitioner must keep in mind that the standard oxygen flowmeter will not be accurate. Flowmeters calibrated for use with helium are available, but these are not essential for administration. A simple correction factor can be utilized with oxygen flowmeters for administration. The correction factor for an 80/20 helium–oxygen mixture is 1.8 and the factor for a 70/30 mixture is 1.6. This conversion means that for every 10 L/min of indicated flow, 1.8 or 1.6 times that amount (18 or 16 L/min) actually leaves the flowmeter. Therefore, to deliver the proper amount of a gas mixture, the therapist must set the flowmeter to the desired flow divided by 1.8 or 1.6, depending on the mixture used.[14]

A harmless side effect associated with the use of helium oxygen therapy is temporary voice disruption, and the patient should be informed of this prior to therapy. Helium therapy is not a widely used modality in respiratory care, however it does have merit and value in the treatment of airway obstruction, such as in asthma, croup, chronic obstructive pulmonary disease, BPD, and postextubation edema.[8]

▰ REFERENCES

 1. AARC clinical practice guidelines for oxygen therapy in the acute care hospital: Respiratory Care 36:1410, 1991.
 2. Bland R: Special considerations in oxygen therapy for infants and children. Am Rev Respir Dis 122(5):45, 1980.
 3. Boyle K, Baker V, Cassaday C: Neonatal pulmonary disorders. In Barnhart SL, Czervinske MP (eds): Perinatal and Pediatric Respiratory Care. Philadelphia, WB Saunders, 1995.
 4. Branson RD: The nuts and bolts of increasing arterial oxygenation: Devices and techniques. Respiratory Care 38:672, 1993.
 5. Burgess W, Chernik V: Respiratory Therapy for Newborn Infants and Children. New York, Thieme-Stratton, 1981.
 6. Clifford SH: The effects of asphyxia on the newborn infant. J Pediatr 18:567, 1941.
 7. Clifford SH: Roundtable discussion of neonatal asphyxia: Proceedings of the tenth annual meeting of the American Academy of Pediatrics. J Pediatr 19:258, 1941.
 8. Gramlich T: Oxygen therapy. In Barnhart SL, Czervinske MP (eds): Perinatal and Pediatric Respiratory Care. Philadelphia, WB Saunders, 1995.
 9. Hoyt AD, Good W, Peterson R: Disorders of the eye. In Taeusch HW, Ballard RA, Avery, ME (eds): Disease of the Newborn. Philadelphia, WB Saunders, 1992.
10. Mishoe SC, Brooks CW, Dennision FH, Hill KV, Frye T: Octave waveband analysis to determine sound frequencies and intensities produced by nebulizers and humidifiers used with hoods. Respiratory Care 40:1120, 1995.
11. Ryerson G, Block A: Oxygen as a drug: Clinical properties, benefits, modes, and hazards of administration. In Burton GG, Hodgkin JE, Ward JJ (eds): Respiratory Care: A Guide to Clinical Practice, 3rd ed. Philadelphia, JB Lippincott, 1991.
12. Salyer JW, Chatburn RL: Patterns of practice in neonatal and pediatric respiratory care. Respiratory Care 35:879, 1990.
13. Scanlan CL: Patterns of cardiopulmonary dysfunction. In Scanlon CL, Spearman C, Sheldon RL (eds): Egan's Fundamentals of Respiratory Care, 6th ed. St. Louis, Mosby-Year Book, 1995.
14. Scanlan CL, Thalken R: Medical gas therapy. In Scanlan CL, Spearman C, Sheldon RL (eds): Egan's Fundamentals of Respiratory Care, 6th ed. St. Louis, Mosby-Year Book, 1995.
15. Schreiber F: Apnea of the newborn and associated cerebral injury: A clinical and statistical study. JAMA 111:1263, 1938.
16. Smith-Wenning K, Smith CC, Zanni RL, Scanlan CL: Neonatal and pediatric care. In Scanlan CL, Spearman C, Sheldon RL (eds): Egan's Fundamentals of Respiratory Care, 6th ed. St. Louis, Mosby-Year Book, 1995.
17. Terry TL: Extreme prematurity and fibroblastic overgrowth of persistent vascular sheath behind each crystalline lens: I. Preliminary report. Am J Ophthalmol 25:203, 1942.

▰ SELF-ASSESSMENT QUESTIONS

 1. Hyaline membrane disease is an example of which type of hypoxia?
    a. hypoxemia
    b. reduced blood flow
    c. hemoglobin deficiency
    d. dysoxia

2. Advantages of nasal cannulas include
    I. well-tolerated
    II. good for long-term use
    III. not easily dislodged
    a. I only   c. I and II
    b. II and III   d. I, II, and III

3. What is the minimum flowrate required with oxygen masks to prevent accumulation of CO_2?
    a. 2 L/min   c. 6 L/min
    b. 4 L/min   d. 8 L/min

4. Nebulizers produce lower sound levels than heated humidifiers when used with oxygen hoods.
    a. true
    b. false

5. Disadvantages of using oxygen tents include
    I. variable FIO_2 concentration
    II. dehydration
    III. danger of asphyxiation
    a. II only   c. II and III
    b. I and III   d. I, II, and III

6. Factors that contribute to the development of retinopathy of prematurity include
    a. arterial oxygen tension   c. maturity of retinal vessels
    b. duration of therapy   d. all of the above

7. _____ is a chronic lung disease that occurs primarily in premature infants who have had prolonged treatment for hyaline membrane disease with oxygen and positive pressure ventilation.
    a. respiratory distress syndrome
    b. absorption atelectasis
    c. retinopathy of prematurity
    d. bronchopulmonary dysplasia

8. Absorption atelectasis generally occurs when FIO_2 greater than _____ is used.
    a. 30%   c. 70%
    b. 50%   d. 90%

9. Which of the following conditions may benefit from the administration of a helium–oxygen mixture?
    a. asthma   c. pneumonia
    b. atelectasis   d. pneumothorax

10. According to the AARC Clinical Practice Guidelines, oxygen therapy for neonates is indicated when the SaO_2 level is less than
    a. 60%   c. 88%
    b. 75%   d. 95%

Chapter 15

Continuous Positive Airway Pressure and Other Forms of Continuous Distending Pressure

BEVERLY J. ERVIN

OBJECTIVES

Having completed this chapter, the reader will be able to:

1 Briefly discuss the history of continuous positive airway pressure (CPAP).

2 Define the terms CPAP, expiratory positive airway pressure, continuous distending pressure, positive expiratory-end pressure, and BiPAP.

3 Summarize the physiologic effects of CPAP in relation to the pulmonary system.

4 Explain the effects of CPAP on the cardiovascular system.

5 Discuss the effects of CPAP on the renal system and on intracranial pressure.

6 List four methods by which CPAP can be administered.

7 Define continuous negative pressure and give indications for its use.

8 Describe the method of operation for BiPAP.

9 Understand the indications for CPAP.

10 List the mechanical and clinical hazards of CPAP therapy.

KEY TERMS

BiPAP
continuous distending pressure (CDP)
continuous negative pressure (CNP)
continuous positive airway pressure (CPAP)

expiratory positive airway pressure (EPAP)
mask CPAP
nasal prongs
physiologic CPAP

Improved outcomes in neonatal intensive care have been realized as the result of innovations in the management of respiratory failure. **Continuous positive airway pressure (CPAP)** was not widely used as a treatment until

1971, when Gregory and associates described its use in the treatment of premature infants with idiopathic respiratory distress syndrome (RDS).[13]

While positive pressure ventilation had been used with these infants, the problems of pulmonary atelectasis persisted. These investigators' observations of such infants, who demonstrated expiratory grunting, led them to believe that the grunting somehow decreased or prevented the atelectasis. When these infants were intubated, the tube itself disrupted the grunting maneuver by preventing exhalation against a closed glottis.

Gregory believed CPAP would duplicate the missing physiologic effect of grunting. With the administration of CPAP, those infants who were given only a 25% chance of survival now obtained an 80% survival rate. As a result, CPAP became an accepted therapy for the treatment of RDS.[6]

The purpose of this chapter is to describe various methods of administering positive pressure and to provide the reader an understanding of its application in the treatment of respiratory distress. Table 15-1 provides a clarification of terms used to describe positive pressure.[5]

◼ EFFECTS ON THE PULMONARY SYSTEM

Table 15-2 summarizes the physiologic effects of CPAP. CPAP increases functional residual capacity (FRC), decreases intrapulmonary shunting, and improves Pao_2. This allows the clinician to decrease the fractional concentration of inspired oxygen (FIo_2) to nontoxic levels. The increase in FRC is due to the expansion of previously collapsed alveoli. The FRC is also increased as a result of the redistribution of lung fluid. The application of CPAP can stabilize the chest wall and provide an adequate FRC as well as decrease the work of breathing.

The importance of the work of breathing in the neonate can be further understood in infants with RDS when it is realized that increases in the work of breathing promote increases in energy expenditure the neonate can ill afford.

Improved oxygenation will also relieve hypoxic vasoconstriction in the pulmonary vascular bed and decrease pulmonary vascular resistance (PVR),

TABLE 15-1 Definition of Terms

TERM	DEFINITION
CPAP	Continuous positive airway pressure. Application of positive airway pressure throughout the respiratory cycle to spontaneously breathing patients.
EPAP	Expiratory positive airway pressure. Application of positive airway pressure during exhalation to spontaneously breathing patients, with airway pressure becoming subatmospheric during inspiration.
CDP	Continuous distending pressure. Application of either positive or negative pressure to maintain increased transpulmonary pressure throughout the respiratory cycle to spontaneously breathing patients.
PEEP	Positive end-expiratory pressure. Application of positive airway pressure during exhalation to a mechanically ventilated patient.

(American College of Chest Physicians: Consensus conference on mechanical ventilation. Chest 104:1835, 1993.)

TABLE 15-2 Physiologic Effects of CPAP

ORGAN SYSTEM	BENEFICIAL EFFECTS	HAZARDS
Pulmonary	Increased FRC	Pneumothorax
	Decreased shunt	Pneumomediastinum
	Increased PaO_2	Pulmonary interstitial emphysema
	Decreased PVR	Increased PVR
	Increased static compliance	Decreased static compliance
	Decreased work of breathing	Increased work of breathing
Cardiovascular		Decreased venous return
		Decreased cardiac output
Other		Secretion of ADH
		Decreased urine output
		Obstruction of lymph drainage through the thoracic duct

resulting in increased pulmonary blood flow, decreased shunting, and increased PaO_2.

There is always a risk of barotrauma when applying any form of positive pressure, including CPAP. The infant must be monitored closely for signs of pneumothorax and pneumomediastinum. Pulmonary interstitial emphysema may also occur.

EFFECTS ON THE CARDIOVASCULAR SYSTEM

The application of CPAP causes an increase in intrathoracic pressure that may decrease venous return to the heart and reduce cardiac output. Infants with RDS possess unstable alveoli because of surfactant deficiency. CPAP helps prevent the resultant collapse of alveoli. With the application of CPAP, functional residual capacity increases and intrapulmonary shunting is decreased, improving ventilation/perfusion (V/Q) matching.[7]

With the institution of CPAP, reduction in PVR occurs as a consequence of improved oxygenation. Application of CPAP causes a reduction in PVR, which reduces the amount of right-to-left shunting through the patent ductus arteriosus or foramen ovale, resulting in increased oxygenation.

EFFECTS ON OTHER BODY SYSTEMS

While CPAP administration may result in a decrease in cardiac output, renal perfusion may also be reduced. CPAP delivery stimulates the hypothalamus to produce increased levels of antidiuretic hormone (ADH), thereby decreasing urine output and renal clearance. In addition, CPAP may also obstruct flow from the thoracic duct, impeding lymph drainage and contributing to fluid overload.

Overdistention of the lungs with CPAP can increase intracranial pressure or cause intraventricular hemorrhage by impeding blood flow from the head. Because of these effects on other body systems, hemodynamic function, including accurate assessment of fluid and electrolyte balance, must be monitored closely in infants being treated with CPAP.[1]

▬METHODS OF ADMINISTERING CPAP

CPAP systems consist of three major components: (1) the basic system used for gas delivery, (2) a resistor valve, and (3) the device to connect the system to the patient. CPAP may be administered by means of an endotracheal (ET) tube, nasal cannula or prongs, nasopharyngeal tube (NP) tube, and face mask. Examples of nasal prongs and a modified ET tube are seen in Figure 15-1.

Endotracheal Tube

The administration of CPAP by means of an ET tube is a relatively safe, reliable method used by many newborn centers. Many infant ventilators provide a CPAP mode that allows warmed humidified gas to be delivered through the ventilator circuit and positive end-expiratory pressure (PEEP) to be generated by the ventilator's mechanical circuitry at the exhalation valve. This is a commonly used and convenient technique. Ventilator alarms may be used to monitor airway pressures, and the ventilator is readily accessible should the patient's condition decline.

Advantages of this system include the fact that the ET tube provides a patent airway and allows access to airway clearance by tracheal suctioning. In addition, the possibility of positive pressure being displaced in the upper airway is diminished. This provides the application of CPAP to the desired site, the alveoli. The disadvantages of this method are those associated with the intubation procedure and the presence of an artificial airway and

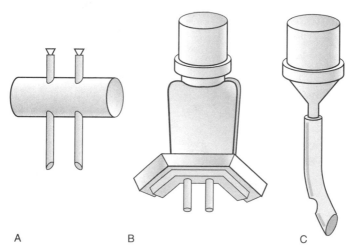

A   B   C

FIGURE 15-1   Examples of devices used to establish nasal CPAP. (*A*) Jackson–Reese tubes; (*B*) Argyle nasal cannula (prongs); (*C*) endotracheal tube modified for nasopharyngeal application (NP tube). (Blodgett D: Manual of Pediatric Respiratory Care Procedures, p 133. Philadelphia, JB Lippincott, 1982.)

include subglottic stenosis, tracheomalacia, mucous plugging and anoxia, oral and nasal mucosa breakdown, and pulmonary infection. Work of breathing may be increased because of the resistance created by the small diameter of the endotracheal tube. Size 3.0 and 3.5 mm inner diameter endotracheal tubes create airway resistance values that are twice the value provided by the infant's upper airway. Increasing the diameter or decreasing the length of the tube decreases the resistance created by the tube.[10] Most of the problems associated with ET tubes can be avoided with proper techniques of insertion and adequate maintenance and monitoring.

Nasal Cannula/Nasal Prongs

Another method of **continuous distending pressure (CDP)** delivery is by means of a specially designed nasal cannula or **nasal prongs**. These nose-pieces are manufactured with a standard 15-mm adaptor for connection to gas delivery systems previously described. In the Argyle device (Sherwood Medical Industries), two short tubes extending into the nares are surrounded by a padded gasket at the base that protects the skin and helps maintain a seal (Fig. 15-2). Major disadvantages of nasal prongs are dislodgment and plugging of the prongs with secretions. Gastric distention is common and placement of a nasogastric tube should be used in conjunction with nasal CPAP.[11]

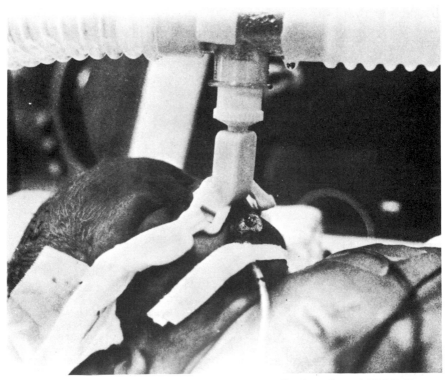

FIGURE 15-2   Argyle nasal prongs in place for application of nasal CPAP. (Reproduced by permission of Sherwood Medical Industries.)

Nasopharyngeal Tubes

Another method involves the use of ET tubes that have been cut off at the patient connector and inserted through the external nares into the nasopharynx (nasopharyngeal or NP tubes). Tube placement is confirmed by direct visualization of the tip of the tube behind the uvula. All of these methods avoid the hazards associated with intubation but have their own limitations.

The use of nasal cannulas or prongs and NP tubes to establish CPAP in the neonate is based on newborns being preferential nose breathers. If the infant fails to breathe through his/her nose (as in crying), or if there is displacement of the prongs, the CPAP is "lost." Correct cannula position is often difficult to maintain, especially in larger, more active infants.

Risks associated with the use of nasal prongs include pressure necrosis and infection. Falsely high pressures may be recorded on the manometer with excessive flows inadvertently entering the openings of the cannula. With the use of prongs, it is difficult to determine the precise amount of pressure actually being delivered to the lungs, as opposed to the upper airway. On the other hand, prongs avoid excessive PEEP levels because the mouth acts as a "pop-off."[14]

NP tubes may provide some advantages over prongs because they are less easily dislodged and may transmit more pressure to the lower airway. Damage to the nasal mucosa may occur because of the presence of the tube, particularly if attached equipment is not well supported.

Face Mask CPAP

Mask CPAP is most often used as a temporary measure to overcome atelectasis after endotracheal tube extubation, or to stabilize the spontaneous breathing of an infant after an apneic episode. An anesthesia face mask is attached to a continuous flow hyperinflation bag with CPAP pressure being regulated by a Mapleson valve. Pressures are monitored by the use of a manometer placed inline. An advantage of mask CPAP is that it has the ability to provide a readily available method of CPAP delivery without the requirement of intubation.

Disadvantages of using the facial mask for CPAP therapy include the fact that it is difficult to provide mouth care to the infant, and many infants will not tolerate having the mask secured to their face. Complications of mask CPAP include facial and ocular tissue trauma, carbon dioxide retention, gastric distention, emesis, aspiration, and cerebral hemorrhage.[2,12,16]

■ CPAP IN THE PEDIATRIC PATIENT

In the pediatric environment, CPAP frequently is used to provide both therapeutic and supportive effects. It is often used preoperatively or postoperatively to support airway structures affected by abnormalities such as subglottic stenosis, cleft palate, laryngeal papillomas, neck tumors, tonsillitis, and epiglottitis. A low level of CPAP, less than 6 to 8 cm H_2O, is sufficient to help support the airways and provide **physiologic CPAP**. The same mechanism applies when CPAP is used to wean a child from mechanical ventilation. A pediatric patient is maintained at a minimum of 2 or 3 cm H_2O to approximate the function of the epiglottis. Caution must be used not to fatigue children by having them breathe through a high-resistance endotracheal tube when they are able to use their own airway. The best course is to extubate the patient as early as possible.

■CONTINUOUS NEGATIVE PRESSURE

Continuous negative pressure (CNP) was initially used on neonates with RDS in the 1960s.[8] The infant's torso would be placed inside a negative pressure chamber with the head extending outside the chamber. Next, a negative pressure (vacuum) was applied to the thorax of the infant. With the onset of CPAP and advanced ventilation capabilities, CNP lost popularity in the 1970s. However, recent studies have revived its application for the treatment of RDS in the neonate.[9]

Other indications for CNP therapy include pulmonary interstitial emphysema and pulmonary artery hypertension due to meconium aspiration syndrome or to other causes. Advantages of this therapy include the avoidance of use of an endotracheal tube and decreased risk of barotrauma. Disadvantages of CNP systems are that they are cumbersome and access to the patient is hindered.[9]

■BiPAP (RESPIRONICS INC.)

The **BiPAP** ventilatory support system is a bi-level positive airway pressure device providing pressure-limited ventilation with PEEP, or **expiratory positive airway pressure (EPAP)**, in response to the spontaneously breathing patient's inspiratory effort.

The BiPAP system uses a nasal mask secured with a headband (Fig. 15-3). This system offers a sensitive response to patient inspiratory effort through the use of a flow transducer. Output is adjusted to assist in inhala-

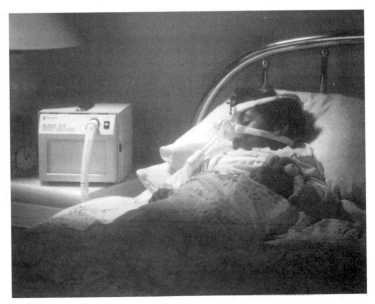

FIGURE 15-3   BiPAP S/T ventilatory support system. (Courtesy of Respironics Inc.)

tion and expiration. This augmentation is supplied by the delivery of two levels of positive pressure. During exhalation, pressure is positive or near ambient. The inspiratory level is positive and always higher than the expiratory level.[3]

The BiPAP system is pneumatically powered and electrically controlled, using a moderate gas pressure supply source that electrically reduces the pressure to the low level supplied to the patient.

Advantages of this system include improved oxygenation and ventilation without the untoward risks of infection and airway trauma seen with other methods of artificial airways. Disadvantages include skin irritation at the site of the mask and difficulty in tolerating mask placement. Indications for its use include chronic respiratory failure, neuromuscular disease, upper airway obstruction, kyphoscoliosis, and hypoventilation.[15]

▬ INDICATIONS AND CLINICAL APPLICATIONS OF CPAP

Indications include the following:

1. The presence of increased work of breathing as indicated by 30% to 40% increases in respiratory rate, substernal and suprasternal retractions, grunting and nasal flaring, the presence of pale or cyanotic skin color, and agitation
2. Inadequate arterial blood gas values, indicated by the inability to maintain a PaO_2 greater than 50 mm Hg with FIO_2 of less than or equal to 0.60 provided minute ventilation is adequate as indicated by a $PaCO_2$ level of 50 mm Hg and a pH greater than or equal to 7.25
3. The presence of poorly expanded and/or infiltrated lung fields on chest radiograph
4. The presence of a condition thought to be responsive to CPAP and associated with one or more of the clinical presentations in RDS, pulmonary edema, atelectasis, apnea of prematurity, recent extubation, tracheal malacia or other similar abnormality of the lower airways, and transient tachypnea of the newborn

▬ MONITORING THE PATIENT ON CPAP

Because the administration of CPAP can cause $PaCO_2$ to fluctuate, blood gases and hemodynamic parameters should be monitored closely. In addition, pulse oximetry is useful in determining the effectiveness of CPAP. Measurements of static lung compliance, FRC at various pressure levels, and tidal volume measurements also help determine the efficacy of CPAP.

Hazards of CPAP

Hazards associated with equipment include the following:

1. Obstruction of nasal prongs from mucus plugging or kinking of the NP tube may interfere with delivery of CPAP and result in a decrease in FIO_2 through entrainment of room air via the opposite naris or mouth.
2. Inactivation of airway pressure alarms

   a. Increased resistance created by turbulent flow through the small orifices of nasal prongs and nasopharyngeal tubes can maintain the pressure of the CPAP system even when decannulation has occurred. This can result in the failure of low airway pressure/disconnect alarms to respond.
   b. Complete obstruction of nasal prongs and NP tubes results in pressurization of the CPAP system without activation of low or high airway pressure alarms.
   c. Activation of a manual breath (commonly available on infant ventilators) may cause gastric insufflation and patient discomfort, particularly if the peak pressure is set inappropriately high.

Hazards and complications associated with the patient's clinical condition include:

   1. Lung overdistention leading to air leak syndromes
   2. Ventilation/perfusion mismatch
   3. CO_2 retention and increased work of breathing
   4. Impedance of pulmonary blood flow with a subsequent increase in pulmonary vascular resistance and decrease in cardiac output
   5. Gastric insufflation and abdominal distention potentially leading to aspiration
   6. Nasal irritation with septal distortion
   7. Skin irritation and pressure necrosis
   8. Nasal mucosal damage due to inadequate humidification[4]

■ AARC CLINICAL PRACTICE GUIDELINES

In the interest of being helpful to the practitioner, the American Association for Respiratory Care (AARC) has compiled and published Clinical Practice Guidelines for the Application of Continuous Positive Airway Pressure to Neonates via Nasal Prongs or Nasopharyngeal Tube.[4] They are reprinted at the end of this chapter with the permission of the AARC and *Respiratory Care*.

■ REFERENCES

   1. Aidinis SJ, Lafferty J, Schapiro HM: Intracranial responses to PEEP. Anesthesiology 45:275, 1976.
   2. Ahumada CA: Continuous distending pressure. In Goldsmith JP, Karotkin EH (eds): Assisted Ventilation of the Neonate, 2nd ed. Philadelphia, WB Saunders, 1988.
   3. Akingbola OA, Servant GM, Custer JR, Palmisano JM: Noninvasive bi-level positive pressure ventilation: Management of two pediatric patients. Respiratory Care 38:1092, 1993.
   4. American Association for Respiratory Care Clinical Practice Guidelines: Application of continuous positive airway pressure to neonates via nasal prongs or nasopharyngeal tube. Respiratory Care 39:817, 1994.
   5. American College of Chest Physicians: Consensus conference on mechanical ventilation. Chest 104:1835, 1993.
   6. Bateman L, Hooper R, Losh T, Miller L: Continuous positive airway pressure. In Barnhart SL, Czervinske MP (eds): Perinatal and Pediatric Respiratory Care. Philadelphia, WB Saunders, 1995.
   7. Carlo W, Martin R: Mechanical ventilation in newborns. In Hillman BC (ed): Pediatric Respiratory Disease: Diagnosis and Treatment. Philadelphia, WB Saunders, 1993.
   8. Chernick V, Vidyasagar D. Continuous negative chest wall pressure in hyaline membrane disease: One year experience. Pediatrics 49:753, 1972.

9. Cvetnic, W. Reintroduction of continuous negative pressure ventilation in neonates: Two year experience. Pediatric Pulmonology 8:245, 1990.
10. Czervinske MP: Continuous positive airway pressure. In Koff PB, Eitzman D, Neu J (eds): Neonatal and Pediatric Respiratory Care, 2nd ed. St. Louis, Mosby-Year Book, 1993.
11. Fiascone JM, Vreland PN, Frantz ID III: Neonatal lung disease and respiratory care. In Burton GG, Hodgkin EJ, Ward JJ (eds): Respiratory Care: A Guide to Clinical Practice, 3rd ed. Philadelphia, JB Lippincott, 1991.
12. Gregory GA: Devices for applying continuous positive airway pressure. In Thiebault DW, Gregory GA (eds): Neonatal Pulmonary Care. Menlo Park, CA, Addison-Wesley, 1979.
13. Gregory GA, Kitterman JA, Phibbs RH, Tooley WH, Hamilton WK: Treatment of idiopathic respiratory distress syndrome with continuous positive pressure. N Engl J Med 248:1333, 1971.
14. Kattwinkel J, Nearman HS, Fanaroff AA, Katona PG, Klaus MH: Apnea of prematurity: Comparative therapeutic effects of cutaneous stimulation and nasal continuous positive airway pressure. J Pediatr 86:588, 1975.
15. Padman R, Lawless S, Von Nessen S: Use of BiPAP by nasal mask in the treatment of respiratory insufficiency in pediatric patients. Pediatric Pulmonology 17:119, 1994.
16. Pape KE, Armstrong DL, Fitzhardinge PM: Central nervous system pathology associated with mask ventilation in the very low birth weight infant: A new etiology for intracerebellar hemorrhages. Pediatrics 58:473, 1976.

■ SELF-ASSESSMENT QUESTIONS

1. The effects of CPAP include
   - I. increased FRC
   - II. increased intrapulmonary shunting
   - III. improved PaO_2
     - a. II only
     - b. I and III
     - c. III only
     - d. I, II, and III

2. What are the major components of a CPAP system?
   - a. resistor valve
   - b. connecting tubing
   - c. gas source
   - d. all of the above

3. What is the effect on work of breathing of a small endotracheal tube when used to administer CPAP?
   - a. decreases
   - b. increases
   - c. no effect

4. Disadvantages of nasal prongs include
   - I. easily dislodged
   - II. gastric distention
   - III. obstruction of nasal prongs
     - a. I only
     - b. II and III
     - c. I and II
     - d. I, II, and III

5. Risks associated with the use of nasal prongs for administering CPAP include all of the following *except*
   - a. pressure necrosis
   - b. infection
   - c. application of incorrect pressure
   - d. excessive PEEP pressure

6. _____ form of CPAP is most often used as a temporary measure to overcome atelectasis after endotracheal tube extubation.
   a. nasal prongs
   b. face mask
   c. endotracheal tube
   d. tracheostomy tube

7. What minimum level of CPAP should be maintained in a pediatric patient to approximate the function of the epiglottis?
   a. 0 to 1 cm H_2O
   b. 2 to 3 cm H_2O
   c. 4 to 5 cm H_2O
   d. 6 to 7 cm H_2O

8. An advantage of using continuous negative pressure for infants is that it
   a. avoids the need for endotracheal intubation
   b. provides easy access to the infant
   c. eliminates the need for supplemental oxygen therapy
   d. allows application of high PEEP levels

9. A form of ventilatory support which provides two levels of positive airway pressure with PEEP is referred to as
   a. CPAP
   b. EPAP
   c. IPAP
   d. BiPAP

10. Complications associated with CPAP include all of the following *except*
    a. ventilation/perfusion mismatch
    b. increased work of breathing
    c. hyperventilation
    d. pulmonary air leaks

▬ APPENDIX

AARC Clinical Practice Guideline

Application of Continuous Positive Airway Pressure to Neonates via Nasal Prongs or Nasopharyngeal Tube

NCPAP 1.0 Procedure
The application of continuous positive airway pressure to neonates and infants by nasal prongs (NCPAP) or by nasopharyngeal tube (NP-CPAP) used in conjunction with a commercially available continuous-flow infant ventilator or a suitably equipped multipurpose ventilator

NCPAP 2.0 Description/Definition:
Continuous positive airway pressure (CPAP) is the application of positive pressure to the airways of the spontaneously breathing patient throughout the respiratory cycle.[1-4] For the most part, neonates are nose breathers; therefore, the application of nasal CPAP is easily facilitated.[5,6] This is accomplished by inserting nasopharyngeal tubes or affixing nasal prongs

Reprinted from *Respiratory Care* (Respir Care 1994;39(8):817–823) to the patient. The device is attached to a warmed and humidified gas from a continuous-flow mechanical ventilator designed for neonates or a suitably equipped multipurpose ventilator, set in the CPAP mode.[7-13] Free-standing systems are sometimes used; however, their use is not addressed in this guideline.

CPAP maintains inspiratory and expiratory pressures above ambient pressure, which should result in an increase in functional residual capacity (FRC) and improvement in static lung compliance and decrease airway resistance in the infant with unstable lung mechanics.[1,3,14-20] This allows a greater volume change/unit of pressure change (ie, greater tidal volume for a given pressure change) with subsequent reduction in the work of breathing and stabilization of minute ventilation (V_E).[9,16,18,19,21-23] CPAP increases mean airway pressure, and the associated increase in FRC should improve ventilation-perfusion relationships and potentially reduce oxygen requirements.[15,16,18,19,21,24-28]

NCPAP 3.0 Settings:
NCPAP or NP-CPAP is applied by trained personnel in acute and subacute care hospitals.

NCPAP 4.0 Indications:
4.1 Abormalities on physical examination—the presence of increased work of breathing as indicated by a 30–40% increase above normal in respiratory rate, substernal and suprasternal retractions, grunting, and nasal flaring;[16,27,29] the presence of pale or cyanotic skin color and agitation[16]
4.2 Inadequate arterial blood gas values—the inability to maintain a PaO_2 greater than 50 torr with FiO_2 of ≤ 0.60 provided aoV_E is adequate as indicated by a $PaCO_2$ level of 50 torr and a pH ≥ 7.25[9,11,14]
4.3 The presence of poorly expanded and/or infiltrated lung fields[16,19] on chest radiograph
4.4 The presence of a condition thought to be responsive to CPAP and associated with one or more of the clinical presentations in 4.1–4.3[18]
    4.4.1 Respiratory distress syndrome[9,11,14]
    4.4.2 Pulmonary edema[30]
    4.4.3 Atelectasis[16]
    4.4.4 Apnea of prematurity[27,31-34]
    4.4.5 Recent extubation[35,36]
    4.4.6 Tracheal malacia or other similar abnormality of the lower airways[9,37,38]
    4.4.7 Transient tachypnea of the newborn[16]

NCPAP 5.0 Contraindications:
5.1 Although NCPAP and NP-CPAP have been used in bronchiolitis,[39] this application may be contraindicated.[40]
5.2 The need for intubation and/or mechanical ventilation as evidenced by the presence of
    5.2.1 Upper airway abnormalities that make NCPAP or NP-CPAP ineffective or potentially dangerous (eg, choanal atresia, cleft palate, tracheoesophageal fistula)[41]
    5.2.2 Severe cardiovascular instability and impending arrest

(continued)

AARC Clinical Practice Guideline *(continued)*

 5.2.3 Unstable respiratory drive with frequent apneic episodes resulting in desaturation and/or bradycardia

 5.2.4 Ventilatory failure as indicated by the inability to maintain P_aCO_2 < 60 torr and pH > 7.25[25]

5.3 Application of NCPAP or NP-CPAP to patients with untreated congenital diaphragmatic hernia may lead to gastric distention and further compromise of thoracic organs.[41]

NCPAP 6.0 Hazards/Complications:

6.1 Hazards and complications associated with equipment include the following.

 6.1.1 Obstruction of nasal prongs from mucus plugging or kinking of nasopharyngeal tube may interfere with delivery of CPAP and result in a decrease in F_iO_2 through entrainment of room air via opposite naris or mouth.

 6.1.2 Inactivation of airway pressure alarms

  6.1.2.1 Increased resistance created by turbulent flow through the small orifices of nasal prongs and nasopharyngeal tubes can maintain pressure in the CPAP system even when decannulation has occurred. This can result in failure of low airway pressure/disconnect alarms to respond.[5]

  6.1.2.2 Complete obstruction of nasal prongs and nasopharyngeal tubes results in continued pressurization of the CPAP system without activation of low or high airway pressure alarms.

  6.1.2.3 Activation of a manual breath (commonly available on infant ventilators) may cause gastric insufflation and patient discomfort particularly if the peak pressure is set inappropriately high.[31]

 6.2 Hazards and complications associated with the patient's clinical condition include

  6.2.1 lung overdistention leading to

   6.2.1.1 air leak syndromes,[42,43]

   6.2.1.2 ventilation-perfusion mismatch,[15]

   6.2.1.3 CO_2 retention and increased work of breathing,[5,44]

   6.2.1.4 impedance of pulmonary blood flow with a subsequent increase in pulmonary vascular resistance and decrease in cardiac output.[30,45]

  6.2.2 gastric insufflation and abdominal distention potentially leading to aspiration.[46]

  6.2.3 nasal irritation with septal distortion.

  6.2.4 skin irritation and pressure necrosis

  6.2.5 nasal mucosal damage due to inadequate humidification.

NCPAP 7.0 Limitations of Device:

7.1 NCPAP and NP-CPAP applications are not benign procedures, and operators should be aware of the possible hazards and complications and take all necessary precautions to ensure safe and effective application.

7.2 NCPAP and NP-CPAP are ineffective during mouth breathing, resulting in loss of desired pressure and decrease in delivered oxygen concentration.[10,47,48]

7.3 NCPAP harnesses and attachment devices are often cumbersome and difficult to secure and may cause agitation and result in inadvertent decannulation.[5,47]

NCPAP 8.0 Assessment of Need:
Determination that valid indications are present by physical, radiographic, and laboratory assessments

NCPAP 9.0 Assessment of Outcome:
CPAP is initiated at levels of 4–5 cm H_2O and may be gradually increased up to 10 cm H_2O to provide the following:[9,17,27,28,47–50]
9.1 Stabilization of F_{IO2} requirement ≤ 0.60 with P_aO_2 levels >50 torr and/or the presence of clinically acceptable noninvasive monitoring of oxygen (P_aCO_2),[7,25,48,49,51] while maintaining an adequate V_E as indicated by P_aCO_2 of 50–60 torr or less and pH ≥ 7.25.
9.2 Reduction in the work of breathing as indicated by a decrease in respiratory rate by 30–40% and a decrease in the severity of retractions, grunting, and nasal flaring.[16,27,29]
9.3 Improvement in lung volumes and appearance of lung as indicated by chest radiograph.[27]
9.4 Improvement in patient comfort as assessed by bedside caregiver.

NCPAP 10.0 Resources:
  10.1 Equipment
      10.1.1 Endotracheal tubes (positioned in the nasopharynx and secured by taping, with placement verified by laryngoscopy or palpation) or commercially available nasal prongs or nasopharyngeal tubes with accompanying harness and accessories may be used for CPAP administration.
      10.1.2 Commercially available continuous-flow infant ventilators equipped with CPAP mode or suitably equipped multipurpose ventilator, intregral or adjunct low and high airway pressure alarms, low and high oxygen concentration alarms, loss of power and gas source alarms may be used.[52]
      10.1.3 Lightweight ventilator circuits with servo-regulated humidification system
      10.1.4 Continuous noninvasive oxygenation monitoring by pulse oximetry or transcutaneous monitor with high and low alarm capabilities is recommended (continuous transcutaneous CO_2 monitoring may also be utilized).[53,54]
      10.1.5 Continuous electrocardiographic and respiratory rate monitor, with high and low alarm capabilities, is recommended.
      10.1.6 Suction source, suction regulator, and suction catheters for periodic suctioning to assure patency of nasal passages and of endotracheal tubes used for NP-CPAP are necessary.[55]
      10.1.7 Resuscitation apparatus with airway manometer and masks of appropriate size should be available.
      10.1.8 Gastric tube for periodic decompression of stomach and chest tubes should be available.
  10.2 Personnel: The application of NCPAP and NP-CPAP should be performed under the direction of a physician by trained personnel who

(continued)

AARC Clinical Practice Guideline *(continued)*

hold a recognized credential (eg, CRTT, RRT, RN) and who competently demonstrate

10.2.1 proper use, understanding, and mastery of the technical aspects of CPAP devices, mechanical ventilators, and humidification systems;

10.2.2 knowledge of ventilator management and understanding of neonatal airway anatomy and pulmonary physiology;

10.2.3 patient assessment skills, with an understanding of the interaction between the CPAP device and the patient and the ability to recognize and respond to adverse reactions and complications;

10.2.4 knowledge and understanding of artificial airway management, training in the procedures of placing endotracheal tubes in the nasopharynx;

10.2.5 the ability to interpret monitored and measured blood gas values and vital signs;

10.2.6 the application of Universal Precautions;[56]

10.2.7 proper use, understanding, and mastery of emergency resuscitation equipment and procedures;

10.2.8 the ability to assess, evaluate, and document outcome (Section 9.0).

NCPAP 11.0 Monoriting:

11.1 Patient-ventilator system checks should be performed at least every 2 to 4 hours and should include documentation of ventilator settings and patient assessments as recommended by the AARC CPG Patient-Ventilator System Checks (MV-SC) and the CPG Humidification during Mechanical Ventilation (HMV).[57,58]

11.2 Oxygen and carbon dioxide monitoring, including

11.2.1 Periodic sampling of blood gas values by arterial, capillary, or venous route[7,9,14,27,28,59,60]

11.2.2 Continuous noninvasive blood gas monitoring by transcutaneous O_2 and CO_2 monitors[27,60]

11.2.3 Continuous noninvasive monitoring of oxygen saturation by pulse oximetry[27,38]

11.3 Continuous monitoring of electrocardiogram and respiratory rate[24,25,27]

11.4 Continuous monitoring of proximal airway pressure (P_{aw}), PEEP, and mean airway pressure ($\overline{P}_{aw}$)[24,25,27]

11.5 Continuous monitoring of FIO_2[24,25,27]

11.6 Periodic physical assessment of breath sounds and signs of increased work of breathing (see Section 4.1)[16,24,25]

11.7 Periodic evaluation of chest radiographs[24,27,56]

NCPAP 12.0 Frequency:

NCPAP and NP-CPAP are intended for continuous use and are discontinued when the patient's clinical condition improves as indicated by successful outcome assessments (Section 9.0).

NCPAP 13.0 Infection Control:
No special precautions are necessary, but Universal Precautions[56] as described by the Centers for Disease Control should be employed
13.1 Disposable nasal CPAP kits are recommended and are intended for single-patient use.
13.2 Ventilator circuits and humidifier chambers should not be changed more frequently than every 48 hours. The Clinical Practice Guideline: Ventilator Circuit Changes, the CDC, and, reported experience[61-64] suggest that use periods of ≥5 days are acceptable when the humidifying device is other than an aerosol generator.
13.3 External surfaces of ventilator should be cleaned according to the manufacturer's recommendations when the device has remained in a patient's room for a prolonged period, when soiled, when it has come in contact with potentially transmittable organisms, and after each patient use.
13.4 Sterile suctioning procedures should be strictly adhered to[5,55]

Perinatal-Pediatrics Guidelines Committee:

Lynne K Bower RRT, Chairman, Boston MA

Sherry L Barnhart RRT, Mattoon IL

Peter Betit BS RRT, Boston MA

Jamie Clink RRT, Dallas TX

Barbara Hendon BA RCP RRT, Wylie TX

Joanne Masi-Lynch BS RRT, Salt Lake City UT

Barbara G Wilson MEd RRT, Durham NC

REFERENCES
1. Duncan AW, Oh TE, Hillman DR. PEEP and CPAP. Anaesth Intensive Care 1986; 14(3):236–250.
2. ACCP-ATS Joint Committee on Pulmonary Nomenclature. Pulmonary terms and symbols. Chest 1975;67(5):583–593.
3. Sedin G. CPAP and mechanical ventilation. Int J Technol Assess Health Care 1991;7 (Suppl 1):31–40.
4. Branson RD. PEEP without endotracheal intubation. Respir Care 1988;33(7):598–610.
5. Czervinske M, Durbin CG, Gal TJ. Resistance to gas flow across 14 CPAP devices for newborns. Respir Care 1986;31(1):18–21.
6. Martin RJ, Carlo WA. Role of the upper airway in the pathogenesis of apnea in infants. Respir Care 1986;31(7):615–621.
7. Wung J-T, Driscoll JM, Epstein RA, Hyman AI. A new device for CPAP by nasal route. Crit Care Med 1975;3(2):76–78.
8. So B-H, Shibuya K, Tamura M, Watanabe H, Kamoshita S. Clinical experience in using a new type of nasal prong for administration of N-CPAP. Acta Paediatr Jpn 1992; 34(3):328–333.
9. Jonson B, Ahlström H, Lindroth M, Svenningsen NW. Continuous positive airway pressure; modes of action in relation to clinical applications. Pediatr Clin North Am 1980; 27(3):687–699.
10. Moa G, Nilsson K. Nasal continuous positive airway pressure: experiences with a new technical approach. Acta Paediatr 1993;82(2):210–211.
11. Kamper J, Ringsted C. Early treatment of idiopathic respiratory distress syndrome using binasal continuous positive airway pressure. Acta Paediatr Scand 1990;79:581–586.
12. Chernick V. Continuous distending pressure in hyaline membrane disease: of devices, disadvantages, and a daring study. Pediatrics 1973;52(1):114–115.

(continued)

AARC Clinical Practice Guideline *(continued)*

13. Caliumi-Pellegrini G, Agostino R, Orzalesi M, Nodari S, Marzetti PG, et al. Twin nasal cannula for administration of continuous positive airway pressure to newborn infants. Arch Dis Child 1974;49:228–230.
14. Kumar A, Falke KJ, Geffin B, Aldredge CF, Laver MB, Lowenstein E, et al. Continuous positive-pressure ventilation in acute respiratory failure: effects on hemodynamics and lung function. N Engl J Med 1970;283(26):1430–1436.
15. Schlobohm RM, Falltrick RT, Quan SF, Katz JA. Lung volumes, mechanics, and oxygenation during spontaneous positive-pressure ventilation: the advantage of CPAP over EPAP. Anesthesiology 1981;55:416–422.
16. Jonzon A. Indications for continuous positive airway pressure and respirator therapy. Int J Technol Assess Health Care 1991;7(Suppl 1):26–30.
17. Bonta BW, Uauy R, Warshaw JB, Motoyama EK. Determination of optimal continuous positive airway pressure for the treatment of IRDS by measurement of esophageal pressure. J Pediatr 1977;91(3):449–454.
18. Schulze A, Madler H-J, Gehrhardt B, Schaller P, Gmyrek D. Titration of continuous positive airway pressure by the pattern of breathing: analysis of flow-volume-time relationships by a noninvasive computerized system. Pediatr Pulmonol 1990;8:96–103.
19. Landers S, Hansen TN, Corbet AJS, Stevener MJ, Rudoph AD. Optimal constant positive airway pressure assessed by arterial alveolar difference for CO_2 in hyaline membrane disease. Pediatr Res 1986;20(9):884–889.
20. Miller, MJ, DiFiore JM, Strohl KP, Martin RJ. Effects of nasal CPAP on supraglottic and total pulmonary resistance in preterm infants. J Appl Physiol 1990;68:141–146.
21. Durand M, McCann E, Brady JP. Effect of continuous positive airway pressure on the ventilatory response to CO_2 in preterm infants. Pediatrics 1983;71(4):634–638.
22. Locke R, Greenspan JS, Shaffer TH, Rubenstein SD, Wolfson MR. Effect of nasal CPAP on thoracoabdominal motion in neonates with respiratory insufficiency. Pediatr Pulmonol 1991;11:259–264.
23. Cogswell JJ, Hatch DJ, Kerr AA, Taylor B. Effects of continuous positive airway pressure on lung mechanics of babies after operation for congenital heart disease. Arch Dis Child 1975;50:799–804.
24. Smith RA, Venus B, Wier DD, Mathru M, Masood S, Goldstein JD, et al. Morphometric changes in a dog model of the adult respiratory distress syndrome after early therapy with continuous positive airway pressure. Respir Care 1987;32(7):525–533.
25. Chatburn RL. Similiarities and differences in the managment of acute lung injury in neonates (IRDS) and in adults (ARDS). Respir Care 1988;33(7):539–553.
26. Gregory GA, Kitterman JA, Phibbs RH, Tooley WH, Hamilton WK. Treatment of the idiopathic respiratory-distress syndrome with continuous positive airway pressure. N Engl J Med 1971;284(24):1332–1339.
27. Speidel BD, Dunn PM. Effect of continuous positive airway pressure on breathing pattern of infants with respiratory-distress syndrome. Lancet 1975;1(7902):302–304.
28. Hegyi T, Hiatt IM. The effect of continuous positive airway pressure on the course of respiratory distress syndrome: the benefits of early initiation. Crit Care Med 1981;9(1):38–41.
29. Gherini S, Peters RM, Virgilio RW. Mechanical work on the lungs and work of breathing with positive end-expiratory pressure and continuous positive airway pressure. Chest 1979;76(3):251–256.
30. Roberton NRC. Prolonged continuous positive airways pressure for pulmonary oedema due to persistent ductus arteriosus in the newborn. Arch Dis Child 1974;49(7):585–587.
31. Ryan CA, Finer NN, Peters KL. Nasal intermittent positive-pressure ventilation offers no advantages over nasal continuous positive airway pressure in apnea of prematurity. AJDC 1989;143(10):1196–1198.
32. Kattwinkel J. Neonatal apnea: pathogenesis and therapy. J Pediatr 1977;90(3):342–347.
33. Kattwinkel J, Nearman HS, Fanaroff AA, Katona PG, Klaus MH. Apnea of prematurity: comparative therapeutic effects of cutaneous stimulation and nasal continuous positive airway pressure. J Pediatr 1975;86(4):588–592.
34. Miller MJ. Carlo WA, Martin RJ. Continuous positive airway pressure selectively reduces obstructive apnea in preterm infants. J Pediatr 1985;106(1):91–94.
35. Engelke SC, Roloff DW, Kuhns LR. Postextubation nasal continuous positive airway pressure: a prospective controlled study. Am J Dis Child 1982;136(4):359–361.
36. Higgins RD, Richter SE, Davis JM. Nasal continuous positive airway pressure facilitates extubation of very low birth weight neonates. Pediatrics 1991;88:999–1003.

37. Neijens HJ, Kerrebijn KF, Smalhout B. Successful treatment with CPAP of two infants with bronchomalacia. Acta Paediatr Scand 1978;67:293–296.
38. Miller RW, Pollack MM, Murphy TM, Fink RJ. Effectiveness of continuous positive airway pressure in the treatment of bronchomalacia in infants: a bronchoscopic documentation. Crit Care Med 1986;14(2):125–127.
39. Beasley JM, Jones SEF. Continuous positive airway pressure in bronchiolitis. Br Med J 1981;283:1506–1508.
40. Smith PG, El-Khatib MF, Carlo WA. PEEP does not improve pulmonary mechanics in infants with bronchiolitis. Am Rev Respir Dis 1993;147:1295–1298.
41. Thompson JE, Farrell E, McManus M. Neonatal and pediatric airway emergencies. Respir Care 1992;37(6):582–599.
42. Yu VYH, Liew SW, Roberton NRC. Pneumothorax in the newborn: changing pattern. Arch Dis Child 1975;50(6):449–453.
43. Chernick V. Lung rupture in the newborn infant. Respir Care 1986;31(7):628–633.
44. Goldman SL, Brady JP, Dumpit FM. Increased work of breathing associated with nasal prongs. Pediatrics 1979;64(2):160–164.
45. Nelson RM, Egan EA, Eitzman DV. Increased hypoxemia in neonates secondary to the use of continuous positive airway pressure. J Pediatr 1977;91(1):87–91.
46. Garland JS, Nelson DB, Rice T, Neu J. Increased risk of gastrointestinal perforations in neonates mechanically ventilated with either face mask or nasal prongs. Pediatrics 1985;76(3):406–410.
47. Tanswell AK. Continuous distending pressure in the respiratory distress syndrome of the newborn: who, when, and why? Respir Care 1982;27(3):257–266.
48. Han VKM, Beverley DW, Clarson C, Sumabat WO, Shaheed WA, Brabyn DG, et al. Randomized controlled trial of very early continuous distending pressure in the management of preterm infants. Early Hum Dev 1987;15:21–32.
49. Richardson CP, Jung AL. Effects of continuous positive airway pressure on pulmonary function and blood gases of infants with respiratory distess syndrome. Pediatr Res 1978;12:771–774.
50. Tanswell AK, Clubb RA, Smith BT, Boston RW. Individualised continuous distending pressure applied within 6 hours of delivery in infants with respiratory distress syndrome. Arch Dis Child 1980;55:33–39.
51. Krouskop RW, Brown EG, Sweet AY. The early use of continuous positive airway pressure in the treatment of idiopathic respiratory distress syndrome. J Pediatr 1975;87(2):263–267.
52. Hayes B. Ventilation and ventilators—an update. J Med Eng Technol 1988;12(5):197–218.
53. Severinghaus JW. Transcutaneous blood gas analysis. Respir Care 1982;27(2):152–159.
54. Hay WW Jr, Brockway JM, Ezyaguirre M. Neonatal pulse oximetry: accuracy and reliability. Pediatrics 1989;83(5):717–722.
55. American Association for Respiratory Care. Clinical practice guideline: endotracheal suctioning of mechanically ventilated adults and children with artificial airways. Respir Care 1993;38(5):500–504.
56. Centers for Disease Control. Update: Universal Precautions for prevention of transmission of human immunodeficiency virus, hepatitis B virus, and other blood-borne pathogens in health care settings. MMWR 1988;37:377–382,387–388.
57. American Association for Respiratory Care Clinical practice guideline: patient-ventilator system checks. Respir Care 1992;37(8):882–886.
58. American Association for Respiratory Care. Clinical practice guideline: humidification during mechanical ventilation. Respir Care 1992;37(8):887–890.
59. American Association for Respiratory Care. Clinical practice guideline: oxygen therapy in the acute care hospital. Respir Care 1991;36(12):1410–1413.
60. Avery GB, Glass P. Retinopathy of prematurity: what causes it? Clin Perinatol 1988;15(4):917–928.
61. American Association for Respiratory Care. Clinical practice guideline: ventilator circuit changes. Respir Care 1994;39(8):797–802.
62. Centers for Disease Control and Prevention. Draft guideline for prevention of nosocomial pneumonia: Part 1. Issues on prevention of nosocomial pneumonia—1994. Part 2: Recommendations for prevention of nosocial pneumonia. Federal Register February 2, 1994 Vol 59, No. 22.
63. Kacmarek RM, English P, Vallende N, Hopkins CC. Extended use of heated neonatal/pediatric ventilator circuits (abstract). Respir Care 1991;36(11):1287.

(continued)

AARC Clinical Practice Guideline *(continued)*

64. Eller R, Kennedy K, Weber P, Nadzam T, Vargo J, Nield M (abstract). The impact of 96-hour ventilator circuit changes on rates of ventilator-associated pneumonia and costs. Respir Care 1993;38(11):1262.

▬BIBLIOGRAPHY

Andersen JB, Olesen KP, Eikard B, Jansen E, Qvist J. Periodic continuous positive airway pressure, CPAP, by mask in the treatment of atelectasis: a sequential analysis. Eur J Respir Dis 1980;61:20–25.

Andréasson B, Lindroth M, Svenningsen NW, Jonson B. Effects on respiration of CPAP immediately after extubation in the very preterm infant. Pediatr Pulmonol 1988;4:213–218.

Fox WW, Berman LS, Downes JJ Jr, Peckham GJ. The therapeutic application of end-expiratory pressure in the meconium apiration syndrome. Pediatrics 1975;56(2):214–217.

Hess D. The use of PEEP in clinical settings other than acute lung injury. Respir Care 1988;33(7):581–595.

Kacmarek RM, Dimas S, Reynolds J, Shapiro BA. Technical aspects of positive end-expiratory pressure (PEEP): Part III. PEEP with spontaneous ventilation. Respir Care 1982;27(12):1505–1518.

Kamper J, Møller J. Long-term prognosis of infants with idiopathic respiratory distress syndrome: follow-up studies in infants surviving after the introduction of continuous positive airway pressure. Acta Paediatr Scand 1979;68:149–154.

Martin RJ, Nearman HS, Katona PG, Klaus MH. The effect of a low continuous positive airway pressure on the reflex control of respiration in the preterm infant. J Pediatr 1977;90(6):976–981.

Okken A, Rubin IL, Martin RJ. Intermittent bag ventilation of preterm infants on continuous positive airway pressure: the effect on transcutaneous P_{O_2}. J Pediatr 1978;93(2):279–282.

Roberton NRC. CPAP or not CPAP? Arch Dis Child 1976;51:161–162.

Stark AR. Disorders of respiratory control in infants. Respir Care 1991;36(7):673–681.

Sturgeon CL Jr, Douglas ME, Downs JB, Dannemiller FJ. PEEP and CPAP: cardiopulmonary effects during spontaneous ventilation. Anesth Analg 1977;56(5):633–641.

Svenningsen NW, Jonson B, Lindroth M, Ahlström H. Consecutive study of early CPAP-application in hyaline membrane disease. Eur J Pediatr 1979;131:9–19.

Weigle CGM. Treatment of an infant with tracheobronchomalacia at home with a light-weight, high-humidity, continuous positive airway pressure system. Crit Care Med 1990;18(8):892–894.

Witte MK, Galli SA, Chatburn RL, Blumer JL. Optimal positive end-expiratory pressure therapy in infants and children with acute respiratory failure. Pediatr Res 1988;24(2):217–221.

Wung J-T, Koons AH, Driscoll JM Jr, James LS. Changing incidence of bronchopulmonary dysplasia. J Pediatr 1979;95(5, Part 2):845–847.

Chapter 16

Mechanical Ventilation of the Infant and Child

BARBARA G. WILSON

OBJECTIVES

Having completed this chapter, the reader will be able to:

1 Classify the function and performance of neonatal/pediatric mechanical ventilators using the following terms: *trigger, limit, control,* and *cycle.*

2 Initiate and develop pathophysiology-based ventilatory management plans to treat neonatal or pediatric respiratory failure.

3 Select ventilator parameters for neonates and pediatric patients, including methods of assessing mechanical ventilation, appropriate to the respiratory care plan.

4 Design a ventilator weaning plan for neonatal/pediatric patients.

5 Discuss the hazards and complications of mechanical ventilation.

6 Assess and interpret airway graphic displays during neonatal/pediatric mechanical ventilation, specifically, pressure, flow, and volume scalars, as well as pressure-volume and flow-volume loops.

7 Evaluate the features of the commercially available infant and pediatric mechanical ventilators to enable selection and application based on patient needs and the ventilatory care plan.

KEY TERMS

baseline variable	pressure-support ventilation
cycle variable	trigger variable
limit variable	ventilator response time
mean airway pressure	volume-control ventilation
patient–ventilator dyssynchrony	volume-support ventilation

Respiratory failure is one of the major causes of morbidity and mortality in infants and children.[19,39] Respiratory care practitioners (RCPs) who provide neonatal and pediatric ventilatory care must possess special knowl-

311

edge of physiology and pathophysiology, as well as of equipment, as a basis for selection and management of all forms of respiratory support. Providing this support requires an understanding of developmental changes in neonatal and pediatric respiratory mechanics: respiratory rate, pattern, inspiratory flow, and tidal volume. These developmental features describe the range of characteristics within which mechanical ventilators must perform. RCPs must also understand the disease process and the respiratory mechanics of the child versus equipment performance to be able to select appropriate ventilatory support and design a care plan unique to each child's clinical scenario.

This chapter will present a comprehensive review of neonatal and pediatric mechanical ventilation including ventilator classification, pathophysiology-based management strategies, equipment selection, and monitoring/assessment techniques. A series of patient case studies will test the reader's ability to design a ventilatory care plan appropriate for the patient.

▬CLASSIFICATION OF MECHANICAL VENTILATORS

Terminology to classify mechanical ventilators has been described by many authors and continues to be an area of confusion for practitioners.[11-13,20,27,31] A classification system should provide a common base of terms to facilitate the understanding, interpretation, and assessment of ventilator performance characteristics. The classification must accurately reflect the pattern of respiratory support a patient receives. This section will present a method of ventilator classification to support the clinical practice of neonatal and pediatric ventilatory care.

A ventilator is designed to alter, transmit, and direct energy in a predetermined way to perform the work of the thorax and lungs. A basic ventilator classification system, proposed by Chatburn, is presented in Table 16-1.[13] This system addresses five basic categories: power input, power transmission, control schemes, output parameters, and alarm systems. Ventilators are powered either by electricity or compressed gas. The transmission of this power is a function of the drive mechanism and control schemes of the ventilator. Clinical application of ventilator classification focuses on the control variables, output parameters, and alarm systems. More specifically, clinicians focus on breath types and breath limits to describe the type of respiratory support a patient may be receiving.[22]

Control Schemes and Variables

Ventilator control variables address the parameters adjusted, measured, or used to manipulate various phases of the ventilatory cycle. The four common types of control variables are flow, pressure, volume, and time. Typically, the control variable remains constant despite changes in ventilatory demand, that is, changes in the patient's compliance and resistance.[28] Each manufacturer develops a control scheme for its ventilator platform to manipulate these variables. Commonalities in these control schemes have developed between ventilators, allowing RCPs to describe ventilatory patterns using common terminology. Using inspiratory flow patterns as an example, it can be seen that third-generation microprocessor technology allows clinicians to select a variety of inspiratory gas flow patterns (waveforms) during various modes of ventilation.[30] The functional performance

---

TABLE 16-1   Ventilator Classification

I. Power input

    A. Pneumatic

    B. Electric

II. Power transmission or conversion (drive mechanism)

    A. External compressor

    B. Internal compressor

    C. Output/control valves

III. Control scheme

    A. Control circuit

    B. Control variables

    C. Phase variables

    D. Conditional variables

IV. Output waveforms

    A. Pressure

    B. Volume

    C. Flow

V. Alarm systems

(Adapted from Chatburn, RL: Classification of mechanical ventilators. Respir Care 37(9): 1009, 1992.)

---

of flow patterns remains constant across manufacturers, but may be produced by different technical control schemes.

Inspiratory flow patterns determine the gas flow characteristic as the mechanical breath is distributed within the patient's lungs. RCPs should consider several factors when selecting an inspiratory flow pattern for a given patient's pulmonary disease. The inflation properties of the lungs, as compared with the mechanical movement of gas into the lungs, is the basis for the pressures generated during inspiration (peak inspiratory and **mean airway pressures**). Pressure increases as volume enters the lungs, meets resistance of the airways, and overcomes the elastic recoil of the lung. Therefore, peak pressure = $(flow)(R_{aw}) + (TV)(Elastance)$. The shape of the inspiratory flow pattern determines the shape of the pressure curve and the peak airway pressure generated during inspiration. Selection of the inspiratory flow pattern, based upon the patient's pulmonary pathophysiology, will improve the effectiveness of ventilation, reduce peak inspiratory pressures, and minimize mean airway pressure.

Figure 16-1 illustrates tracings typical of the inspiratory flow patterns available with mechanical ventilators.

Sine wave: Nonconstant flow produces an inspiratory pattern in which flow increases during the early phase of inspiration, peaks at midinspiration, then decreases until end-inspiration.

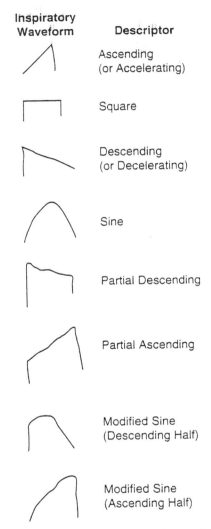

FIGURE 16-1 Waveform display of flow patterns for mechanical ventilation. (Rau JL: Inspiratory flow patterns: The shape of ventilation. Respir Care 38:132,1993.)

Square wave: A square wave pattern is produced by a constant flow of gas throughout inspiration.

Ascending wave: Ascending flow patterns produce a ramp pattern with low flow at beginning inspiration, linear increases in flow throughout inspiration, and peak flow at end-inspiration.

Descending flow: Descending flow is a waveform characterized by peak flow at the beginning of inspiration and linear decreases until end-inspiration.

Ascending flow patterns deliver the highest flow at end-inspiration, when the effects of airway resistance and elastance are highest, producing the highest peak pressures compared with other flow patterns. Descending flow patterns generate the highest airway pressures due to flow at beginning inspiration, when lung volume and elastance are low. Flow then decreases throughout inspiration as delivered volume increases. Therefore, peak pressures are lower overall, but mean airway pressure is higher with this flow pattern. In general, peak pressure increases and mean airway pressure decreases as the highest point of flow in the pattern moves from the beginning to the end of the inspiratory cycle.

In clinical situations where patients have high airway resistance (asthma, tracheal stenosis, airway obstruction), peak airway pressures can be reduced by avoiding flow patterns with characteristically high peak flow rates. Square-wave or partial-descending flow patterns generate lower peak pressures than descending flow patterns in this scenario. Lung diseases characterized by low compliance (acute respiratory distress syndrome, infant respiratory distress syndrome) benefit from descending flow patterns in which peak pressures are reduced but mean airway pressure is increased. Clinicians should monitor I:E (inspiratory time to expiratory time) ratios when selecting flow patterns and adjust peak flow to maintain suitably short inspiratory times.

Phase Variables

Factors that affect the phases of the ventilatory cycle are called phase variables.[4] These factors address the initiation, duration, and termination of inspiration and expiration. All ventilators measure variables associated with the delivery of the mechanical breath (time, pressure, volume). Inspiration begins when one of these variables, historically time or pressure, reaches a preset value called the **trigger variable.** Several newer neonatal and pediatric ventilators offer flow triggering; these ventilators sense changes in flow, thereby increasing the sensitivity of the ventilator in matching the patient's spontaneous demands and decreasing response time of breath delivery. Therefore, mechanical breaths may be pressure, time, or flow triggered. Some neonatal ventilators trigger inspiration via an external sensor taped to the abdomen of the infant to sense respiratory movement and initiate inspiration. Under these conditions, the mechanical breath could be considered an impedance trigger.

The **cycle variable** determines when inspiration ends. This variable is used as a feedback signal to terminate gas flow and allow the patient to passively exhale. Time is currently the standard cycle variable and, therefore, most ventilators are considered time cycled.

Limit variables prevent selected ventilatory parameters from exceeding predetermined values and impose safety checks on the ventilator system. During inspiration, pressure, volume, and flow increase above end-expiratory values. Limit variables allow the clinician to control the upper limits of pressure, volume, or both to preserve the size of the mechanical breath a patient receives, hence the description "pressure limited" and "volume limited." A **baseline variable** describes the variable controlled during the expiratory phase of the ventilatory cycle. The most commonly manipulated expiratory variable is pressure. This pressure is most often positive (positive end-expiratory pressure, continuous positive airway pressure), but may be negative in the case of negative pressure ventilation or negative end-expiratory pressure (NEEP) applied to facilitate expiration in the face of increased airway resistance (for a discussion of active exhalation during high-frequency oscillatory ventilation [HFOV], see Chap. 24).

Ventilatory Modes

Using this terminology, a system develops to describe ventilatory modes and breathing patterns used during mechanical ventilation. Ventilatory modes may include spontaneous breaths and mechanical breaths, or a combination of both.

Spontaneous breaths may be supported with continuous positive airway pressure (CPAP), a mode that maintains a constant positive airway pressure above baseline throughout inspiration and expiration. A preset expiratory pressure limit prevents the patient from exhaling down to atmospheric pressure at end-expiration. Raising the expiratory pressure above atmospheric pressure traps a volume of gas in the lungs proportionate to the pressure applied and to lung compliance. This gas volume augments the expiratory reserve volume (ERV) of the lung and increases the functional residual capacity (FRC). Continuous or demand flow during inspiration maintains airway pressure above atmospheric pressure. CPAP mode can be used alone or in conjunction with mechanical breaths.

Pressure-support (PS) ventilation is also a spontaneous breathing mode that can be used alone or in combination with other modes (synchronized intermittent mandatory ventilation, CPAP). A preset level of inspiratory pressure is delivered above the baseline pressure with each spontaneous effort. PS is initiated when pressure or flow is dropped during inspiration to the preset threshold. Flow then accelerates into the breathing circuit, increasing proximal airway pressure to the preset pressure level, with the breath being terminated at 25% of peak flow. The tidal volume delivered in this mode will vary with changes in endotracheal tube diameter, lung compliance, airway resistance, and PS settings. Inspiratory time can be fixed or variable during PS, depending upon the ventilator design.

Volume-support (VS) ventilation combines the benefits of PS ventilation with the safety of a volume guarantee during spontaneous breathing. The Siemens 300 ventilator monitors airway resistance and compliance of the lung and adjusts the PS level using a predetermined algorithm to deliver a preset volume.

Mechanical breaths may be control or assist-control breaths. Control breaths deliver a preset ventilator rate to the patient. Inspiratory and expiratory times are fixed in this mode and dependent upon ventilator rate and I:E ratio. The patient may not breathe spontaneously or trigger additional mechanical breaths in control mode. Control ventilation is best achieved by sedating or paralyzing the patient to prevent spontaneous breathing. Assisted breaths deliver a patient-triggered ventilator rate in excess of the control rate with each spontaneous effort. Machine "sensitivity" determines the degree of effort a patient must exert to cycle the ventilator into inspiration; ideally, this should be adjusted to -0.5 to -1.5 cm H_2O of pressure or 0.1 to 0.3 LPM of flow to minimize work of breathing.

Control and assisted breaths may be volume or pressure limited. Patients may receive **volume-control ventilation**, in which a predetermined breath rate is delivered and breaths are volume limited, or volume-assist ventilation, in which mechanical breaths are also volume limited, but the patient triggers breaths in excess of the preset rate. A patient may also receive pressure-control ventilation, in which a preset breath rate is delivered along with a preset pressure limit. Pressure-assist ventilation describes a breathing pattern in which the patient may trigger the breath rate in excess of a preset rate and breaths are pressure limited. Pressure-regulated volume control combines the attributes of pressure-control and pressure-assist ventilation with a volume guarantee. In this mode, the ventilator monitors the airway resistance and compliance of the lungs and adjusts the inspiratory pressure level via a predetermined algorithm to deliver a preset volume limit.

Intermittent mandatory ventilation (IMV) and synchronized intermittent mandatory ventilation (SIMV) modes combine mechanical breaths with spontaneous breathing, in which the spontaneous volume and rate are a function of the patient's inspiratory effort and stimulus to breathe. Flow for spontaneous breathing may be provided by a continuous flow of oxygen through the breathing circuit, a demand valve, or a combination of both. If positive end-expiratory pressure (PEEP) is applied with continuous and demand flow, the spontaneous breaths become CPAP breaths. Pressure support may also be administered in conjunction with SIMV, as previously described. SIMV differs from IMV by synchronizing the initiation of the mechanical breaths with the patient's spontaneous effort, in order to prevent stacking of mechanical and spontaneous breaths. The development of SIMV for small infants with adequate trigger sensitivity and response time has been an area of active research and development by ventilator manufacturers.

Ventilator classification according to this system may seem cumbersome and challenging to some practitioners. However, this system addresses new advances in ventilator operation and provides a method of describing new technology. Neonatal ventilators have traditionally been classified as continuous-flow, time-cycled, pressure-limited IMV systems. Using this new classification system, the mechanical breaths produced by neonatal ventilators would be considered flow controlled, time triggered, time cycled, and pressure controlled. The spontaneous breaths provided by these ventilators would be flow-controlled, positive expiratory pressure (CPAP) breaths.

Recent advances in neonatal ventilator design now provide the option of volume-controlled SIMV.[1] Fine calibration and measurement of smaller volumes facilitates volume-assist mechanical SIMV breaths with CPAP or pressure support of the spontaneous breaths.[2,9,37] Mechanical breaths are pressure or flow triggered, time cycled, and volume assist breaths. Spontaneous breaths are flow-controlled CPAP or flow-variable pressure-support breaths.

Some adult ventilator manufacturers have recently extended the range of pressure, flow, and volume the ventilator can deliver in an attempt to crossover into the pediatric population. The primary differences between neonatal/pediatric and adult ventilators are the ranges of flow, volume, trigger sensitivity, and response time a ventilator can deliver. Neonatal/pediatric ventilators deliver lower flows and volumes at faster rates, with faster response times to enhance trigger sensitivity. Neonatal ventilators provide continuous and variable flow at preset values and therefore offer a variety of waveform patterns. The variable flow patterns of neonatal/pediatric ventilators allow pressure, volume, or both to vary in response to the pneumatic characteristics of the patient's lungs. Therefore, pressure-control and pressure-assist ventilation are now available on a neonatal/pediatric ventilator. This improves the performance of these ventilators in the face of decreased compliance by decreasing peak inspiratory pressures and increasing mean airway pressure to recruit collapsed alveoli. Table 16-2 contains the common classifications of neonatal/pediatric ventilators.

■INITIATING MECHANICAL VENTILATORY SUPPORT

Providing ventilatory support to infants and children requires careful attention to the physiologic balance between the respiratory and cardiac systems.[10,35] The pulmonary and systemic circulations are physically connected in series with the lungs and chest wall surrounding the heart and great vessels, directly exposing both organ systems to changes in intrathoracic pressure. Changes in intrathoracic pressure as a result of ventilatory interventions affect cardiovascular performance by altering cardiac output, that is, increases in intrathoracic pressure cause decreases in cardiac preload and afterload as a result of respiratory intervention.[26] The pulmonary circulation of neonates and children is also highly reactive to changes in oxygenation. Pulmonary vascular resistance can quickly increase to life-threatening levels because of arterial desaturation.[15] Most infants and children recover from these episodes, but children with marginal physiologic reserves or severe illness could suffer serious consequences. Any abnormality that interrupts the delicate balance between the respiratory and cardiac systems, be it disease or treatment, can cause a cascade of worsening physiologic and clinical outcomes because alterations in performance of one system can cause alterations in the other. As ventilatory strategies and interventions are considered and undertaken, RCPs must anticipate the physiologic responses and adapt the care plan based on patient response.

Given these complex interactions, a single,standardized respiratory support strategy is not appropriate. Strategies must address specific pathologic conditions, age, weight, and activity of the patient. The goal of mechanical ventilation is to improve oxygen delivery to meet metabolic demand and eliminate carbon dioxide while reducing work of breathing

TABLE 16-2   Classification of Modes of Mechanical Ventilation

MODE	MANDATORY BREATH VARIABLES			SPONTANEOUS BREATH SUPPORT
	Trigger	*Cycle*	*Limit*	
CMV (continuous mechanical ventilation)	Time	Time	Volume	Not applicable
A/C (assist/control ventilation)	Time	Time	Volume	Not applicable
	Pressure	Time	Volume	Not applicable
IMV	Time	Time	Volume	CPAP
SIMV	Time	Time	Volume	
	Pressure	Time	Volume	

TABLE 16-3   Ventilator Management Goals

Reestablish end-expiratory lung volume and patient–ventilator synchrony.

Prevent pulmonary overdistention and intrinsic PEEP.

Minimize inspiratory airway pressures.

Administer the lowest FIo_2 possible.

Initiate weaning as soon as indicated.

---

for a patient (Table 16-3). The physiologic interplay between the respiratory and cardiac systems directly affects the delivery and utilization of oxygen and elimination of carbon dioxide (CO_2). Ventilatory support should meet these goals while minimizing the deleterious effects of the interventions on the performance of the cardiorespiratory system. The approach should be simple, meet the needs of the patient, and provide the greatest benefit at the lowest risk of complication. Table 16-4 lists indications for mechanical ventilation by patient population.

Ventilator management strategies should target the altered physiologic parameters. This information is obtained from thorough patient assessment, including chest x-ray film interpretation, laboratory data, and an understanding of the primary diagnosis and resultant pathophysiology. General categories of physiologic disturbance are inadequate oxygen delivery and inadequate CO_2 elimination.[24,25] A general ventilator management algorithm for children with these disturbances is outlined in Figure 16-2. Figure 16-3 provides a specific ventilator management algorithm for inadequate oxygen delivery as a result of respiratory disease. Figure 16-4 provides a specific ventilator management algorithm for inadequate oxygen delivery as a result of cardiac disease. Inadequate oxygen delivery for premature infants and term infants with pulmonary hypertension are treated separately in Figures 16-5 and 16-6 because of the differences in pathophysiology.

If the primary cause of decreased oxygen delivery is arterial hypoxemia as a result of respiratory disease, ventilatory support becomes a primary patient management intervention (see Fig. 16-3). Arterial hypoxemia may

---

TABLE 16-4   Indications for Mechanical Ventilation

Infants and Children
Arterial hypoxemia ($Sao_2 < 90\%–92\%$)

Severe upper airway obstruction

Cardiovascular instability

Apnea and bradycardia

	INFANTS	CHILDREN
Alveolar hypoventilation (pH < 7.20)	>60 mm Hg	>50 mm Hg
Increased work of breathing (RR)	>70–80 bpm	>40 bpm

Inadequate Oxygen Delivery—Respiratory Disease
Decreased Oxygen Content

↓

Possible Causes:

Cardiac Disease (R-to-L intracardiac shunt)

Respiratory Disease (ventilation/perfusion mismatch due to
intrapulmonary shunt or alveolar hypoventilation)

Respiratory Disease

Alveolar Hypoventilation

Goal: Increase effective ventilation, maintain acid–base status WNL
Ventilation Strategy: Restore EELV and TV

Synchronous Mechanical Ventilation—Volume Limited

Delivered TV 8 to 10 mL/kg (term infants and children)

Rate to maintain $Paco_2$ and pH WNL

Flo_2 to maintain Spo_2 > 92%

PEEP titrated to best compliance and hemodynamics

Keep PIP < 35 cm H_2O

Avoid: Overdistention, dyssynchrony, PEEPi

FIGURE 16-2   General management algorithm for inadequate oxygen delivery.

be the result of hypoventilation or ventilation/perfusion mismatch due to atelectasis and reduction of end-expiratory lung volume. The diagnosis of significant intrapulmonary shunting is made by determining the alveolar-to-arterial oxygen gradient ($AaDo_2$). When hypoventilation occurs due to atelectasis or increased physiologic deadspace, the ventilatory strategy should be focused on restoring adequate lung volume via increased tidal volume and PEEP. If decreased lung compliance is the cause of the hypoxemia, ventilator strategy is again aimed at restoring lung volume, while minimizing lung injury due to pulmonary overdistention (volutrauma) or barotrauma.

Using the algorithm in Figure 16-4, if inadequate oxygen delivery is the result of an intracardiac shunt (congenital heart disease), ventilatory interventions play a more minor role in patient management and are aimed at reducing the work of breathing for the patient and improving pulmonary and systemic blood flow. The presence of a cardiac anomaly may be diagnosed with a 100% oxygen challenge. If the FIo_2 is increased to 1.00 and the hypoxemia remains unresponsive to oxygen therapy, the shunt is most likely a result of a cardiac defect. Bedside echocardiography will confirm the diagnosis and identify the specific disturbance. The ventilator strategy for these patients is dependent upon the quantity of pulmonary blood flow produced by the anomaly. If there is insufficient pulmonary blood flow, ventilator management is directed at decreasing pulmonary vascular resistance, increasing right ventricular function via mild respiratory alka-

Inadequate Oxygen Delivery—Respiratory Disease
Decreased Oxygen Content
↓
Possible Causes:
Cardiac Disease (R-to-L intracardiac shunt)
Respiratory Disease (Ventilation perfusion mismatch due
to intrapulmonary shunt or alveolar hypoventilation)

Respiratory Disease
Increased Intrapulmonary Shunt due to:
Atelectasis
Decreased EELV
Decreased lung compliance
↓
Ventilator strategy depends upon pathophysiology:
Atelectasis: Increase TV
Decrease EELV: restore FRC with PEEP
Increase lung compliance: Increase TV and FRC with PEEP
↓
Atelectasis and Decreased EELV
Goal: Restore adequate lung volume
Ventilation Strategy: Increase tidal volume and EELV
Synchronous Mechanical Ventilation—volume limited
Delivered TV 8 to 10 mL/kg (term infants and children)
Rate to maintain $Paco_2$ and pH WNL
FIo_2 to maintain Spo_2 > 92%
PEEP titrated to best compliance and hemodynamics
Keep PIP < 35 cm H_2O
Avoid: overdistention, dyssynchrony, PEEPi
(Localized Area of Atelectasis: Consider Tx bronchoscopy)

Decreased Lung Compliance
Goal: Improve lung compliance, restore adequate lung volume, minimize lung injury
Ventilation Strategy: Recruit lung volume, improve oxygenation using low-stretch ventilation
Synchronous Mechanical Ventilation
Delivered TV 8 to 10 mL/kg (term infants and children)
Rate to maintain $Paco_2$ and pH WNL
FIo_2 to maintain Spo_2 > 92%
PEEP titrated to best compliance and hemodynamics
Keep PIP < 35 cm H_2O
Assess respiratory mechanics to avoid: overdistention, dyssynchrony, PEEPi
↓
Failure to improve: decreasing compliance, FIo_2 > .60
P_{aw} > 15 cm H_2O, PIP > 35 cm H_2O
↓
Initiate pressure-limited ventilation with decelerating flow pattern
Titrate PEEP to best compliance and hemodynamics
Sedate for dyssynchrony, consider paralysis
to decrease O_2 consumption, if O_2 delivery is compromised
Initiate permissive hypercapnia—limit PIP to 35 cm H_2O
(Maintain pH > 7.25)
Optimize Hgb and HCT
Support CO with volume and inotropic Tx
↓
Failure to improve: decreased compliance, failure to wean FIo_2 or P_{aw}
length of ventilation approaching 5 to 7 days
or hemodynamically unstable
↓
ECLS

FIGURE 16-3 Specific management algorithm for inadequate oxygen delivery resulting from respiratory disease.

Inadequate Oxygen Delivery—Cardiac Disease Decreased Oxygen Content
↓
Possible Causes:
Cardiac Disease (R-to-L intracardiac shunt)
Respiratory Disease (ventilation/perfusion mismatch due to
alveolar hypoventilation or intrapulmonary shunt)

Cardiac
Congenital Heart Disease
↓
Perform 100% O_2 challenge
Severe hypoxemia not responsive to O_2
↓
Cardiac echo confirms Dx
↓
Goal: Improve oxygen delivery
Flo_2 administered to maintain Spo_2 characteristic of anomaly
Decrease work of breathing to decrease O_2 consumption—intubate and ventilate
Improve pulmonary and systemic blood flows—inotropic Tx
Maintain or increase hemoglobin and hematocrit
↓
Ventilator strategy depends upon type of anomaly:
1. Decreased pulmonary blood flow
2. Increased pulmonary blood flow
↓
Insufficient Pulmonary Blood Flow:
Goal: Improve pulmonary blood flow by decreasing PVR
and increasing RV function by decreasing P_{aw}
Ventilator Strategy: Mild respiratory alkalosis, low P_{aw}
Delivered TV 8 to 10 mL/kg
Slow ventilatory rate to decrease mean intrathoracic pressure
(Increase tidal volume to maintain $Paco_2$ goal, if necessary)
Keep PIP <35 cm H_2O
PEEP 0 to 2 cm H_2O (lowest setting possible)
Flo_2 to maintain Spo_2 appropriate to the anomaly
↓
If P_{aw} required to maintain oxygen delivery
interferes with hemodynamics in the face of inotropic Tx
↓
Consider HFJV to lower P_{aw} and maintain ABGs

Excessive Pulmonary Blood Flow:
Goal: Decrease pulmonary blood flow by increasing PVR, Increase systemic blood flow (CO)
Ventilation Strategy: Mild respiratory acidosis, increase P_{aw}
Delivered TV 8 to 10 mL/kg
Ventilatory rate to maintain $Paco_2$ 55 to 65, pH > 7.25
Keep PIP <35 cm H_2O
Increase PEEP to increase mean intrathoracic pressure (<10 cm H_2O)
Sedate child to prevent spontaneous breathing
Flo_2 to maintain Spo_2 appropriate to the anomaly
↓
Consider inspired CO_2 Tx or hypoxic gas Tx
Optimize (increase) Hgb and HCT
↓
Inotropic Tx as appropriate

FIGURE 16-4 Specific management algorithm for inadequate oxygen delivery related to cardiac disease.

Premature Infant
Inadequate Oxygen Delivery

Early Intervention Strategy:
Labor and Delivery: infants < 1250 g
birth weight or evidence of
surfactant deficiency:
↓
Prophylactic surfactant in DR

No Early Intervention:
History, physical, and CXR confirm
RDS

↓
Decreased EELV
Hypoxemia

O_2 to maintain Spo_2 > 92%

↓
Hypoxemia resolves, wean Flo_2
Mild hypoxemia and CO_2 retention

↓
Wean PIP as TV improves
Wean Flo_2

↓
Reassess after 8 hours for
surfactant re-dose:
MV with Flo_2 0.40 and
Pao_2 < 80 mm Hg and
RDS on CXR

↓
Extubate to NCPAP when ready

↓
Hypoxemia continues
Increased WOB due to RR

↓
Nasal CPAP + 4 to 6 cm H_2O
Flo_2 < 0.60

↓
Hypoxemia continues

↓
Intubate, initiate MV
Settings:
Delivered TV: term 8 to 10 mL/kg
LBW 6 to 8 mL/kg
VLBW 4 to 6 mL/kg
Rate: adjust to maintain pH > 7.25
Flo_2: titrate to Spo_2 92–95%
PEEP: titrate to best Cdyn, Spo_2, BP

↙ ↘

Respiratory acidosis
Increase TV (PIP)
Assess respiratory
mechanics
R/O overdistention

Hypoxemia
Increase Flo_2, if > 0.60
Increase PEEP

Increase Ti
Assess respirative mechanics for
synchrony, ?sedation

↓
Overdistention on AGA

↓
Observe PIP, if > GA
↙

↘
Institute permissive hypercapnia
↓
Rescue surfactant therapy
RDS confirmed on CXR,
Flo_2 0.40 and Pao_2 ≤ 80 mm Hg
↓
Observe delivered TV
Monitor $TCCo_2$ or $ETCo_2$
↓
Adjust TV as Cdyn increases
Wean Flo_2 for SPo_2 > 92%
↓
Reevaluate Ti as spontaneous breathing
increases to assure synchrony
↓
Re-dose as indicated (Q 6 to 8 hours)
MV with Flo_2 0.40 and Pao_2 ≤ 80 mm Hg
and RDS on CXR

FIGURE 16-5   Management algorithm for inadequate oxygen delivery in the premature infant.

losis and low mean airway pressure, or both. If there is excessive pulmonary blood flow, the ventilator strategy is focused on increasing pulmonary vascular resistance to divert blood away from the lungs toward systemic blood flow via respiratory acidosis and increasing mean airway pressure. FIo_2 is administered to maintain an SpO_2 appropriate for the type of cardiac anomaly prior to repair.

If inadequate oxygen delivery occurs in a newborn, special consideration should be given to gestational age and body weight. Premature infants less than 1250 g with evidence of surfactant deficiency often receive exogenous surfactant in the delivery room. Other infants may receive surfactant as a rescue therapy for failure to respond to conventional mechanical ventilation. The ventilatory strategy for these infants is targeted at restoring lung volume with PEEP and adequate tidal volume delivery. Additional doses of surfactant may be administered every 4 to 6 hours if Pao_2 is less than 80 mm Hg with FIo_2 greater than 0.40. A low-stretch tidal volume strategy with permissive hypercapnia may also be utilized for those infants with severe respiratory failure (see Fig. 16-5).[18,29]

Term infants with inadequate oxygen delivery are susceptible to rapid changes in pulmonary vascular resistance due to a highly reactive pulmonary capillary bed. Ventilatory goals for these hypoxemic neonates should include mild respiratory alkalosis to promote pulmonary vasodilation. Restoration of end-expiratory lung volume is achieved through elevated mean airway pressure. Severely hypoxemic infants should be mildly sedated to decrease oxygen consumption. Hemoglobin and hematocrit should also be optimized to improve oxygen delivery. Surfactant can also be administered to term infants with radiologic findings consistent with respiratory distress syndrome. High-frequency ventilation or extracorporeal membrane oxygenation (ECMO) should be considered when maximal medical management fails (see Fig. 16-6).

Synchronous and Patient-Triggered Ventilation

Patient–ventilator synchrony is defined as the matching of ventilator-delivered breaths to patient-demanded breaths during assisted or supported ventilation.[34] Infants breathe synchronously with ventilator rates and inspiratory times set similar to the infant's native rate and inspiratory time,[31] regardless of the ability of the baby to trigger the ventilator. However, this requires ventilatory rates of 85 to 100 breaths per minute (bpm) and inspiratory time (Ti) close to 0.3 seconds. Other methods of achieving patient–ventilator synchrony in small infants include sedation or paralysis. To achieve truly synchronous ventilation in this population, the RCP must utilize newer ventilator technologies and recognize ventilator parameter deficiencies in relation to the patient's spontaneous need and adjust the flow pattern, trigger, cycle, or limit to improve the interaction.[2,3,6]

Patient-triggered ventilation is a relatively new practice in neonatal and pediatric ventilatory care.[2,5,7,21,32,34] Several methods of sensing spontaneous breathing efforts in small infants have been introduced to facilitate synchronous ventilatory support. Table 16-5 describes the characteristics of available patient-triggered systems, as adapted from Graham Bernstein.[8] **Patient–ventilator dyssynchrony** occurs when patient efforts to breathe go unmatched by ventilatory support. Dyssynchrony can cause infants to actively exhale against a closed expiratory valve of the ventilator and

Term Infant
Inadequate Oxygen Delivery—Severe Hypoxemia

Decreased pulmonary blood flow due to increased PVR
History, physical exam, CXR has ruled out CHD and CDH
↓

Titrate FIo_2 to maintain Spo_2 > 95%, postductal
↓

FIo_2 1.00, hypoxemia continues with increased RR and HR
↓

Intubate and institute synchronous mechanical ventilation
Goal: Mild respiratory alkalosis ($Paco_2$ 30–32, pH > 7.5)
   Adjust PIP to deliver TV 8–10 mL/kg,
   Keep PIP < 35 cm H_2O
   FIo_2 1.00, continue to monitor postductal Spo_2
   PEEP: titrate to best compliance and hemodynamics
   Rate: titrate to mild respiratory alkalosis ($Paco_2$ 30 to 32, pH > 7.5)
↓

Hypoxemia continues
↓

Sedate infant to decrease O_2 consumption
Optimize Hgb and HCT
Reassess hemodynamics to maintain cardiac output and BP
Reassess respiratory mechanics and PEEP
↙   ↘

Pao_2 < 50, despite maximal CMV Hemodynamically stable ↓	Pao_2 > 50, hemodynamics stable Assess patient for surfactant Tx ↓
Assess patient for surfactant Tx Administer, if indicated	As patient stabilizes with time, Spo_2 will rise and stabilize (> 98%), slowly wean FIo_2 (2–5%) increments
↓	↓
Hypoxemia continues	When FIo_2 ≤ 0.60, wean P_{aw} slowly in 1 to 2 cm H_2O increments every 4 to 6 hours, maintain EELV on CXR @ 8–9th rib
↙ ↘	
HFV Transfer to ECLS center	
↓	↓
Use high EELV strategy ?Wean FIo_2—No? ↓	Allow synchronous spontaneous breathing when P_{aw} < 15 cm H_2O ↓
Hypoxemia continues ↓	Proceed with weaning to extubation
Assess CXR ? 9th rib level—Yes? ↓	
Hypoxemia continues or CV unstable ↓	
ECLS	

FIGURE 16-6 Management algorithm for inadequate oxygen delivery in the term infant with severe hypoxemia.

TABLE 16-5 Characteristics of Available Patient-Triggered Ventilator Systems

PTV SYSTEM	SENSOR	RESPONSE TIME	MODES	FEATURES
Infant Star and Star Sync	Graseby capsule	52 ± 13 msec	SIMV A/C	Displays spontaneous Ti and RR. Audible signal during inspiration aids in capsule placement. No sensitivity setting.
Bear Cub NVM-1 monitor and CEM	Hot wire anemometer	65 ± 15 msec	SIMV A/C	NVM-1 displays TV, VE, airway leak. NVM-1 alarm limits difficult to set/disable. Large deadspace volume for VLBW babies.
Babylog 8000	Hot wire anemometer	95 ± 24 msec	SIMV A/C	Sensor built in to circuit Y. Fully integrated, easy to use. Graphic display of pressure or flow waveforms. Displays TV, VE, airway leak.
Bird VIP and Partner IIi monitor	Variable orifice pneumotach	30–70 msec	SIMV A/C	Partner IIi displays TV and VE, airway leak. Graphic display of flow, pressure, volume waveforms. Termination sensitivity option. Leak compensation.
Sechrist IV HP CR monitor and SAVI module	Chest leads	40–80 msec	A/C	CR gram aids correct lead placement and sensitivity setting. Terminates positive pressure on active exhalation.

(Adapted from Bernstein G: Synchronous and patient-triggered ventilation in newborns. Neo Respir Dis 3(2):1, 1993.)

results in increased imposed work of breathing for the patient. Any ventilatory support below that demanded by the patient results in significant imposed work of breathing. Increasing work of breathing may result in worsening PaO_2 and $PaCO_2$ values due to increased oxygen consumption and carbon dioxide production. Not only does this interfere with gas exchange and ventilatory management, it also results in poor weight gain and pulmonary air leak syndrome. Successful patient-triggered ventilator systems facilitate ventilator weaning, increase patient weight gain and growth, and decrease morbidity associated with continuous mechanical ventilation in small babies.[14,16,17]

■ SET VENTILATOR PARAMETERS

General guidelines for selecting individual ventilator parameters can be made within the context of a pathophysiologic approach to ventilatory management. Adequate tidal volume delivery must be assured for all ventilated patients. Whether pressure-limited or volume-limited ventilation is selected, tidal volume must be measured at the endotracheal tube (ETT) to distinguish the set from the delivered tidal volume. Generally, tidal volumes of 10 mL/kg for children, 8 to 10 mL/kg for term infants, 6 to 8 mL for low-birth-weight infants, and 4 to 6 mL/kg for very low-birth-weight infants should be delivered at the ETT. The peak inspiratory pressure (PIP) required to deliver a selected tidal volume must be assessed simultaneously. PIPs should not be allowed to exceed 35 cm H_2O in term infants and children. As a guideline, premature infants should not have PIPs that exceed their gestational age in weeks (*e.g.*, a 24-week gestational age infant should not have a PIP greater than 24 cm H_2O) to reduce the risk of pulmonary barotrauma or volutrauma. The balance between delivered tidal volume and PIP is very important and must be carefully considered in all patient groups to provide adequate lung expansion without deleterious side effects.

Ventilator Rate. The ventilator rate is prescribed in combination with tidal volume to provide adequate alveolar ventilation for the patient. This is generally achieved by maintaining $Paco_2$ between 40 and 48 mm Hg in children with normal lungs. $Paco_2$ may be allowed to increase further in children with chronic pulmonary disease or those at risk for pulmonary barotrauma. The $Paco_2$ values tolerated with a "permissive hypercapnic" approach are higher than previously recommended and may increase further if pH remains greater than 7.25. Permissive hypercapnia is a valuable ventilator management strategy that allows the RCP to use smaller tidal volumes and lower peak inspiratory pressures to prevent pulmonary barotrauma and volutrauma in the face of severe decreases in lung compliance. This approach appears to be well tolerated by infants and children, with no adverse effects being described in the literature.[18,29]

A relatively larger tidal volume strategy with low preset ventilatory rates may be used in surgical pediatric patients to correct atelectasis, maintain end-expiratory lung volume, minimize mean airway pressure, and preserve hemodynamic performance. Neonatal ventilatory strategies are aimed at lower inspiratory volumes and faster ventilator rates to limit the toxic effects of peak inspiratory pressure on developing lung tissues.

Fraction of Inspired Oxygen (FIo₂). The fraction of inspired oxygen should be adjusted to maintain the arterial oxygen saturation (SpO_2 = 92% to 95%) and oxygen delivery for the patient. FIo_2 should be analyzed continuously with high and low alarm limits set on the analyzer to prevent inadvertent hypoxemia or hyperoxemia. Oxygen is a drug with toxic effects. Host tolerance, FIo_2, and duration of administration are important considerations in oxygen therapy. Aggressive efforts should be made to wean oxygen below 60% (or to maintain Pao_2 below 100 mm Hg in premature infants) to prevent oxygen toxicity.

Positive End-Expiratory Pressure (PEEP). PEEP is produced by closing the ventilator expiratory valve prematurely and trapping a volume of expiratory gas, which increases expiratory pressure above baseline. The volume of gas trapped in the lung is proportionate to the pressure setting and the patient's lung compliance. PEEP restores end-expiratory lung volume; improves oxygenation, lung compliance, and distribution of ventilation in low-lung-compliance states; and decreases airway collapse. The best PEEP level required by any patient is determined by performing a PEEP titration study. In this technique, PEEP is increased incrementally with 10 to 15 minutes between increases while lung compliance is measured along with indicators of cardiac output and oxygenation via pulse oximetry. The PEEP value that produces the best SpO_2 with the best lung compliance and hemodynamics is the best PEEP.

PEEP levels can become toxic to patients if end-expiratory lung volume is increased to the point of pulmonary overdistention. These levels can be observed on the pressure–volume curve on an airway graphics monitor (see the later section on monitoring). Such an increase of end-expiratory volume increases deadspace ventilation and may compromise hemodynamic performance. Rapid changes in lung compliance may require frequent PEEP titration studies.

Inspiratory Time. Inspiratory time is selected by the bedside clinician to facilitate patient comfort and synchronous breathing during mechanical ventilation. The patient's age and breathing pattern and the time constant of the lung are considerations in the selection of inspiratory time. Recommended inspiratory times by age group are as follows:

Low-birth-weight infants	0.25–0.5 seconds
Term infants	0.5–0.6 seconds
Toddlers	0.5–0.75 seconds
Children	1.0–1.5 seconds
Adults	1.0–2.0 seconds

Following selection of an appropriate inspiratory time, expiratory time is adjusted to achieve the set mechanical rate. Total cycle time (TCT) is the period of time allotted for one complete inspiratory and expiratory cycle. I:E ratio is an expression of the set inspiratory time and the remaining expiratory cycle time. Recommended I:E ratios vary greatly with ventilator rate. Ratios of 1:2 or 1:3 are most desirable; ratios should certainly be no lower than 1:1 in assisted ventilation to allow adequate time for exhalation and to prevent air trapping.

Peak Flow. Peak flow should be titrated to the spontaneous demands of the patient or to maintain a selected set inspiratory pressure. Peak inspiratory pressures during volume-limited ventilation are directly related to peak flow adjustments (increasing the peak flow causes an increase in peak inspiratory pressure). Good ventilatory technique achieves a balance of inspiratory work of breathing, patient comfort, and airway pressures.

■ ASSESSMENT OF MECHANICAL VENTILATION

Methods for monitoring mechanical ventilation span the spectrum from physical assessment and direct observation to continuous electronic surveillance of mechanical and physiologic parameters. The RCP must incorporate all facets of ventilatory monitoring into a comprehensive, responsive care system which reduces morbidity and length of mechanical ventilation and improves patient outcome. Physical examination has increasing clinical relevance and is often the deciding factor between monitor error and true change in patient status. Its role is increasing as RCPs take direct responsibility for the execution of patient management protocols. Noninvasive techniques to assess gas exchange and pulmonary mechanics supplement physical assessment data and provide a continuous data stream, with alarms, to identify changes in ventilatory status and alert caregivers. Appropriate integration and interpretation of all assessment data is essential for efficient, cost-effective, high-quality ventilatory care.

Ventilator monitoring can be classified into intermittent and continuous methods. Intermittent methods include ventilator parameter assessment, chest x-ray, and arterial or capillary blood gas analysis. Continuous monitoring includes noninvasive respiratory monitoring techniques such as transcutaneous blood gas analysis, pulse oximetry, capnography, and airway graphic analysis. These topics are presented in other sections of this text and will be presented here as they relate to ventilatory management.

Intermittent Ventilator Monitoring

Ventilator Parameters. Ventilator parameters should be measured and recorded by personnel experienced in neonatal/pediatric ventilatory care at least every 4 hours.

Spontaneous tidal volume and respiratory rate: Spontaneous tidal volume and respiratory rate reflect lung compliance, respiratory muscle strength, and work of breathing.

Mechanical tidal volume and set rate: Assessment of mechanical tidal volume and preset rate assures delivery of the prescribed alveolar ventilation and facilitates detection of endotracheal or ventilator circuit leaks.

Peak airway pressure: Peak inspiratory pressures during volume-limited ventilation are a reflection of set volume, inspiratory flow, airway resistance, lung compliance, and endotracheal tube size. Airway pressures should be measured at the patient, not at the ventilator, to determine the effects of ventilatory support on the patient's lung. Peak inspiratory pressures will vary with changes in the patient's pulmonary condition. The presence of airway secretions, bronchospasm, tubing kinks, pneumothorax, agitation, and decreased lung compliance will increase peak inspiratory pressures. Decreases in peak pressures reflect leaks around the endotracheal tube/ventilator circuit or improvement in airway resistance and compliance. Peak pressure is *not* an indicator of changes in patient condition during pressure-limited ventilation. However, leaks in the ventilator circuit and endotracheal tube may be observed as decreases in peak pressure in this mode.

Mean airway pressure: Mean airway pressure is an important indicator of the degree of mechanical ventilation required to achieve adequate ventilation and oxygenation. Mean airway pressure is a function of tidal volume, inspiratory time, peak inspiratory pressure, peak flow, flow pattern, ventilator rate, and PEEP.

Barotrauma and volutrauma to the lung increase as peak and mean airway pressures increase. Ventilatory parameters should be adjusted to provide adequate alveolar ventilation and oxygenation at the lowest mean airway pressure. Mean airway pressures greater than 15 cm H_2O are considered elevated and should be examined for possible reduction by utilizing alternate ventilatory strategies or modes. Plateau pressure (P_{plat}) or end inspiratory pressure (EIP) is obtained by recording the pressure following a breath hold maneuver in constant flow, volume-limited ventilation. Plateau pressure reflects the compliance of the lung during static gas flow and eliminates the effects of airway resistance. Plateau pressures in excess of 35 cm H_2O have been reported as significant in adults, indicating a need for alternate ventilatory strategies.[1] However, these data have yet to be thoroughly investigated in neonatal and pediatric populations, and this number is offered as a guideline.

Ventilator Alarm Systems. Ventilator alarm systems, which alert caregivers to changes in the patient–ventilator system, have developed dramatically with the advent of microprocessor technology. Input power alarms notify clinicians of changes in electrical or pneumatic supplies. Control circuit alarms notify the clinician of incompatible parameters or indicate that some aspect of the ventilator self-test has failed. Output alarms indicate unacceptable levels of ventilator output such as pressure limits (high and low) for peak airway, mean airway, and end-expiratory pressures, as well as failure of the airway pressure to return to baseline in an acceptable period of time; volume limits (high and low) and minute ventilation limits (high and low); time limits (high and low) for breath rate and inspiratory and expiratory time; and gas concentration (high and low). Alarm limits should be adjusted to alert caregivers to valid changes in patient condition that require direct attention and action, but not to alarm needlessly and desensitize intensive care personnel to the need to respond.

Chest X-ray. The chest x-ray is one of the most commonly ordered procedures in the intensive care unit. A scientific comparison of physical examination of the chest with chest x-ray film assessment in a pulmonary intensive care unit demonstrated that chest x-rays films are more sensitive than the clinician's examination in detecting significant problems.[32] Of the routine x-ray films in this study, 24% showed an abnormality that resulted in a change of management by the caregivers. The abnormalities noted included endotracheal tube and central line malposition, new or advancing pulmonary infiltrates, and unsuspected pneumothorax. These findings were more common in smaller children. Repositioning resulted from assessment of 35% of the x-ray films done for endotracheal tube placement and 44% of those done for central line placement. Daily chest x-ray films are, therefore, valuable assets in monitoring and assessing the patient receiving mechanical ventilation.

Capillary and Arterial Blood Gas Analysis. The need for routine laboratory analysis of blood gas values has been reduced in neonatal pediatric cares with the use of noninvasive monitoring. However, monitor correlation and assessment of pH and co-oximetry still require periodic laboratory assessment.

Continuous Ventilatory Monitoring

Transcutaneous O_2 and CO_2 Monitoring. Neonatal critical care has demonstrated the most enthusiasm for transcutaneous blood gas determination. These monitors estimate partial pressure of O_2 and CO_2 electrochemically via electrodes attached to the skin. The greatest benefits of this technology are continuous monitoring with alarms and the reduction in the frequency of blood gas measurement and, hence, blood replacement in small infants. Transcutaneous monitoring has been limited by the need for frequent calibration of electrodes, cost of supplies, occasional burns induced by the warming electrode, inaccuracy when the skin is not perfused, inaccuracies in older patients, and the development of pulse oximeter technology.

Pulse Oximetry. Oxygen saturation of normal hemoglobin as determined by the pulse oximeter correlates very closely to the oxygen saturation as determined by co-oximetry when the patient's saturation is between 70% and 100% in the well-perfused, normothermic person.[10] Many medical procedures, transfers, and high-risk conditions put infants and children at risk for arterial oxygen desaturation. Using continuous pulse oximetry, these events can be detected early, the intervention accomplished, and the morbidity to the patient prevented without complex equipment and maintenance. Clinicians should verify pulse rate accuracy in the assessment of pulse oximetry values to avoid misinterpretation in the face of motion artifact, so often observed in children.

Capnography and End-Tidal CO$_2$. Capnography is the graphic waveform produced by variations in CO_2 concentration throughout the respiratory cycle as a function of time. End-tidal CO_2 ($ETCO_2$) is defined as the peak CO_2 value during the expiratory phase of respiration. It is dependent on adequate pulmonary capillary blood flow to alveoli, which in turn depends on adequate right and left heart function. In neonatal/pediatric ventilatory care, the mainstream measurement devices utilize low deadspace adapters (less than 1.2 mL). These perform without removing a volume of gas from the ventilator circuit, which could potentially decrease delivered minute ventilation. Practical uses of $ETCO_2$ monitoring include assessing the adequacy of alveolar ventilation during mechanical ventilation, checking patient–ventilator system function, decreasing blood gas sampling, ensuring endotracheal tube patency, and monitoring respiratory function of spontaneously breathing children. Capnography can be used to great advantage in mechanically ventilated patients if the waveform is displayed and analyzed along with numeric data. Mechanical failures can be detected, the adequacy of respiratory support analyzed, and changes in the mode of ventilation made to maximize the efficiency of ventilation, decrease the patient's work of breathing, and improve patient–ventilator synchrony.[23,36]

Airway Graphic Analysis (AGA). Prior to the introduction of waveform graphics with neonatal and pediatric populations, ventilator monitoring was restricted to readings from the ventilator's controls, digital monitors, mechanical gauges, and physical and laboratory assessment. Detailed analysis of the patient–ventilator interface was impossible. Airway graphic monitors are now available via mobile bedside units (VenTrak-Novametrix Medical Systems, Bicore-Allied Medical Systems) or as components of ventilator designs (Bird Products Corp., Drager Inc.). The placement of finely calibrated pneumotachometers at the endotracheal tube has facilitated measurement and display of pressure, volume, and flow within flow ranges suitable to even the smallest premature infant. AGA offers unique information regarding ventilator performance, breath type selection, patient pathophysiology, and the interactions produced within the patient–ventilator system. It can be used to study the characteristics of ventilator operation (trigger, cycle, limit, and flow pattern) versus the pathophysiology of the patient's lungs (decreased compliance, airway resistance). This includes analysis of ventilator interventions, clinical events, and alarm conditions via trending data. Using this technology, it is possible to shape the form of ventilatory support to improve patient–ventilator synchrony, reduce work of breathing, and calculate a variety of physiologic parameters related to respiratory mechanics.

The most commonly reported waveforms are pressure, flow, and volume; they are often called scalar graphics. Convention dictates that positive values (tracings above the baseline) correspond to inspiration and negative values (tracings below the baseline) correspond to expiration, that horizontal axes represent time in seconds, and that vertical axes represent the measured variable in its common units of measurement. Optimal neonatal and pediatric measurements are obtained when the pneumotachometer is positioned between the patient and the ventilator circuit Y. Flow sensors should be capable of measuring a wide range of flows and reasonably resistant to motion artifact, moisture, and respiratory secretions. Figure 16-7 is an airway graphic tracing of a continuous flow, pressure-limited ventilation. Scalar displays of all three graphics for a 10-second period of time are taken directly from an actual monitor screen.

Airway Pressure (P_{aw}). There is an increase in airway pressure during inspiration to a maximal point (PIP), with a short inspiratory plateau where pressure remains constant. The PIP is determined by patient and circuit compliance, airway resistance, and the delivered tidal volume and inspiratory flow rate. The inspiratory plateau demonstrates the period of time when the pressure limit has been reached prior to the termination of the set inspiratory time. Note that inspiration on the pressure scalar begins from a PEEP baseline. No spontaneous breathing efforts are noted between mechanical breaths. Although resistance of the endotracheal tube is a component of the pressure graphic, pressures reported are generally considered airway pressure.

Flow Graphics (V). The flow graphic has two distinct parts, inspiratory flow and expiratory flow, and each should be analyzed separately. The inspiratory flow graphic represents the magnitude, duration, and flow delivery pattern of the mechanical breath. Similarly, an inspiratory flow graphic of a spontaneous breath would represent the magnitude, duration, and flow demand of the patient. Note that changes in flow delivery and inspiratory time alter the shape of the flow graphic, resulting in a positive slope at the beginning of inspiration and a negative slope at end-inspiration (see Fig. 16-7). A square-wave, constant-flow pattern occurs during early inspiration. Note the downward sloping of the flow pattern at end-inspiration. This "decay" in flow pattern occurs during the inspiratory pressure plateau and begins to simulate a decelerating flow pattern. Expiratory flow returns to baseline prior to initiation of the next mechanical breath, indicating completion of exhalation.

The characteristic of the inspiratory flow graphic is determined by the characteristics of the patient's inspiratory demand, the ventilatory support provided to meet that demand, and lung compliance. The expiratory flow

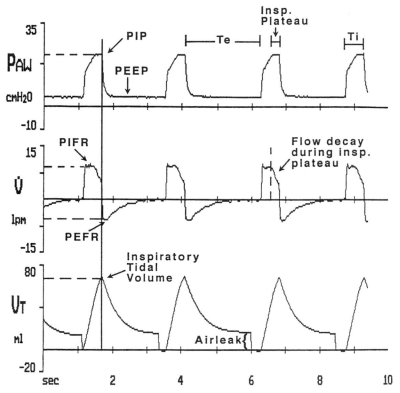

FIGURE 16-7 Scalar graphics in pressure-limited, constant-flow ventilation with normal lungs.

graphic is a passive movement and is demonstrated below the baseline. The magnitude, duration, and pattern of the expiratory graphic are determined by the compliance and resistance of both the patent's lung and ventilator circuit. Important features of the ventilator circuit that affect the flow graphic include the size and length of the endotracheal tube, the internal diameter and length of the ventilator circuit, resistance of the expiratory valve, and distensibility of the circuit itself. The characteristics of the ventilator circuit that affect the expiratory flow pattern are generally fixed; changes in the expiratory flow curve may, therefore, be attributable to changes in the patient's compliance and resistance or activity. Increased airway resistance due to obstructive disease or secretions may result in decreased peak expiratory flow, increased duration of flow, or failure of flow to return to baseline.

Volume (TV). Tidal volume increases proportionately with airway pressure. Note that peak airway pressure, termination of inspiratory flow, and maximal inspiratory tidal volume delivery occur at the same time (note the cursor line in Fig. 16-7). Expiratory volume does not return to baseline, indicating that expiratory volume is less than inspiratory volume. Typically, inspiratory and expiratory volume should be equal. However, it

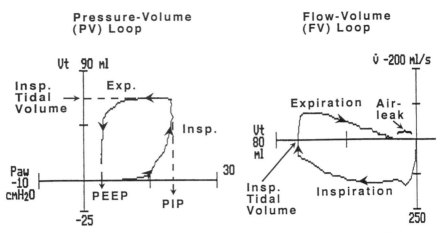

FIGURE 16-8 Pressure-volume and flow-volume loops in pressure-limited, constant-flow ventilation in normal lungs.

is not uncommon in infants and children with uncuffed endotracheal tubes for the expiratory volume to be less than inspiratory volume. An actual % leak can be calculated and reported under these conditions and may aid in the clinical assessment of the patient.

In summary, by reading down the individual breath displays, it is possible to assess variations in airway pressure, flow, and volume and to examine the time sequence of ventilatory events. In addition to plotting the scalar parameters individually, two parameters can be graphically plotted against each other. This results in pressure-volume and flow-volume loops, which can be helpful in assessing work of breathing, patient–ventilator synchrony, and overdistention of the lung.

Figure 16-8 displays the pressure-volume and flow-volume loops from a continuous-flow, pressure-limited breath.

Pressure-Volume Loop. Inspiration begins from the PEEP baseline on the horizontal axis and increases to the set pressure limit within the set inspiratory time. PIP is read at end-inspiration from the horizontal axis. A reduction in both volume and pressure occur during expiration. Volume does not return to zero because of the leak, as previously described. The TV, PIP, and PEEP are determined by inspection. Dynamic compliance (delivered TV/[PIP – PEEP]) is the slope of the line connecting PEEP and PIP. Alterations in the shape of the inspiratory limb of the pressure-volume loop from this normal appearance will provide insight into changes in lung compliance and the presence of pulmonary abnormalities (*e.g.*, atelectasis or overdistention).

Flow-Volume Loop. Inspiratory flow begins from the zero point and is displayed below the horizontal axis as a square-wave, constant-flow pattern. Peak inspiratory flow is read from the vertical axis. Again, note the decay in the square wave during the inspiratory plateau period. Expiratory flow occurs above the horizontal baseline, but terminates early and does not return to the zero point, indicating an air leak. Peak expiratory flow is read from the vertical axis. The early termination of the expiratory flow graphic, described here as a leak, could also be a result of pneumotach inaccuracy at low flow and volumes or gas trapping. To insure accurate graphic interpretation, the clinician must assure that the measurement device (pneumotach) is rated for the range of flow and volume to be measured, that is, a neonatal pneumotach is used for neonatal volumes and flows. Inspiratory and expiratory TV are read at the point where the graphic crosses the horizontal baseline.

As the RCP becomes familiar with normal airway graphic displays for pressure-limited and volume-limited ventilation, detection of ventilatory abnormalities becomes easier and more meaningful to ventilator management. Abnormalities can include patient–ventilator dyssynchrony, gas trapping, increased expiratory resistance, and pulmonary overdistention.

Figure 16-9 demonstrates the types of patient–ventilator dyssynchrony that can be detected using airway graphics. Patient–ventilator dyssynchrony, defined earlier in this chapter as the mismatching of ventilator-delivered breaths to patient-demanded breaths during assisted or supported ventilation, may be alleviated by recognizing ventilator parameter deficiencies using AGA and adjusting the flow pattern, trigger, cycle, or limit to improve the patient–ventilator interaction. Patient–ventilator dyssynchrony should be considered in all cases of patient agitation and weaning difficulty. Clinicians must become expert at differentiating the causes

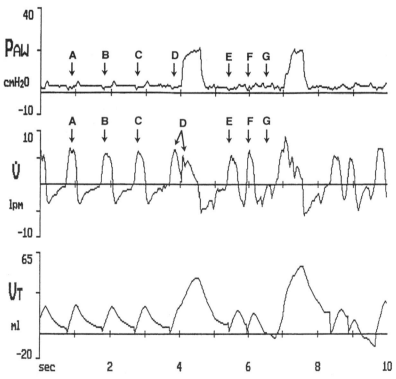

FIGURE 16-9   Patient–ventilator dyssynchrony as a result of inadequate trigger sensitivity.

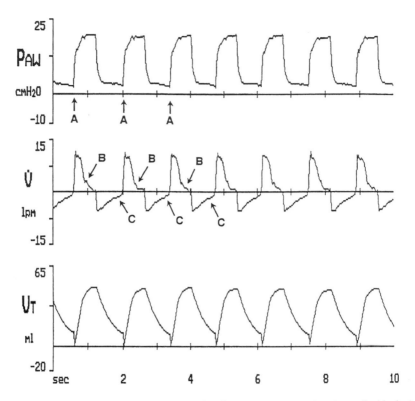

FIGURE 16-10 Gas-trapping as a result of premature termination of exhalation.

of patient–ventilator dyssynchrony and developing an interventional ventilator management system to facilitate synchronous breathing.

Gas-trapping (Fig. 16-10) is a result of premature termination of the expiratory phase of breathing, or incomplete exhalation at high respiratory rates or under conditions of increased expiratory resistance. Airway pressure, volume, and flow do not return to baseline before the initiation of the next supported breath. Although the patient may have inspiratory synchrony, expiratory synchrony is also an important consideration. Gas trapping results in the development of intrinsic PEEP and can alter the cardiovascular stability and work of breathing.

Increased expiratory resistance (Fig. 16-11) due to airway obstruction is readily identified with airway graphics. Prolonged expiratory flow on the flow scalar indicates a resistance to exhalation. Increased expiratory resistance can be a result of bronchospasm, large airway obstruction (foreign body, kink or obstruction of the endotracheal tube), or expiratory valve failure.

Pulmonary overdistention (Fig. 16-12) is defined as an abrupt decrease in compliance at the termination of inspiration or an increase in inspiratory pressure without a significant increase in delivered inspiratory pressure. Overdistention occurs when the volume limit of some components of the lung has been exceeded. As the ventilator attempts to deliver the mechanical breath, airway pressures increase with little volume being delivered. This

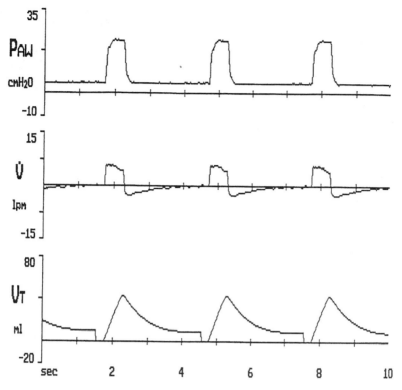

FIGURE 16-11 Prolonged exhalation as a result of increased expiratory resistance.

results in a decrease in dynamic compliance, with the inspiratory loop having a reduced slope and terminal peaking. Overdistention leads to volutrauma, barotrauma, and increased pulmonary vascular resistance.

Table 16-6 presents common ventilatory abnormalities observed with airway graphic analysis, as well as ventilator strategies for correction. Improved ventilator monitoring capabilities via airway graphic analysis are essential to the appropriate assessment of ventilator performance and

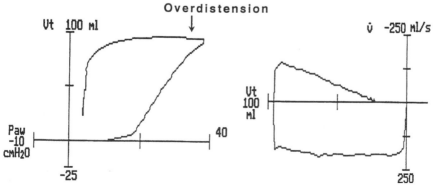

FIGURE 16-12 Pulmonary overdistention.

patient management. Graphics monitoring provides dynamic real-time information with which the clinician can generate and test hypotheses of patient–ventilator management, assess the response to intervention, and provide instantaneous feedback at the bedside. Using these tools, practitioners may be able to reduce laboratory assessments, sedation requirements, and the duration of mechanical ventilation.

▬ WEANING FROM MECHANICAL VENTILATION

The goal of mechanical ventilation changes significantly as the patient progresses from the acute phase of respiratory failure to the resolution phase, during which successful weaning and extubation become critical. In acute respiratory failure, lung compliance and end-expiratory lung volume (EELV) are decreased. The ventilatory goals during this phase are to restore lung volume, improve oxygen delivery, and minimize ventilator-induced lung injury. During the weaning phase of mechanical ventilation, lung volumes, compliance, and oxygenation are improving. The goal of mechanical ventilation changes during the resolution phase is to facilitate effective spontaneous breathing as ventilatory support is reduced. Therefore, patient–ventilator synchrony becomes an essential component of the ventilator weaning care plan as sedation is decreased and the patient

TABLE 16-6   Airway Graphic Abnormalities and Suggested Ventilator Strategies

AIRWAY GRAPHIC ABNORMALITY	VENTILATOR STRATEGY FOR CORRECTION
Patient–ventilator dyssynchrony	
1. Inadequate trigger sensitivity	Maximize sensitivity. Change from pressure to flow trigger. Leak compensation (Bird VIP).
2. Excessive inspiratory time	Decrease set inspiratory time to eliminate inspiratory plateau. Termination sensitivity (Bird VIP).
3. Inadequate flow support	Increase set inspiratory flow. Decrease inspiratory time. Change from constant flow to variable flow pattern.
4. Inadequate pressure support	Titrate pressure support level to inspiratory demand and delivered tidal volume.
Gas-trapping	Decrease inspiratory time. Increase expiratory time. Termination sensitivity (Bird VIP).
Increased expiratory resistance	Check circuit for obstruction, kinks, etc. Suction airway. Assess placement of endotracheal tube. Consider use of bite block. Administer bronchodilator. Tracheobronchial malacia (only): titrate PEEP to stint open airway.
Pulmonary overdistention	Decrease set tidal volume. Decrease set inspiratory pressure. Optimize PEEP.

becomes more alert and interactive. RCPs must be able to balance rapidly changing pulmonary pathophysiology, patient demand and comfort, and ventilator performance to successfully reduce ventilatory support without increasing work of breathing to a point of fatigue and failure. A systematic approach must be established which addresses sedation, ventilatory synchrony, and rapid assessment of patient physiology.

Patient–ventilator synchrony is a function of synchronizing the inspiratory as well as the expiratory phases of the breathing cycle with the patient. In infants and children, inspiratory synchrony focuses on the type of trigger, trigger sensitivity, ventilator response time, endotracheal tube effects, and flow pattern. Trigger sensitivity is the effort required to initiate an assisted breath and is directly proportional to the inspiratory work of breathing. Trigger sensitivity is a function of the type of mechanical trigger (pressure vs. flow), location of the sensor (proximal vs. distal), and endotracheal tube effects. The recent addition of several new types of inspiratory triggers and microprocessor technology for small infants and children has increased the sensitivity and response time for detection of small inspiratory efforts. Proximal sensing (at the patient) removes the mechanical effects of the ventilator circuit and expiratory valve from the sensor system, facilitating detection of smaller efforts more rapidly.

Ventilator response time is the time from the inspiratory effort to the onset of flow. The average response time for neonates is currently 30 to 70 msec, based on the manufacturer's algorithm, microprocessor interaction, and type of trigger mechanism. Endotracheal tube effects, specifically leaks due to uncuffed tubes and increased airway resistance as a function of ETT diameter, greatly influence trigger sensitivity. As new technologies improve trigger sensitivity, leaks resulting from uncuffed endotracheal tubes can cause autocycling. The ventilator trigger system may sense the drop in baseline pressure or flow due to the ETT leak as an inspiratory effort and deliver a falsely "assisted" breath. One ventilator manufacturer has added a leak compensation feature (Bird VIP, Bird Products Corp.), which titrates additional flow into the ventilator circuit to maintain the PEEP baseline in the face of airway leaks in an effort to preserve trigger response.

The flow pattern delivered during spontaneous breathing is very important. Fixed flow (constant flow, square wave form) is helpful during acute respiratory failure to preserve mean airway pressure and improve oxygenation. However, during weaning, variable flow patterns (decelerating or sine wave form) are more effective at matching the variable spontaneous demand of the awake and alert patient. The flow pattern of pressure support ventilation is increasingly successful at satisfying the spontaneous efforts of small infants and children. Pressure support also reduces the resistance associated with breathing through small endotracheal tubes and may supplement spontaneous tidal volume as respiratory muscle strength increases. Again, ETT leaks can limit the usefulness of this breath type. If the termination point of the PS breath cannot be reached owing to ETT leak, inspiratory time may be dramatically increased. Clinicians should select variable flow termination points or time limits for the PS breath to improve cycling accuracy without compromising tidal volume or flow delivery. Airway graphic displays are irreplaceable in fine tuning this type of ventilatory support.

Assessment of expiratory synchrony is often overlooked as a factor in ventilator weaning. Expiratory synchrony is a function of end-expiratory lung volume (EELV), premature termination of exhalation (intrinsic PEEP), and expiratory resistance. EELV is affected by the set PEEP and lung compliance. If EELV is too low, lung compliance and tidal volume decrease further, while respiratory rate increases from baseline to preserve minute ventilation. This creates a breathing pattern (inadequate TV, increased RR), characteristic of "failure to wean." If EELV is too high, pulmonary overdistention occurs and alveolar deadspace and $PaCO_2$ increase, another characteristic of failure to wean. In either scenario, an inappropriate ventilator strategy (insufficient or excessive PEEP) precipitated the weaning failure. Therefore, EELV should be titrated to the best compliance and lung expansion for the patient, without overdistention observed on the P-V curve of airway graphics or chest x-ray film.

If EELV or tidal volume are inadequate for a patient, the patient's normal compensatory response is increased respiratory rate to maintain alveolar ventilation. As frequency increases, premature termination of exhalation, the failure of flow, pressure, and volume to return to baseline prior to the next assisted breath, occurs. As many as 33% of all weaning infants experience premature termination of exhalation during weaning.[38] The gas trapping and intrinsic PEEP produced under these conditions can interfere with trigger sensitivity, increase work of breathing, and compromise hemodynamic status by increasing mean intrathoracic pressure. The key to minimizing the development of intrinsic PEEP is to provide adequate tidal volume (*i.e.*, adequate pressure support) and EELV (*i.e.*, PEEP), such that the patient has a normal respiratory rate and adequate expiratory time to facilitate completion of exhalation. Consideration of the cycle mechanism for the breath is also helpful; flow-cycled breaths match inspiratory time with patient demand better than time-cycled breaths and improve expiratory synchrony by decreasing inspiratory time.

Finally, increased expiratory resistance can significantly increase imposed work of breathing for a patient. It may be a function of mechanical or physiologic factors. Poorly functioning exhalation valves or breathing circuits can create an obstruction to exhalation. Bronchospasm or airway secretions may also pose physical obstruction to exhalation and prolong the expiratory phase. Troubleshooting or replacing ventilator components, good tracheobronchial hygiene, and aerosolized bronchodilator therapy reduce excessive expiratory resistance. However, the RCP should approach these corrections in a systematic manner, measuring the outcomes of individual interventions before proceeding to the next. Table 16-7 lists common problems associated with failure of weaning strategies and offers suggestions for intervention and correction.

Management of sedation in mechanically ventilated infants and children requires an established protocol approach that is uniformly applied to all patients. The Duke pediatric intensive care unit currently uses the modified Ramsay sedation scale, which describes behavior patterns for children as an assessment tool for determining level of sedation. Table 16-8 describes the components of the six-point scale, while Table 16-9 provides patient behavior examples at the various levels of sedation.

Weaning patients are maintained at level 2 to 3 on the modified Ramsay scale, which facilitates spontaneous breathing yet keeps the patient

TABLE 16-7 Common Problems Associated With Weaning Failures

PROBLEM	SUGGESTED INTERVENTION/CORRECTION
Patient cannot appropriately trigger the ventilator-assisted breath.	Increase sensitivity setting. Change to flow trigger. Initiate leak compensation. Utilize airway graphics to identify problem.
Ventilatory support too low to overcome work of breathing of ETT and/or circuit.	Select variable flow pattern. Initiate pressure support ventilation, titrate PS to reduce work of breathing.
Flow dyssynchrony occurs in constant flow mode.	Decrease inspiratory time. Increase set flow. Change to variable flow pattern.
Inadequate tidal volume.	Increase pressure support such that PS tidal volume is 33–50% of mandatory breath tidal volume.
Inadequate end-expiratory lung volume (EELV).	Titrate PEEP to best compliance, assess lung volume on chest x-ray film.
Intrinsic PEEP in circuit.	Assess adequacy of EELV and TV. Decrease inspiratory time. Select flow cycled breath type. Use airway graphics to optimize ventilatory adjustments.
Increased expiratory resistance.	Trouble shoot ventilator to rule out mechanical problem (*i.e.,* expiratory valve). Assess patient for bronchospasm, administer aerosolized bronchodilator and assess outcome. Perform tracheal suctioning to rule out secretions as a possible cause of airway obstruction.

comfortable. Sedation is administered via continuous drip instead of bolus to prevent incidence of oversedation and maintain a consistent level of comfort. The Ramsay's score is assessed every hour by the bedside nurse, who then titrates sedation following physician orders to maintain the prescribed level of comfort. This approach individualizes the sedation to the needs of the patient throughout the day and night. It reduces incidental agitation and somnolence as sedation is administered more consistently. It also decreases nursing and respiratory care time by maintaining the child in a predictable, consistent level of behavior as mechanical ventilation is decreased, and it optimizes opportunity to continuously wean across a 24-hour period. This sedation procedure, coupled with synchronous ventilation, has been very successful in decreasing the length of mechanical ventilation and weaning failures in the patient population.

In summary, successful weaning is based on careful assessment of changing pathophysiology, patient comfort and sedation levels, and synchronization with the ventilator system as spontaneous breathing increases. Patient–ventilator synchrony is a function of optimizing inspiratory as well as expiratory factors. Inspiratory synchrony is achieved with

TABLE 16-8   Modified Ramsay Scale

Light

1 = Anxious and agitated, restless, or both

2 = Cooperative, oriented, and tranquil

3 = Responds to commands only

Deep

4 = Brisk response to light glabellar tap or loud auditory stimulus

5 = Sluggish response to a light glabellar tap or loud auditory stimulus

6 = No response to a light glabellar tap or loud auditory stimulus

selection of an adequate trigger sensitivity, ventilator response time, and flow pattern. Expiratory synchrony is achieved with adequate end-expiratory lung volume, absence of intrinsic PEEP, and minimal expiratory resistance. In cases of failure to wean, these factors should be investigated and corrected to keep the management plan on track.

Extubation Criteria

Extubation criteria for infants and children are not as well defined as they are for adults because of the wide ranges of age and physiology. Institutions and individual intensive care units should develop specific criteria for their unique patient population based on experience and practice standards. Elements to assess for readiness to extubate are listed in Table 16-10. Chest x-ray films should demonstrate resolving pulmonary processes and adequate lung inflation. Respiratory mechanics should demonstrate reasonable return of lung compliance, airway resistance, oxygenation, and CO_2 elimination prior to the decision to extubate.

If the child is old enough to perform a maximal inspiratory effort, adult standard values apply. Weight gain during the intubation period is very

TABLE 16-9   Description of Patient Type by Ramsay Sedation Score

1 = Patient bucking the ventilator due to anxiety and stress from ICU environment.

2 = Patient undergoing a neurological assessment or being weaned from ventilator.

3 = Patient mildly sedated to the point of tolerating a previously bothersome endotracheal tube or a patient being weaned from the ventilator.

4 = Patient will appear asleep but is able to respond briskly to verbal stimulation or external stimuli such as a postoperative patient.

5 = Patient who needs to be deeply sedated for a procedure or to decrease oxygen consumption.

6 = Patient who needs to be unresponsive for minor surgical or invasive procedure such as chest tube insertion or endoscopy.

TABLE 16-10   Elements to Assess to Determine Readiness for Extubation

---

Chest radiograph

Respiratory mechanics

    Cdyn, R_{aw}, MIP

    Oxygenation, CO_2 Elimination

Weight gain

Respiratory secretions

Hemodynamics

Level of consciousness/sedation

Airleak at ETT

---

important in the assessment of small infants and children. Greater than 15% increase in body weight during the intubation period is indicative of increased body water. Increased body water decreases chest wall compliance and dynamic compliance of the lungs and could precipitate loss of end-expiratory lung volume following extubation. Gentle diuretic therapy may be helpful in returning this value to normal, keeping BUN and creatinine within normal limits. The extubatable child must be able to control respiratory secretions following extubation. This requires a balance of consciousness, sedation, and the ability to cough and clear secretions, and is related to the overall volume and character of secretions. Blood pressure and perfusion should be adequate without significant inotropic therapy (less than 5 µg/kg/min). Children with a history of upper airway obstruction (croup, epiglottitis) must be evaluated for the presence of an air leak at the ETT prior to extubation.

■HAZARDS AND COMPLICATIONS OF MECHANICAL VENTILATION

As with all medical therapies, the toxic effects of ventilatory support must be identified and monitored on a regular basis. The common side effects of mechanical ventilation in infants and children include patient–ventilator dyssynchrony, pulmonary overdistention and resultant pulmonary barotrauma and volutrauma, gas trapping and intrinsic PEEP, elevated peak inspiratory and mean airway pressures (P_{aw} > 35 cm H_2O, MAP > 15 cm H_2O), oxygen toxicity (FIo_2 > 0.60) and failure to wean when criteria have been met (Table 16-11). In addition, patients may experience ventilator-acquired pneumonia, hyperventilation or hypoventilation, airway complications from prolonged intubation, and hemodynamic complications as a result of excessive ventilatory settings. If assessment of these parameters is incorporated into the respiratory care plan of the ventilated patient, much of the morbidity associated with mechanical ventilation can be avoided. Table 16-11 summarizes these side effects, listing associated morbidity.

TABLE 16-11 Side Effects of Mechanical Ventilation and Associated Morbidity

SIDE EFFECT	ASSOCIATED MORBIDITY
Patient–ventilator dyssynchrony	Increased work of breathing Failure to grow and gain weight Increased sedation requirements Failure to wean from ventilator
Pulmonary overdistention	Barotrauma and/or volutrauma Air leak syndromes
Intrinsic PEEP	Increased work of breathing Barotrauma and/or volutrauma
Excessive airway pressures (P_{aw} and MAP)	Barotrauma and/or volutrauma Air leak syndromes
$FIO_2 > .60$	Oxygen toxicity
Failure to wean	Prolonged length of mechanical ventilation, increased risk for ventilator-associated pneumonia

SUMMARY

Ventilatory support for infants and children requires a through understanding of cardiorespiratory physiology and pathophysiology as a basis for the development of management strategies and equipment selection. Using the principles presented in this chapter, the role of the RCP moves from setting up and checking the ventilator to developing and monitoring ventilatory care plans designed to achieve physiologic endpoints. These endpoints include restoring adequate tidal and end-expiratory lung volumes, relieving hypoxemia, improving patient–ventilator synchrony, and reducing work of breathing and ventilator-induced lung injury. This comprehensive ventilatory care approach results in improved patient outcome, reduced length of ventilation, and limited extubation failures.

If abnormal convalescence does occur, the RCP must determine the primary cause through careful patient assessment. Revisions in the care plan are then made to reflect the assessment findings and changes in the targeted parameters. Knowledge of this type of physical assessment and strategic planning are essential skills which all RCPs must develop. In the case of perinatal/pediatric patients, the RCP must possess unique knowledge, skills, and experience to achieve a highly specialized level of independent clinical expertise. Specialized education and training is necessary to assure that treatment protocols are current and revised periodically based on new clinical research and practice. This chapter presents the fundamental principles of ventilatory care to support these practice goals. The educational foundation it provides must be supported with consistent clinical experience and supplemented by a quality improvement program which provides feedback on ventilatory practices and patient outcome. Only then will the pediatric patient with respiratory failure be adequately served by our profession.

Neonatal/Pediatric Ventilators

Bear Cub With NVM-1 Volume Monitor and Enhancement Module
Allied Healthcare Products, Inc. Riverside, CA (Fig. 16-13).

Operation. The Cub operates in the time-cycled, pressure-limited mode with assist/control, IMV, and CPAP breath types. Ventilator rate is adjustable from 1 to 150 bpm. Inspiratory time is adjustable from 0.1 to 3.0 seconds. A constant-flow, square-wave pattern is adjustable from 3 to 30 LPM. FIo_2 is adjustable from 0.21 to 1.00. Pressure limit may be selected from 0 to 72 cm H_2O. Maximum working pressure is 87 cm H_2O. Automatic compensation for inadvertent PEEP. Manual breath at preset parameters.

Special Features. The NVM-1 monitor, with sensor placed at the endotracheal tube, accurately measures inspiratory and expiratory tidal volume, respiratory frequency, % tube leakage, and minute ventilation. Deadspace of the sensors varies with ETT size from 1.5 mL (2.0-mm tube) to 2.1 mL (5.0-mm tube). The Bear Cub Enhancement Module (CEM) offers synchronized ventilation by measuring patient effort as a change in flow via the NVM monitor and signalling the CEM which, in turn, signals the ventilator to deliver an assisted breath. It also provides a 1-, 2-, or 3-breath backup in CPAP mode, which is initiated if the patient's breathing interval fails to exceed the interval selected (2 to 10 seconds). Gas inputs for air and oxygen are required to be between 30 and 75 psig.

Monitors and Indicators. The Bear Cub has a proximal airway pressure manometer and digital inspiratory and expiratory times, ventilator rate, mean airway pressure, and I:E ratio displays. Visual alerts show low oxygen and air pressures, low inspiratory pressure, loss of PEEP/CPAP, pro-

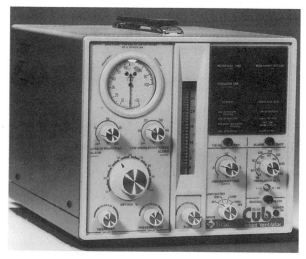

FIGURE 16-13 Bear Cub (Allied Healthcare Products, Inc., Riverside, CA).

longed inspiratory pressure, ventilator inoperative, low air inlet pressure, low oxygen inlet pressure, and rate/time incompatibility.

Alarms. *Ventilator:* Alarm loudness is adjustable at the back of the ventilator. Activating the alarm silence lasts 30 seconds. Visual and audible low inspiratory pressure alarm is adjustable from off to 50 cm H_2O, as is a low PEEP/CPAP alarm adjustable from off to 20 cm H_2O. Ventilator inoperative visual and audible alarms indicate electrical power failure, disconnect, or failure to cycle. Rate/time incompatibility and low gas inlet pressures are also audible and visual alarms. *NVM-1 Monitor:* Indicates visual and audible low and high minute volume, apnea, % tube leak, and patient disconnect. The CEM alarms indicate system failure, patient episode, proximal disconnect, and an obstructed expiratory tube.

Bird VIP With Partner IIi Volume Graphics Monitor and Flow Synchronization
Bird Products Corp, Palm Springs, CA (Fig. 16-14)

Operation. The VIP operates in the time-cycled, pressure-limited, or volume-limited modes, offering SIMV/CPAP and assist/control breath types in each mode. Pressure support is available in the SIMV volume-limited

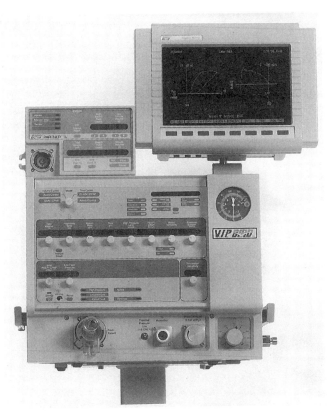

FIGURE 16-14 Bird VIP with Partner IIi volume and graphics monitors and flow synchronization option (Bird Products Corp., Palm Springs, CA).

mode, from 1 to 50 cm H_2O. The ventilator is designed to deliver a tidal volume from 20 mL to 995 mL in the volume-limited mode. A constant-flow, square-wave pattern is produced in both the pressure- (3 to 40 LPM) and volume- (3 to 100 LPM) limited modes. Pressure support utilizes a variable flow pattern. Sensitivity may be pressure triggered at 1 to 20 cm H_2O in both modes or flow triggered in the pressure-limited mode (0.2 to 5.0 LPM). FIO_2 is adjustable from 0.21 to 1.00. An over-pressure relief valve is adjustable from 0 to 130 cm H_2O. Manual breaths can be delivered individually at preset values. Demand flow is available at 0 to 120 LPM at a sensitivity setting of 1 cm H_2O. Gas inputs for air and oxygen are required to be between 40 and 75 psig. Electrical power inputs are published in the manufacturer's information. Ventilator components (base ventilator, Partner IIi, graphics monitor) are modular and may be purchased separately and moved between machines. Flow synchronization is available as a software upgrade.

Special Features. Use of the Partner IIi volume monitor with the neonatal flow sensor allows measurement of delivered tidal volume at the patient and an adjustable flow trigger with less than 1 mL of mechanical dead-space. Termination sensitivity (TS) is available in the pressure-limited mode. TS allows the clinician to adjust the cycle parameter from a set time to 5% to 25% of peak inspiratory flow, thereby decreasing the effects of excessive set inspiratory time and improving patient–ventilator synchrony. A leak compensation feature proportionately adds flow (0 to 10 LPM, based on sensitivity selection) into the circuit to compensate for ETT or circuit leak and maintain a stable PEEP baseline. The Bird graphics monitor displays real-time scalar traces of pressure, flow, and volume as well as pressure-volume and flow-volume curves and trend information.

Monitors and Indicators. Breath rate, inspiratory time, I:E ratio, peak inspiratory pressure, and mean airway pressure are available as scrolling values or may be individually selected for continuous monitoring. Power, external DC battery source, patient effort, demand flow, and a proximal pressure manometer are also displayed.

Alarms. High pressure limit is adjustable from 3 to 120 cm H_2O, low peak pressure is adjustable from off to 3 to 120 cm H_2O, low PEEP/CPAP is adjustable from -9 to 24 cm H_2O; high prolonged pressure, apnea interval, low inlet gas pressure, and circuit failure are available.

Newport Breeze E150
Newport Medical Instruments, Inc., Newport Beach, CA (Fig. 16-15)

Operation. The Breeze operates in the time-cycled, pressure-limited, or volume-limited modes, offering SIMV, assist/control, and spontaneous breath types in each mode. Sigh breaths can be selected in the volume-limited, assist/control mode. The sigh breath size is determined by increasing inspiratory time by 50%; they can occur every 100 breaths. Inspiratory time is adjustable from 0.1 to 3.0 seconds. Flow ranges from 3 to 120 LPM. Rate can be selected from 1 to 150 bpm. Tidal volume is adjustable from 10 to 2000+ mL. PIP is adjustable from 0 to 60 cm H_2O, PEEP/CPAP may be increased from 0 to 60 cm H_2O. Spontaneous flow range is 0 to 50+

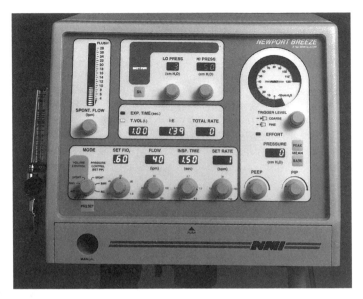

FIGURE 16-15 Newport Breeze E150 (Newport Medical Instruments, Inc., Newport Beach, CA).

LPM. Sensitivity is adjustable from -9 to 60 cm H_2O. Pressure over range is adjustable from 0 to 120 cm H_2O. A nebulizer gas supply is also available. Manual breaths are operator controlled and may be pressure or volume pressure preset. Internal battery with 1 hour minimum, rechargeable to 18 hours maximum.

Special Features. Duo flow allows clinician to adjust inspiratory flow of the mechanical breath to match time constants of the lung and then tailor the spontaneous flow for maximum patient comfort and minimal work of breathing. The Navigator graphics monitor is a stand-alone airway graphics monitor and flow sensor that can be used to measure pressure, volume, and flow at the patient Y. It displays scalar and loop graphics as well as data screens of calculated mechanics parameters.

Monitors and Displays. Set FIO_2, mechanical and spontaneous flow rate, mechanical and total breath rate, set low and high pressure alarms, set tidal volume, expiratory time, I:E ratio, peak and mean airway pressures, PEEP/CPAP, trigger level selected.

Alarms. *Audible and visual:* High pressure (10 to 120 cm H_2O), low pressure (3 to 99 cm H_2O), apnea (5, 10, 15, 30, 60 seconds), low CPAP, and low battery. *Audible only:* Gas supply source and power failures. Alarm silence duration is 60 seconds.

Newport Wave E200
Newport Medical Instruments, Inc., Newport Beach, CA (Fig. 16-16)

Operation. The Wave operates in the pressure- or volume-limited modes, with constant or decelerating wave patterns, SIMV, assist control, and

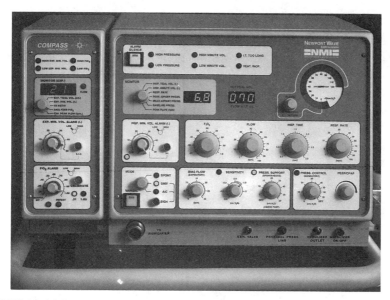

FIGURE 16-16 Newport Wave E200 (Newport Medical Instruments, Inc., Newport Beach, CA).

spontaneous breath types. Pressure support is available from 0 to 60 cm H_2O. Sigh breaths can be selected in the volume-limited, assist/control mode. The sigh breath size is determined by increasing inspiratory time by 50%, with occurrence at every 100 breaths. Inspiratory time is adjustable from 0.1 to 3.0 seconds, with inspiratory pause of 0%, 10%, 20%, and 30% inspiratory time. Breath rate is adjustable for 1 to 100 bpm. Inspiratory pressure is adjustable from 1 to 75 cm H_2O, PEEP/CPAP from 0 to 45 cm H_2O. Bias flow is adjustable from 0 to 30 LPM. Sensitivity is 0.50 to 5 cm H_2O. Pressure over relief is also adjustable from 0 to 120 cm H_2O. A manual breath option is operator controlled at preset volume or pressure limits.

Special Features. Master–slave feature allows two Waves to be synchronized for independent lung ventilation.

Monitors and Displays. Set and inspiratory tidal volume, minute volume, respiratory rate, peak and mean airway pressure, PEEP/CPAP, and peak flow.

Alarms. *Audible and visual:* High and low pressure, high and low minute ventilation, prolonged inspiratory time, and ventilator inoperative status. *Audible only:* Gas supply and power source failures. Alarm silence is 60 seconds.

Sechrist IV-100B
Sechrist Industries, Inc., Anaheim, CA (Fig. 16-17)

Operation. The Sechrist operates in a time-cycled, pressure-limited mode with a constant-flow, square-wave pattern in the (S)IMV and CPAP modes.

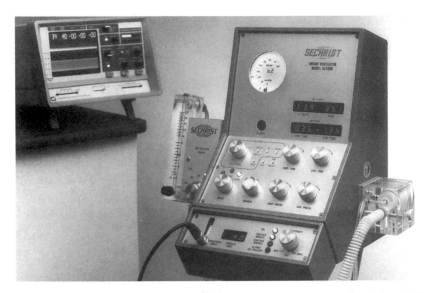

FIGURE 16-17 Sechrist IV-100B SAVI (Sechrist Industries, Inc., Anaheim, CA).

An airway pressure waveform selection control allows adjustment from square to sine waveform. An expiratory pressure adjustment from -2 to 20 cm H_2O allows correction for inadvertent PEEP as a function of ventilatory settings. Manual breath button delivers preset pressure breath. Flow is adjustable from 0 to 32 LPM to 40 LPM (flush) via a side-mounted flowmeter. The blender delivers variable FIo_2 from 0.21 to 1.00. Inspiratory and expiratory times are adjustable from 0.10 to 2.90 and 0.30 to 60.0 seconds respectively. Breath can be set from 1 to 150 bpm. An I:E ratio indicator displays ratios from 1:0.1 to 1:99. The external exhalation valve block may be used for neonates as well as pediatric patients and is detachable for cleaning.

Special Features. The Sechrist SAVI system provides patient-triggered ventilation. Synchronized ventilation is accomplished via thoracic impedance by relaying respiration information from the respiratory channel of a standard ICU cardiac monitor. The analog respiratory waveform output provides the electronic signal for onset of patient inspiratory effort. SAVI then sends a trigger signal to the IV-100B to initiate the preset inspiration. The SAVI also signals patient active exhalation based on impedance time or change, terminating the breath based upon patient breathing pattern. A sensitivity control knob adjusts SAVI capture of impedance signals. The trigger rate display may indicate 1 to 300 bpm. Response time is listed as 15 msec.

Monitors and Displays. Visual readout of breath rate, I:E ratio, and inspiratory and expiratory time are located above controls on the ventilator face. An audible and visual alarm indicator is also present.

Alarms. Alarms function independently from the microprocessor: low pressure, failure to cycle, source gas failure, power failure, apnea, or prolonged inspiration. Inspiration is terminated at 4 seconds if the microprocessor fails. Alarm delay is adjustable from 3 to 60 seconds. An alarm mute is set at 25 seconds + 5 seconds. A separate, adjustable safety pressure relief valve is located on the back of the ventilator.

Infant Star Series 100, 200, 500, 950
Infrasonics, Inc., San Diego, CA (Fig. 16-18)

Operation. The Infant Star family of ventilators operates in the time-cycled, pressure-limited (S)IMV, assist/control, and CPAP modes, with constant-flow, square-wave patterns. Various features are added as the series number increases to add clinical value and performance capabilities to the ventilator. The 100 and 200 series are low-cost ventilators that apply Infrasonic technology in limited fashion to meet specific patient scenarios. As with all ventilator selection, purchasers must decide which features best meet the needs of their patient population. The Infant Star 500 will be presented here, as it offers the full range of performance characteristics. The 950 is presented in the chapter on high frequency ventilation (see Chap. 24). Ventilator rate is adjustable from 1 to 150 bpm. Peak inspiratory pressure ranges from 5 to 90 cm H_2O. PEEP/CPAP ranges from 0 to 24 cm H_2O. Inspiratory time is adjustable from 0.1 to 3.0 seconds. Set flow rate for the mandatory breath ranges from 4 to 40 LPM. Background flow varies from 2 to 30 LPM in 2-L increments, with demand flow variable up to 40 LPM. FIo_2 is adjustable from 0.21 to 1.00. Gas source requires 45 to 90 psig. A heated exhalation block prevents water conden-

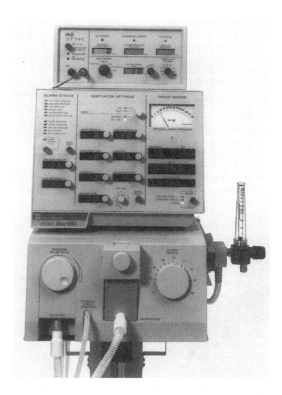

FIGURE 16-18 Infant Star Series 950 (Infrasonics, Inc., San Diego, CA).

sation and expiratory valve obstruction. A manual breath option delivers single breath at preset values.

Special Features. The Star Sync Module utilizes the Graseby's capsule, which is a small abdominal pressure sensor attached to the infant, to detect spontaneous breaths and synchronize mandatory breaths to provide true SIMV. It is operational in all modes.

Monitors and Displays. Proximal and mean airway pressures, I:E ratio, expiratory time, and duration of positive pressure.

Alarms. High and low inspiratory pressures, low PEEP/CPAP, airway leak, insufficient expiratory time, low air and oxygen source pressure, low battery, and external power loss. The ventilator inoperative alarm and error code system identifies the following obstructive tube alarms: AO1 (high inspiratory pressure), AO2 (obstructed expiratory limb), AO3 (high expiratory resistance), AO4 (high PEEP/CPAP), and AO5 (obstructed inspiratory limb or proximal pressure line).

Babylog 8000
Drager Inc., Chantilly, VA (Fig. 16-19)

Operation. The Babylog operates in a time-cycled, pressure-limited mode with a constant-flow, square-wave pattern in the SIMV, assist/control, and CPAP modes. A flow sensor is placed at the ETT which allows measurement of bidirectional tidal volume, flow triggering, apnea, and obstruction monitoring. Inspiratory time is adjustable from 0.1 to 2.0 seconds,

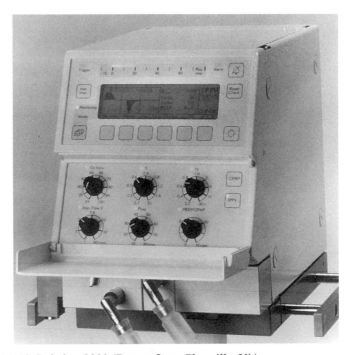

FIGURE 16-19 Babylog 8000 (Drager Inc., Chantilly, VA).

expiratory time is adjustable from 0.2 to 30 seconds. Inspiratory and expiratory flow are adjustable from 1 to 30 LPM. FIo_2 is adjustable from 0.21 to 1.00. Gas supply requires 40 to 70 psig.

Special Features. A digital valve array allows adjustable flow patterns via the VIVE operating mode (variable inspiratory and variable expiratory flow) to enable clinicians to adjust inspiratory and expiratory flow separately to meet the demands of the mechanical breath versus the spontaneous breath. A built-in graphics screen displays single breath pressure or flow airway graphics from the flow sensor, as well as measured ventilator parameters.

Monitors and Displays. Graphic display of pressure and flow. Measured values for minute volume, mechanical and spontaneous tidal volume, leak, FIo_2, and trend data.

Alarms. FIo_2, air and oxygen source pressure, high and low airway pressure and PEEP/CPAP, apnea, high and low minute volumes.

Servo 300

Siemens-Elema AB, Solna, Sweden (Fig. 16-20)

Operation. The SV300 operates in the time-cycled, pressure-limited, or volume-limited modes with constant flow, square wave, or variable flow, and decelerating wave patterns with SIMV, assist/control, and CPAP modes. Pressure support is also available in SIMV volume-limited or pressure-limited modes. New modes are introduced with this ventilator which have a volume guarantee to pressure control (pressure-regulated volume control [PRVC]) and pressure support (volume support [VS]) ventilation. Pressure (-17 to 0 cm H_2O) or flow (8 mL/sec to 33 mL/sec) trigger is available in all flow ranges (infant, child, adult). Ventilator frequency varies by mode: in CMV rate is adjustable from 5 to 150 bpm; in SIMV rate is adjustable from 0.5 to 40 bpm. Inspiratory time is a function of the percent of cycle time and is continuously adjustable. Pause time is also adjusted as a percent of cycle time. Inspiratory pressure and pressure support are adjustable from 0 to 100 cm H_2O. PEEP can be increased from 0 to 50 cm H_2O above baseline. Inspiratory rise time, in percent of cycle time, moves the point where peak flow is delivered during decelerating flow. Tidal volume can be adjusted from 2 to 40 mL, with preset minute volume of 0.2 to 60 LPM. FIo_2 is adjustable from 0.21 to 1.00. A pause hold is available in inspiration or expiration.

Special Features. An oxygen breath control delivers FIo_2 1.00 for 20 breaths or a maximum of 1 minute. *New modes:* PRVC, VS, and SIMV with pressure-control and pressure-support breaths.

Monitors and Displays. Set ventilator parameters are displayed in red, while actively monitored patient parameters are displayed in green on the face of the ventilator. *Frequency:* set and delivered; *Pressure:* peak, mean, pause, PEEP; *Volume:* inspiratory and expiratory tidal volume, inspiratory and expiratory minute volume; inspiratory time, FIo_2, flow rates, and I:E ratio.

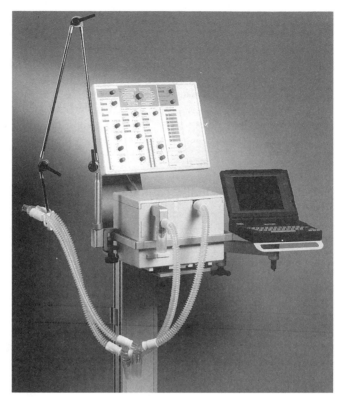

FIGURE 16-20 Servo 300 (Siemens-Elema, AB, Solna, Sweden).

Alarms. High airway pressure is adjustable from 15 to 120 cm H_2O, oxygen concentration alarms at measured values ± 6%. Expired minute ventilation alarms high and low and is adjustable in the various patient ranges (neonatal to adult). The apnea alarm is preset for the patient range: neonate, 10 seconds; pediatric, 15 seconds; and adult, 20 seconds. High and low gas supply alarms are also present, as are indicators of battery usage and technical malfunction. An alarm silence is preset for 2 minutes. There is a visual alarm reset indicator which is activated when an alarm parameter has been violated.

▬REFERENCES

1. ACCP Consensus Conference on Mechanical Ventilation. Chest 106(2):6561, 1994.
2. Amitay M, Etches PC, Finer NN, Maidens JM: Synchronous mechanical ventilation of the neonate with respiratory disease. Crit Care 21(1):118, 1993.
3. Asselin JM, Winn T, Durand DJ et al: Study of flow-synchronized ventilation with the VIP Bird Ventilator. Respir Care 38(11):1252, 1993.
4. Bandy KP, Hicks JJ, Donn SM. Volume-controlled ventilation for severe neonatal respiratory failure. Neo Intens Care June:70, 1992.
5. Bernstein G, Mannino FL, Heldt GP et al: Prospective randomized multicenter trial comparing synchronized and conventional intermittent mandatory ventilation (SIMV vs. IMV) in neonates. Part 2. J Pediatr 128(4):453, 1996.
6. Bernstein G, Cleary JP, Heldt GP et al: Response time and reliability of three neonatal patient-triggered ventilators. Am Rev Respir Dis 148:358, 1993.

7. Bernstein G: Synchronous and patient-triggered ventilation in newborns. Neo Intens Care Sept/Oct:54, 1993.
8. Bernstein G: Synchronous and patient-triggered ventilation in newborns. Neo Respir Dis 3(2):1, 1993.
9. Bing D, Mammel M: Accuracy of neonatal tidal volume measurement devices. Respir Care 40:1193, 1995.
10. Black DR, Wilson BG, Meliones JN: The role of cardiorespiratory interactions in respiratory care. Respir Care 41:123, 1996.
11. Branson RD, Chatburn RL: Technical description and classification of modes of ventilator operations. Respir Care 37:1026, 1992.
12. Chatburn RL: A new system for understanding mechanical ventilators. Respir Care 36:1123, 1991.
13. Chatburn RL: Classification of mechanical ventilators. Respir Care 37:1009, 1992.
14. Cleary JP, Bernstein G, Mannino FL et al: Improved oxygenation during synchronized intermittent mandatory ventilation in neonates with respiratory distress syndrome: A randomized, crossover study. J Peds 126(3):407, 1995.
15. Drummond WH, Gregory GA, Heymann MA et al: The independent effects of hyperventilation, tolazoline, and dopamine on infants with persistent pulmonary hypertension. J Pediatr 98:603, 1981.
16. El-Khatib MF, Chatburn RL, Potts DL, et al: Mechanical ventilators optimized for pediatric use decrease work of breathing and oxygen consumption during pressure support ventilation. Crit Care Med 22(12):1942, 1994.
17. Govindaswami B, Heldt GP, Bernstein G et al: Reduction in cerebral blood flow velocity (CBFV) variability in infants < 1500 g during synchronized ventilation (SIMV). Pediatr Res 33:1258A, 1993.
18. Kacmarek RM, Hickling KG: Permissive hypercapnia. Respir Care 38(4):373, 1993.
19. Loda FA, Glezen WP, Clyde WA Jr: Respiratory disease in group day care. Pediatrics 49:428, 1972.
20. Loh L, Venn PJH: Classifying mechanical ventilators. Br J Med Nov:466, 1987.
21. MacDonald KD, Wagner WR: Infant synchronous ventilation. J Respir Care Pract Aug/Sept:21, 1992.
22. MacIntyre NR: Patient–ventilator interactions: dys-synchrony and imposed work loads. In Fulkerson WJ, MacIntyre NR (eds): Problems in Respiratory Care. Philadelphia, JB Lippincott, 1991.
23. Meliones JN. Chiefetz IM, Wilson BG: The use of airway graphic analysis to optimize mechanical ventilation strategies. Palm Springs, CA, Bird Products Corporation, 1995.
24. Meliones JN, Wilson BG, Leonard RL, Spitzer AR: Pathophysiology-based approach to neonatal respiratory care. In Dantzker DR, MacIntyre NR, Bakow ED (eds): Comprehensive Respiratory Care. Philadelphia, WB Saunders, 1995.
25. Meliones JN, Martin LD, Barnes SD, Wilson BG, Wetzel RC: Respiratory support. In Nichols DG et al (eds): Critical Heart Disease in Infants and Children. St. Louis, CV Mosby, 1995.
26. Meliones JN, Snyder R, DeKeon M et al: Effects of ventilation on diastolic filling after cardiac surgery. JACC 19:52a, 1992.
27. Mushin WW: Physical aspects of automatic ventilators: Basic principles. In Mushin WW, Rendell-Baker, W, Thompson PW, Mapleson WW (eds): Automated Ventilation of the Lung, 3rd ed. Oxford, Blackwell, 1980.
28. Rau JL: Inspiratory flow patterns: The shape of ventilation. Respir Care 38:132, 1993.
29. Reynolds EM, Ryan DP, Doody DP: Permissive hypercapnia and pressure-controlled ventilation as treatment of severe adult respiratory distress syndrome in a pediatric burn patient. Crit Care Med 21(6):944, 1993.
30. Servant GM, Nicks JJ, Donn SM, Bandy KP et al: Feasibility of applying flow-synchronized ventilation to very low birthweight infants. Respir Care 37:249, 1992.
31. Smallwood RW: Ventilators-classifications and their usefulness. Anaesth Intensive Care 14:251, 1986.
32. South M, Morlet CJ: Synchronous mechanical ventilation of the neonate. Arch Dis Child 61:1190, 1986.
33. Stain D, Kinasewitz G, Verren L, George R: Value of routine daily chest x-rays in the medical intensive care unit. Crit Care Med 13:534, 1985.
34. Visveshwara N, Freeman B, Peck M et al: Patient-triggered synchronized assisted ventilation of newborns: Report of a preliminary study and three years' experience. J Perinatology 11(4):347, 1991.

35. Wilson BG: Ventilatory support for children with congenital heart disease. NBRC Horizons 21(3):1, 1995.
36. Wilson BG, Chiefetz IM, Meliones JN: The use of airway graphic analysis to optimize mechanical ventilation in small infants and children. Palm Springs, CA, Bird Products Corporation, 1996.
37. Wilson BG: Direct measurement via an inline pneumotach is necessary to determine effective tidal volume in children. Respir Care 40(11):1172, 1995.
38. Wilson BG, Meliones JN: Continuous airway graphics analysis (AGA) reduces intrinsic PEEP during mechanical ventilation. Crit Care Med 24(1):A128, 1996.
39. Wohl MEB, Mead J: Age as a factor in respiratory disease. In Cherniak V (ed): Kendig's Disorders of the Respiratory Tract in Children. Philadelphia, WB Saunders, 1990.

▄SELF-ASSESSMENT QUESTIONS

The following case studies demonstrate the application of the management algorithms from this chapter. The reader should develop a ventilator management plan for each case study which includes the goals of mechanical ventilation; type of ventilator, mode, and settings; monitoring strategy; and discussion of the pathophysiology. Be sure that all strategies include a plan to minimize ventilator-induced lung injury and synchronized ventilation, when appropriate.

CASE 1: A premature infant with respiratory distress syndrome has a ground-glass appearance with air bronchograms on chest x-ray (CXR), decreased lung volume, and alveolar collapse (decreased functional residual capacity) due to surfactant deficiency. Develop an algorithm that addresses the hypoxemia and establishes end-expiratory lung volume. Peak inspiratory pressures should be minimized to reduce the incidence of barotrauma and volutrauma on underdeveloped lung tissue.

CASE 2: A 10-year-old child with severe asthma is intubated in an outlying hospital for severe respiratory failure. Patient assessment reveals hyperinflated lungs on CXR, respiratory acidosis, hypoxemia, and incomplete exhalation with gas trapping on airway graphic analysis. The ventilatory strategy should target relief of the hyperinflation and incomplete exhalation, while medical therapies treat the bronchospasm.

CASE 3: A newborn with congenital heart disease has a lesion causing excessive pulmonary blood flow preoperatively. Physicians are concerned with improving oxygen delivery to the tissues, while reducing the work of breathing for this patient. Develop a ventilator management plan that will help balance pulmonary blood flow against systemic blood flow.

CASE 4: A 6-month-old infant weighing 5 kg who has chronic lung disease is admitted to the PICU following abdominal surgery to place a permanent feeding tube. There is no arterial access in this patient. The surgeon would like to maintain mechanical ventilation overnight and extubate the child in the morning. The child is awakening from anesthesia and appears comfortable. Develop a ventilator management plan that allows for weaning the mechanical ventilation, facilitates spontaneous breathing, adequately monitors the child without repeated capillary blood gases, and allows extubation in the morning. In your plan, describe the specific criteria that must be met prior to elective extubation for this child.

Chapter 17

Pharmacology

BETH A. ZICKEFOOSE

OBJECTIVES

Having completed this chapter, the reader will be able to:

1. Describe the fundamental principles of pharmacokinetics and pharmacodynamics and the differences that exist between pediatric and adult patients.

2. Calculate appropriate pediatric drug dosages.

3. Compare and contrast sympathomimetic bronchodilators and anticholinergic bronchodilators.

4. Discuss the actions and effects of xanthines and identify an acceptable serum concentration.

5. Discuss the use of mucolytic agents and cromolyn sodium in the pediatric patient.

6. Describe the role of corticosteroids in asthma management.

7. Identify decongestants, antihistamines, expectorants, and antitussives in pediatric cough–cold formulations.

8. Describe the use of respiratory stimulants in the neonatal patient.

9. Discuss the use of ribavirin and pentamidine in the pediatric patient.

KEY TERMS

adrenergic	pharmacodynamics
anticholinergic	pharmacokinetics
antitussive	potency
corticosteroids	stereoisomerism
efficacy	sympathomimetic
expectorant	therapeutic index
mucolytic	

Pharmacology can be defined as the study of drugs. Drugs are chemicals which interact with living tissue to produce therapeutic effects.

To administer a pharmacologic agent to a pediatric population, the health care practitioner must realize that pediatric and adult patients vary greatly. Of all medications approved by the Food and Drug Administration (FDA), only 25% are indicated for use in pediatric patients.[15] This chapter presents agents utilized in pulmonary care of infants and children, and will highlight factors pertinent to pediatric respiratory care.

Two fundamental concepts of pharmacology must be understood in order to properly administer drugs in clinical practice. **Pharmacokinetics** addresses how drugs enter the body, reach the site of action, and are eventually eliminated. **Pharmacodynamics** reflects the actions and effects of drugs.

▬ PHARMACOKINETICS

Absorption

Pharmacokinetic principles commence with drug absorption. All routes of drug administration, with the exception of intravenous, involve varying degrees of absorption to allow the drug to enter the systemic circulation. The amount of time necessary for the drug to reach circulation is usually dependent on the thickness of the absorptive membrane. For example, oral and topical administration require the drug to diffuse through epithelial membranes, which delays absorption. Intramuscular routes allow a moderate rate of absorption since the drug needs only to diffuse through loosely joined epithelial cells of capillary walls. Inhalation routes provide for rapid absorption because of the ease of diffusion across the alveolar–capillary membrane.

Drug absorption varies greatly in infants and neonates. There is a vast difference in their gastric emptying rates as well as increased absorption

---

TABLE 17-1 Comparison of Rated Drug Absorption of Various Routes of Administration

ROUTE	RATE OF ABSORPTION
Oral	Slow
Subcutaneous	Slow
Intramuscular	Moderate
Intravenous	Immediate
Sublingual	Rapid
Transtracheal	Rapid
Inhalation	Rapid
Intracardiac	Immediate

(Bledsoe BE, Bosker G, Papa FJ: Prehospital Emergency Pharmacology, 3rd ed. Englewood Cliffs, NJ: Prentice-Hall, 1992.)

through the skin. A complete comparison of drug absorption rates is shown in Table 17-1.

Distribution

Following absorption, a drug is distributed throughout the body via the circulatory system. Drugs with a fast onset of action are able to pass easily through interstitial spaces to reach the target organ. Other drugs have a delayed onset. Some of these drugs may be distributed and retained in fatty tissues (*e.g.*, diazepam) or be bound to calcium ions in bones and cartilage (*e.g.*, tetracycline). In the case of diazepam and tetracycline, only small amounts of the drug actually reach the intended target tissue. Drugs will also tend to bind with plasma proteins, thereby diminishing distribution. For this reason, scientists calculate the percentage of protein binding when establishing dosage recommendations.

Biotransformation

Biotransformation refers to chemical changes of the drug molecule into active or inactive metabolites. Although it is often assumed that drugs are in an active form when administered, many drugs are actually inactive. These agents must be converted into their active form before they can achieve the desired effect. For example, the antiinflammatory drug prednisone is at first inactive. However, it soon undergoes hepatic biotransformation to prednisolone, its active metabolite. The liver and microsomal system of enzymes of the gut wall are the principal sites for biotransformation. Drug metabolism is slower in infants and may be greatly impaired in the premature infant, which would interfere with biotransformation of many agents.

Elimination

The final factor in pharmacokinetics involves elimination of the drug from the body. This is accomplished most often via renal excretion, or by alternate routes such as the liver, intestines, or lungs.

A drug's half-life ($T^1/_2$) is the time necessary for the serum concentration to decrease by 50%. Clinically, $T^1/_2$ denotes the drug's elimination time. Regardless of the peak serum concentration or the route of administration, a specific drug's $T^1/_2$ will always remain constant. For example, in Figure 17-1, the time concentration curve illustrates a half-life of approximately 2 hours. Following a single dose, five half-lives must pass before the drug may be considered completely eliminated. Conversely, stable serum concentrations can be achieved following five doses, providing each is administered after one half-life.[8]

▬PHARMACODYNAMICS

Pharmacodynamics is concerned with the actions and effects drugs produce on the body. The *effects* are defined as the physiologic changes that a drug produces. The *action* is the mechanism by which it produces this effect.

All drugs produce a variety of effects. The term *primary* describes the effects that are desired. For example, a patient with bronchospasm may be treated with a bronchodilator. The indications for the drug (bronchospasm) are usually the opposite of the primary effect of the drug

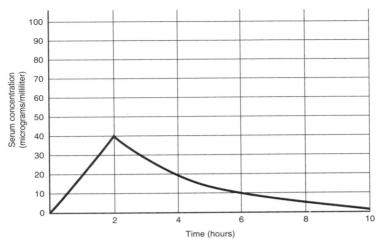

FIGURE 17-1 Time concentration curve for a drug with a half-life of 2 hours. Note that after 4 hours the serum concentration is one-half of the concentration present at 2 hours.

(bronchodilation). Secondary effects are considered undesirable and are often referred to as *side effects* or *adverse effects*. Terms such as **efficacy** describe the intensity of the drug's primary effect. **Potency** is often used erroneously as a synonym for efficacy when it is actually referring to the amount of drug required to achieve the desired effect.

For a drug to be effective, there has to be a minimal concentration of it in the body. A concentration below the therapeutic level will not produce the desired response. However, if the drug concentration rises too high, it may enter a toxic or even fatal range. Typically, the goal is to keep the patient's drug serum concentration within the therapeutic level using the lowest possible dosage (Fig. 17-2).

The **therapeutic index** of a drug reflects its safety. It is calculated as the ratio of effective and toxic dosages.[5] For example, if the effective dosage is 10 mg but a dose of 200 mg is toxic, the therapeutic index would be 20. In other words, the toxic dose is 20 times the effective dose. Drugs such as Narcan, an opioid antagonist, have a high therapeutic index. Thus, Narcan is considered a safe drug with little possibility of overdose. However, digoxin's therapeutic index is only 2 or 3. This illustrates that by simply doubling the recommended dose, the patient is at significant risk for toxicity.

The desired effect is produced by a drug's mechanism of action. This action is caused by drug molecules binding to protein receptors located on the surface of cell membranes. Drugs can interact with a receptor in one of two manners: agonist and antagonist. If it binds with a receptor and causes a response, the drug is an agonist. An antagonist is a drug that also binds with the receptor but initiates no response. However the mere presence of the antagonist on the receptor denies other drugs or even normal body neurohormones access to the receptor. Clinically, antagonists are called *blockers*.

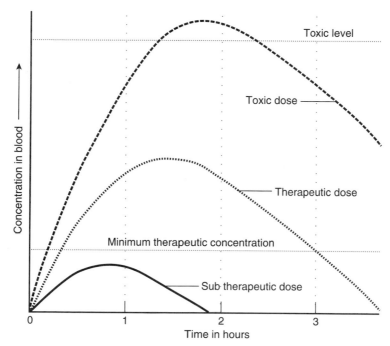

FIGURE 17-2 Comparison of blood levels following subtherapeutic, therapeutic, and toxic doses of the same drug. (Bledsoe BE, Bosker G, Papa FJ: Prehospital Emergency Pharmacology, 3rd ed. Englewood Cliffs, NJ, Prentice-Hall, 1992.)

Calculating Pediatric Doses

Owing to the vast differences between pediatric and adult patients concerning pharmacokinetics and pharmacodynamics, it is not recommended that pediatric dosing regimens simply be extrapolated from adult data. However, established pediatric dosages are often not provided on the product information sheets. The following rules will give fractions of the adult dose based on age, weight, or body surface area (BSA).[17]

Various formulas are available for converting adult dosages to safe dosages for infants and children. Fried's rule and Young's rule are based on the child's age and assume that a child of 12½ years of age would receive a full adult dose (Box 17-1). Clark's rule is based on weight and

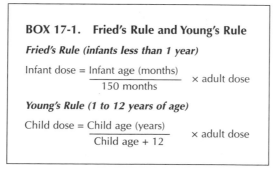

BOX 17-1. Fried's Rule and Young's Rule

Fried's Rule (infants less than 1 year)

$$\text{Infant dose} = \frac{\text{Infant age (months)}}{150 \text{ months}} \times \text{adult dose}$$

Young's Rule (1 to 12 years of age)

$$\text{Child dose} = \frac{\text{Child age (years)}}{\text{Child age} + 12} \times \text{adult dose}$$

BOX 17-2.　Clark's Rule

$$\text{Child dose} = \frac{\text{Child weight (lbs)}}{150\text{ lbs}} \times \text{adult dose}$$

---

assumes that when a child reaches 150 lb, the full adult dose should be given (Box 17-2). The most accurate method of calculating a pediatric dose is by using the BSA rule (Box 17-3).

■ AUTONOMIC CONTROL OF LOWER AIRWAYS

The patency of bronchi and bronchioles is largely determined by the tone of the smooth muscle in the walls of the airways. The tone is sustained by a balance between the parasympathetic and sympathetic divisions of the autonomic nervous system. Bronchial smooth muscle cells are innervated directly by parasympathetic neurons that travel within the vagus nerve. These neurons release acetylcholine, which activates muscarinic receptors leading to bronchoconstriction. In contrast, sympathetic fibers do not innervate bronchial smooth muscle cells directly. Instead, they terminate in the parasympathetic ganglia and act to inhibit the parasympathetic influences just described. Bronchial smooth muscle cells contain β_2-adrenergic receptors that mediate bronchodilation when epinephrine is released from the adrenal medulla.[3]

■ BRONCHODILATORS

Patients who suffer from asthma and other bronchospastic disorders are exquisitely sensitive to imbalances in these autonomic pathways. Strategies for producing bronchodilation are based on administering drugs that either mimic sympathetic influences or block parasympathetic influences on smooth muscle tone.

Sympathomimetic Bronchodilators

The most commonly used drugs in respiratory care are the adrenergic **sympathomimetic** agents. These drugs "mimic" the sympathetic nervous system, causing bronchodilation. Their efficacy is based on the ability to activate β_2 receptors on bronchial smooth muscle cells, leading to their relaxation.

The molecular structure of **adrenergic** bronchodilators has been modified throughout the last few decades. Agents such as epinephrine have activity at all the adrenergic receptors (α, β_1, and β_2). For example, when epinephrine is administered, it attaches at (1) α receptors causing vasoconstriction; (2) β_1 receptors causing tachycardia; and (3) β_2 receptors causing bronchodilation. Because the effects mediated by α and β_1 recep-

---

BOX 17-3.　BSA Rule

$$\text{Child dose} = \frac{\text{Child BSA} \times \text{m}^2}{1.73\text{ m}^2} \times \text{adult dose}$$

---

tors may be undesirable, chemists have successfully modified the molecular structure of bronchodilators such as epinephrine to enhance β_2 receptor affinity. These modifications have spawned development of β_2-selective agents such as metaproterenol and terbutaline.

The molecular structure of bronchodilators also determines their manner of termination. Many of these agents are terminated by catechol-o-methyltransferase (COMT), an enzyme found in the gut wall and liver. For this reason, these drugs cannot be administered orally (P.O.) but are effective by inhalation or injection. Other drugs are terminated only by an enzyme called monoamine oxidase (MAO). Owing to this enzyme's slower activity, these drugs will have a longer duration of effect. Drugs terminated only by MAO can be administered orally. This makes these drugs popular with pediatricians, who routinely prescribe oral bronchodilators for outpatient treatment of bronchospasm.

Sympathomimetic bronchodilators have comparable efficacy in relieving bronchospasm but differ in their potency and dosage formulations. Refer to Table 17-2 for a concise list of popular bronchodilators and their administration routes, dosages, and adverse effects.

The principal effect of sympathomimetic bronchodilators is smooth muscle relaxation. However, they also provide additional beneficial effects. Activation of β receptors on mast cells causes a membrane stabilizing effect that slows the release of inflammatory mediators. Also, β-receptor activation has been shown to enhance the mucociliary transport system.[23]

There are negative secondary effects of sympathomimetic bronchodilators that also must be addressed. Skeletal muscle tremor is the most common effect associated with these agents.[4] This may be due to either an excitatory influence within the central nervous system (CNS) or a direct activation of β receptors found within skeletal muscle. Cardiovascular side effects may include tachycardia, alterations in blood pressure, and palpitations. Relaxation of vascular smooth muscle lowers peripheral resistance which may lead to reflex increases in heart rate and cardiac output. Adverse effects of commonly used bronchodilators are summarized in Table 17-2.

Racemic Epinephrine (Vaponefrin, Micronefrin)

Organic molecules demonstrate a peculiar property known as **stereoisomerism**. While all molecules of a given substance contain the same atoms, chemical bonds between atoms can twist or rotate, which alters their structural arrangement. This allows molecules of a given substance to exist as mirror images, or isomers, of one another. One isomer is called *levo* and the other, *dextro*.

Racemic epinephrine is a 2.25% mixture containing a 50:50 ratio of levo and dextro isomers. It is only half as powerful as pure epinephrine. Since it has mild efficacy as a bronchodilator, racemic epinephrine is used most frequently for its decongestant effect in the treatment of laryngeal edema and stridor accompanying laryngotracheobronchitis, or postextubation edema.[23] The recommended pediatric dose is 0.05 mL/kg, with a maximum dose of 0.5 mL aerosolized with 2 cc of normal saline as needed.

Anticholinergic Bronchodilators

Anticholinergic drugs offer an alternate mechanism for bronchodilation and can be used alone or in conjunction with traditional adrenergic bron-

TABLE 17-2 Common Bronchodilators Used With Infants and Children

GENERIC NAME (TRADE)	ROUTE	DOSAGE	ADVERSE EFFECTS
Albuterol (Proventil, Ventolin) 0.5%	Aerosol	Neonate: 0.05–0.15 mg/kg every 4–6 hours Pediatric: 1.25–2.5 mg every 4–6 hours	Palpitations, tremor, nausea, headache
	P.O.	0.1 mg/kg every 8 hours up to a maximum of 12 mg/day	
	MDI	1–2 puffs every 4–6 hours	
Metaproterenol (Metaprel, Alupent) 5%	Aerosol MDI	0.1–0.3 mL every 4–6 hours 1–3 puffs every 3–4 hours, maximum of 12 puffs per day	Tremor, nervousness, palpitations, headache
	P.O.	0.3–0.5 mg/kg every 6–8 hours to a maximum of 20 mg dose	
Isoetharine (Bronkosol)	Aerosol	0.1–0.2 mg/kg every 4–6 hours	Tachycardia, tremor, headache, nausea
	MDI	1–2 puffs every 4–6 hours	
Isoproterenol (Isuprel)	Aerosol	0.05 mg/kg every 4 hours 1.25 mg maximum	Tachycardia, palpitations, headache, tremor
Terbutaline (Brethine, Breathaire)	Aerosol	0.5–1.5 mg every 4–6 hours	Tachycardia, nervousness, tremor, insomnia
	MDI	2 puffs every 4–6 hours	
	P.O.	0.15 mg/kg TID with maximum of 5 mg daily	
Atropine	Aerosol	0.05 mg/kg every 6–8 hours, 0.25 minimum, 1 mg maximum	Dry mouth, tachycardia, bradycardia, fever, blurred vision, urinary retention, mucus plugging
Iprutropium bromide (Atrovent)	Aerosol MDI	* 1–2 puffs every 6–8 hours	Dry mouth, cough, headache, nausea, dizziness, blurred vision

Key: P.O. = orally; MDI = metered dose inhaler; TID = 3 times per day.
*Safety and efficacy not yet established for children under 12 years of age.
(Barnhart SL, Czervinske MP: Perinatal and Pediatric Respiratory Care. Philadelphia, WB Saunders, 1995.)

chodilators. By blocking cholinergic receptors on bronchial smooth muscle, the negative influence of parasympathetic bronchoconstriction is diminished. Atropine is a potent anticholinergic bronchodilator that is often used for short-term relief of bronchospasm. Adverse effects include dry mouth, urinary retention, mydriasis (dilation of pupils), tachycardia, and, more importantly, the potential for inhibiting and drying of secretions.

Ipratropium bromide (Atrovent) is a newer agent having a quaternary structure which limits its absorption from the respiratory tract. This results in reducing the systemic side effects observed with atropine, such as the inhibition of salivation and depressed mucociliary action, while still allowing local effects.[17] It is less effective than sympathomimetic bronchodilators for managing acute episodes of bronchospasm but is useful for chronic maintenance.[6,9,10] One study in asthmatic children between the ages of 6 and 14 years showed a reduction of symptoms while using ipratropium bromide.[14] However, the safety and efficacy of aerosolizing ipratropium bromide for children less than 12 years of age still remains to be established.[4]

Xanthine Bronchodilators

The methylxanthines are naturally occurring plant extracts that include caffeine, theobromine, and theophylline. These agents produce an excitatory influence on the CNS and a staggering number of pharmacological influences on the cardiovascular, respiratory, and gastrointestinal systems (Table 17-3). Theophylline has been used in the treatment of bronchospasm for over 50 years, but during the past decade its risk/benefit ratio has been challenged. Controversy has been spawned by clinical trials demonstrating less efficacy than traditional bronchodilators, significant risk for toxicity, and an inability to define precisely its mechanism of action.

Although theophylline is known to improve asthmatic symptoms in cases unresponsive to traditional bronchodilators, the mechanism for its beneficial effects continues to puzzle researchers. For years it was proposed that theophylline inhibited phosphodiesterase, the enzyme responsible for the breakdown of cAMP. By inhibiting this enzyme, the intracellular levels of cAMP are elevated, thereby promoting bronchodilation and mast cell stability. The problem with this theory is that this influence is not achievable at therapeutic serum concentrations; it only occurs with serum levels well into the toxic range. Nevertheless, patients benefit from lower serum concentrations. Newer theories have focused on three additional possibilities: (1) adenosine inhibition; (2) release of catecholamine; (3) inhibition of prostaglandins.[23] It is not unreasonable to predict that the eventual mechanism for theophylline's efficacy will be based on a composite of these theories.

While the actions of theophylline are being clarified, its beneficial and toxic effects have been more clearly defined. In addition to bronchodilation, theophylline inhibits the release of inflammatory mediators, improves mucociliary clearance, improves diaphragmatic strength, and stimulates the CNS. The improvement of diaphragmatic strength has been useful in preventing respiratory failure following extubation of low-birth-weight infants.[21] The CNS stimulation makes this a popular pharmacologic

TABLE 17-3 Common Side Effects of Methylxanthines

NEUROLOGIC	CARDIOVASCULAR	GASTROINTESTINAL	RENAL, OTHER
Tremor	Tachycardia	Nausea/vomiting	Diuresis
Headache	Hypotension	Diarrhea	Hypokalemia
Nervousness	Shock	Hematemesis	Rhabdomyolysis
Disorientation	Cardiac arrest		Acid–base disturbance
Seizures			

agent to treat apnea of prematurity.[18] The sum of these influences accounts for its pivotal role in the chronic maintenance of patients suffering moderate and severe forms of asthma and obstructive diseases.

Unfortunately, theophylline toxicity is not uncommon, particularly in children, and is among the top causes of drug therapy-related hospitalizations each year. Toxic effects generally follow a dose-response pattern and have been categorized as grades 1 through 4 according to severity.[19] For example, grade 1 symptoms are mostly gastrointestinal in nature (*e.g.*, nausea, diarrhea), whereas grade 4 symptoms are immediately life threatening (*e.g.*, status seizures, ventricular fibrillation). Therapeutic and toxic serum concentrations are well defined, and for this reason careful attention must be given to monitoring theophylline serum levels.

There are many different brands of theophylline, including time-released agents such as Theo-dur and Theo-dur Sprinkle, intended for small children and infants (Table 17-4). An ethylenediamine salt of theophylline, aminophylline, is the most commonly used intravenous formulation. Only 79% to 86% of the molecular weight of aminophylline preparations is actually theophylline, and calculations must be adjusted to administer dosages comparable to pure theophylline. For example, aminophylline dihydrate contains only 79% theophylline. To be equivalent to 100 mg of theophylline, one must administer 127 mg of this particular aminophylline preparation.

The maximum effects of theophylline are generally appreciated with serum concentrations ranging between 10 and 20 µg/mL. Levels less than 5 µg/mL provide no clinical effects, and toxicity begins to appear when levels exceed 20 µg/mL. Newer theories are now recommending that 5 to 15 µg/mL might be a safer and more effective range.[13,20] Restlessness, nausea, and tremors are generally the first side effects to appear, followed by cardiac arrhythmias and convulsions as levels exceed 30 µg/mL. Therefore, it is vital to monitor serum concentrations frequently during the initial phase of treatment and periodically thereafter. It is significant that many drugs can alter otherwise normal concentrations of theophylline, and concurrent use of such drugs requires special attention to theophylline levels (Table 17-5).

TABLE 17-4 Commonly Used Methylxanthine Preparations

GENERIC	BRAND
Theophylline	Bronkodyl
	Slo-bid Gyrocaps
	Slo-Phyllin
	Theobid
	Theo-Dur
	Theo-Dur Sprinkle
Aminophylline	Aminophylline, et al.

TABLE 17-5 Selected Drugs That Alter Theophylline Serum Concentrations

Agents That Decrease Theophylline Levels		
Barbiturates	Rifampin	Ketoconazole
Phenytoin	Sympathomimetics	Smoking
Agents That Increase Theophylline Levels		
Beta blockers	Glucocorticosteroids	Quinolones
Calcium channel blockers	Ephedrine	Oral contraceptives
Cimetadine	Influenza vaccine	Erythromycins
Agents That May Increase or Decrease Theophylline Levels		
Carbamazepine	Isoniazid	Furosemide

MISCELLANEOUS RESPIRATORY AGENTS

Hydration and Mucolytics

Although adequate hydration is the most effective way to facilitate secretion removal, other methods are sometimes necessary. Bland aerosols utilizing sterile water or hypotonic or isotonic saline can be aerosolized continuously or intermittently to prevent thickening of secretions. Hypertonic saline is only indicated when sputum induction is necessary and should be used cautiously. Patients with diseases such as cystic fibrosis may benefit more, however, from a mucolytic agent.

As the suffix -*lytic* suggests, **mucolytics** are agents that break down various substances comprising mucus, such as glycoproteins and other proteins. The actions of these agents allow mucus to be expectorated more easily, and hence, their primary indication is thickened and inspissated secretions.

Probably the most popular mucolytic agent is N-acetylcysteine (Mucosil, Mucomyst). This agent acts by breaking down disulfide bonds in mucoprotein, thereby decreasing the viscosity of mucus and facilitating expectoration. It can be administered as an aerosol or directly instilled into an endotracheal or tracheostomy tube for hygiene purposes.

N-acetylcysteine is available as 10% and 20% concentrations. Although the 20% solution may be more potent, it carries a higher risk of side effects such as bronchospasm.[23] Because the usual dosage of this more concentrated form is 3 to 5 mL, it is often combined with a bronchodilator to reduce the risk of bronchospasm.

Two percent sodium bicarbonate is another mucolytic agent which increases the bronchial pH. This action weakens side chains in the mucus molecule, and therefore reduces mucus viscosity.[17] The dosage and side effects are similar to those for N-acetylcysteine. This agent is contraindicated, however, in the patient who is severely sodium-restricted. It is also contraindicated in the case of severe metabolic alkalosis.

As with any mucolytic agent, care must be taken to observe all patients for signs of sudden airway obstruction caused by secretions that are loosened and subsequently plug. Suction equipment should be available for all patients with reduced cough mechanisms or artificial airways.

Pulmozyme

Recombinant human DNase (Pulmozyme) was approved in 1993 to be used in patients with cystic fibrosis (CF) to improve pulmonary function and reduce the frequency of respiratory infections. Sputum of the CF patient contains a large amount of deoxyribonucleic acid (DNA) from bacterial cell death. This vast amount of extracellular DNA tends to thicken the airway secretions. Pulmozyme hydrolyzes this DNA, thereby reducing sputum viscosity. Clinical studies have confirmed a significant decrease in congestion and dyspnea and modest improvements in pulmonary function (FEV$_1$ increased 10% to 15%).[16] Most patients benefit from one aerosol of 2.5 mg per day. Safety and efficacy is not yet known for children under 5 years of age.

Cromolyn Sodium

Cromolyn sodium (Intal) acts to stabilize mast cell membranes, thereby preventing the release of inflammatory mediators, including histamine. It is indicated only for prophylaxis of mild to moderate asthma and has very little effect during the acute allergic episode. A therapy regimen of 6 to 12 weeks is necessary to prevent airway hypersensitivity.

Cromolyn sodium is most commonly administered via a nebulized solution or metered dose inhaler (MDI). Children older than 5 years of age receive 20 mg every 6 hours. Children between the ages of 2 and 5 years receive 20 mg every 6 to 8 hours. Dosage via MDI is two puffs, four times a day.[7,12]

Aerosolized Corticosteroids

In addition to bronchodilators, **corticosteroids** are among the most potent agents utilized in the management of asthma.[2] The predominant effect is a reduction of airway inflammation. Additional effects include a decrease in mucus secretion and airway edema. The mechanism of action involves a reduction in the synthesis of inflammatory mediators including leukotrienes and prostaglandins. This action suppresses the vascular changes responsible for inflammation. Steroids also act by increasing the number and responsiveness of β receptors.[20]

Three forms of inhaled corticosteroids are available in the United States. The MDI formulations include (1) flunisolide (Aerobid), (2) beclomethasone diproprionate (Vanceril), and (3) triamcinolone acetonide (Azmacort). The MDI formulation allows for topical administration that reduces, but does not eliminate, the adverse effects common to systemic administration.

The most significant adverse effect of systemically administered corticosteroids is the suppression of the adrenal axis steroid production. Children may experience impaired bone formation and growth retardation. Administration via inhalation does reduce these effects significantly, but this route introduces a risk for dry throat and oropharyngeal candidiasis.[1] Children benefit greatly from the use of an MDI spacer. This, along with instructions regarding proper inhalation technique, will help the child coordinate inspirations as well as reduce the local effects. The child should be instructed to rinse the mouth following dosing to prevent oral candidiasis. Table 17-6 lists the most commonly utilized antiinflammatory agents, their recommended dosages, and adverse effects.

TABLE 17-6 Inhaled Corticosteroids

GENERIC NAME	DOSAGE	ADVERSE EFFECTS
Flunisolide (Aerobid)	MDI = 1–2 puffs every 12 hours	Dry throat, oral candidiasis, dysphonia, impaired growth, impaired bone formation
Beclomethasone dipropionate (Vanceril)	MDI = 1–2 puffs every 6–8 hours	Dry throat, oral candidiasis, dysphonia, impaired growth, impaired bone formation, nasal irritation
Triamcinolone acetonide (Azmacort)	MDI = 1–2 puffs every 6–8 hours	Nasal irritation, cough

(Barnhart SL, Czervinske MP: Perinatal and Pediatric Respiratory Care. Philadelphia, WB Saunders, 1995.)

COUGH AND COLD AGENTS

All upper respiratory infections, including the common cold, lead to inflammatory changes within mucous membranes lining the sinuses, throat, and nasal passages. Vasodilation, increased vessel permeability, and glandular secretions contribute to the familiar symptoms such as congestion, rhinorrhea, throat irritation, and cough. The following four drug classes are used for the symptomatic relief of the common cold, and are available over-the-counter or by a physician's written prescription: (1) decongestants, (2) antihistamines, (3) expectorants, and (4) antitussives. Each of these drugs is aimed at reducing specific cold symptoms and may be used alone or as part of a combination regimen. Table 17-7 provides a list of specific ingredients of the various pediatric cough–cold agents discussed below.

Decongestants

Decongestants are α-adrenergic (sympathomimetic) drugs that shrink mucous membranes via a vasoconstrictive effect. Subsequently, upper airway passages are opened, thereby improving airflow and reducing the work of breathing. They are available in topical or systemic forms. Topical administration provides immediate relief. Unfortunately, repeated use of topical agents can lead to rebound nasal congestion. This rebound effect has been attributed to the spray's repeated irritation of the nasal mucosa, and to down-regulation or an actual reduction in the number of α receptors that follows their repetitive stimulation.[11] In either case, overzealous use of nasal sprays leads to the patient being "hooked" and driven to use the agent with even greater frequency in order to remain symptom free. Rebound nasal congestion is rarely associated with systemic use, however the systemic route is associated with influences such as elevated blood pressure. For this reason, decongestants must be used cautiously by hypertensive patients.

Antihistamines

Contrary to popular belief, histamine has little significance in producing the symptoms associated with the common cold. Although it is a well-known inflammatory mediator and plays a significant role in allergic

TABLE 17-7 Ingredients of Various Pediatric Cough–Cold Agents

BRAND	DECONGESTANT	ANTIHISTAMINE	EXPECTORANT	ANTITUSSIVE
Pedia Care (cough–cold)	Pseudoephedrine	Chlorphenir-amine		Dextro-methorphan
Naldecon EX	Phenylpropa-nolamine		Quaifenesin	
Naldecon DX	Phenylpropa-nolamine		Quaifenesin	Dextro-methorphan
Vicks Formula 44E			Quaifenesin	Dextro-methorphan
Triaminic Cold	Phenylpropa-nolamine	Chlorphenir-amine		
Triaminic DM-cough	Phenylpropa-nolamine			Dextro-methorphan
Triaminic Expectorant DH	Phenylpropa-nolamine	Pyrilamine	Quaifenesin	Hydrocodone
Sudafed	Pseudoephedrine			
Neo-Synephrine	Phenylephrine			
Benedryl		Diphenhy-dramine HCL		
Phenergan		Promethazine HCL		
Pediacof Syrup	Phenylephrine	Chlorphenir-amine	Potassium iodide	Codeine
Robitussin Pediatric Cough				Dextro-methorphan
Dorcol Pediatric Formula	Pseudoephedrine		Quaifenesin	Dextro-methorphan
Beneylin Pediatric				Dextro-methorphan

forms of rhinitis, the influence of antihistamines is short-lived and insignificant during the pathogenesis of the common cold.[22] In addition to their actions on histamine receptors, all antihistamines block cholinergic receptors. This anticholinergic influence promotes the drying of secretions and allows for symptomatic relief. However, this "drying up" effect may be a concern for patients with underlying pulmonary disease because it may reduce the ability to clear mucus from the lower airways. In such patients, adequate hydration is essential.

Within the CNS, histamine and acetylcholine function as excitatory neurotransmitters. By blocking histamine and cholinergic receptors, antihistamines produce drowsiness, which may provide much-needed rest for the cold sufferer. However, in cases where sedation must be avoided, water-soluble antihistamines may be preferred because they do not pass through the blood–brain barrier. Examples of water-soluble antihistamines include terfenadine (Seldane) and astemizole (Hismanal).

Expectorants

Expectorants are agents that stimulate the production of a thinner, less adhesive mucus, thereby increasing the clearance of these secretions from the respiratory tract. It is important to note that adequate hydration via an increase in water intake is by far the best expectorant available.

One of the most commonly used expectorants is guaifenesin. When taken orally, guaifenesin is believed to stimulate the gastric vagal reflex which subsequently produces a watery, less viscid secretion that is much more mobile. This agent is the active ingredient in medicines such as Robitussin and Naldecon EX.

Inorganic iodide also has known expectorant and mucolytic effects on the respiratory system. Potassium iodide (SSKI) is a saturated oral solution that is available only by prescription.

Antitussives

Antitussives are agents that suppress the cough reflex mediated via the medulla. Antitussive agents are usually opioids (such as codeine and hydrocodone), or opioid derivatives (such as dextromethorphan).

Antitussives offer relief from the annoying, dry, hacking cough produced by cold viruses. However, they must be used cautiously in the patient with underlying pulmonary diseases. If copious bronchial secretions are present, suppression of the cough reflex is not usually indicated. One possible exception is when excessive coughing is causing sleep deprivation. It is also important to note that antitussive agents should not be used simultaneously with expectorants. This combination creates a situation wherein secretions are mobilized but the cough reflex required to clear them is depressed.

▰ RESPIRATORY STIMULANTS

Respiratory stimulants are agents that increase ventilatory drive. There are no drugs currently available that selectively stimulate the respiratory centers, so drugs that are claimed to be respiratory stimulants are actually generalized CNS stimulants or analeptics. Doxapram (Dopram) is the most commonly used stimulant because of its relative safety, having the greatest margin between the dose that stimulates ventilation and that which precipitates convulsive seizures.[17] Doxapram can be used for management of postoperative respiratory depression, but may require repeated dosing because it is short acting following bolus doses. Doxapram has been found to improve tidal volume more than respiratory rate, and is occasionally used in continuous intravenous drips to counter apnea in neonates. As discussed previously, methylxanthines also excite the CNS. Therefore aminophylline is also used in the prevention of apnea in the premature infant.

▰ AEROSOL ANTIVIRAL AGENTS

Ribavirin (Virazole) is an antiviral aerosol formulation that has been approved for the management of bronchiolitis and pneumonia caused by respiratory syncytial virus (RSV). While its mechanism of action is not completely understood, ribavirin is known to be a virostatic agent that disrupts viral protein synthesis by inhibiting ribonucleic acid (RNA).

Ribavirin has very specific directions for dosing and administration. It is recommended for continuous aerosol administration via an oxygen mask, hood, or tent with a Viratek SPAG-2 (small particle aerosol generator) device. This large-volume nebulizing system aerosolizes a 2% solution over 12 to 18 hours per day, for 3 to 7 days. Due to precipitation and crystalline blockage of the expiratory valve of ventilator circuitry, ribavirin must be used cautiously when nebulized to patients receiving continuous mechanical ventilation.[5]

Adverse effects of ribavirin include worsening of the patient's respiratory and cardiovascular status. Health care personnel have also reported adverse effects from exposure to aerosolized ribavirin such as eye irritation and headache. Protective goggles are recommended for health care personnel during administration of ribavirin. Ribavirin has been found to be teratogenic in animal studies; consequently, pregnant health care workers should avoid exposure to the ribavirin aerosol.

During the last decade, there have been many attempts to develop guidelines and delivery systems to help minimize environmental exposure of the caregiver to ribavirin. Clinical trials are being performed to evaluate the effectiveness of scavenger systems and containment canopies. Expiratory filters are recommended for the ventilator circuitry when patients are receiving mechanical ventilation. Health care workers should utilize universal precautions when working with patients during dosing hours and interrupt the ribavirin therapy prior to direct patient care.

▬PENTAMIDINE ISETHIONATE

The aerosolization of the antiprotozoal agent pentamidine isethionate (Nebupent) is indicated in the treatment and prophylaxis of *Pneumocystis carinii* pneumonia, a common opportunistic respiratory infection in the immunocompromised and acquired immunodeficiency syndrome (AIDS) patient. Pentamidine's mechanism of action is thought to be the inhibition of RNA, DNA, and protein synthesis.

Owing to side effects such as coughing and bronchial irritation, care must be taken to protect the health care professional from unnecessary exposure to pentamidine. The FDA has approved aerosolization with the Respirgard II nebulizer, a unit that has a series of one-way valves and an expiratory filter. Scavenger systems and strict isolation during aerosolization are also being investigated as methods to reduce second-hand exposure.

The current recommended pediatric dose for aerosolized pentamidine is 300 mg in 6 mL sterile water once a month. Children who are old enough to comply with the aerosol administration technique may benefit from the therapy, though its use has not been completely evaluated in children.

▬REFERENCES

1. Ambromowicz M (ed): Drugs for asthma. Medical Letter on Drugs and Therapeutics 37:1, 1995.
2. Barnes PJ: A new approach to the treatment of asthma. N Engl J Med 321:1517, 1989.
3. Barnes PJ: Autonomic control of airway function in asthma. Chest 5s:45s, 1991.
4. Barnhart SL, Czervinske MP: Perinatal and Pediatric Respiratory Care. Philadelphia, WB Saunders, 1995.

5. Bills GW, Soderberg RC: Principles of Pharmacology for Respiratory Care. New York, Delmar Publishers, 1994.
6. Easton PA et al: A comparison of the bronchodilating effects of beta-2 adrenergic agent (albuterol) and an anticholinergic agent (ipratropium bromide) given by aerosol alone or in sequence. N Engl J Med 315:735, 1986.
7. Fisons Pharmaceuticals, Fisons Corporation: Intal nebulizer solution package insert. Rochester, NY, January, 1992.
8. Gilman AG, Rall TW, Nies AS, Taylor P (eds): Goodman and Gilman's The Pharmacological Basis of Therapeutics. New York, Pergamon Press, 1990.
9. Gross NJ: Ipratropium bromide. N Engl J Med 319:486, 1988.
10. Higgins RM, Stradling JR, Lane DJ: Should ipratropium bromide be added to beta-agonists in treatment of acute severe asthma? Chest 94:718, 1988.
11. Hoffman BB, Lefkowitz RJ: Catecholamines and sympathomimetic drugs. In Gilman AG, Rall TW, Nies AS, Taylor P (eds): Goodman and Gilman's The Pharmacological Basis of Therapeutics, 8th ed. New York, Pergamon Press, 1990.
12. Johnson KB: Drug doses. In Johnson KB (ed): The Harriet Lane Handbook, 13th ed. St. Louis, CV Mosby, 1993.
13. Kelly HW, Hill MR: Asthma. In DiPiro JT, Talbert RL, Hayes PE, et al (eds): Pharmacotherapy: A Pathophysiologic Approach. New York, Elsevier, 1992.
14. Mann NP, Hiller EJ: Ipratropium bromide in children with asthma. Thorax 37:72, 1982.
15. Nahata MC: Pediatrics. In DiPiro JT, Talbert RL, Hayes PE, et al (eds): Pharmacotherapy: A Pathophysiologic Approach. New York, Elsevier, 1992.
16. Ramsey BW, Astley SJ, Aitken ML, et al: Efficacy and safety of short-term administration of aerosolized recombinant human deoxyribonuclease in patients with cystic fibrosis. Am Rev Respir Dis 148(1):145, 1993.
17. Rau JL Jr: Respiratory Care Pharmacology, 4th ed. St. Louis, Mosby-Year Book, 1994.
18. Roberts R: Pharmacologic approaches to the prevention and treatment of bronchopulmonary dysplasia. Respir Care 31:581, 1986.
19. Sessler CN. Theophylline toxicity: Clinical features of 116 consecutive cases. Am J Med 88:567, 1990.
20. Smith L: Childhood asthma: Diagnosis and treatment. Curr Probl Pediatr 23:271, 1993.
21. Viscardi R: Efficacy of theophylline for prevention of post-extubation respiratory failure of very low birth weight infants. J Pediatr 107:469, 1985.
22. West S et al: A review of antihistamines and the common cold. Pediatrics 56:100, 1975.
23. Witek TJ Jr, Schachter EN (eds): Pharmacology and Therapeutics in Respiratory Care. Philadelphia, WB Saunders, 1994.

SELF-ASSESSMENT QUESTIONS

1. Following a single dose, _____ half-lives must pass before the drug is considered eliminated from the body.
   a. two
   b. three
   c. five
   d. seven

2. A drug's therapeutic index is a ratio indicating
   a. safety
   b. efficacy
   c. potency
   d. intensity

3. If the average adult dose for Albuterol is 0.5 cc, utilizing Young's rule, what is the recommended dosage for a 3-year old?
   a. 0.1 cc
   b. 0.2 cc
   c. 0.3 cc
   d. 0.4 cc

4. Which of the following is the most common adverse effect of sympathomimetic bronchodilators?
   a. tachycardia
   b. palpitations
   c. hypertension
   d. skeletal muscle tremors

5. Racemic epinephrine is used in the treatment of
   a. laryngeal edema
   b. postextubation edema
   c. laryngeal tracheobronchitis stridor
   d. all of the above

6. Ipratropium bromide elicits its effect by blocking _____ receptors.
   a. β_1
   b. sympathetic
   c. parasympathetic
   d. α

7. Which of the following is not an effect produced by theophylline?
   a. bronchodilation
   b. mast cell degranulation
   c. improved diaphragmatic strength
   d. central nervous system stimulation

8. Recombinant human DNase was approved for use in patients with
   a. cystic fibrosis
   b. pneumonia
   c. respiratory distress syndrome
   d. asthma

9. In order to prevent airway hypersensitivity, _____ weeks of cromolyn sodium therapy is recommended.
   a. 1 to 2
   b. 2 to 5
   c. 4 to 8
   d. 6 to 12

10. Ribavirin is indicated in the treatment of
    a. asthma
    b. bacterial pneumonia
    c. RSV bronchiolitis
    d. cystic fibrosis

Chapter 18

Bronchial Hygiene Therapy

KIM V. HILL

OBJECTIVES

Having completed this chapter, the reader will be able to:

1 List the procedures that are included in bronchial hygiene for the newborn and child.

2 Describe the correct drainage position for each segment of the lungs.

3 Explain monitoring of the patient during drainage.

4 Describe the rationale for the use of percussion and vibration.

5 List the various types of devices that may be used for percussion and vibration in the newborn and child.

6 Describe the proper procedure for percussion and vibration in the newborn and child, including monitoring of the patient.

7 State the desired effects of chest physical therapy procedures and explain how these effects may be assessed.

8 Discuss the use of bland aerosols in the newborn and child with cardiorespiratory disease.

9 Describe the procedures used to administer aerosol therapy to the newborn and child.

10 Describe positive expiratory pressure therapy and list the indications and hazards.

11 Describe autogenic drainage and its application in children.

12 Describe a flutter valve device and its application in children.

13 Describe the use of incentive spirometry and intermittent positive pressure breathing for pediatric patients.

KEY TERMS

autogenic drainage	percussion
dry powder inhaler	postural drainage
flutter valve	small particle aerosol generator
positive expiratory (PEP) therapy	vibration

Bronchial hygiene therapy refers to the procedures used to prevent and treat the accumulation of secretions in the airways of the infant and child and to aid in the maintenance of airway patency. Specific measures used to accomplish these goals include various techniques of chest physical therapy (positioning or postural drainage, percussion of the chest wall, and vibration of the chest wall), administration of bland aerosol solutions to loosen secretions, administration of pharmacologic aerosols to either thin secretions or promote bronchodilation by relaxing bronchial smooth muscle, positive expiratory pressure therapy, and inflation therapy. There is much controversy regarding the most effective and least harmful methods of chest physical therapy and the efficacy of various bland and pharmacologic aerosols. Specific procedures vary from region to region and even among institutions in proximity to one another, with little scientific rationale for any particular mode of therapy. Recent advances in the continuous monitoring of the child's cardiopulmonary status using pulse oximeters and transcutaneous monitors have helped to identify procedures that may be unduly stressful to the newborn and child. Careful evaluation of the effectiveness of these procedures in infants and children is of utmost importance and should guide their use.

In infants and children with normal lung pathology, clearance of secretions is the result of two processes: mucociliary clearance and cough.[11] The mucociliary escalator moves secretions toward the larger airways where they can be removed by effective coughing procedures. In order to cough effectively, the patient must be able to take a deep breath and generate sufficient gas flow during expiration.

Various pulmonary disorders can cause alterations in these normal clearance mechanisms. In cystic fibrosis, for example, the solute concentration in mucus is altered as a result of increased sodium reabsorption and decreased chloride secretion on the surface of the respiratory epithelium.[10] This leads to drying of the ciliary layer so that mucus transport is reduced.[11] Abnormalities of the ciliary system, called dyskinetic cilia syndromes, are also possible, leading to further reductions in mucus clearance.[13]

A decreased ability to cough may result from damage to the airway, such as in asthma or infection. In postoperative or trauma patients, pain during breathing will also decrease the ability or willingness of the patient to take the deep breaths necessary for the cough to be effective. Deep breathing can also be limited by neuromuscular conditions, such as muscular dystrophy, cerebral palsy, or poliomyelitis.

The procedures used to provide bronchial hygiene for infants and children include chest physical therapy, positive expiratory pressure therapy, autogenic drainage, and the use of flutter valves. Bronchial hygiene therapy should always be followed by coughing; suctioning of the airway may be necessary if the patient cannot cough effectively. Aerosol therapy and inflation therapy will also be discussed in this chapter, as they are valuable in achieving and maintaining bronchial hygiene.

■CHEST PHYSICAL THERAPY

The techniques of chest physical therapy (CPT) are designed to use specific positioning of the patient to drain the various segments of the lungs and percussion and vibration of the chest wall in an attempt to mobilize secretions into the larger airways, where they can be removed by coughing or suctioning. The goal of CPT is to increase the mobilization and removal of secretions.[19] Patients who benefit the most from CPT include children with cystic fibrosis and bronchiectasis, although patients with asthma, pneumonia, bronchiolitis, and neuromuscular conditions, as well as postoperative patients, may receive CPT for specific episodes of secretion retention or reduced cough effectiveness.[19]

Postural Drainage

Specific positioning of the patient to enlist gravity in facilitating secretion removal is referred to as **postural drainage**. This approach relies on a thorough knowledge of the anatomy of the airways and lungs. Drainage positions for the various segments and lobes are illustrated in Figure 18-1. The decision about which segments and lobes should be drained is based upon physical findings and the chest x-ray film whenever possible.

Postural drainage should begin with drainage of the affected areas, followed by prophylactic drainage of the remaining segments if time and the patient's condition allow. When postural drainage is accompanied by percussion and vibration, each segment should be treated for 2 to 5 minutes.[14,19] If percussion and vibration are contraindicated or not tolerated by the patient, each segment should be drained for up to 15 minutes.[2] While positioned for postural drainage, the patient's vital signs should be carefully monitored and the patient should be observed for any signs of breathing difficulty, including skin color, use of accessory muscles, or retractions. The use of continuous monitoring devices such as pulse oximeters and the EKG can assist in evaluation of the patient's tolerance of each procedure and position. At the conclusion of the therapy session, sputum production and breath sounds should be carefully evaluated.

Percussion

In addition to placing the child in various drainage positions, some attempt is usually made to accelerate movement of secretions into the major airways to increase the rate of removal of the secretions from the lungs through gravity drainage. The two techniques used to loosen secretions are referred to as percussion and vibration. **Percussion**, which is also referred to as *cupping* or *clapping*, involves striking the chest wall over the area to be drained with some device that will trap air between itself and the chest wall. This allows a force to be applied to the chest without directly striking the chest wall with a flat surface, which is very likely to cause injury and discomfort.

In pediatric patients, the cupped hand is commonly used to apply percussion to the chest wall (Fig. 18-2). Care should be taken not to percuss over the spine, sternum, abdomen, lower ribs, sutured areas, drainage tubes, kidneys, or liver.[14] The objective is to create a "popping" sound while percussing the chest, generating a percussive wave which travels through the chest wall to loosen secretions. It takes practice to develop the right technique; continuous communication with the patient will assist the practitioner in finding a method that is effective and avoids injury.

In the infant, the chest cage is so small that direct percussion with the practitioner's hand is usually difficult, and various devices have been developed to substitute for the cupped-hand technique. Many institutions have devised their own "percussors," such as medication cups with the rim

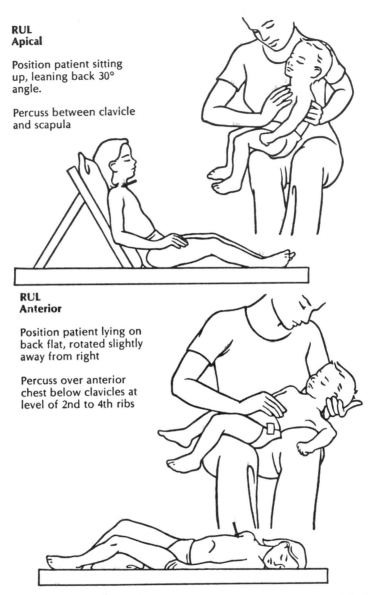

RUL
Apical

Position patient sitting
up, leaning back 30°
angle.

Percuss between clavicle
and scapula

RUL
Anterior

Position patient lying on
back flat, rotated slightly
away from right

Percuss over anterior
chest below clavicles at
level of 2nd to 4th ribs

FIGURE 18-1   Postural drainage positions for infants and children. (Blodgett D: Manual of Pediatric Respiratory Care Procedures. Philadelphia, JB Lippincott, 1982.) (*Continues.*)

padded, resuscitation masks with the bag connection occluded, bulb syringes cut in half and padded, and rubber feeding nipples. Mechanical percussors are also available, as are commercial variations of the "padded cup." One example of the commercial variety is the Palm Cup (DHD Medical Products, Canastota, NY), which is illustrated in Figure 18-3. These devices are available in various sizes, the smallest of which works quite well on the newborn chest.

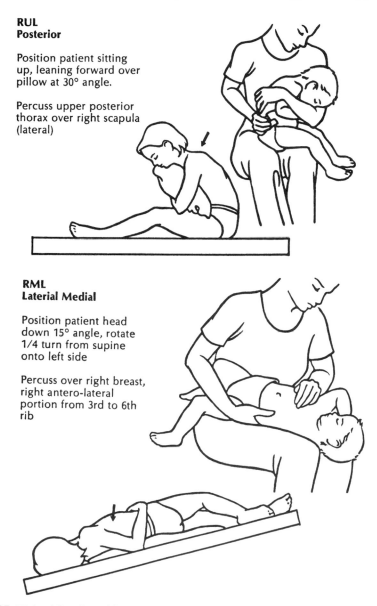

RUL
Posterior

Position patient sitting up, leaning forward over pillow at 30° angle.

Percuss upper posterior thorax over right scapula (lateral)

RML
Lateral Medial

Position patient head down 15° angle, rotate 1/4 turn from supine onto left side

Percuss over right breast, right antero-lateral portion from 3rd to 6th rib

FIGURE 18-1   (Continued.)

Percussion should not be viewed as a routine or harmless technique to be applied indiscriminately in the treatment of newborns and children with cardiorespiratory disorders. Patients who are critically ill and unstable will not usually tolerate this technique. Stabilization of the acute disease process should be the first priority in these patients. Once stabilization has been achieved, percussion may be very helpful in the treatment of retained secretions, bronchitis and bronchiolitis, atelectasis, or pneumonia.

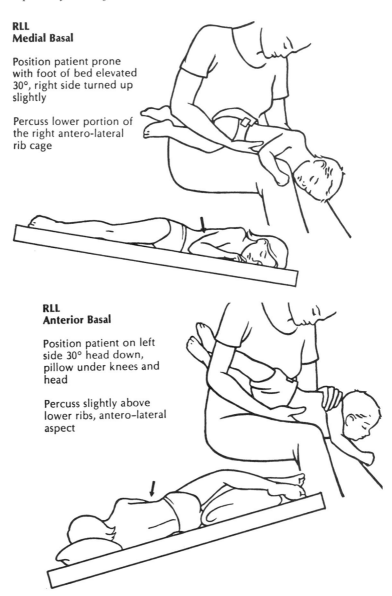

**RLL
Medial Basal**

Position patient prone with foot of bed elevated 30°, right side turned up slightly

Percuss lower portion of the right antero-lateral rib cage

**RLL
Anterior Basal**

Position patient on left side 30° head down, pillow under knees and head

Percuss slightly above lower ribs, antero–lateral aspect

FIGURE 18-1   (Continued.)

Vibration

Vibration refers to rapid movement of the chest wall rather than distinct clapping or percussion. Several techniques are useful in performing vibration, including placing the fingertips on the chest wall, tensing the muscles of the forearm, and rapidly vibrating the fingertips (Fig. 18-4). Vibration is applied only during the expiratory phase of each breath, so that movement of secretions may be enhanced by expiratory air flow. An older child can be asked to "hiss" or use pursed-lip breathing during exhalation to prolong the expiratory time. Vibration should be performed during three or four

RLL
Lateral Basal

Position patient lying on abdomen rotate 1/4 to left, 30° head down

Percuss right lateral thorax at level of 8th rib.

RLL
Posterior Basal

Position patient lying prone with head down 30°, pillow under hips

Percuss just above 11th to 12th rib on right posteriorly

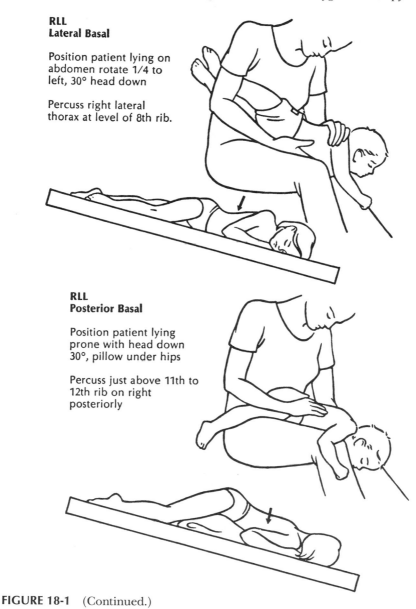

FIGURE 18-1   (Continued.)

breaths following drainage and/or percussion of each lung segment. Mechanical vibrating devices are also available, and electric toothbrushes are a common substitute seen in many neonatal intensive care units.

Modification of Chest Physical Therapy Procedures
In some situations, postural drainage, percussion, and vibration should be modified in order to avoid the complications and hazards that have been associated with these procedures (Table 18-1). CPT should be coordinated with other therapy, such as aerosol bronchodilators or inflation therapy, for

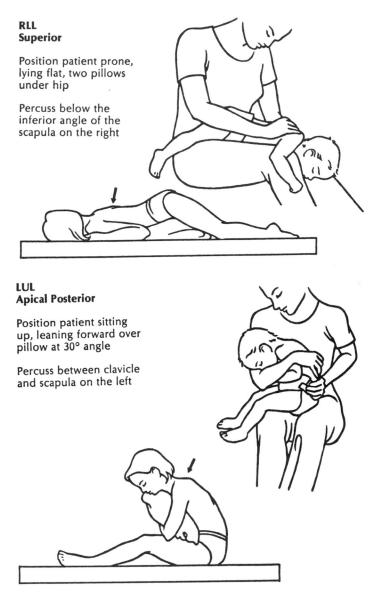

RLL
Superior

Position patient prone, lying flat, two pillows under hip

Percuss below the inferior angle of the scapula on the right

LUL
Apical Posterior

Position patient sitting up, leaning forward over pillow at 30° angle

Percuss between clavicle and scapula on the left

FIGURE 18-1 (Continued.)

maximum effectiveness. The use of sedatives or analgesics will also improve the patient's tolerance for painful or uncomfortable positions. The duration of therapy will depend upon the patient's condition and his or her ability to tolerate the procedure. Some patients may require periods of rest between drainage positions, or the therapy sessions can be divided into shorter time periods. The practitioner should reassure the child both before and during therapy in order to reduce anxiety.

Percussion may be extremely painful following surgery or insertion of drainage tubes. In these cases, postural drainage alone may be beneficial

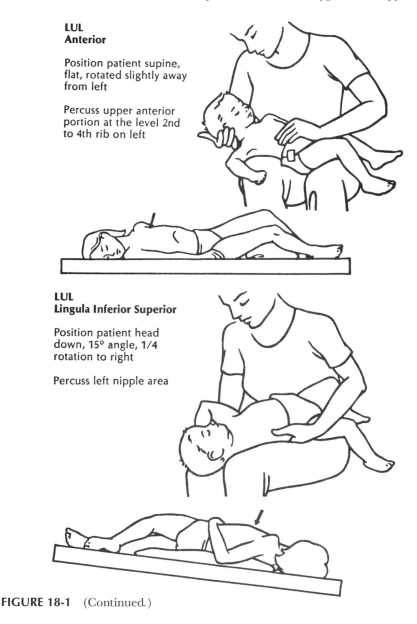

LUL
Anterior

Position patient supine, flat, rotated slightly away from left

Percuss upper anterior portion at the level 2nd to 4th rib on left

LUL
Lingula Inferior Superior

Position patient head down, 15° angle, 1/4 rotation to right

Percuss left nipple area

FIGURE 18-1 (Continued.)

in improving secretion clearance. Mechanical vibration devices are often better tolerated than direct percussion with the practitioner's hands.

Many patients may not tolerate the Trendelenburg position required for draining certain segments of the lower lobes. This includes patients with gastroesophageal reflux, recent intracranial trauma or surgery, increased intracranial pressure, abdominal distention, hypertension, and cardiopulmonary failure.[14] The bed can be left flat and supplemental oxygen administered to improve their tolerance. CPT should also be avoided for 1 to 2 hours after meals or feedings.

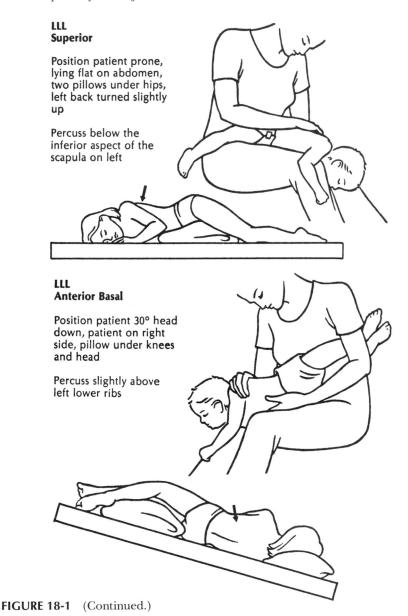

LLL
Superior

Position patient prone, lying flat on abdomen, two pillows under hips, left back turned slightly up

Percuss below the inferior aspect of the scapula on left

LLL
Anterior Basal

Position patient 30° head down, patient on right side, pillow under knees and head

Percuss slightly above left lower ribs

FIGURE 18-1 (Continued.)

Evaluating the Effectiveness of Chest Physical Therapy

The major desired effects of CPT techniques include an increase in removal of secretions, improvement of ventilation and oxygenation, and improvement of atelectasis and pneumonia. Although there is not clear consensus about the effectiveness of CPT or evidence of superiority of one method over another, careful evaluation of the effectiveness of the procedure in each patient is necessary.[2,7] Chest physiotherapy has been shown to improve pulmonary function and increase mucus clearance in some patients, while other studies have shown no significant advantage to

LLL
Lateral Basal

Position patient lying on
abdomen, head down
30°, rotate 1/4 onto right

Percuss left lateral thorax
at 8th rib level

LLL
Posterior Basal

Position patient lying
prone, 30° head down,
pillow under hips

Percuss just above 11th
and 12th ribs on left

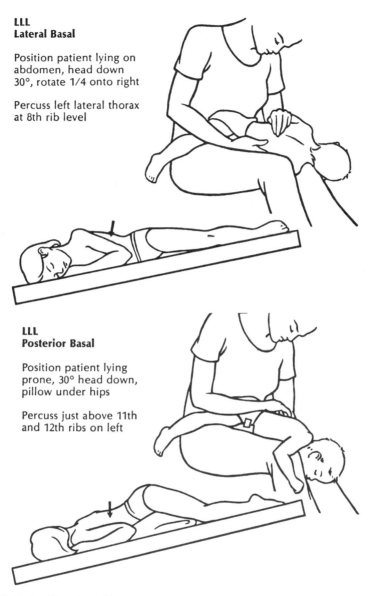

FIGURE 18-1 (Continued.)

CPT over other forms of therapy.[8] CPT is indicated for and seems beneficial in cystic fibrosis and following extubation in neonates, and it may offer some benefit in asthma, bronchitis, bronchiectasis, and atelectasis. It does not appear to be of benefit in pneumonia or bronchiolitis or in the routine care of postoperative patients.[8]

The American Association for Respiratory Care (AARC) Clinical Practice Guideline for Postural Drainage Therapy recommends that each patient be evaluated to determine the need for and effectiveness of CPT (Table 18-2). Careful assessment of the response of the infant and child

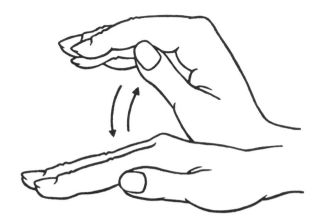

FIGURE 18-2 Hand position used for percussion of the chest in pediatric patients. (Blodgett D: Manual of Pediatric Respiratory Care Procedures. Philadelphia, JB Lippincott, 1982.)

to CPT will help to avoid indiscriminate and inappropriate use of this modality. CPT should only be ordered when a clear indication exists and the practitioner can document an improvement in the patient following therapy.

Autogenic Drainage

Autogenic drainage (AD) is a series of controlled breathing exercises designed to improve mucus clearance, particularly in patients with cystic fibrosis and bronchiectasis.[11] The patient begins by breathing at low lung volumes (in the expiratory reserve volume [ERV] range) in order to loosen secretions from the small airways. The volume of ventilation is then increased, with the patient breathing within the normal tidal volume range but exhaling into the ERV range. Breathing at this ventilating volume helps to collect secretions in the middle-size airways. Finally, the patient breathes at high lung volumes (above tidal volume) to expel the secretions.

While this particular approach to bronchial hygiene does not require any additional equipment, it does involve considerable teaching and coaching by respiratory care practitioners. The patient must be able to control his or her breathing at the various lung volumes; different forms of biofeedback have been developed to facilitate this.[11] Patients are generally able to perform the procedure with regular practice. Since no equipment or medication is needed, the exercises can be done safely and frequently in outpatient settings.

Flutter Valves

The **flutter valve** device was developed in Switzerland and combines positive expiratory pressure therapy with high-frequency oscillations at the airway opening.[11] The device (Fig. 18-5) consists of a tube with a loosely supported steel ball at one end which is covered by a perforated cap. The patient exhales into the tube, generating a positive expiratory pressure of 10 to 25 cm H_2O. During exhalation, the ball flutters in the tube, creating oscillations which are transmitted back to the airways. The patient is

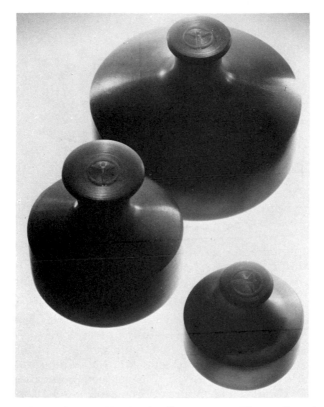

FIGURE 18-3 Several sizes of "Palm Cup" percussors. The smallest size is suitable for use in the newborn. (Courtesy DHD Medical, Canastota, NY.)

able to control the pressure and oscillations. The positive expiratory pressure and oscillations help to facilitate removal of secretions.

▄AEROSOL THERAPY

Aerosol therapy is indicated for humidification of the tracheobronchial tree, for bronchial hygiene therapy, and for delivering medications.[9] It is essential to provide adequate humidification of inspired gases to the infant and pediatric patient, especially in intubated patients, since the upper airway has been bypassed. Heated humidifiers, such as cascade or wick types that provide 100% relative humidity, are excellent for providing humidity to the infant and pediatric patient. Aerosol generators, particularly high-volume aerosols such as those produced by ultrasonic nebulizers, can provide a significant amount of fluid to the infant, and the risk of fluid overload with these devices is considerable. Therefore, caution should be taken when using aerosol generators and they should only be used if a substantial liquid volume or medication deposition is required.[9]

Effective delivery of aerosolized medications depends upon the delivery device and its location relative to the patient. Aerosol particle size, the patient's ventilatory pattern, and upper airway anatomy all influence

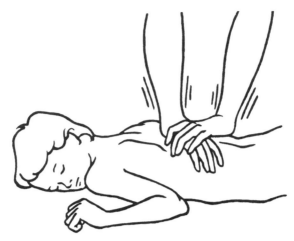

FIGURE 18-4   Technique for performing vibration of the chest wall. (Blodgett D: Manual of Pediatric Respiratory Care Procedures. Philadelphia, JB Lippincott, 1982.)

aerosol deposition in the patient's airway.[6] The AARC has developed Clinical Practice Guidelines (CPGs) to assist the practitioner in selecting the proper delivery device for the neonatal and pediatric patient. Selecting the appropriate delivery device is essential for the administration of bland and therapeutic aerosols. Factors such as patient cooperation, coordination, and understanding all play an important role in selection of the most appropriate device.[6]

According to the AARC Clinical Practice Guidelines, there are four types of aerosol generators: small volume nebulizers, large-volume nebulizers, metered dose inhalers, and dry powered inhalers.

A small volume nebulizer (SVN) or jet nebulizer is a device that is powered by a 50 psig gas source or compressor that utilizes the Bernoulli prin-

---

TABLE 18-1   Hazards and Complications of Chest Physical Therapy

Hypoxemia

Increased intracranial pressure

Acute hypotension during procedure

Pulmonary hemorrhage

Pain or injury to muscles, ribs, or spine

Vomiting and aspiration

Bronchospasm

Dysrhythmias

(American Association for Respiratory Care Clinical Practice Guideline: Postural drainage therapy. Resp Care 36:1418, 1991.)

TABLE 18-2   Assessment of Need and Outcome of Chest Physical Therapy

ASSESSMENT OF NEED	ASSESSMENT OF OUTCOME
Excessive sputum production	Change in sputum production
Effectiveness of cough	Patient subjective response to therapy
History of pulmonary problems treated successfully with CPT	Change in ventilator variables suggesting improved compliance and resistance
Decreased breath sounds, crackles, rhonchi	Change in breath sounds
Change in vital signs	Change in vital signs
Abnormal chest x-ray film consistent with atelectasis, mucus plugging, or infiltrates	Change in chest x-ray film
Deterioration in arterial blood gas values or oxygen saturation	Change in arterial blood gas values or oxygen saturation

(American Association for Respiratory Care Clinical Practice Guideline: Postural drainage therapy. Resp Care 36:1418, 1991.)

ciple to produce an aerosol. This device has a small reservoir for medication and is connected to the gas source with small-bore tubing. For children older than 3 years of age, the aerosol is inhaled by the patient through a mouthpiece and flexible reservoir tubing. A face mask is recommended for children younger than 3 years of age.[6]

A large volume nebulizer (LVN) is used to deliver large volumes of aerosol continuously over an extended period of time. LVNs are powered by a 50 psig gas source or compressor, usually in conjunction with an aerosol mask, tracheostomy collar, or face tent.[6] The use of LVN in the neonatal intensive care unit should be prohibited, especially in conjunction with oxygen hoods, because the sound levels produced with these devices can be damaging to the infant's ears and lead to hearing loss.[16]

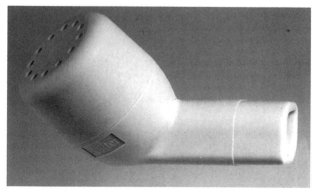

FIGURE 18-5   FLUTTER valve device. (Courtesy of VarioRaw, a subsidiary of Scandipharm, Inc.)

A metered dose inhaler (MDI), or "puffer," is a device that incorporates both medication and a propellant in a small canister to provide an aerosol. Proper use of an MDI requires that the aerosol be discharged at the beginning of inspiration and inhaled by the patient. In infants and pediatric patients, this is a challenging procedure. Special spacer devices with one-way valves have been developed especially for the pediatric patient for administering medication by MDI. These devices incorporate a holding chamber similar to that used with the adult patient, except that a mask is attached to the end to help administer more of the drug to the child. Spacer/holding chambers enhance delivery of the aerosol by providing a reservoir and help decrease the velocity of the aerosols and particle size discharged from the MDI. Spacers also eliminate the need for coordination of inspiration and simultaneous actuation of the MDI and increase delivery of medication to the patient. These devices are appropriate for use in patients younger than 3 years of age who are unable to use a mouthpiece. Each discharge from the MDI provides one dose of the medication contained within the canister.[6]

Dry powder inhalers (DPI) are breath-initiated devices that utilize capsules containing a single dose of a drug, along with a carrier substance to aid in the delivery of the medication. The capsule is placed inside a spinhaler or rotohaler and punctured, and the patient is then instructed to inhale. Their inspiratory flow rate draws the dry powder from the device into the airway. This device is recommended for use in children who have inspiratory flow rates greater than 50 L/min and are 6 years of age and older.[6]

The **small particle aerosol generator** (SPAG) is a jet nebulizer that produces an aerosol with a particle size of approximately 1.3 microns. It is designed specifically for delivery of the antiviral agent ribavirin (Virazole). The SPAG unit includes a nebulizer and drying chamber, each with a flowmeter. The flowmeter for the nebulizer should be set between 6 and 10 L/min and the drying chamber flow set between 3 and 8 L/min. The pressure regulator should be set to 25 psig. Ribavirin can be delivered by mask, oxyhood, or mist tent, or inline with a ventilator circuit.

Caution should be taken with administration of this drug because of the possibility of harmful side effects. Ribavirin is teratogenic in small mammals. This risk is of concern to health care workers. The drug should be administered with a scavenging system. A scavenging system is one that includes a double enclosure where two high-flow vacuum systems aspirate ribavirin from the system through high-efficiency particulate air filters and remove it from the environment.[12]

Equipment and Administration

All aerosolized drugs are administered with SVNs, which are powered from a flowmeter that may be attached to any 50 psig gas source. They may also be powered from a small compressor. Whenever possible, they should be attached to a blender for precise control of inspired oxygen. Using oxygen as a nebulization source may result in the administration of excessive oxygen concentration, which has been shown to have toxic effects even for short periods of time in premature infants. Using air as a power source may result in hypoxemia during the treatment. Aerosolization of the drugs should occur within 5 to 10 minutes. Liquid output of these nebulizers is low, and intermittent use should not result in significant addition of fluid to the infant.

Bland Aerosol Therapy

Intermittent bland aerosol therapy finds little use in the treatment of the newborn. It is, of course, essential that adequate humidification of inspired gas be achieved, particularly if the infant is intubated. A heated humidifier, such as a cascade- or wick-type, is best suited to supply the humidity needed. Aerosols, particularly high-volume aerosols such as those produced by ultrasonic nebulizers, can provide a significant amount of fluid to the infant, and the risk of fluid overload with these devices is appreciable. Adequate humidification of inspired gas should alleviate the need for bland aerosol therapy to facilitate secretion removal in the infant and child.

Bland aerosol administration, including the delivery of sterile water or hypotonic, isotonic, or hypertonic saline, may have some beneficial effects in the treatment of the neonatal and pediatric patient.

According to the AARC Clinical Practice Guidelines, indications for bland aerosol administration include laryngotracheal bronchitis, subglottic edema, postextubation edema, preoperative management of the upper airway, presence of a bypassed upper airway, and the need for sputum induction.[5]

Bland aerosol therapy should be avoided if the patient has bronchoconstriction or any history of upper airway hyperresponsiveness, because the side effects associated with therapy may produce bronchospasm.[5] Hazards associated with the use of bland aerosols are listed in Table 18-3.

The effectiveness of bland aerosols as mucolytic agents has not been established, and they should not be considered substitutions for humidification or hydration.[5] Care should also be taken when delivering bland aerosol therapy, as aerosols have the potential for carrying microorganisms that can be transported into the respiratory tract, thereby increasing the patient's risk for pulmonary infections.[9]

■POSITIVE EXPIRATORY PRESSURE THERAPY

Positive expiratory pressure (PEP) therapy is a technique used for bronchial hygiene that aids in the mobilization of secretions from the airway in patients with large volumes of sputum production (greater than 30 mL per day).[15] PEP mask therapy was developed in the 1970s and has been introduced in the United States as an alternative to chest percussion and drainage. Some researchers even suggest that PEP therapy is more effective than incentive spirometry and intermittent positive pressure breathing

---

TABLE 18-3   Hazards Associated With the Use of Bland Aerosol Therapy

Wheezing or bronchospasm

Bronchoconstriction when artificial airway is employed

Infection

Overhydration

Patient discomfort

Caregiver exposure to droplet nuclei of potentially infectious organisms

---

(American Association for Respiratory Care Clinical Practice Guideline: Bland aerosol administration. Resp Care 38:1196, 1993.)

TABLE 18-4   Steps for Performing PEP Mask Therapy

1. Assemble equipment, select appropriate expiratory resistor.
2. Sit with elbows resting comfortably on table, with mask applied tightly but comfortably over nose and mouth.
3. Use diaphragmatic breathing, take in a larger-than-normal breath but not to TLC.
4. Exhale actively but not forcefully, maintaining a PEP of 10 to 20 cm H_2O. Exhalation should be about 2 to 3 times longer than inspiration.
5. Perform 10 to 20 PEP breaths, then remove mask and perform 2 to 3 "huff" coughs.
6. Cough to raise secretions as needed.
7. Repeat steps 2 to 6 several times (4 to 8 times) for a complete PEP session.

(Mahlmeister MJ, Fink JB, Hoffman GL, Fifer LF: Positive-expiratory-pressure mask therapy: Theoretical and practical considerations and a review of the literature. Resp Care 36:1218, 1991.)

in cases of postoperative atelectasis. It also can be used in conjunction with aerosol bronchodilators.[15]

PEP therapy is administered using a transparent mask, a t-piece with a one-way valve, an adjustable fixed-orifice expiratory resistor capable of developing 10 to 20 cm H_2O during passive exhalation, and an inline manometer to monitor airway pressure during therapy (Fig. 18-6). The patient is instructed to inspire a larger-than-normal tidal volume through the one-way valve and exhale against the expiratory resistor. The patient should perform 10 to 20 breaths, remove the mask, and then perform a series of huff coughs to expectorate secretions. The steps in performing PEP mask therapy are listed in Table 18-4.

Huff coughing involves a modified forced expiratory technique (FET) that is accomplished by exhaling moderate to high lung volumes through an open glottis. The patient should be instructed to take a slow, deep breath with a 1 to 3 second breath hold, and then perform short, quick, forced exhalations with the glottis open.[15]

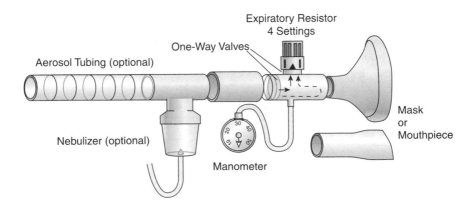

FIGURE 18-6   Mask system for PEP therapy.

TABLE 18-5 Indications for PEP Therapy

To reduce air trapping in asthma and COPD

To aid in mobilization of retained secretions (in cystic fibrosis and chronic bronchitis)

To prevent or reverse atelectasis

To optimize delivery of bronchodilators in patients receiving bronchial hygiene therapy

(American Association for Respiratory Care Clinical Practice Guideline: Use of positive airway pressure adjuncts to bronchial hygiene therapy. Resp Care 38:516, 1993.)

The indications for PEP therapy are listed in Table 18-5. There are no absolute contraindications to the use of PEP therapy, however, practitioners should evaluate each patient individually for the onset of side effects or hazards that could potentially develop from the administration of PEP therapy. Patients should be evaluated for the ability to tolerate an increased work of breathing; the presence of elevated intracranial pressure; hemodynamic stability; recent facial, oral, or skull surgery or trauma; or acute sinusitis.[3] The hazards of PEP therapy are listed in Table 18-6.

Considerations in Administering PEP Therapy

An appropriate-sized resistor is very important for proper technique and delivery of the treatment. A therapeutic goal of 10 to 20 cm H_2O and exhalation with an I:E ratio of 1:3 or 1:4 is desirable. Most patients can achieve these goals with resistors with a diameter of 2.5 to 4.0 mm. Care should be taken not to administer PEP therapy during periods of disease exacerbation. It is better to increase the frequency of the therapy rather than the duration. PEP therapy performed longer than 20 minutes can lead to fatigue. Aerosol therapy by SVN or MDI can be administered immediately before or in conjunction with PEP therapy to enhance secretion mobilization.

PEP therapy is an alternative method of secretion mobilization that can be utilized when risks prevent chest percussion and drainage from being per-

TABLE 18-6 Hazards of PEP Therapy

Increased work of breathing that may lead to hypoventilation and hypercarbia

Increased intracranial pressure

Cardiovascular compromise

  Myocardial ischemia

  Decreased venous return

Air swallowing, with increased likelihood of vomiting and aspiration

Claustrophobia

Skin breakdown and discomfort from mask

Pulmonary barotrauma

(American Association for Respiratory Care Clinical Practice Guideline: Use of positive airway pressure adjuncts to bronchial hygiene therapy. Resp Care 38:516, 1993.)

formed or tolerated. PEP therapy has fewer limitations than CPT and can be easily performed by the patient with proper training. Patients with cystic fibrosis can benefit greatly from this therapy because it can be self-administered and also done in the home with other bronchial hygiene therapy.

▬ INCENTIVE SPIROMETRY

Incentive spirometry (IS) has been used for lung expansion for many years. IS, or sustained maximal inspiration (SMI), was designed to mimic the naturally occurring sighs inherent in everyone. The patient is encouraged to take slow, deep breaths using devices that provide visual reinforcement for the patient, followed by a 3- to 5-second breath hold. This therapy promotes good breathing.

The objectives of IS are to increase transpulmonary pressure, increase inspiratory volumes, improve inspiratory muscle performance, and simulate pulmonary hyperinflation so that airway patency can be maintained. It is also useful in preventing and reversing atelectasis.[1]

Indications

The primary indication for IS is to treat atelectasis, but it is also advantageous in the prevention of atelectasis in cases of abdominal and thoracic surgeries and major surgeries that require general anesthesia. Patients with neuromuscular disease or dysfunctional diaphragms may also benefit from the use of IS.[18] The indications for IS are listed in Table 18-7.

Contraindications, Hazards, and Complications

IS is contraindicated in patients who cannot cooperate or be instructed or supervised in the appropriate use of the device. IS is also contraindicated in patients with an inadequate vital capacity (less than 10 mL/kg) or inspiratory capacity (less than one third of predicted value).[1] For IS to be effective in the pediatric population, the child must be able to cooperate and understand the procedure to accomplish breathing goals that exceed the child's normal tidal volume.[17]

IS can be ineffective for many patients who are not closely supervised. Hyperinflation, barotrauma, and discomfort from poor pain control can all occur with unsupervised therapy. These hazards can be avoided by proper teaching and supervision of the therapy by a trained practitioner.[17] Hypoxia caused by interruption of oxygen therapy may occur, but this can be prevented by use of a nasal cannula during therapy. Fatigue can be avoided by proper instruction and patient coaching.[17] Exacerbation of bronchospasm can be prevented by pretreatment with a bronchodilator.

Assessment of Therapy

Documentation for IS is very similar to documentation for all therapy and should include date, time, vital signs, breath sounds, inspired volume or flow achieved, number of goals achieved, cough and sputum production, patient tolerance, and any adverse reactions. IS is considered to be effective if atelectasis is prevented or reversed and improved inspiratory muscle performance is achieved.[17] Specific signs of improvement include decreased respiratory rate, resolution of fever, normal heart rate, absence of crackles,

TABLE 18-7 Indications for Incentive Spirometry

Presence of conditions predisposing to the development of pulmonary atelectasis

    Upper-abdominal surgery

    Thoracic surgery

    Surgery in patients with COPD

Presence of pulmonary atelectasis

Presence of a restrictive lung defect associated with quadriplegia or dysfunctional diaphragm

(American Association for Respiratory Care Clinical Practice Guideline: Incentive spirometry. Resp Care 36:1402, 1991.)

improvement of previously absent or diminished breath sounds, normal chest x-ray film, and improved oxygenation and lung volumes.[1]

Equipment

There are several different brands of incentive spirometers. Most of these devices are disposable, but a few nondisposable units are available. Each IS device is either volume oriented or flow oriented. Volume-oriented devices, in which a goal is determined and the patient inhales until the preset volume is met, are the most commonly used. Flow-oriented devices incorporate a float or ball mechanism in which the patient's peak inspiratory flow rate must be sufficient to raise the ball or float. This can be difficult for some patients, thus accounting for the popularity of volume-oriented devices. Although there are differences in the orientation of the devices, there is no clinical evidence that supports the preference of one type over another.[1]

■ INTERMITTENT POSITIVE PRESSURE BREATHING

Intermittent positive pressure breathing (IPPB) is used for short-term treatment or intermittent mechanical ventilation for improving lung expansion, delivering medications, and assisting ventilation.[4]

Indications

In the past, IPPB has been given for a broad range of clinical conditions, even without clinical evidence supporting its use. IPPB subsequently became a misused and overused treatment modality and, because of this, there are some negative connotations associated with it. In 1980, the Respiratory Care Committee of the American Thoracic Society developed guidelines for the use of IPPB in certain clinical situations. More recently, the AARC developed Clinical Practice Guidelines describing the specific use and indications for IPPB. Clearly, IPPB should not be used for all patients, but it can be very beneficial when indicated.[18]

In pediatric patients, the hazards and complications that could develop from administration of IPPB make this an unpopular choice and ineffective therapy. Therefore, IPPB is not widely used for these patients.[17] The specific indications for IPPB are listed in Table 18-8.

TABLE 18-8 Indications for IPPB

Need to improve lung expansion

   Presence of atelectasis unresponsive to other therapy

   Inability to clear secretions

Need for short-term ventilatory support

Need to deliver aerosol medication

(American Association for Respiratory Care Clinical Practice Guideline: Intermittent positive pressure breathing. Resp Care 38:1189, 1993.)

Contraindications and Hazards

The only absolute contraindication for IPPB therapy is the presence of an untreated pneumothorax. Other situations should also be carefully evaluated before instituting IPPB therapy, including an intracranial pressure greater than 15 mm Hg; unstable hemodynamic values; recent facial, oral, or skull surgery; tracheoesophageal fistula; recent esophageal surgery; hemoptysis; nausea; air swallowing; active tuberculosis; radiographic evidence of pulmonary blebs; and hiccups.[4] The complications and hazards associated with the administration of IPPB are listed in Table 18-9.

Special Considerations in Pediatric Patients

The respiratory care practitioner should thoroughly explain the procedure and equipment to the patient prior to beginning therapy to alleviate any fears or apprehension. The therapist should also demonstrate how the machine will operate during the treatment and allow the child to hear the sounds made by the machine itself.

Monitoring IPPB Therapy

The child should be closely monitored and supervised during each treatment. Vital signs and breath sounds should be documented before, during, and after each treatment. The goal of IPPB therapy is to generate tidal volumes at least 25% greater than the patient's spontaneous volume.

TABLE 18-9 Complications and Hazards of IPPB

Increased airway resistance	Impaction of secretions
Barotrauma, pneumothorax	Psychological dependence
Nosocomial infections	Impedance of venous return
Hypocarbia	Exacerbation of hypoxemia
Hemoptysis	Hypoventilation
Hyperoxia with O_2 as gas source	Mismatch of ventilation and perfusion
Gastric distention	Airtrapping, auto-PEEP, overdistended alveoli

(American Association for Respiratory Care Clinical Practice Guideline: Intermittent positive pressure breathing. Resp Care 38:1189, 1993.)

Exhaled volume should be evaluated before and during therapy. If the volume delivered with IPPB is no greater than the child's spontaneous volume, the therapy is of little use and should be discontinued.[17]

REFERENCES

1. American Association for Respiratory Care Clinical Practice Guideline: Incentive spirometry. Resp Care 36:1402, 1991.
2. American Association for Respiratory Care Clinical Practice Guideline: Postural drainage therapy. Resp Care 36:1418, 1991.
3. American Association for Respiratory Care Clinical Practice Guideline: Use of positive airway pressure adjuncts to bronchial hygiene therapy. Resp Care 38:516, 1993.
4. American Association for Respiratory Care Clinical Practice Guideline: Intermittent positive pressure breathing. Resp Care 38:1189, 1993.
5. American Association for Respiratory Care Clinical Practice Guideline: Bland aerosol administration. Resp Care 38:1196, 1993.
6. American Association for Respiratory Care Clinical Practice Guideline: Selection of an aerosol delivery device for neonatal and pediatric patients. Resp Care 40:1325, 1995.
7. Andersen JB, Falk M: Chest physiotherapy in the pediatric age group. Resp Care 36:546, 1991.
8. Eid N, Buchheit J, Neuling M, Phelps H: Chest physiotherapy in review. Resp Care 36:270, 1991.
9. Fink JB, Jue PK: Humidity and aerosol therapy for pediatrics. In Barnhart SL, Czervinske MP (eds): Perinatal and Pediatric Respiratory Care. Philadelphia, WB Saunders, 1995.
10. Hardy KA: Advances in our understanding and care of patients with cystic fibrosis. Resp Care 38:282, 1993.
11. Hardy KA: A review of airway clearance: New techniques, indications, and recommendations. Resp Care 39:440, 1994.
12. Hess DR, Branson RD: Humidification: Humidifiers and nebulizers. In Branson RD, Hess DR, Chatburn RL (eds): Respiratory Care Equipment. Philadelphia, JB Lippincott, 1995.
13. Le Mauviel L: Primary ciliary dyskinesia. West J Med 155:280, 1991.
14. Lewis R: Chest physical therapy. In Barnhart SL, Czervinske MP (eds): Perinatal and Pediatric Respiratory Care. Philadelphia, WB Saunders, 1995.
15. Mahlmeister MJ, Fink JB, Hoffman GL, Fifer LF: Positive-expiratory-pressure mask therapy: Theoretical and practical considerations and a review of the literature. Resp Care 36:1218, 1991.
16. Mishoe SC, Brooks CW Jr, Dennison FH, Hill KV, Frye T: Octave waveband analysis to determine sound frequencies and intensities produced by nebulizers and humidifiers used with hoods. Resp Care 40:1120, 1995.
17. Rosen HK: Lung volume expansion therapy. In Barnhart SL, Czervinske MP (eds): Perinatal and Pediatric Respiratory Care. Philadelphia, WB Saunders, 1995.
18. Scanlan CL, Realey A, Earl L: Lung expansion therapy. In Scanlan CL, Spearman C, Sheldon RL (eds): Egan's Fundamentals of Respiratory Care, 6th ed. St. Louis, Mosby-Year Book, 1995.
19. Scott AA, Koff PB: Airway care and chest physiotherapy. In Koff PB, Eitzman D, Neu J (eds): Neonatal and Pediatric Respiratory Care, 2nd ed. St. Louis, Mosby-Year Book, 1993.

SELF-ASSESSMENT QUESTIONS

1. Patients who may benefit from chest physical therapy include those with
   a. cystic fibrosis
   b. asthma
   c. bronchiolitis
   d. all of the above

2. Manual techniques used to loosen secretions include
   a. percussion
   b. auscultation
   c. vibration
   d. a and c

3. Desired effects of chest physical therapy include
   a. increased removal of secretions
   b. improvement of atelectasis
   c. improved ventilation and oxygenation
   d. all of the above

4. _____ is a series of controlled breathing exercises designed to improve mucus clearance.
   a. huff coughing
   b. PEP therapy
   c. autogenic drainage
   d. postural drainage

5. Effective delivery of aerosolized medications depends upon all of the following *except*
   a. delivery device
   b. age of the patient
   c. location of the device relative to the patient
   d. ventilatory pattern

6. A _____ is a breath-initiated device that utilizes capsules containing a single dose of a drug, along with a carrier substance to aid in the delivery of the medication.
   a. metered dose inhaler
   b. small volume nebulizer
   c. SPAG
   d. dry powder inhaler

7. The airway pressure during exhalation while performing PEP therapy should be
   a. 0 to 5 cm H_2O
   b. 5 to 10 cm H_2O
   c. 10 to 20 cm H_2O
   d. 20 to 30 cm H_2O

8. The primary indication for incentive spirometry is
   a. treatment of atelectasis
   b. prevention of atelectasis
   c. removal of secretions
   d. improvement of oxygenation

9. The goal of IPPB is to generate tidal volumes of at least _____% more than the patient's spontaneous tidal volume.
   a. 15
   b. 25
   c. 35
   d. 50

10. The only absolute contraindication to IPPB therapy is
    a. recent facial surgery
    b. intracranial pressure greater than 10 mm Hg
    c. hemoptysis
    d. untreated pneumothorax

Chapter **19**

Airway Care

PATRICK ROTH

OBJECTIVES

Having completed this chapter, the reader will be able to:

1 List the types of equipment that can be used to suction the infant's airway.

2 Describe the major complications of suctioning and discuss the procedures that can be utilized to prevent complications.

3 State suction pressure ranges when suctioning the newborn.

4 Describe the procedure for insertion of the catheter and monitoring of the infant during nasopharyngeal and oropharyngeal suctioning.

5 Discuss the procedure for orotracheal and nasotracheal suctioning.

6 Describe the procedure for determining appropriate catheter size and insertion distance when suctioning through an endotracheal tube.

7 Discuss the consequences of using catheters that are too large and of inserting catheters too far into the airway.

8 Describe the procedures for insertion and withdrawal of suction catheters when suctioning through an endotracheal tube.

9 Describe the instillation process and state two solutions that can be instilled.

10 List the indications for endotracheal intubation.

11 Describe the equipment needed for endotracheal intubation.

12 Describe how to choose the correct endotracheal tube size for a newborn and child.

13 Describe the procedure used for orotracheal and nasotracheal intubation.

14 List the major reasons for choosing the oral or nasal route.

15 Discuss the "7-8-9" rule.

16 Explain how the anatomy of the infant's airway differs from that of the adult.

17 Discuss the monitoring of the infant during the intubation procedure.

18 Describe the ways in which tube position is monitored after intubation.

19 Discuss the complications associated with intubation.

20 Describe the indications and procedure for extubation.

21 Discuss the differences between cuffed and uncuffed tubes and when to use each.

22 Discuss indications for tracheostomy.

KEY TERMS

7-8-9 rule
flow-inflating resuscitator
Macintosh blade
Miller blade
nasopharyngeal airway

oropharyngeal airway
self-inflating resuscitator
sniffing position
stylet
vallecula

Establishing and maintaining the newborn or pediatric airway is one of the most important aspects of care that may be delivered. The relatively small diameter and the flexibility of the airway are factors that make obstruction more likely.

▬PHARYNGEAL SUCTION

In the stable infant without an artificial airway, secretions must be removed by suctioning. Because of their age or mental capability, infants are often unable to clear their own secretions. In this situation, the practitioner should use suction to clear the secretions for the patient. Suction is also indicated following any therapy delivered to improve pulmonary status (*e.g.*, medicated aerosol, chest percussion and drainage).

Suction Equipment

In preparation for suctioning, you will need to gather the following equipment:

- Suction regulator
- Suction circuit
- Catheter in appropriate size
- Water-soluble lubricant
- Manual resuscitation device (bag) and mask with an oxygen source

The clinician will also need personal protective equipment that is appropriate for the situation, with goggles and gloves as the minimum. Portable suction is another option when a central vacuum system is unavailable.

Technique for Nasopharyngeal and Oropharyngeal Suction

Once the equipment is assembled, the patient should be preoxygenated with blow-by oxygen to prevent desaturation and the complications that accompany it. If suctioning nasally, the catheter should be lubricated with water-soluble jelly and inserted into the nares. The catheter should be directed straight into the nares, so it will follow the natural curve of the pharynx.

Infants are preferential nose breathers. Great care should be taken upon insertion of the catheter to prevent damage to the mucosa. Respiratory difficulty can develop as a result of swelling of the nasal mucosa. The suction catheter is advanced until resistance is felt: do not force the catheter past an obstruction. Suction pressure should be 80 to 100 mm Hg for the neonatal patient and 100 to 120 mm Hg for the pediatric patient.[1,2,12] Suction is applied continuously upon removal. Normal saline may be added for thick nasal and upper airway secretions. Administering a few drops in the nares before suction helps to thin secretions. The patient should also be oxygenated after the procedure. A cardiac monitor and/or pulse oximeter may also be helpful in monitoring this type of patient for bradycardia or desaturation.

Oropharyngeal suction differs in both route of entry and the depth of insertion of the catheter. During either procedure, the goal is to stimulate a cough. The suction catheter must be in a good position to retrieve any mucus that is expectorated to this level of the airway. Once the airway is cleared of secretions, the catheter is removed.

NASOTRACHEAL SUCTION

Equipment for nasotracheal suction is the same as that for pharyngeal suction, with the addition of the cardiac monitor, pulse oximeter, and laryngoscope. Direct visualization of the vocal cords is often used in nasotracheal or orotracheal suctioning.

Nasotracheal suction is used to attempt to clear secretions from the lower respiratory tract that the patient is unable to handle on his or her own. Because of its invasive nature, the risk of complications is higher than with pharyngeal suction. The procedure not only removes secretions, but also removes gas volume from the lungs. The procedure is done as needed for a short time until secretion clearance is under control or an artificial airway is indicated.[1]

With adult patients, the catheter is advanced on inspiration until the clinician determines it is in the trachea or resistance is felt. The catheter is pulled back approximately 1 cm, and suction is applied for no more than 10 seconds. Blind nasotracheal suction is not done routinely in children for the following reasons:

1. Children frequently have a strong vagal response to stimulation of the upper airway. The risk of bradycardia must be carefully considered.
2. A child's airway is relatively more anterior than the adult airway, making blind nasotracheal suctioning very difficult, if not impossible, to accomplish in the typical child.

SUCTIONING THROUGH AN ENDOTRACHEAL TUBE

Once an artificial airway is placed in a child, patency is an important issue to consider. Endotracheal (ET) tubes can obstruct even with adequate care owing to the small internal diameter. Suctioning should be performed as needed. Clinical indications for suctioning are O_2 desaturation, bradycardia, deteriorating breath sounds, increasing CO_2 as measured with a transcutaneous monitor; restlessness; or increasing peak inspiratory pressures on the ventilator.

The equipment needed includes everything that has been mentioned earlier. The clinician will need to be more aware of monitoring devices during endotracheal suctioning. Even the most stable of patients can have problems in response to suction. For this reason alone, endotracheal suctioning is considered to be a two-person procedure.

Before suctioning, the patient should be preoxygenated for 3 to 5 minutes. This may be accomplished by increasing the FIO_2 on the ventilator by at least 0.10 to 0.20. The patient may also be manually ventilated as another option. The FIO_2 could be increased to 1.0, but in premature children there is always concern when high levels of oxygen are administered on even a short-term basis.

Once preoxygenation is complete, the patient can be suctioned. This should be accomplished using a suction catheter with an outside diameter no greater than one half the inside diameter of the ET tube.[10] A simple calculation to determine this is shown in Box 19-1. In the example shown, a patient is intubated with an ET tube that has an inside diameter (ID) of 5.5 mm. When this patient is suctioned, the largest suction catheter to be used would be an 8.0 French because that is the size closest to that determined by the formula. The practitioner should use the largest appropriate catheter in order to clear the airway in the quickest, most efficient manner possible.

Suctioning through the ET tube is a sterile procedure, so the practitioner must take care not to contaminate the catheter. The catheter is inserted into the ET tube to a predetermined depth. That depth is determined by adding the length of the ET tube to the length of the ET tube adapter. The total length is the point to which the suction catheter can be advanced safely (Fig. 19-1). Ideally, the catheter is advanced to approximately the end of the tube or a little farther. In patients who have airway lesions (e.g., burns), extreme care should be taken not to advance the catheter beyond the end of the ET tube for routine care. Taking care to suction to the correct depth will prevent mucosal damage. Once the catheter has been advanced to the proper position, suction is applied as the catheter is applied.

Suction pressures should be 80 to 100 mm Hg for neonatal patients and 100 to 120 mm Hg for pediatric patients.[1,2,12] Once continuous suction is applied, the catheter is twirled between the thumb and forefinger to prevent mucosal damage. The procedure should not last more than 10 seconds with each pass of the catheter. The patient is then reoxygenated manually or via the ventilator for at least 1 minute. For the patient on maximum ventilator support, inline suction devices or adapters are available to facilitate suctioning without interruption of the support being delivered (Fig. 19-2).

Normal saline is frequently used to thin secretions and loosen mucus plugs for removal. A few drops (1–5 cc) of the solution are instilled

---

BOX 19-1 Calculation of Correct Suction Catheter Size

$$\text{Maximum diameter (French)} = \frac{\text{Inside diameter (mm)} \times 3}{2}$$

Example:

$$\text{Maximum diameter (French)} = \frac{5.5 \times 3}{2}$$

$$= \frac{16.5}{2}$$

$$\text{Maximum diameter (French)} = 8.25$$

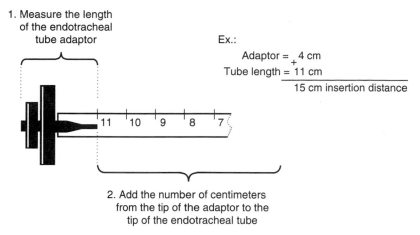

1. Measure the length of the endotracheal tube adaptor

Ex.:

$$\begin{array}{r} \text{Adaptor} = 4 \text{ cm} \\ + \\ \underline{\text{Tube length} = 11 \text{ cm}} \\ 15 \text{ cm insertion distance} \end{array}$$

11 10 9 8 7

2. Add the number of centimeters from the tip of the adaptor to the tip of the endotracheal tube

FIGURE 19-1 Method of determing proper insertion depth of a suction. (Reproduced by permission. Whitaker KB: Comprehensive Perinatal and Pediatric Respiratory Care. Albany, NY, Delmar Publishers, 1992.)

through the airway. The amount to be instilled is dependent on the size of the patient. A 2% solution of sodium bicarbonate is an alternative thinning agent for thick secretions. The patient is ventilated to distribute the fluid throughout the lungs and then suctioned as previously explained.

■ SUCTIONING THROUGH THE TRACHEOSTOMY TUBE

Suctioning the patient with a tracheostomy tube differs very little from suctioning a patient with an ET tube. There are, however, some problems associated with the location of a tracheostomy tube. In babies with chubby chins and in those who are moving a great deal, it is difficult to complete the procedure in a sterile manner. As is the case when suctioning using an ET tube, the procedure should be performed by two people.

The other significant difference is the depth of insertion of the catheter. Because the tracheostomy tube is shorter, the catheter should not be inserted as deeply. Once the length of the tracheostomy tube is known, the

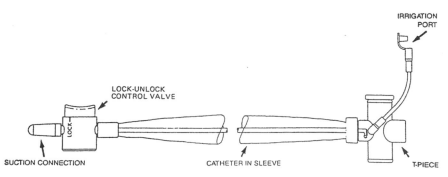

IRRIGATION PORT

LOCK-UNLOCK CONTROL VALVE

SUCTION CONNECTION

CATHETER IN SLEEVE

T-PIECE

Ballard closed suction system. (Courtesy of Ballard, Midvale, UT)

FIGURE 19-2 Inline suction catheter. (Fluck RR Jr, Hess DR, Branson RD: Airway and suction equipment. In Branson RD, Hess DR, Chatburn RL: Respiratory Care Equipment. Philadelphia, JB Lippincott, 1995, p. 139.)

clinician may follow the same procedure used to determine the depth of insertion for an ET tube. Once again, this will prevent mucosal damage, which may complicate the care of the long-term patient.

▬POSTSUCTION ASSESSMENT OF THE PATIENT

Observation of the patient's status following the procedure is essential. The clinician must assess the patient after suctioning. After a short recovery time, the patient should show signs of improvement. Assessment of the patient's breath sounds, color, heart rate, respiratory rate, oxygenation, and ventilation should be done. The color and consistency of the secretions should also be noted and recorded. Further treatment may be indicated by the results of the assessment of the patient.

▬OROPHARYNGEAL AIRWAY

The **oropharyngeal (oral) airway** is designed to maintain a patent airway. It is shaped so that it protrudes down behind the tongue, keeping it away from the posterior wall of the pharynx. The airway is constructed of a flange, a short bite block, and an open air channel (Fig. 19-3). This particular airway is placed in unconscious infants or children. Postsurgical patients will frequently have these in place upon arrival to the recovery room.

The oropharyngeal airway is inserted into the side of the patient's mouth, then rotated 90 degrees until in position. This technique avoids damage to the patient's soft palate. Care should be taken not to push the tongue into the back of the throat.

To determine the correct airway size for each patient, the practitioner should hold the airway up to the patient's cheek. The properly sized airway should reach from the corner of the mouth to the angle of the jaw. If the airway is too small or inserted incorrectly, the tongue will obstruct the airway.

When the patient begins to regain consciousness, he or she will push the airway out with the tongue. The oral airway in a patient who is even minimally alert can induce vomiting as a result of its placement, so close observation is necessary. While the airway is in place, the head and jaw should also be kept in good position in order to maintain a patent airway.

▬NASOPHARYNGEAL AIRWAY

The **nasopharyngeal (nasal) airway** also maintains the patency of the airway in the posterior pharynx between the tongue and the posterior wall of the throat and is often tolerated by the semi-alert patient (Fig. 19-4). This airway is made of a soft, pliable latex material. The nasal airway is also used to facilitate suctioning of the upper airway in patients with large amounts of upper airway secretions who require frequent suctioning. These airways are prone to obstruction, so the clinician will need to pay close attention to keeping the airway patent in these patients. This can be accomplished through suctioning or removing the airway to clear the obstruction and then replacing it. These procedures should be done as needed.

The nasal airway prevents damage to the nasal mucosa during repeated suctioning. Nasal airways are placed in the nares. The airways should be as large as possible without causing blanching of the skin at the opening. The airway should be changed every 8 hours.

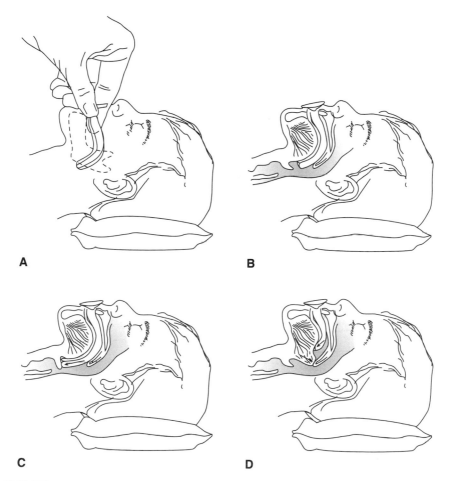

FIGURE 19-3 Oropharyngeal airway insertion. The appropriate size can be esti-mated by holding the airway next to the child's face. (**A**): the tip of the airway should end just behind the angle of the mandible (broken line), resulting in proper align-ment with the glotic opening (**B**). If the oral airway inserted is too large, it will align posterior to the angle of the mandible (**C**) and obstruct the glottic opening by push-ing the epiglottis down (**C, arrow**). If the oral airway is inserted too small, the tip will align well above the angle of the mandible (**D**) and exacerbate airway obstruction by pushing the tongue into the oropharynx (**D, arrows**). (American Heart Association: Textbook of Pediatric Advanced Life Support. Dallas, TX, AHA, 1994.)

ENDOTRACHEAL INTUBATION

At some point in the course of treating a critically ill child, intervention is necessary to maintain the airway. There are several reasons for intubating patients to support their pulmonary status.

Most commonly, a decrease in pulmonary function is an indication for intubation and mechanical ventilation. Respiratory failure in children often is the result of primary airway obstruction with fatigue. Acute respiratory failure occurs when patients have a $Paco_2$ of 50 to 60 mm Hg with a pH lower than 7.30 or a Pao_2 less than 60 with an FIo_2 of less than 0.60.[9] These arter-ial blood gas values are considered sufficient criteria for intubation and mechanical ventilation.

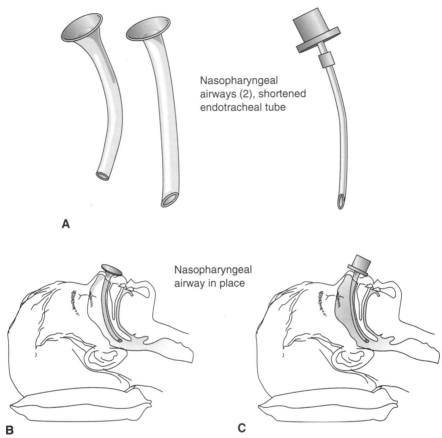

FIGURE 19-4 (*A*) Nasopharyngeal airway. A shortened endotracheal tube may be substituted (to reduce resistance). (*B*) Placement of a nasopharyngeal airway. (*C*) Cut-off endotracheal tube used as a nasopharyngeal tube. Note that the standard 15 mm adapter must be firmly reinserted into the endotracheal tube. (American Heart Association: Textbook of Pediatric Advanced Life Support. Dallas, TX, AHA, 1994.)

Second, intubation is indicated for patients with such upper airway ob-structions as severe croup or epiglottitis. These patients need a patent airway until the infectious process subsides. Patients with tracheomalacia, tracheal stenosis, or enlarged tonsils and adenoids may also need intubation until sur-gical intervention or some other way of stabilizing the airway is possible.

Intubation may also be warranted for airway protection. If a patient loses cough or gag reflexes, he or she is at risk for aspiration. Drug over-dose and head injury are two common situations in which these protective reflexes may be lost.

The insertion of an ET tube will also facilitate bronchial hygiene. The patient with large amounts of secretions is more easily suctioned by this route. The patient with recurrent lobar atelectasis is also more easily man-aged with an airway in place.

Finally, the endotracheal tube placed during resuscitation may be used as a route for administration of drugs. During cardiac arrest, when there is no vascular access, resuscitation drugs should be given via the ET tube until an intravenous (IV) or intraosseous (IO) catheter is established.[3]

Equipment for Intubation

The equipment needed for intubation is listed in Table 19-1. The manual resuscitator will either be **self-inflating** or **flow-inflating**. The flow-inflating bag requires some practice to operate. The bag consists of an oxygen source, an adjustable valve to control overflow, and a reservoir bag. The flow must be adjusted properly so as to offer adequate gas for ventilation and washout of exhaled gases in the reservoir. The valve needs to be adjusted appropriately for adequate ventilation without causing pulmonary barotrauma. Even though the flow-inflating bag requires more attention, some centers believe the advantages are considerable. First, the bag is capable of delivering the FIO_2 that is used to power the bag, so that delivery of 100% oxygen is possible. Second, the bag is capable of delivering positive end-expiratory pressure or continuous positive airway pressure. Finally, the compliance of the small patient's chest is more easily sensed by the clinician.

The self-inflating bag offers the option of ventilating the patient when an oxygen source is not needed or immediately available. A minimum FIO_2 of 0.85 will be delivered with a self-inflating bag set up according to the manufacturer's specifications. Many of the bags available have options for the addition of a reservoir to increase the delivered FIO_2. PEEP devices are also available for self-inflating bags that are designed without this option.

An institution's choices with respect to manual resuscitation bags seem to be made on an individual basis. One study that compared self-inflating and flow-inflating bags described advantages of both. The author suggested that the use of self-inflating bags could be supported on the basis of problems of practitioner competency in the operation of flow-inflating bags.[6]

Other equipment at the bedside includes a mask of appropriate size, adhesive tape and benzoin for securing the tube, Yankauer suction or a larger suction catheter (12 or 14 French) for clearing the upper airway, and a sterile suction kit to suction the ET tube once it is in place.

TABLE 19-1 Equipment for Endotracheal Intubation

Oxygen source

Manual resuscitation bag

Mask

Endotracheal tubes in appropriate size

Magill forceps

Stylet

Laryngoscope handle and blade

Suction equipment

Adhesive tape

Benzoin

$ETCO_2$ detector

EKG monitor

Pulse oximeter

Stethoscope

The laryngoscope consists of a handle and a blade. The availability of large and small handles and personal preference usually dictate which handle is used. The small handle is less cumbersome when intubating smaller patients, so it is used more commonly.

Blades are available in sizes 0 through 4, and are chosen in relation to the size of the patient. A straight 0 blade is used for intubating neonates. With larger patients, the larger blades are used. All sizes of blades fit both sizes of handles.

Whether a **Miller** (straight) or **Macintosh** (curved) blade is used is often a matter of personal preference. The technique utilized with each blade varies in accomplishing visualization of the vocal cords. The straight blade is used to directly lift the epiglottis (Fig. 19-5). Some clinicians will insert the straight blade deeper, and then back out until the epiglottis falls. They will then pick up the epiglottis and visualize the vocal cords.

The curved blade fits into the **vallecula**, which is the space above the epiglottis. As pressure is applied, the epiglottis moves up and out of the way, leaving the vocal cords exposed for visualization.

A **stylet** is a plastic-coated metal rod that is inserted into the ET tube to stiffen it as it is passed into the trachea. It should be available to give the ET tube support and the capability to be shaped for orotracheal placement. Some patients have variations of their airway that require bending the tube to maneuver it through the vocal cords. The stylet can give the tube some rigidity that it does not naturally have. The stylet is placed in the ET tube so it does not extend beyond the end of the tube, where it could cause damage to the mucosa or trachea.

An end-tidal CO_2 ($ETCO_2$) detector or capnometer should be used immediately after intubation to confirm placement of the tube in the trachea.[4,5,13] When the detector is initially placed inline between the resuscitation bag and the ET tube, it will be purple in color. As the patient is ventilated manually and exhaled gas passes through the detector, a yellowish color indicates the presence of CO_2, meaning that the endotracheal tube

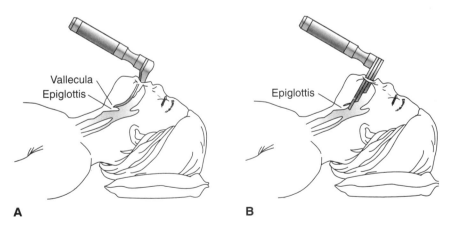

Vallecula
Epiglottis

Epiglottis

A   B

FIGURE 19-5 Laryngoscope blade in proper position for intubation. Position of laryngoscope blade when using (*A*) a curved blade versus (*B*) a straight blade. Note that a straight blade may often be used in the same manner as a curved blade, i.e., its tip placed in the vallecula. (American Heart Association: Textbook of Pediatric Advanced Life Support. Dallas, TX, AHA, 1994.)

has been placed into the trachea. If the tube has been placed in the esophagus, the detector will not change color, since esophageal air contains no CO_2. The use of a CO_2 detector provides a quick check while waiting for a chest x-ray film to ensure placement.

Most important to this process is selection of the ET tube. Prior to intubation, the size of the tube must be determined. Premature infants and newborns up to 6 months of age will require a 3.0- or 3.5-mm ID tube, and infants from 6 to 12 months of age will require a 3.5- to 4.0-mm ID tube. For patients 1 year of age and older, a simple formula may be used (Box 19-2).

Another method of determining tube size is by looking at the patient's little finger. The outside diameter of the ET tube will approximate the size of the little finger at the first knuckle. Both of these methods for determining tube size provide reference points. Because patients vary in size, these methods do not give absolute sizes, but they do offer a good estimate.[11] These methods are not exact, so there should be tubes 0.5 mm smaller and larger at the bedside. Although the other tubes are usually not used, the procedures where they are needed will proceed in a much smoother fashion.

ET tubes are available with and without cuffs, so the decision of which type of tube to use must also be made. Current recommendations are that uncuffed ET tubes should be used for children less than 8 years old.[3] The cricoid cartilage is the narrowest point in the airway until the child is approximately 8 years old. A seal is maintained around the tube at the cricoid cartilage with an uncuffed tube. As a child grows, the vocal cords become the narrowest point in the airway, and the seal is then achieved with a high-volume, low-pressure ET tube cuff. Minimal-leak technique should be employed when using cuffed tubes to minimize the chance of tracheal damage that can result from overinflation of the cuff.

Orotracheal Route of Intubation

Intubation by the oral route is preferred in an emergency situation for the neonatal and pediatric patient. Before the procedure begins, the patient should have continuous EKG monitoring and pulse oximetry in place. All equipment should be assembled and functioning.

BOX 19-2 Calculation of Correct Endotracheal Tube Size for Infants 1 Year of Age and Older

Inside diameter (mm) $= \dfrac{16 + \text{age in years}}{4}$

Example: 4-year-old child:

$$= \dfrac{16 + 4 \text{ years old}}{4}$$

$$= \dfrac{20}{4}$$

Correct inside diameter $= 5.0$ mm

The patient is preoxygenated for 1 to 3 minutes before the intubation. The time frame for preoxygenation will be dictated more by clinical status of the patient. Generally, the more clinically stable the patient, the shorter the amount of time needed for preoxygenation. Preoxygenation is accomplished by replacing the 21% oxygen of the functional residual capacity (FRC) with 100% oxygen.[7] This will allow more time for intubation to be performed before hypoxia and associated complications set in.

While preoxygenation is occurring, sedation and muscle relaxants are administered for ease of intubation. In neonates, control can be accomplished without sedation or muscle relaxants, but older infants and children are less easily controlled for elective intubation. Although cooperation in the procedure is possible when working with adults, it is out of the question in pediatric care. Pharmacological intervention makes the procedure much easier and smoother and minimizes trauma to the airway. Although specific types of sedation and muscle relaxation are beyond the scope of this discussion, the clinician performing the intubation must be aware that the disease process will affect the choice of drugs. For example, agents that may cause an increase in intracranial pressure would be contraindicated for a patient with head injury.

Once the patient has been sedated, the intubation may proceed. The patient is placed in the "sniffing" position, which is accomplished by elevating the head and neck to a plane above the shoulders, usually by placing a rolled towel under the head (see Fig. 19-5). The laryngoscope is placed in the right side of the mouth, and the tongue is swept to the left side of the mouth with the blade. Pressure is exerted upward and forward with the laryngoscope at a 45-degree angle. The patient's teeth or maxillary ridge should not become the fulcrum for a prying laryngoscope blade. Damage to teeth or unerupted teeth can result. Once visualization of the vocal cords occurs, the ET tube is introduced into the right side of the mouth. If the patient has a small mouth, a second person may pull the right cheek aside to allow more space to visualize. The ET tube is then advanced through the cords.

Uncuffed tubes have either single or double black lines to assist in obtaining correct depth of insertion. The tube should be advanced until the line is at the level of the vocal cords. Ideally, this places the tube at midtrachea. A cuffed tube is advanced until the cuff is through the cords. The centimeter markings at the teeth or lip should be noted as a reference point for tube position and the tube should be secured. Care should be taken during positioning as a small amount of movement in some infants can result in a right mainstem intubation or an accidental extubation.

While intubation is being attempted, the assisting person needs to monitor oxygen saturation, heart rate, and the length of time of the procedure. Each attempt should take no longer than 30 seconds. If the attempt extends beyond 30 seconds, the procedure should be interrupted and the patient manually ventilated to reoxygenate.

Once the tube is in place and usually before it is taped, the chest is auscultated for equal breath sounds. In older children, auscultation over the stomach helps rule out esophageal intubation. If unequal breath sounds are heard, the tube should be pulled back 1 to 2 cm at a time until equal breath sounds are noted.

Chest expansion should be symmetrical, and an $ETCO_2$ monitor should be placed inline. The $ETCO_2$ monitor will give accurate results in most cases.

It is often impossible to determine any results in a full cardiac arrest situation as these devices are dependent upon perfusion and CO_2 production.[4,5]

The ET tube should now be secured in place, usually with tape, although there are commercial fixation devices available. After the tube is secured, a chest x-ray film is essential to determine tube placement.

Depth of orotracheal tube insertion in neonates can follow the **"7-8-9" rule**: the 7-cm mark should be at the lip for a 1-kg infant; the 8-cm mark should be at the lip for a 2-kg infant; and the 9-cm mark should be at the lip for a 3-kg infant.[14] This is an approximation, and a chest x-ray film is still needed to confirm good position.

Once tube placement is confirmed, the airway will need to be checked for any variation in placement. After some time, tubes can change position as a result of the patient being moved, tape becoming loose, and medical procedures being performed. If a cuffed tube is used, the cuff will need to be checked on a regular basis. Minimal-leak technique should be utilized, and the cuff pressure should be measured to ensure that overinflation does not occur.

Nasotracheal Route of Intubation

Intubation by the nasal route is very similar to the procedure used for the oral route. The ET tube is frequently smaller by a half size than the size that would be used orally. If possible, the larger of the nares is used to insert the tube. Before insertion, the tube should be lubricated with a water-soluble jelly to decrease the potential for mucosal damage. The tube is then inserted and advanced until it can be seen in the airway. Visualization of the vocal cords is accomplished by the same method as previously described. The clinician may use Magill forceps to guide the tip of the tube through the vocal cords. A second person may assist by advancing the tube. The rest of the procedure is the same as for an oral intubation.

Blind nasal intubation in children is not worth attempting, owing to the anterior and cephalad position of the larynx. The risk of damage is too great and the chances of success are minimal.

Complications of Intubation

Intubation, like any other procedure, comes with its complications. Trauma to upper airway tissue, perforation of the pharynx and larynx, pneumothorax, and esophageal intubation are all problems that may arise.

There is also the possibility of vagal stimulation, which will cause bradycardia or arterial hypotension. Bronchospasm or laryngospasm may result in hypoxia, cardiac dysrhythmias, or hypotension. The most common complication of pediatric intubation is accidental extubation, which occurs at a rate of 3% to 13%.[9]

▬EXTUBATION

The patient will need to be evaluated for extubation as recovery occurs. The disease process that necessitated intubation should have either been reversed or improved; the patient should be hemodynamically stable as measured by cardiac output, capillary refill, urine output, and/or blood pressure; and pulmonary status should have improved to the point where the patient has an adequate tidal volume and minute volume while breathing spontaneously. The gag, swallow, and cough reflexes should be intact. The patient should also have an oxygen saturation of 95% or greater on an FIO_2 of less than 0.40. Once the patient meets these criteria, then the decision to extubate can be made.[8,9]

If the extubation is planned, the patient can be given dexamethasone at a dose of 0.5 to 0.6 mg/kg to help prevent upper airway swelling secondary to the intubation. Ideally, the first dose of dexamethasone is given 4 to 8 hours before the extubation is attempted.[10a,12a] This use of steroids has become an accepted treatment for this situation, but further study is needed to determine the ideal dosage.

In preparing for extubation, the equipment for possible reintubation should be at the bedside. There should also be equipment for oxygen delivery once the endotracheal tube is removed. Finally, racemic epinephrine and a small-volume nebulizer should be available in case the patient is stridorous and could benefit from this therapy.

Once prepared for extubation, the patient is manually ventilated for hyperoxygenation. The oropharynx may be suctioned as well as the ET tube. The tube is held, and the tape is released. A large manual breath is given, and the tube is pulled out at peak inspiration. The patient may hold his or her breath or have some laryngospasm. The patient should then be placed on oxygen, and the FIO_2 should be titrated for appropriate saturation.

Complications noted after extubation may include a sore throat and hoarseness. Stridor can also develop up to 8 hours postextubation. Treatment for the patient with stridor includes parenteral steroids, aerosolized racemic epinephrine, or short-term helium–oxygen therapy.

■ TRACHEOSTOMY

Tracheostomy is an option for those patients who will have long-term pulmonary problems. The indications for a tracheostomy are listed in Table 19-2.

Patient comfort is enhanced with a tracheostomy, while decreasing chances of laryngeal damage. With some special tracheostomy tubes or adjuncts, the patient has the potential for better communication and speech than with an endotracheal tube.

The tracheostomy has complications specific to it over and above those of having an artificial airway in place.[12] Obviously the upper airway is bypassed, so the humidification, air warming, and filtering functions of the airway are eliminated, and the risk of infection is increased. The patient can also be decannulated accidentally. An extra tracheostomy tube of the same type and size should always be with the patient.

Due to their smaller size, pediatric tracheostomy tubes are made with a single cannula and may be cuffed or uncuffed. The tube has no inner can-

---

TABLE 19-2   Indications for Tracheostomy

Long-term ventilation

Airway obstruction

Subglottic stenosis

Tracheomalacia

Laryngeal cleft

Facilitation of pulmonary hygiene

nula to remove for cleaning or weaning. The tubes may also be custom made to better function in children who have special airway needs.

Rare complications include hemorrhage at the surgical site postoperatively, erosion into the innominate vessels, and laryngeal nerve injury. Structural problems such as tracheal scarring or stenosis can also result from the tracheostomy tube.

Tracheostomy care generally includes cleaning and care of the site. The tracheostomy tube is held in place by some type of tie around the back of the neck. The skin under the tie must be cared for, or breakdown will occur. Scheduled changing of the tracheostomy tube itself should also be included.

REFERENCES

1. American Association for Respiratory Care: Clinical practice guidelines for nasotracheal suctioning. Respiratory Care 37:898, 1992.
2. American Association for Respiratory Care: Clinical practice guidelines for endotracheal suctioning of mechanically ventilated adults and children with artificial airways. Respiratory Care 38:500, 1993.
3. American Heart Association: Textbook of Pediatric Advanced Life Support. Dallas, TX, AHA, 1990.
4. Bhende MAS, Thompson AE, Cook DR: Validity of a disposable end-tidal CO_2 detector in verifying endotracheal tube placement in infants and children. Ann Emerg Med 21:142, 1992.
5. Einarson O, Rochester CL, Rosenbraun S: Airway management in respiratory emergencies. Clin Chest Med 15:13, 1994.
6. Kanter RK: Evaluation of mask bag ventilation in resuscitation of infants. Am J Dis Child 14:1761, 1987.
7. McDonald TB, Berkowitz RA: Airway management and sedation for pediatric transport. Ped Clin North Am 40:381, 1993.
8. Oakes D: Neonatal/Pediatric Respiratory Care: A Critical Care Pocket Guide. Old Towne, ME, Health Educator Publications, 1989.
9. Pettignano R, Pettignano MM: Airway management. In Barnhart SL, Czervinske MP (eds): Perinatal and Pediatric Respiratory Care. Philadelphia, WB Saunders, 1995.
10. Plevak DJ, Ward JJ: Airway management. In Burton GG, Hodgkin JE, Ward JJ (eds): Respiratory Care: A Guide to Clinical Practice, 3rd ed. Philadelphia, JB Lippincott, 1991.
10a. Postma DS, Prazma J, Woods CI, Sidman J, Pilsbury HC: Use of steroids and a long-acting vasoconstrictor in the treatment of postintubation croup. Arch Otolaryngol Head Neck Surg 113:844,1987.
11. Pullerits J: Routine and special pediatric airway equipment. Intern Anesth Clinics 30:109, 1992.
12. Slonin NB, Schneider S, Weng T, Fields L: Pediatric Respiratory Therapy: An Introductory Text. New York, Glen Educational Medical Service, 1974.
12a. Tibballs J, Shann FA, Landau LI: Placebo-controlled trial of prednisolone in children intubated for croup. Lancet 340:745, 1992.
13. Todres D: Pediatric airway control and ventilation. Ann Emerg Med 22:440, 1993.
14. Tochen M: Orotracheal intubation in the newborn infant: A method for determining depth of tube insertion. J Pediatrics 95:1050, 1979.

SELF-ASSESSMENT QUESTIONS

1. Which of the following are necessary when suctioning an infant by the pharyngeal route?
   I. suction regulator
   II. catheter of the appropriate size
   III. manual resuscitation device
   IV. oxygen source
   a. I only
   b. II and III
   c. I and IV
   d. I, II, III, and IV

2. Suction pressures utilized in neonatal patients should be in the range of _____ mm Hg.
   a. 20 to 40
   b. 40 to 60
   c. 60 to 80
   d. 80 to 100

3. Clinical indications for suctioning the infant include all of the following *except*
   a. oxygen desaturation
   b. improving breath sounds
   c. bradycardia
   d. restlessness

4. For suctioning an infant with a size 3.0-mm ID ET tube, what size suction catheter should be used?
   a. 4 French
   b. 6 French
   c. 8 French
   d. 10 French

5. Which of the following should be assessed after suctioning the child?
   I. breath sounds
   II. heart rate
   III. respiratory rate
   IV. color
   a. II only
   b. I and III
   c. II and IV
   d. I, II, III, and IV

6. To determine the correct size of oropharyngeal airway to use for a child, the airway should extend from the corner of the mouth to the
   a. tragus of the ear
   b. corner of the eye
   c. angle of the jaw
   d. tip of the nose

7. What minimum FIO_2 is delivered from a self-inflating manual resuscitation bag powered with 100% oxygen?
   a. 0.50
   b. 0.70
   c. 0.85
   d. 1.00

8. Indications for tracheostomy in the newborn and child include
   a. long-term ventilation
   b. laryngeal cleft
   c. tracheomalacia
   d. all of the above

9. What size of endotracheal tube should be used for an 8-year-old child?
   a. 4-mm ID
   b. 6-mm ID
   c. 8-mm ID
   d. 10-mm ID

10. A 2-kg neonate is intubated with a size 3.5-mm ID tube. The 8-cm mark on the tube is at the level of the infant's lip. What action should be taken by the practitioner?
   a. advance the tube until the 9-cm mark is at the lip
   b. withdraw the tube until the 7-cm mark is at the lip
   c. cut off the end of the tube
   d. leave the tube in its current position

Chapter 20

Cardiopulmonary Resuscitation of the Infant and the Child

M. DEE JOHNSON

OBJECTIVES

Having completed this chapter, the reader will be able to:

1 Discuss the equipment and supplies that should be available in the delivery room for resuscitation of the neonate.

2 Describe the methods of immediate evaluation and management of the neonate in the delivery room.

3 Review the use of the Apgar score in the evaluation of the neonate suffering from asphyxia.

4 Discuss the importance of the management of fluids, temperature, and electrolytes in the successful care of the infant or child being resuscitated.

5 Discuss the use of medications in the management of the infant or child being resuscitated.

6 Describe cardiopulmonary resuscitation of the infant or child according to American Heart Association guidelines.

7 Describe the procedure for removal of an obstruction in the choking infant or child.

8 Describe the use of mouth-to-mask and bag–mask ventilation in the infant or child.

9 Discuss the use of the laryngoscope and intubation of the neonate or infant.

10 Discuss the procedures to be used in the evaluation of the infant or child for stabilization and follow-up care in the clinical setting.

KEY TERMS

cardiopulmonary resuscitation
Heimlich maneuver
introitus
PALS
pressors

self-inflating resuscitation bag
side-by-side method
"sniffing" position
tactile stimuli

415

▬RESUSCITATION OF THE NEONATE OR INFANT

The successful resuscitation of the neonate (infant in the first 28 days of life) or the infant requires quick and decisive action on the part of the resuscitation team. In the delivery room, situations can arise suddenly and demand the prompt response of the physician, nurse and respiratory therapists present. All of the personnel should be knowledgeable in perinatal physiology, skilled in resuscitation techniques, and familiar with all delivery room equipment and techniques.

Recognition of the Neonate in Distress

Often, high-risk deliveries are anticipated by the staff and arrangements are made to have the appropriate personnel present prior to the delivery. One report, however, pointed out that only 56% of deliveries requiring immediate neonatal resuscitation were anticipated.[3] There are several common categories of complications for the infant in the delivery room. Complications most commonly arise in the premature infant and the term infant who suffers from asphyxia at birth.

Only a small percentage of term infants require aggressive resuscitation at birth. For numerous reasons, a higher percentage of premature infants require resuscitation. The heart rate is often the first sign of distress. The neonate will show immediate signs of bradycardia, apnea, and lack of neuromuscular tone with accompanying low Apgar scores. The Apgar score of less than or equal to 3 at 1 minute is a positive indicator of the need for resuscitation. If the need for resuscitation is apparent, it should be started immediately and not delayed for the Apgar assessment at 1 minute. Even when the 1-minute score reflects stability, the infant should be carefully reevaluated at 5 minutes of age. Some infants who appear fine at birth deteriorate rapidly. Of those children who are aggressively treated with resuscitation methods, a majority will survive and develop normally.

Other common complications for the neonate include maternal complications contributing to a difficult birth, lack of adequate fetal blood flow, and complications that present during labor and delivery. Problems for the mother occur when she has demonstrated a history of any of the complications listed in Table 20-1. These complications will require monitoring of the mother and anticipation of an infant in distress. Lack of fetal blood flow can result from numerous causes. Immediate attention must be given to prevent complications that may occur as a result of a lack of oxygen and nutrients to the neonate. Complications experienced during delivery can lead to stress being placed on the infant during birth.

Although various progressive methods of evaluation of oxygenation and perfusion of the infant usually begin before the actual delivery occurs, rapid, thorough, and continuous assessment must begin immediately at birth. Resuscitation is necessary for any infant who, for any reason, cannot establish adequate ventilation for effective gas exchange or maintain adequate circulation to perfuse major organ systems within the first few minutes after delivery.

Preparation of Equipment

Equipment and supplies must be present and properly operating and the personnel should be familiar with the location and operation of each piece of equipment in the delivery room. An area within each delivery

---

TABLE 20-1   Complications Requiring Resuscitation of the Newborn

---

Maternal Complications
> Use of drugs that cross the placenta (*e.g.,* cocaine, crack)
>
> Acute attack of asthma
>
> Congestive heart failure or anomalies
>
> Lack of prenatal care
>
> Development of preeclampsia or eclampsia
>
> Acute exacerbation of a respiratory disease
>
> Maternal hypertension
>
> Accidental trauma to the mother (car, fire, fall, personal injury)
>
> Multiple births

Lack of Fetal Blood Flow to the Neonate
> Prolapse of the umbilical cord
>
> Kinking or knotting of the umbilical cord
>
> Insufficient organ development in utero
>
> Placenta previa/abruptio placenta
>
> Asphyxia of the fetus

Complications During Delivery of the Neonate
> Improper positioning of the infant
>
> Presence of sexually transmitted diseases
>
> Inability to pass through the birth canal
>
> Passage of meconium
>
> Failure of the cardiovascular/respiratory systems

---

room should be set up for infant care within a few feet of the delivery site, complete with oxygen supply, suction apparatus, radiant warmer, a table that allows access to the infant from at least three sides, and storage space for all infant resuscitation equipment, supplies, and drugs.

Recommendations for equipment, supplies, drugs, and fluids for the storage area or carts are listed in Table 20-2.

Equipment should be prepared before the delivery whenever possible. The radiant warmer and transport incubator should be turned on; all suction and oxygen apparatus should be set up and functional; and estimated sizes of laryngoscope blades, endotracheal (ET) tubes, catheters, and other equipment should be set up and available. The resuscitation bag, either a gas-inflated bag or a self-inflating bag, should be readied and set up with the appropriate flow of oxygen.

Self-inflating resuscitation bags (averaging 250 mL) refill themselves after being compressed because of the elasticity of the material and the shape of the bag itself. The bag contains room air (delivering 21% oxygen) unless a 100% oxygen gas source is added, as well as some type of reservoir device. The reservoir device is filled with 100% oxygen so that when the bag is squeezed the patient will receive a breath that is equal to or greater than 80% oxygen. Most of these bags are equipped with a pop-off

---

TABLE 20-2   Supply List for Emergency Resuscitation in the Delivery Room

---

Equipment and Supplies

Radiant warmer

Transport incubator

Oxygen source with flowmeter

Bubble humidifier with connective tubing

Suction device with manometers (2)

Suction catheters (5, 6, 8, 10 Fr)

Bulb syringe

Cardiotachometer with ECG oscilloscope/leads

Neonatal resuscitation bag/manometer

Face masks (sizes 0–4)

Oral airways (sizes 000–0)

Endotracheal tubes (sizes 2.5–4.0)

Laryngoscope/blades (00–1) with extra bulbs and batteries

Stylet, scissors, gloves

Stethoscope

Tape (1/2 and 3/4 size)

Rolled diaper

Tincture of benzoin

Umbilical artery catheters (sizes 3.5–5.0)

Sterile umbilical artery catheterization tray

Needles (18, 21, 25 gauge)

Syringes (sizes 3, 5, 10 cc)

Sterile cord clamp

Three-way stopcock

Y-connector

Infant feeding tubes for gastric depression (sizes 5 and 8 Fr)

Alcohol wipes

Iodophor solution

Gauge sponges

Dextrostix

Hematocrit tubes

Laboratory tubes

Blood gas syringes

Dry, warmed blankets

Medications and Fluids

Atropine 0.02 mg/kg

Sodium bicarbonate 4.2% solution

Dextrose in water 10% and 50%

Epinephrine 1:10,000

Albumin 5%/Normal Saline

Naloxone 0.02 mg/mL to 5 years or 0.1 mg/kg to age 5 years

Heparin

Ringer's lactate

Sterile water

Normal saline

---

to prevent the delivery of excessive pressure to the infant. The pop-off is set at a pressure of 35 to 50 cm H_2O.[2] Because of the pressures necessary for the initial breaths, a device may be needed to bypass this pop-off. Use of an inline manometer is recommended to monitor airway pressures. The gas-inflated anesthesia bag is inflated by use of an attached gas source (usually 100% oxygen) and a Mapleson valve, which provides a port for a pressure manometer to be attached so that airway pressures may be monitored during positive pressure breaths. Patient lung compliance is more easily assessed with the use of the gas-inflated bag since resistance to inflation can be felt during compression of the bag.

All equipment, supplies, and medication should be checked on a routine basis as well as before and after each resuscitation effort. This is necessary to ensure that all equipment is functioning properly, all supplies are present and can be easily located, and outdated medications are replaced.

Resuscitation Techniques

In order to begin to resuscitate the neonate, infant, or child, the qualified personnel must be familiar with the steps of **cardiopulmonary resuscitation** (CPR). The ABCs of CPR include assessing and evaluating the airway, breathing, and circulation of the victim. There are specific steps for the infant and child that differ according to the size of the victim and the structure of the airway. Table 20-3 shows a comparison of the techniques and the proper sequence for the administration of CPR.

The neonate in the delivery room is in a unique situation since breathing has not taken place prior to delivery. As the infant's head is delivered, the mouth is cleared first to prevent aspiration of pharyngeal contents with the first breath and the nose is then suctioned, both with a bulb

TABLE 20-3   Summary of Resuscitation Maneuvers in Infants and Children

MANEUVER	INFANT (<1 YEAR)	CHILD (1 TO 8 YEARS)
Airway	Head-tilt/chin-lift (unless trauma present)	Head-tilt/chin-lift (unless trauma present)
	Jaw thrust	Jaw thrust
Breathing		
Initial	2 breaths at 1 to 1 1/2 s/breath	2 breaths at 1 to 1 1/2 s/breath
Subsequent	20 breaths/min	20 breaths/min
Circulation		
Pulse check	Brachial/femoral	Carotid
Compression area	Lower third of sternum	Lower third of sternum
Compression with	2 or 3 fingers	Heel of 1 hand
Depth	Approximately 1/2 to 1 in	Approximately 1 to 1 1/2 in
Rate	At least 100/min	100/min
Compression-ventilation ratio	5:1 (pause for ventilation)	5:1 (pause for ventilation)
Foreign-body airway obstruction	Back blows/chest thrusts	Heimlich maneuver

(American Heart Association, Emergency Cardiac Care Committees: Guidelines for cardiopulmonary resuscitation and emergency cardiac care. JAMA :268, 2257, 1992.)

syringe. If meconium is present, more aggressive suctioning should be performed (see Chap. 9). When fully delivered, the infant should be held at the level of the vaginal opening (**introitus**) while being dried off with warmed towels. Drying will help maintain the infant's body temperature and at the same time stimulate the initiation of ventilation. Holding the infant at the level of the introitus will optimize blood flow between placental and infant circulations while the umbilicus is still intact.

When the infant has begun to breathe and pulsations in the umbilical cord have subsided, the cord may be clamped and cut.[1] At this time, the infant should be placed on a radiantly warmed bed with the head tilted slightly downward and the infant lying on his or her side. The airway may be further cleared with gentle suctioning of the mouth and nose with the bulb syringe. After the 5-minute Apgar score has been obtained and assuming that all vitals signs are stable, a suction catheter may be inserted through each nostril into the hypopharynx to rule out choanal atresia, and then through the mouth into the esophagus and stomach. If difficulty or resistance is encountered, the possibility of esophageal atresia or tracheal–esophageal fistula should be investigated by inserting a suction catheter, normally an 8 or 10 French (see Chap. 12). Once the catheter is in the stomach, if more than 25 mL of fluid is removed, the presence of a small bowel obstruction should be suspected.[1] Negative pressure should not exceed 100 mm Hg (136 cm H_2O) for a maximum of 5 seconds with each pass. When this procedure has been completed and the infant is stable, he or she may be wrapped in a warm blanket and given to the parents.

When the neonate does not respond and resuscitation is necessary, he or she should be placed on an open bed under a radiant warmer in a supine position with the neck in a neutral position. A rolled-up towel can be placed under the neonate's shoulders in order to help maintain the proper head position. Stimulation of the infant at this point should be limited to two attempts.

Assessing responsiveness and ventilation, establishing a patent airway, and preventing aspiration are of primary and intermediate concern. Apnea is the most common type of respiratory disorder in the neonate. After determining unresponsiveness by using **tactile stimuli** (pinching of the side or toes), the airway will need to be opened using the head-tilt/chin-lift method in order to determine if there is an obstruction of the airway by the tongue. In relation to the size of the airway, the tongue of a newborn is 25% larger at birth than it will be in the adult and is more likely to cause obstruction. The resuscitator's ear should be close to the mouth and nose of the neonate in order to hear the passage of air while watching the chest and abdomen for signs of movement (Fig. 20-1). Following a lack of response, two breaths are delivered for 1 to $1\frac{1}{2}$ seconds per inflation with a pause between breaths. The rescuer places his or her mouth over the infant's mouth and nose to deliver the necessary breaths (Fig. 20-2). The volume of air should be only enough to make the chest rise.

Artificial respirations can also be delivered using bag–mask ventilation (using 100% oxygen) or by breathing through a mask covering the mouth and nose of the neonate. The proper-sized mask is one that covers the bridge of the nose to the cleft of the chin, making an airtight seal.

Artificial respirations should not be performed rapidly as gastric distention will result which could make it harder to inflate the lungs. Venti-

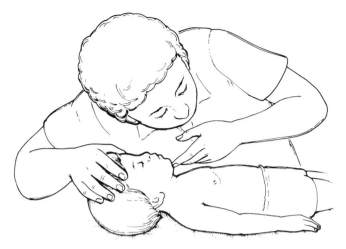

FIGURE 20-1 Determining breathlessness while maintaining head-tilt/chin-lift.

lation is considered adequate if there is bilateral chest expansion and breath sounds are heard when the chest is auscultated.

The detection of the presence of a heart rate and circulation of the blood is the next step. The heart rate can be determined by auscultation of the apical pulse using a stethoscope, grasping the umbilical stump to feel for pulsation, or placing 2 or 3 fingers on the inside of the infant's upper arm to assess the brachial artery (Fig. 20-3). If a pulse is present, only rescue breathing is required at a rate of 20 times a minute.

Chest compressions should be performed if (1) the heart rate is less than 60 beats per minute, or (2) the heart rate is between 60 and 80 beats per minute and the chest is not rising despite adequate ventilation with 100% oxygen for approximately 30 seconds.[1] Proper hand position is achieved by placing the index finger on an imaginary line across the nipples; placing the next two fingers on the sternum, making sure that they

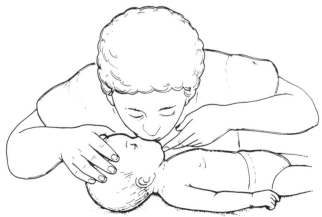

FIGURE 20-2 Rescue breathing with an airtight seal around the mouth and nose.

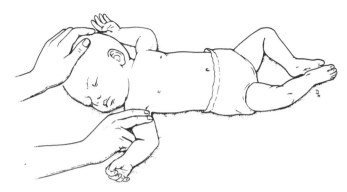

FIGURE 20-3 Locating the brachial pulse in an infant.

are not directly over the tip of the sternum; and then lifting the index finger (Fig. 20-4). Compressions should be at a depth of $1/2$ to 1 inch at a rate of at least 100 times per minute. The ratio of compressions to breaths is 5:1 (five compressions to one breath).

A second method of delivering compressions is the **side-by-side method**, in which the thumbs are placed on the sternum just below the nipple line and the fingers encircle the chest cavity (Fig. 20-5).

Once bag–mask ventilation and compressions have begun on the infant, assessment is made by evaluating responsiveness and the return of color, respirations, and normal heart rate. When the neonate is found to have less-than-adequate ventilation with bag–mask ventilation, there is an indication for the immediate intubation of the trachea. Endotracheal intubation should be considered if the infant has been delivered through thick or particulate meconium or has aspirated blood.[1] In this situation, intubation and thorough suctioning should be done before any other measures of resuscitation, especially bag–mask ventilation, in order to prevent further aspiration of these substances. A second indication is if an obstruction appears to be preventing adequate bag–mask ventilation. In this situation, the ET tube will usually bypass the obstruction and allow for adequate ventilation.

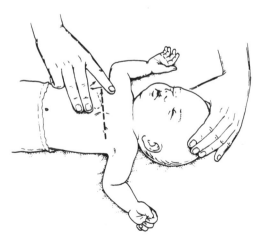

FIGURE 20-4 Locating finger position for chest compression in an infant.

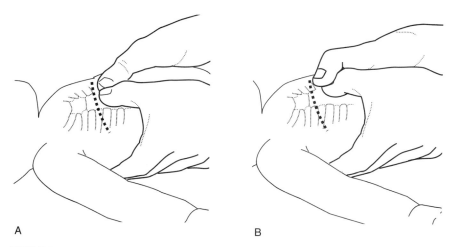

A   B

FIGURE 20-5 (**A**) Side-by-side thumb placement for chest compressions in newborns. (**B**) Overlapping thumb used for very small newborns.

Intubation is also indicated when the infant being ventilated with a bag–mask system has not shown significant improvement in heart rate and color or demonstrated a return of spontaneous breathing after a few minutes of assisted ventilation or when cardiac compression becomes necessary. Size of the ET tube may be determined by matching the diameter of the neonate's little finger to the diameter of the tube or by correlating the diameter with the birth weight (Table 20-4). When intubation is performed, suction should be turned on and available at all times. This will allow for immediate clearance of the airway and visualization of the vocal cords. Oxygen should be administered at all times during the procedure to prevent any additional complications.

Endotracheal intubation is much more likely to be successful on the first attempt if the following steps are taken before the initial laryngoscopy:

TABLE 20-4 Appropriate Sizes of Equipment for Resuscitation of the Newborn

	WEIGHT IN GRAMS				
	<1000	*1000–1250*	*1250–2500*	*2500–3000*	*>3000*
Oral airway	000	000	00	0	0
Endotracheal tube (mm)	2.5–3.0*	3.0	3.0	3.0–3.5	3.5–4.0
Suction catheter (French)	5	5 or 6	6	6 or 8	8
Mask for bag–mask resuscitation	0	0	0–1	1	1–4
Laryngoscope blade	00–0	0–1	0–1	0–1	1

*A 2.5-mm ET tube should not be used unless absolutely necessary, as it is difficult to suction and frequently occludes.

1. Select the proper size and prepare the ET tube, carefully inserting a stylet. In addition to the size selected, have a tube one size larger and one size smaller on hand. A stylet provides rigidity and appropriate curvature of the ET tube to facilitate rapid intubation, but it is important that the tip not project beyond the distal tip of the tube.
2. Choose a laryngoscope handle and blade, lock in place, and check that the light is bright enough and that the bulb is screwed tightly in place.
3. Make sure that suctioning equipment is set up and functioning properly and that a sterile suction catheter is attached and ready for use.
4. Properly position the infant's head in the **"sniffing" position** by keeping the head midline and the neck slightly extended. This allows the practitioner to obtain a straight line axis of the pharynx and the trachea. Slight elevation of the occipital skull will facilitate this. Gentle pressure exerted over the larynx (Selleck's maneuver) may also help the operator to visualize the opening to the airway.
5. Adequately hyperinflate and hyperoxygenate the infant for at least 10 seconds before attempting intubation. After 30 seconds (or sooner if bradycardia occurs), the intubation attempt should be stopped so that the infant may be reventilated with 100% oxygen using bag–mask ventilation.

Once the tube is in place and secured, ventilation can be resumed with a volume that allows for adequate chest movement and breath sounds heard on auscultation. There should be a return of color, a rise in heart rate to 120 to 160 beats per minute, and a progressive return of spontaneous breathing and chest movement. Overventilation may result in gastric distention, aspiration, or pneumothorax.

Infants who do not respond rapidly to stimulation, ventilation, intubation, and cardiac compressions need to receive fluid and drugs through a central line that is placed as quickly as possible. The preferred placement of the central line is into the umbilical artery or, if that is not possible, into the umbilical vein. Although umbilical artery catheterization may be more difficult to perform, it offers several advantages: (1) it allows for direct and continuous measurement of blood pressure; (2) arterial blood samples may be easily obtained; and (3) it may be left in place for several days to allow for continued monitoring and fluid or drug infusion in the postresuscitation management period. An umbilical venous catheter is usually removed immediately after resuscitation to prevent possible infection and clotting of the portal vein.

Initial drug therapy and fluid administration are directed toward correcting acidosis, hypoglycemia, hypovolemia, and hypotension.

Epinephrine is commonly used for neonates who remain in asystole or whose heart rates remain under 80 beats per minute despite intubation, ventilation, and chest compressions. A 1:10,000 concentration is used for neonates at a dose of 0.01 to 0.03 mg/kg (0.1 to 0.3 mL/kg) which can be given intravenously or directly through the ET tube. The intravenous route is preferred for neonates since dosage by ET tube can cause low plasma concentrations. The alpha adrenergic properties of the drug will cause vasoconstriction which elevates perfusion pressures during compressions, delivering more oxygen to the heart and brain. The infant should experience an increase in heart rate following the administration of epinephrine. If this does not occur, the dose may be repeated every 3 to 5 minutes.

If metabolic acidosis persists, sodium bicarbonate can be given. The recommended concentration of sodium bicarbonate is 0.5 mEq/mL of a 4.2% solution. Sodium bicarbonate and calcium are used in the acute phase of resuscitation to treat hyperkalemia and severe hypocalcemia. It should be administered slowly and the neonate should be observed for adverse effects.

Volume expanders or **pressors** are indicated to treat hypovolemia in the neonate, which is common if there is an acute blood loss or if the infant fails to respond to resuscitation. This is frequently a problem in the premature infant, possibly because their umbilical cords are clamped early in order to proceed with resuscitation measures. Hypovolemia is considered in those who have undergone delivery complicated by partial umbilical cord occlusion, accidental placental transection during cesarean section, placental abruption, or any maternal bleeding before or during delivery.

At physical examination, these infants may appear gray, pale, or mottled and usually have poor perfusion and capillary filling pressures manifested by cold, cyanotic extremities and weak or absent peripheral pulses. Hypovolemia should be suspected if mean arterial pressures are low, if systolic pressure decreases more than 5 mm Hg with inspiration, or if the central venous pressure is less than 4 cm H_2O. Volume expansion can be achieved by using whole blood matched to the mother's blood, 5% albumin with normal saline, or 10 mL/kg of normal saline or Ringer's lactate. The volume expander is given rapidly through the intravenous route over a 5 to 10 minute period. Care should be taken not to overexpand the intravascular volume because this may result in hypertension and subsequent intracranial hemorrhage. The presence of central venous and arterial lines greatly facilitates optimal fluid management in these infants.

Naloxone hydrochloride is given to the neonate for reversal of respiratory depression that is induced by narcotics given to the mother within 4 hours of delivery. The initial dose of 0.1 mg/kg of a 1 mg/mL or 0.4 mg/mL solution may be repeated every 2 to 3 minutes as needed. Naloxone hydrochloride should not, however, be given to infants of mothers who are chronically addicted to narcotic drugs because it may precipitate narcotic withdrawal in these infants, leading to further complications.

Hypoglycemia in the neonate is defined as a blood glucose level of less than 30 mg/dL in the full-term infant and less than 20 mg/dL in the infant weighing less than 2500 g. These abnormally low blood glucose levels occur frequently in the asphyxiated newborn because their glucose stores are easily depleted under stress. Untreated hypoglycemia may rapidly cause death secondary to cardiac failure or hypotension. Hypoglycemia can be treated by a rapid infusion of glucose via an intravenous bolus of 1 mL/kg of 50% dextrose followed by continuous infusion of 10% dextrose at 4 mL/kg/h.

Treatment of Foreign Body Obstruction

The method of assessing breathing and circulation of the neonate is used for an infant up to the age of 1 year. The other common problem that can cause preventable death is foreign body airway obstruction. According to the Journal of the American Medical Association, two thirds of the victims of death caused by foreign body aspiration are infants under the age of 1 year. Airway obstruction can be caused by infectious conditions such as croup or epiglottitis (see Chap. 10) but it is more commonly the result of an object being lodged in the airway. If obstruction is suspected, the rescuer delivers up to 5 back blows with the infant in a prone position resting on the rescuer's forearm with the head positioned lower than the trunk of the body. While holding the head firmly, the rescuer turns the infant over in a supine position by sandwiching the infant between his or her arms. Five quick, downward chest thrusts are then delivered in the same location as that used for delivering chest compressions (Fig. 20-6). If there is no response, the procedure is repeated until the infant dislodges the object or becomes unconscious.

If the infant becomes unconscious, the steps are repeated, but attempts to ventilate after the five chest thrusts are now added. A sweep of the mouth is never done unless the object is visible and easily removed. This is to prevent any unnecessary trauma to the oral mucosa. Once the object has been dislodged or the rescuer is able to deliver a breath, the steps for assessing circulation can be initiated and CPR can be started if necessary.

Stabilization and Follow-Up Care

After resuscitation and stabilization, the neonate or infant is usually transported to an intensive care unit for close observation and careful monitoring of vital signs. Care should be taken to provide a neutral thermal environment; deliver warmed, humidified oxygen; monitor vital signs every 15 minutes for the first hour, maintaining a systolic blood pressure over 40 mm Hg; and continue infusion of a volume expander solution such as Ringer's lactate. An arterial blood gas reading should be obtained to determine ventilation and oxygenation levels, and a Dextrostix should be used to monitor the level of glucose. Noninvasive monitors, such as a pulse oximeter and transcutaneous oxygen monitor or capnography, are used if available. Early recognition of complications can prevent the infant from suffering any additional complications.

▪ RESUSCITATION OF THE CHILD

The causes of pediatric cardiopulmonary arrest requiring resuscitation are different from those of the neonate and infant. Pediatric cardiopulmonary arrest is rarely caused by an interruption in cardiac function unless there is underlying congenital cardiac disease.

The congenital cardiac defect will be defined by a dysrhythmia that is ventricular in nature. If the rhythm is not asystole, it will be either bradycardic or tachycardiac or a ventricular fibrillation. The irregular beat will have an effect on the cardiac output of the child and ultimately lead to an arrest.

The causes most often associated with respiratory failure are injury or shock. Shock can be diagnosed in the early stages by assessment of heart rate, peripheral pulses, and skin temperature, which is cool in most cases but will be warm if the patient is septic. Survival rates approach 50% after prompt resuscitation in children with respiratory arrest alone.[1]

Pediatric resuscitation guidelines are to be used in children ages 1 to 8 years. The common causes of injury vary greatly within this age group; much attention has been paid to prevention of serious injury. The six most common types of childhood injuries are motor vehicle passenger injuries, pedestrian injuries, bicycle injuries, submersion, burns, and firearm injuries.[1] Injuries related to motor vehicles, submersion, and burns are more common in children under the age of 4, whereas pedestrian injuries, bicycles, and firearms cause more trauma for children from the ages of 5 to 8 years.

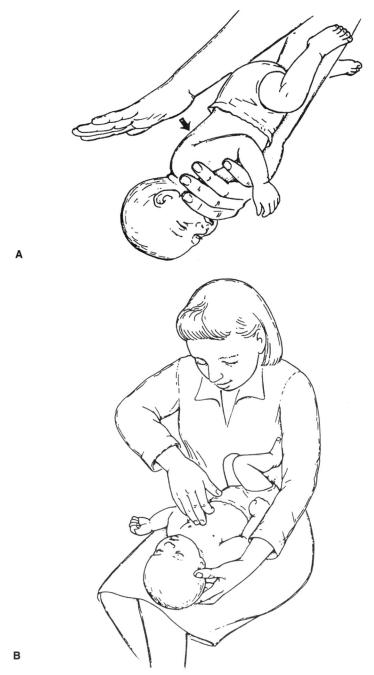

FIGURE 20-6 (*A*) Back blow in an infant. (*B*) Chest thrust in an infant.

Recognition of a Child in Distress

Recognition of the child in distress is often the responsibility of the care-giver or those individuals who are with the child at the time of an injury in which a progressive deterioration of mental status occurs. The child may demonstrate signs of tachycardia initially or may immediately show the more serious sign of impending distress, bradycardia. If the child is bradycardic, immediate attention to the trauma must begin.

Deterioration in respiratory function or possible respiratory arrest should be anticipated in infants or children who demonstrate any of the following signs: an increased respiratory rate or effort; inadequate respiratory rate, effort, or chest excursion; decreased breath sounds; diminished level of consciousness or response to pain; poor skeletal muscle tone; or cyanosis. Early shock is diagnosed by evaluation of heart rate, presence and volume (strength) of peripheral pulses, and adequacy of end-organ perfusion.[1]

Preparation of Equipment

Equipment and supplies should be readily available for resuscitation of the child. To properly treat the child, oxygen and complete supplies, suction apparatus, laryngoscope and blades, ET tubes, chest board, resuscitation bag, and other equipment will need to be assembled and tested for proper functioning. A list of pediatric equipment and drugs can be found in Table 20-5.

Oxygen at 100% should be administered as soon as available with a mask of the appropriate size. The mask should provide an airtight seal without any pressure to the eyes. The resuscitation bag for a child should be able to hold a minimum of 450 mL; for larger children, an adult bag holding a min-

---

TABLE 20-5   Supply List for Emergency Resuscitation of the Child

Equipment and Supplies	Medications and Fluids
Oxygen source with flowmeter	Adenosine 0.1–0.2 mg/kg
Bubble humidifier with connective tubing	Atropine 0.02 mg/kg, range 0.1 mg to max 0.5 mg
Suction device with manometer	Bretylium 5 mg/kg
Suction catheters (8, 10, 12, 14 Fr)	Sodium bicarbonate 8.4%–1 mEq/kg or 0.3 × kg × base deficit
Face masks (sizes 4–adult)	Dopamine 2–20 µg/kg per minute
Oral airways (sizes 1–6)	Dobutamine 2–20 µg/kg per minute
Endotracheal tubes (sizes 3.5–7)	Epinephrine
Laryngoscope/blades (1–4) with extra bulbs and batteries	1:10,000 IV/IO @ 0.01 mg/kg
Stylet, scissors, gloves	1:10,000 ET tube @ 0.1 mg/kg initially, up to 0.2 mg/kg
Stethoscope	Albumin 5%/Normal Saline
Tape (1/2 and 3/4 sizes)	Naloxone 0.04 mg/mL
Chest board	Lidocaine 1 mg/kg
Medical antishock trousers (MAST)	Glucose 2–4mL/kg of 25%
Defibrillator/leads	Ringer's lactate
Syringe (size 10 cc)	Sterile water
Alcohol wipes	Normal saline
Blood gas syringes	Heparin
Tonsil-tipped suction device	

imum of 800 mL may be necessary. These bags should not have a pop-off and if there is one present it should be bypassed. An oxygen reservoir should be added and supplied with 10 to 15 liters per minute of oxygen in order to deliver an oxygen percentage in the range of 60% to 95%.[2] Ventilations should be delivered in a manner that minimizes gastric distention.

Drug therapy is directed toward correcting hypoxia and the decreased cardiac output, increasing contractility of the heart, and reversing bradycardia. Peripheral intravenous access is the desired route of administration of drugs, although drugs can be administered through the ET tube. Pediatric advanced life support (**PALS**) guidelines also recommend the use of the intraosseous route if the peripheral veins are not available.[1]

For cardiac arrest of the child, epinephrine is considered a first-line drug to treat both asystole and bradycardia. Epinephrine also enhances the contractile state of the heart, stimulates spontaneous contractions, and increases the vigor and intensity of ventricular fibrillation, making the fibrillation more amenable to termination by electrical defibrillation. Epinephrine can be administered either intravenously or through the ET tube. Doses are listed in Table 20-5. Adenosine is used to treat symptomatic supraventricular tachycardia (SVT). Atropine can be used to treat persistent bradycardia, poor perfusion, or hypotension in the child.

Blood glucose should be carefully monitored in the child and glucose should only be given if the child suffers from shock or respiratory failure where hypoglycemia can be documented. Volume expanders such as Ringer's lactate, normal saline, or albumin 5% should be given to the child immediately and used to flush drugs through the intravenous line as well as to prevent hypovolemia.

Sodium bicarbonate, although not a first-line resuscitation drug, is used to treat metabolic acidosis in the child as well as in the infant. It can be administered through either the intravenous or intraosseous route using 1 mL/kg of an 8.4% solution, and the child is monitored for any side effects. The most common side effect is the development of metabolic alkalosis.

Dopamine is used to treat shock and is administered intravenously at a rate as low as 2 µg/kg per minute to a maximum of 20 µg/kg per minute. It should increase the blood pressure as well as the urine output of the child. Dobutamine is given to increase myocardial contractility, which should aid in the correction of a low cardiac output. The dosage for dobutamine is the same as for dopamine.

Resuscitation Techniques

The sequence of resuscitation for a child is similar to that of an adult victim. The first step is to determine unresponsiveness in the child by shaking gently and calling to the child while surveying the scene for possible signs of trauma to the neck or cerebral spinal cord.

If there is no response, breathing should be immediately assessed. The head-tilt/chin-lift method is used to provide a patent airway. This method will prevent the tongue from obstructing the airway (Fig. 20-7). When injury to the neck is suspected, the jaw-thrust maneuver can be attempted by placing one hand on each side of the angle of the jaw and lifting the mandible upward (Fig. 20-8). The rescuer should observe the chest for signs of breathing and attempt to feel air movement. If breathing is absent, two rescue

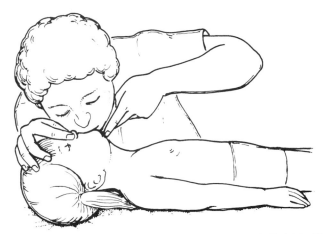

FIGURE 20-7   Mouth-to-mouth seal while maintaining head-tilt/chin-lift position.

breaths are delivered slowly (1 to 1½ seconds each) with a pause between breaths. This is done by placing the rescuer's mouth over the victim's mouth and pinching the victim's nose closed. Seeing the rise of the chest with each breath will ensure adequate ventilation while decreasing the possibility of any gastric distention or air trapping.

The next step is to check for a pulse, preferably at the carotid site (Fig. 20-9). In the hospital the femoral pulse is often used for assessment. If a pulse is detected, rescue breathing is continued at a rate of 1 breath every 3 seconds. The rescuer should stop each minute to assess the victim. If there is no pulse and no breathing, compression of the chest is started at a ratio of five compressions to one breath (80 to 100 compressions per minute). Compressions should be between 1 and 1½ inches deep, which should be approximately one third to one half of the depth of the chest of the child. To locate proper hand position, the rescuer traces the lower margin of the rib cage to the xiphoid process and places an index finger over the notch. The heel of the hand is placed next to the index finger parallel to the sternum (Fig. 20-10). The other hand is used to stabilize the head. Table 20-3 compares infant and child CPR.

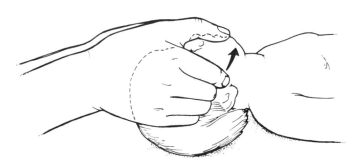

FIGURE 20-8   Jaw-thrust.

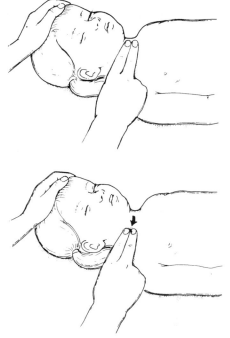

FIGURE 20-9 Locating and palpating the carotid artery pulse.

If the child is not responding to CPR, the use of 100% oxygen and bag–mask ventilation should be considered. If adequate oxygen is not delivered, the child can develop metabolic acidosis and multiple organ failure. Supplying oxygen will help to compensate for the low levels being delivered to the tissues as a result of a decreased cardiac output. If possible, the oxygen should be humidified to avoid the further trauma to the airways caused by dried or retained secretions. The child will need to be assessed for the proper size mask so that an airtight seal can be provided

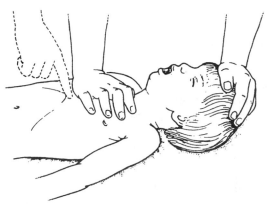

FIGURE 20-10 Locating hand position for chest compression in a child.

TABLE 20-6   Suggested Sizes for Endotracheal Tubes and Suction Catheters*

AGE	INTERNAL DIAMETER OF TUBE, MM	SUCTION CATHETERS
Newborn	3.0	6 Fr
6 months	3.5	8 Fr
18 months	4.0	8 Fr
3 years	4.5	8 Fr
5 years	5.0	10 Fr
6 years	5.5	10 Fr
8 years	6.0	10 Fr
12 years	6.5	10 Fr
16 years	7.0	10 Fr
Adult female	7.5–8.0	12 Fr
Adult male	8.0–8.5	14 Fr

*Endotracheal tube selection for a child should be based on the child's size, not age. One size larger and one size smaller should be allowed for individual variations. (American Heart Association, Cardiac Care Committees: Guidelines for cardiopulmonary resuscitation and emergency cardiac care. JAMA:268, 2263, 1992.)

without putting any pressure on the eyes. A self-inflating bag that provides at least 450 mL, without a pop-off valve, is preferred for the child.

If the child still does not respond, endotracheal intubation should be considered. Indications for endotracheal intubation include (1) inadequate central nervous system control of ventilation, (2) functional or anatomic airway obstruction, (3) excessive work of breathing leading to fatigue, and (4) need for high peak inspiratory pressure or positive end-expiratory pressure to maintain effective alveolar gas exchange.[1] Table 20-6 lists the proper sizes of ET tubes for the child. Uncuffed tubes are recommended for children under 8 years. The correct size can be determined using the formula:

$$\text{Size} = \frac{\text{age in years} + 16}{4}$$

Proper techniques for intubation of children are the same as those for infants, and they have been described previously.

If the child suffers from a foreign body aspiration, the abdominal thrust (**Heimlich maneuver**) is used to remove the object. The rescuer stands behind the victim and encircles the victim's chest with his or her arms. The fist of one hand is placed with the thumb side against the victim's abdomen in the midline, half way between the naval and the xiphoid process. The other hand is used to grab the fist and exert a series of swift, upward movements to relieve the object (Fig. 20-11). After a series of thrusts, the victim should be assessed.

The abdominal thrusts continue until the object is dislodged or the victim becomes unconscious. At this point, the victim is placed on the ground in a supine position and assessed for breathing. If the object is vis-

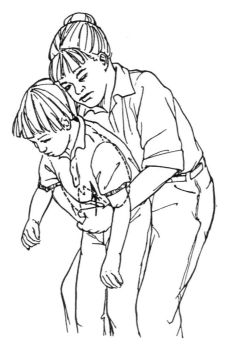

FIGURE 20-11   Abdominal thrusts with victim standing or sitting (conscious).

ible in the pharyngeal area, it should be removed immediately and the victim assessed. If the initial attempt to open the airway is unsuccessful (head-tilt/chin-lift), the rescuer should make a second attempt to open the airway and deliver a breath. After an unsuccessful second attempt at ventilation, the rescuer should straddle the victim and deliver five abdominal thrusts using the heel of one hand placed above the naval but below the rib cage on the midline of the chest, with the second hand placed on top of the first (Fig. 20-12). A finger sweep of the mouth for the object is not indicated unless the rescuer can see the object and remove it easily. After each series of five abdominal thrusts, the rescuer should attempt to ventilate the unconscious victim before repeating the Heimlich maneuver. Assessment of the carotid pulse and the delivery of chest compressions cannot begin until the airway has been opened.

Stabilization and Follow-Up Care
The postresuscitation care of the child will involve continued stabilization of the child, transport of the child to an area where proper care can be given, and the prevention of further trauma to the child. Assessing vital signs, auscultating the chest, noting appropriate responses to questions, and monitoring for side effects of drug therapy will be an ongoing process. Neurological, renal, and hepatic assessment can be made at this time. A medical history should be obtained.

A pulse oximeter probe should be attached to the patient's finger to monitor oxygen saturation levels and an arterial blood gas measurement should

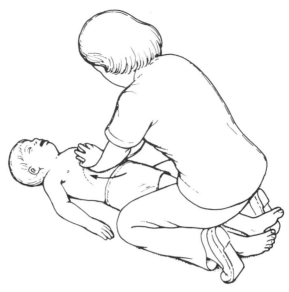

FIGURE 20-12   Chest thrust in a child.

be obtained to assess proper ventilation. An EKG can be obtained to check heart function. A nasogastric or orogastric tube may be required to prevent or relieve gastric distention. If an intraosseous line was placed during resuscitation, it should be replaced with an intravenous line at this time.

▬REFERENCES

1. American Heart Association, Emergency Cardiac Care Committees: Guidelines for cardiopulmonary resuscitation and emergency cardiac care. JAMA 268:2251–2281, 1992.
2. McPherson SB: Respiratory Care Equipment, 5th ed. St. Louis, Mosby Year Book, 1995.
3. Malinowski C: Neonatal resuscitation program and pediatric advanced life support. Respiratory Care 40:575, 1995.

▬BIBLIOGRAPHY

American Heart Association: Currents in emergency cardiac care. In Interim Training Guidelines for Pediatric Resuscitation, 1992. Dallas TX, American Heart Association.

Barnes TA: Clinical practice guidelines for resuscitation in acute care hospitals. Respiratory Care 40:346, 1995.

Barnes TA: Emergency ventilation techniques and related equipment. Respiratory Care 37:673, 1992.

Barnhart SL, Czervinske MP: Perinatal and Pediatric Respiratory Care. Philadelphia, WB Saunders, 1995.

Boudin KM: Strategies for maintaining ACLS skills in hospitals. Respiratory Care 40:550, 1995.

Byrne PJ, Tyebkhan JM, Laing LM: Ethical decision-making and neonatal resuscitation (reprinted from Seminars in Perinatology). Neonatal Intensive Care 8:34, 1995.

Burchfield DJ: Medication use in neonatal resuscitation: Epinephrine and sodium bicarbonate. Neonatal Pharmacology Quarterly 2:25, 1993.

Greenberg MD: Emergency vascular access: The use of intraosseous infusion. Physician Assistant 19:59, 1995.

Hazinski MF: Advances and controversies in cardiopulmonary resuscitation in the young. Journal of Cardiovascular Nursing 6:74, 1995.

Hazinski MF: New guidelines for pediatric and neonatal cardiopulmonary resuscitation and advanced life support. Part 1. Basic CPR for adults and children. Pediatric Nursing 12:373, 1986.

Interim training guidelines for neonatal resuscitation: Currents in emergency cardiac care. AHA 3(4):26, 1992.

Keddington RK: Emergency cardiac care: New pediatric guidelines. RN 57:44, 1994.

The Pediatric Code. American Journal of Nursing Co., VHS videocassette.

Perlson R: Safe and successful delivery-room intubation and resuscitation of meconium-stained newborns by respiratory therapists. Respiratory Care 35:1228, 1990.

Peters SJ: Commentary on what dose of epinephrine is being used in pediatric resuscitation? Results of a survey. ENA'S Nursing Scan in Emergency Care 9:4, 1993.

Pratt JL: Pediatric emergency care and resuscitation. Current Opinion in Pediatrics 5:289, 1993.

Sloman M: Paediatric cardiopulmonary resuscitation. Nursing Times 84:50, 1988.

Soud T: Airway, breathing, circulation, and disability: What is different about kids? Journal of Emergency Nursing 18:107, 1992.

Whitaker K: Comprehensive Perinatal and Pediatric Respiratory Care. Albany, Delmar Publishers, 1992.

■SELF-ASSESSMENT QUESTIONS

1. The physician, nurse, and therapist are preparing for a premature delivery. Why would you set up a radiant warmer?
   a. to help provide tactile stimuli
   b. to provide access to the baby from at least three sides
   c. to help improve fetal lung compliance
   d. to access stored resuscitation equipment

2. When the neonate is first born, what is the benefit of holding the baby at the level of the introitus initially?
   a. optimizing blood flow to the infant
   b. stabilizing of ventilations
   c. preventing hypothermia
   d. aid in the release of glucose from the tissues

3. The second Apgar score has been obtained and all vital signs appear to be normal at this time. The next step would be to evaluate for
   a. choanal atresia
   b. presence of meconium
   c. gastric distention
   d. signs of hypothermia

4. In order to prevent hypovolemia and dehydration of the neonate from developing, you would suggest all of the following *except*
   a. albumin 5%
   b. Ringer's lactate
   c. normal saline
   d. atropine

5. The use of epinephrine is recommended to treat asystole or bradycardia for the infant and child during resuscitation. It can be administered through an intravenous site or down the ET tube. Low plasma level may result with the use an ET tube
   a. for infants only
   b. for children only
   c. for both infants and children
   d. It is not given through the ET tube for either infants or children.

6. According to the American Heart Association, you cannot begin to start CPR on either an infant or child until
   a. you have called for assistance
   b. unresponsiveness has been determined
   c. you can deliver breaths to a patent airway
   d. you have attended and completed a CPR class

7. When the rescuer observes a choking child, the first step is to ask if he or she is choking. Once this has been confirmed, the rescuer should
   a. quickly call for assistance
   b. administer four back blows between the shoulder blades
   c. stand behind the victim and find the correct position to begin abdominal thrusts
   d. attempt to ventilate the victim

8. When a therapist is administering bag–mask ventilation to either the infant or child, all of the following are considerations *except*
   a. picking the appropriate-sized mask
   b. quickly attaching an oxygen gas source
   c. choosing the appropriate-sized bag
   d. having a pop-off set at 25 cm H_2O pressure

9. What is the proper position for the head of a neonate during intubation?
   a. sniffing position
   b. head hyperextended to 60 degrees
   c. neck neutral using the jaw-thrust maneuver
   d. tilted position

10. Once the child has been stabilized and a patent airway is in place, the therapist will have time to evaluate pertinent data. In order to avoid aspiration and relieve gastric distention, what is used?
    a. pulse oximeter
    b. intravenous line
    c. nasogastric tube
    d. intraosseous line

Chapter 21

Home Care of the Newborn and Child

LAURA BEVERIDGE

OBJECTIVES

Having completed this chapter, the reader will be able to:

1 Discuss the need for effective discharge planning.

2 Identify the composition and role of the discharge planning team.

3 Describe the indications for home oxygen therapy.

4 Explain the components of an adequate prescription for home oxygen therapy.

5 Compare and contrast the various types of home oxygen equipment and delivery systems available.

6 Describe the home assessment to be performed before oxygen therapy in the home is begun.

7 Discuss the ways in which infants receiving home oxygen therapy should be monitored.

8 Describe the problems and safety measures associated with the use of oxygen in the home setting.

9 Discuss the importance of physician orders and communication in relation to home oxygen therapy.

10 Describe the uses of aerosol and humidity therapy in the home.

11 Describe the methods and delivery systems used for home aerosol and humidity therapy.

12 Discuss the monitoring of the patient on aerosol and humidity therapy at home.

13 Describe the problems and safety measures associated with the use of aerosols and humidity at home.

14 Discuss the various types of infant apnea that may require monitoring in the home.

15 Explain the process of discharge planning for infant apnea.

16 Describe a typical home support system for the family.

17 State the criteria for discontinuation of home monitoring.

18 Discuss patient selection and discharge criteria for mechanical ventilation in the home.

(continued)

OBJECTIVES (Continued)

19 Describe the steps in discharge planning for home mechanical ventilation patients.

20 Discuss the monitoring of home ventilator patients.

KEY TERMS

apparent life-threatening event
  (ALTE)
apnea monitoring
discharge planning
liquid oxygen system

oxygen concentrator
rooming in
sudden infant death syndrome
  (SIDS)

Advances in medical treatment and technology have had a dual impact on the changing scope of neonatal and pediatric home care. Increasing numbers of infants and children are surviving complicated pregnancies, extreme prematurity and its sequelae, congenital anomalies, life-threatening infections, trauma, and numerous chronic disease states (*e.g.*, neuromuscular, neurological). Technology available in the home setting has progressed so dramatically that many survivors of theses scenarios are now able to leave the stresses of the hospital environment and enter the normalcy of their own home. Respiratory care has no doubt played the largest role in these changes over the last few years.

Along with the increasing number of young patients who might potentially benefit from home care has come the overwhelming pressures to control spiraling health care costs by moving patients out of hospitals as quickly as possible. This trend mandates the evolution of an efficient and organized care plan incorporating a wide variety of disciplines and requiring thorough education of the family and caregivers.

▄ DISCHARGE PLANNING

As the need to control health care costs has evolved, **discharge planning** has become a specialty that can best be described as a coordinated process resulting in a plan of continued care once the patient leaves the hospital. The plan of care must encompass the medical, emotional, psychological, and social needs of the patient and family and ensure that all needs can and will be met upon the patient's release. The ultimate goal of any discharge plan should be the normalization of life for the infant or child while providing for all special needs that exist or might arise in the course of care. Without this as a goal, the entire process, regardless of complexity, would fail the patient entirely.

Several criteria must be met before a patient can be released into the home setting. Before discharge planning is initiated, parents and caregivers must be willing to care for the child at home. In most cases, there must always be at least two caregivers who are willing to take on this responsibility. This ensures that one person does not collapse under the strain of physical demand, emotional stresses, and sleep deprivation. Once this is established, all caregivers should be made aware of the dramatic changes that will occur in their once-private lives.

The home must be assessed for environmental safety (*e.g.*, cleanliness, temperature, access), adequate space, and electrical safety. Many homes will require rewiring, repair, and sometimes even renovations before the child can be released to the home.

Financial considerations can have the greatest impact on the discharge process. In many situations, parents must leave jobs and encounter an avalanche of medical expenses. Insurance companies and governmental funding agencies do not always approve home care without much time and consideration.[3]

Other criteria for patient selection include, but are not limited to, the following:

- Access to professional caregivers (nurses, respiratory care practitioners [RCPs], occupational therapists, physical therapists) from organizations that are well-qualified (preferably accredited by the Joint Commission on the Accreditation of Healthcare Organizations [JCAHO])
- Proximity to the hospital, physician offices, etc.
- Access to transportation
- Telephone service
- Access to 911 emergency systems
- Community support services

Team Planning

Discharge planners are the individuals who bring the puzzle together by coordinating the numerous members of the home care team. They are responsible for arranging needed services and assisting families in locating outside agencies.[7] In most areas of the country, this qualified discharge planner is a social worker or nurse. However, some institutions have realized that respiratory therapists make excellent discharge planners because of their extensive clinical and technical knowledge.

The discharge planning team will consist of practitioners from many different disciplines (Table 21-1). This interdisciplinary team has a responsibility to work together, thus ensuring the patient's comfort and safety at home. It is helpful for the discharge planner to have each member of the team identify goals for the patient in order to bridge gaps and allow members to complement each other.[7] This attempt to facilitate the planning process is important in pediatric care because of the anxiety and stress on the parents and family members.

The Role of the Respiratory Care Practitioner

The RCP is the individual who is best prepared by far in the many facets of managing the patient who needs oxygen, apnea monitoring, mechanical ventilation, tracheostomy management, and other related modalities. The input from these professionals is invaluable in the entire discharge process and it is imperative that their involvement begin upon initiation of this plan.

The hospital-based RCP is already knowledgeable regarding the patient's needs and clinical course (*e.g.*, arterial blood gas baselines, ven-

---

TABLE 21-1   Members of the Discharge Planning Team

Physician

Nurse

Social worker

Respiratory care practitioner
(hospital and home medical equipment company)

Physical therapist

Occupational therapist

Dietitian

Psychologist/family counselor

Clergy

Child life specialist

Case manager

Speech therapist

---

tilator settings, history of apnea/bradycardia) and has an understanding of how this patient can best be cared for in the home setting.

The home care RCP can work closely with the hospital-based RCP in gathering this information and selecting the proper equipment for the home. Parent caregiver education is often shared by the hospital and home care company. The longer the home care team has to become acquainted with the patient, the easier the transition will be for everyone involved. One of the common hurdles in discharge planning is failure to provide this important interactive time.

Once the patient is home, the RCP most often becomes the person with whom the family develops the deepest trust and relationship. After all, this is the professional that best understands the technology in the child's home and provides ongoing assessment and education long after other individuals on the team have served their functions.

Selection of Home Medical Equipment Providers

As home care evolves, the standard of care continues to improve. There is a strong argument that home medical equipment (HME) providers should meet JCAHO requirements before a discharge planner involves them in pediatric cases. This would ensure that the provider meets certain criteria (Table 21-2) and that patients receive the same protection in the home as in the hospital.

Patient Discharge

The discharge planning process will vary in complexity depending on the patient's needs. It is beyond the scope of this chapter to cover every aspect of the process, but it is important to establish final guidelines which should be met before patient discharge can occur:

1. The infant or child must have been stable for a reasonable period of time (the physician and other members of the team must agree on a definition of "reasonable").

TABLE 21-2 JCAHO Criteria for Home Medical Equipment Providers

Credentialed respiratory care practitioners

24-hour call with quick response time

Quality equipment and up-to-date technology with ongoing monitoring of proper function and preventive maintenance plans

Ongoing assessment of pertinent information (oximetry, vital signs, appearance, social needs, environment, equipment needs, medical needs, caregiver capabilities, etc.)

Protection of patient rights and responsibilities

Ongoing education of parents/caregivers

Ongoing communication with physicians concerning patient status and needs

Assistance with insurance billing

2. Parents and caregivers must feel comfortable with their ability and education in all areas of patient care training.
3. The patient's home must be prepared by obtaining all needed supplies and equipment, appropriate repairs, and safety devices (*e.g.*, smoke alarm, fire extinguisher), and by organizing living space for easy access upon arrival.
4. All professional caregivers and support services have been notified with a time frame for the patient's release.
5. All arrangements for transport needs have been met, including equipment (*e.g.*, oxygen, suction, ventilator) and personnel (*e.g.*, nurse, RCP, EMT).
6. The family has been instructed on any last-minute changes in patient prescriptions or physician orders as well as appointment schedules for physician follow-up.

In summary, discharge planning involves many variables, but it provides a smooth transition into the child's home environment. Normalization of daily activities and family interaction in the home setting contributes to the overall happiness and well being of pediatric patients. The respiratory care practitioner has a great impact on this discharge process and provides families with ongoing support, assessment, and information.

OXYGEN THERAPY

Indications

Long-term oxygen therapy is based on the infant's or child's inability to maintain adequate Pao_2 on room air. The American College of Chest Physicians and the National Heart Lung and Blood Institute reviewed oxygen therapy at the National Conference of Oxygen Therapy in 1984.[9] The First Denver Consensus Conference in 1986 and the Second Denver Consensus Conference in 1987 made recommendations that further defined the present guidelines now used by Medicare.[9] Medicare guidelines (Table 21-3) are used by some third-party payers as a general rule for pediatric patients, but are not rigidly adhered to in every case.

TABLE 21-3　Medicare Guidelines for Reimbursement of Oxygen Therapy

PaO_2 AND SaO_2	MEDICARE QUALIFICATION
$PaO_2 \leq 55$ mm Hg $SaO_2 \leq 88\%$	Patient will qualify under Medicare guidelines
$PaO_2 = 56–59$ mm Hg $SaO_2 = 89\%$	Patient will qualify if there is accompanying cor pulmonale, polycythemia, CHF, or P pulmonale
$PaO_2 \geq 60$ mm Hg $SaO_2 \geq 90\%$	Patient will qualify in some cases with a thorough statement from the physician

Methods and Delivery

Supplying oxygen in the home is actually complicated in comparison to hospital delivery. There are additional variables to be considered such as patient mobility, distance to the patient's home, the risk of power outages, daily activities, and space availability in the home. The RCP must effectively gather the needed information and carefully design the system that will best meet the needs of the child. Systems used for home delivery include cylinders, liquid oxygen, and concentrators.[9] Combinations of these systems are frequently used to meet patient needs.

Oxygen Cylinders

The most commonly used cylinders in the child's home are the H, E, D, and B cylinders (Fig. 21-1). The D and B cylinders are easily carried in shoulder bags which lighten a patient's load when carrying a diaper bag, apnea monitors, and infant carriers. The E cylinder can be pushed in its cart for ambulating or used as a backup for concentrators. The H cylinder is appropriate for continuous use, but it is the author's opinion that concentrators or liquid systems are a better option. Although all cylinders should be secured, the H cylinder is large and still creates a greater risk in the home of small children. The lengths of time these cylinders will last at 2 L/min are listed in Table 21-4.

Cylinders are the least expensive choice when used for the low liter flows which are frequently seen in pediatric patients.

Liquid Oxygen

Thermos-type reservoirs (Dewier flasks) containing liquid oxygen stored at $-297°$ F can be used in the home and provide for greater portability and ease.[9] These units can hold 18 to 55 L of liquid oxygen, with each liter of liquid oxygen evaporating into 860 L of gaseous oxygen. A 30-L unit will last 215 hours at 2 L/min, or approximately 9 days. Even when the system is turned off, the liquid oxygen will continue to evaporate slowly into the atmosphere at a rate of 1 to 2 lb/day. The rate of evaporation varies with different units and must be taken into account when calculating the length of use. The amount of oxygen lost by evaporation will increase at higher temperatures. Units should always be stored in open areas to prevent the creation of an oxygen-enriched space. Portable units which come in several sizes are filled from the base unit. These portable units create a lighter load for parents while providing for extended lengths of use (Table 21-5).

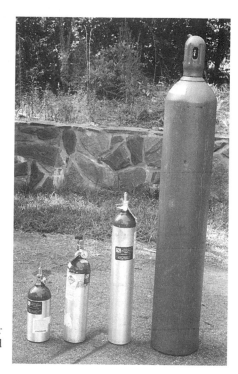

FIGURE 21-1 Oxygen cylinders for home use. Shown are sizes B, D, E, and H (from left to right).

Patients living in areas in which power outages occur more often than usual are excellent candidates for a **liquid oxygen system**. Homes with small rooms are easily overheated by oxygen concentrators. Liquid oxygen systems will reduce the amount of heat created as well as reduce the power bill for families who might already be in a financial crunch.

Oxygen Concentrators

An **oxygen concentrator** (Fig. 21-2) is an electrically powered device that provides a constant source of oxygen from ambient air. A molecular sieve bed in the concentrator separates oxygen from nitrogen, trace gases, and

TABLE 21-4   Duration of Cylinder Flow at 2 L/min (beginning with full cylinder)

CYLINDER TYPE	VOLUME OF FULL CYLINDER (L)	DURATION OF CYLINDER FLOW (HOURS)
B	266	1.75
D	400	2.6
E	680	4.6
H	7700	52

TABLE 21-5   Portable Liquid Unit Duration

VOLUME OF UNIT (L)	DURATION OF FLOW (HOURS)	OVERALL WEIGHT (LB)
≈0.4	3	≈6
≈0.8	6	≈11
≈1.6	11	≈12

water vapor. Oxygen concentrations vary depending on liter flow, the type of unit, and the cleanliness of the sieve bed and filters. Table 21-6 provides an overview of manufacturer's acceptable output ranges. As flow rates to the patient are increased, the delivered oxygen concentration decreases. This decrease is rarely a clinical problem because the concentration varies only a small amount with the prescribed oxygen flow rates.

The oxygen output from concentrators must be analyzed on a periodic basis to ensure adequate FIO_2 delivery. Several new units have built-in analyzers to alert the patient and caregivers when FIO_2 decreases. Internal and external filters must also be cleaned or changed to protect the sieve beds and compressor.

Concentrators are usually on wheels and can be moved around the child's house. If extension tubing is added, the therapist or technician

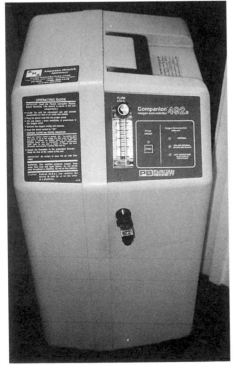

FIGURE 21-2   Puritan-Bennett Companion 492 oxygen concentrator.

TABLE 21-6 Output From Oxygen Concentrators

UNIT	FLOW RATE (L/MIN)	Flo$_2$ (%)
PB 590	1–4	95 ± 3
	5	90 ± 3
AirSep	≤6	90 ± 3
Devilbiss	1	94 ± 3
SolAiris	2–4	95 ± 3
	5	93 ± 3

must use a flow meter at the patient end of the tubing to check for flow accuracy. It is possible that the concentrator flow rate will need to be increased to deliver the ordered flow rate to the patient through this longer length of tubing.

Backup oxygen must be provided for patients on concentrators in case of machine or power failure. The amount of backup oxygen available should be at least two to three times the estimated response time for the HME provider to the patient's home.

Home Assessment and Monitoring

Assessment and monitoring of the patient is performed by respiratory care practitioners employed by the HME provider. Many companies are now accredited by JCAHO for both equipment management and clinical services. Monitoring of equipment operation and safety includes frequent checks of various parameters (Table 21-7). Check-off lists are beneficial for initial set-up (Fig. 21-3) and can be completed by the RCP or trained company service technicians.

Clinical monitoring services are performed by the credentialed RCP and include ongoing assessment of the child's clinical parameters including (1) pulse oximetry; (2) vital signs; (3) patient appearance; (4) medication changes; (5) diet changes; (6) environmental factors affecting the child's health; (7) psychosocial factors affecting parents, caregivers, and the patient; and (8) the need for additional education and instruction.

Strong assessment skills and communication of pertinent findings to the physician will prevent most patients from being seen in emergency rooms or from being readmitted to hospitals on a frequent basis. As RCPs continue to demonstrate these skills, it will become easier for third-party payers to realize that respiratory care services are integral to the home care process. At this point, home respiratory care companies are reimbursed for rental or purchase of oxygen equipment only. Clinical services are provided by companies that have a commitment to the provision of thorough and quality patient care.

Problems and Safety

The potential for problems and safety concerns with the infant or child on oxygen is enormous. Ongoing assessment and monitoring as previously

---

TABLE 21-7   Equipment Maintenance Checklist

Ongoing checks of oxygen purity

Electrical checks

Tracking hours of use

Proper filter changes

Environmental adequacy

Delivery of portable oxygen

Filling of liquid units

Delivery and change out of supplies

---

described will reduce these concerns and improve overall care. Key issues which should be an ongoing focus include the following:

Compliance with the physician's order. Is the patient on the correct liter flow? Is the patient receiving oxygen continuously if ordered? Will the patient tolerate the selected delivery method?

Adequate oxygen supply. Is the patient receiving liquid refills on a timely basis? Is there an adequate backup oxygen supply? Is there enough portable oxygen for trips to the physician or for family outings?

Smoking in the vicinity of the patient oxygen supply. Surprisingly, family members have been known to smoke around a child on oxygen. Thorough education and instruction on this issue is extremely important to the child's health and safety.

Environmental factors. Is the home kept reasonably clean and free of excessive dust? Are temperature extremes affecting the child's well being?

Electrical problems. Are parents and caregivers careful with power cords? Is there any one electrical circuit overload that could pose a fire risk? Are frequent power surges or power outages occurring? Is the family able to pay their increased monthly power bill due to the extra equipment?

Educational needs. There is so much for families and caregivers to remember on a daily basis. Does the family need additional instruction on clinical or equipment issues? Are equipment manuals still present for family reference? Are instruction sheets still available? Are there additional pamphlets, articles, or books that would be of interest to the parents or caregivers?

Fire safety. Is the equipment kept away from open flames and heaters? Are there smoke alarms and fire extinguishers in the house? Are parents using 100% cotton clothing instead of fabrics that can be highly flammable?

Ongoing problems should be well documented in the patient progress notes. If problems are too overwhelming for the family or if the child's

OXYGEN CONCENTRATOR

Goal: The patient/caregiver(s) will be properly trained in all aspects of the equipment provided and understand its purpose.

Names of person(s) receiving instructions and identify primary caregiver(s):

_____

_____

Location _____ Date _____

General Information:

☐ Ensure appropriate person(s) in addition to patient are present during instructions

☐ Provide patient/caregiver(s) with a Patient Instruction Manual and advise all present to read it carefully.

☐ Patient/caregiver(s) understand doctor's prescription.

☐ Patient/caregiver(s) provided with Augusta Health Alliance 24-hour telephone number. Instructed to call for problems, concerns, or additional services as needed.

☐ Advise patient/caregiver(s) that no one should attempt to make repairs or adjustments to equipment.

Safety Information and Precautions:

☐ Explain all warnings, cautions, and notes found in the Patient Instructional Manual concerning the operation of the equipment.

☐ Explain all fire and safety rules associated with the equipment use.

☐ Patient knows to post NO SMOKING signs.

☐ Advise patient/caregiver(s) of need for smoke alarm/fire extinguisher. Comments: _____

☐ Check outlet for proper grounding. If outlet is not properly grounded, patient/caregiver(s) aware of potential hazards associated with use of medical equipment. Comments: _____

☐ Patient verbalizes understanding of electrical safety.

☐ Advise that persons who have not read the Patient Instruction Manual should not operate the equipment.

☐ Environment suitable for medical equipment. Comments: _____

Oxygen Concentrator:

☐ Patient/caregiver(s) familiarized with ON/OFF button, flow meter adjustment, oxygen outlet, external filters, power cord, reset button, OCI features (if applicable).

☐ Patient/caregiver(s) can demonstrate proper operation and knows *NOT* to alter liter flow without prior approval from physician.

☐ Concentrator properly positioned. Patient/caregiver(s) understands to keep at least 8-inch distance around concentrator.

☐ Patient/caregiver(s) know to avoid plugging other appliances into same outlet.

FIGURE 21-3 Initial equipment checklist for an oxygen concentrator. (*Continues.*)

☐ Emphasize the importance of cleaning outside filter every other day. Patient/caregiver(s) understands to check filter daily for dust/dirt build up, understands filter cleaning procedure. Extra outside filter provided.

☐ In the event of concentrator failure, patient/caregiver(s) has been instructed to transfer to gaseous oxygen system and notify Augusta Health Alliance immediately.

☐ Patient/caregiver(s) has been provided with a back-up system and can properly demonstrate its use (read manometer, turn ON/OFF, knows when to call for replacement cylinder, proper storage when not in use, and how to change out).

☐ Patient/caregiver(s) provided with Guide Sheet/Magnet with cleaning schedule, type of equipment, cylinder duration. Informed of follow-up visit within next 48–72 hours. Advised of monthly therapist visits.

☐ Received set-up packet (Patient Rights and Responsibilities, No Smoking signs, Better Breather book, copy of Rental Sales Contract, Release of Medical Information).

☐ Patient/caregiver(s) understands insurance/billing procedure, provided with Augusta Health Alliance contact source and telephone number for billing questions.

Comments:

_____

_____

_____

_____

FIGURE 21-3 (Continued.)

care is affected, it might be necessary to readmit the patient. The physician should be informed of these problems even if they are not entirely clinical in nature.

Physician Orders and Communication

The original referral form or admission intake form will reflect the information needed to provide the necessary equipment and to ensure third-party coverage. Oxygen is a drug and requires detailed orders as would any other drug prescribed by a physician. The prescription should include the following details:

- Patient name, address, phone number, and age
- Contact source (parents, caregivers, other family members)
- Diagnosis
- Oxygen requirement (L/min or FIO_2)
- Delivery device
- Length of time oxygen is needed
- Reimbursement information

An original plan of treatment will be completed by the physician reflecting the ordered equipment and supplies (Fig. 21-4). This plan should also address saturation guidelines which are acceptable. The RCP will then inform the physician if these saturations fall outside of the set guidelines.

Progress notes are helpful communication tools, especially if they reflect any changes in the family's ability to cope with the child's care. In many cases, the respiratory care practitioner will be the only person assessing and evaluating the patient on a regular basis. The physician will rely on this information when making additions or changes to the original orders. Third-party reimbursement will also depend on thorough and ongoing documentation since it provides proof of continued oxygen equipment needs. Frequency and form of communication will vary with

---

PLAN OF TREATMENT

Dear Doctor:

Please review this Plan of Treatment, make any changes you deem necessary, sign and return to Augusta Health Alliance.

Patient: _____

Address: _____

Diagnosis: _____

Secondary Diagnosis: _____

Prescription: _____

Augusta Health Alliance's pulmonary assessment includes vital signs, pulse oximetry, and breath sounds/chest assessment. These will be performed:

☐ PRN

☐ Other: _____(specify frequency)

Augusta Health Alliance will contact the physician when the patient is not compliant with written prescription, the patient is in an unsafe/unhealthy environment which adversely affects his/her care, or when:

Oxygen saturation is below _____%

Please describe any precautions or limitations that would affect the plan of care:

☐ DNR

☐ CO_2 Retainer—Baseline CO_2 _____ mm Hg.

Physician's signature: _____ Date: _____

Physician's name: _____

Address: _____

_____

Phone: _____

FIGURE 21-4   Original plan of treatment.

each patient and should be discussed with the physician during discharge planning.

In summary, pediatric oxygen therapy is safe and effective when performed by qualified home care companies and respiratory care practitioners. Thorough education of families, well-maintained equipment, current technology, effective monitoring tools, ongoing assessment, and good communication skills will ensure that the patient is receiving quality care in the home setting.

■AEROSOL AND HUMIDITY THERAPY

Techniques and equipment used for aerosol therapy in the home are similar to those used in the hospital setting. As described in the previous oxygen therapy discussion, thorough referral information, appropriate documentation of patient visits, monitoring of therapy, and assessment of the patient are all necessary for care of the child at home.

Aerosol therapy is used in the home to administer pharmacologic agents (*e.g.*, bronchodilators, cromolyn sodium) or to provide continuous or intermittent bland aerosol for mobilization of secretions. Intermittent bland aerosol is frequently used to promote a cough or to decrease edema in the upper airway. Continuous aerosol therapy is most commonly ordered for tracheostomy patients who require additional humidification of the airway owing to a bypass of the critical upper airway mucosa. Heating of the aerosol will improve aerosol delivery but increase the risk of airway burns, as well as adding additional electrical risk to the home. This is a topic that requires discussion with the physician. If the child has fewer secretion problems, it is much safer to administer the aerosol without heating. A physician's order for aerosol therapy should include the following:

- Type of therapy (intermittent versus continuous)
- Frequency and duration
- Medication or solution
- Cool versus heated
- Type of aerosol delivery system
- Related monitoring
- FIo_2 (if oxygen is ordered)

Methods and Delivery

An air compressor is needed to power the nebulizer and create adequate aerosol output since the luxury of a piped-in compressed air system does not exist in the home setting. Patient delivery devices are usually the same as those used in the hospital. These include aerosol masks, tracheostomy masks, face tents, t-tubes, and nebulizer circuits with mouthpieces (see Chap. 14).

For continuous aerosol therapy, the same total flow guidelines used in the hospital must also be applied in the home. To ensure adequate flow, look for aerosol output from exhalation ports during patient inspiration. To optimize aerosol density, decrease total flow as much as possible while still providing adequate flow to the patient.

Many patients also require continuous oxygen delivery in addition to aerosol therapy. Oxygen can be bled or entrained into the circuit and analyzed for proper FIO_2. High flow rates from the air compressor will greatly reduce the FIO_2. If the patient requires higher FIO_2, it is possible that two flow systems (concentrators or liquid units) will be needed to supply the patient's oxygen needs.

Air compressors are simple and easy to use. Manufacturer's instructions for maintenance and proper use must be closely followed.

Home Assessment and Monitoring

Clinical effects of aerosol therapy should be monitored closely in the pediatric patient. The same information gathered by RCPs in the hospital will be needed to assess and monitor the child at home. The RCP has even greater responsibility for effectively evaluating the patient receiving home therapy since the patient will not likely be seen by a physician on a frequent enough basis to identify problems such as atelectasis or thickening of secretions. Progress notes to the physician should reflect sputum characteristics, viscosity of secretions, abnormal findings on auscultation and percussion, oxygen saturations, and any vital sign or physical changes in the patient since the last assessment. As in the hospital setting, practitioners in the home setting realize the importance of notifying a physician immediately when findings warrant. Obviously, some pediatric patients will have tracheostomies, and as the child grows, the tracheostomy tube will become too small and require replacement. Continual evaluation of the tube size and airway patency is essential.

Problems and Safety

Taking proper steps to provide extensive education and thorough monitoring will minimize potential problems in the home. Issues about which home RCPs should be aware include the following:

Medication delivery. Are parents administering the correct dosage of albuterol, cromolyn sodium, and other aerosolized drugs? Are treatments given at the proper frequency as ordered by the physician?

Equipment maintenance. Are filters kept clean by the caregivers? Is the compressor creating too much heat or noise? Are caregivers keeping the compressor several inches from the wall or other objects? Are instructions and equipment information kept in a handy place?

Infection control. Is equipment being cleaned properly and changed on a regular basis? Are families using proper suctioning technique? Are water drainage bags properly placed to prevent moisture buildup? Is tracheostomy care done properly on a regular basis?

Nebulizer heaters. Is temperature closely monitored? (Airway burns are of special concern in children.) Avoid continuous heating of the aerosol if secretions can be controlled without it.

Hydration concerns. Are caregivers filling nebulizers properly? Are tracheostomy patients having problems with thick secretions? Is there a manual resuscitator nearby to aid in thorough lavage and suctioning as well as for emergencies? Are there any signs that the child is being overhydrated by continuous aerosol production?

Fire hazards. Are electrical outlets secure and not overloaded? Is there adequate ventilation to prevent overheating of the compressor?

Tracheostomy concerns. Is there a suction unit nearby at all times? Do caregivers know how to care for the tracheostomy site? Has the child grown enough to require a larger tracheostomy tube? Is there an extra tube nearby?

As in other home situations, the family is usually the primary care source and this carries enormous responsibility. Proper planning and family education is imperative to ensure the patient's comfort, care, and safety.

▬ APNEA (CARDIORESPIRATORY) MONITORING

Apnea and associated bradycardia can result in oxygen desaturation and death. Electronic home monitoring is frequently used in managing infants at increased risk for prolonged apnea, prolonged bradycardia, and **sudden infant death syndrome (SIDS)**. These monitors are designed to trigger visual and audible alarms when apneic episodes and heart rate changes exceed preselected limits as ordered by the physician.

Premature and term infants can be at risk for apnea and bradycardia for a variety of reasons. Recommendations for home monitor use include the following:

- Premature infants who displayed a history of apnea/bradycardia prior to hospital discharge
- Siblings of two or more SIDS victims
- Infants exhibiting central hypoventilation
- Infants with a history of an **apparent life-threatening event (ALTE)**. Any witnessed episode that is characterized by apnea, changes in color or muscle tone, choking, or gagging is labeled as an ALTE.[1]
- Infants with sleep apnea syndrome due to neurological disorders or upper airway malformations[11]
- Infants and children with tracheostomies
- Mechanically ventilated infants with moderate to severe cases of respiratory syncytial virus are also frequently monitored because of the increased chance of upper airway obstruction.[1,2,8,11]

Apnea monitors facilitate early hospital discharge, allowing the infant to develop in a normal home environment. A home monitoring program is cost effective and is, therefore, usually covered by third party reimbursement.

Sudden Infant Death Syndrome

A diagnosis of SIDS is made only after a thorough postmortem examination and investigation fail to explain the specific cause of death.[1] SIDS claims an estimated 7000 infants per year in the United States and is responsible for 40% of all infant mortality in the 1 month to 1 year age range.[2] Although the literature has identified numerous risk factors for SIDS (Table 21-8), there is still no research that has been able to identify any specific factor that would allow a prospective population of infants to be studied.[4] The control group would be too large and much too expensive to initiate an apnea monitoring program.

Infants with a history of apnea or ALTEs might be at an increased risk for SIDS.[8] However, apnea of prematurity and SIDS have not been proven

TABLE 21-8 Risk Factors Associated With SIDS

Apnea	Low Apgar scores
Prematurity	Low socioeconomic status
Sibling of SIDS victim	Maternal age <20 yrs
Low birth weight	Small for gestational age
Maternal drug use	Upper respiratory infections
Maternal smoking	History of ALTEs
BPD	Winter months
Males	Prone positioning of infant
Complications during pregnancy (anemia, etc.)	

to be directly related. As monitor use has increased with apnea of prematurity and apnea of infancy, the overall death rate from SIDS has not changed dramatically. On the other hand, ALTEs have been shown to be predictors of SIDS if no cause for the ALTE can be identified.[4,6]

Many ALTEs are shown to be a result of gastroesophageal reflux, upper airway obstruction, congenital anomalies of the airway, congenital heart disease, infection, and other specific causes and can therefore be treated properly to alleviate any risks of reoccurrence. Infants with a history of two or more ALTEs have as much as a threefold increase in sudden infant death even when home monitors are used.[8]

Methods and Delivery

At the present time, the most widely used method of home apnea monitoring is impedance pneumography (see Chap. 8).[5] The standards for today's home monitors also include the capability of recording and storing information about respiratory wave forms, heart rate trending, and patient/caregiver compliance information reflecting monitor use. Many new monitors also record electrocardiograms and can be interfaced with oximeters to record corresponding saturation changes.

Downloading of information from these monitors allows the home respiratory care practitioner to look at waveforms and graphs and to deliver information to the physician (Fig. 21-5). Case managers involved in third-party reimbursement are finding downloaded information a useful tool in establishing continued medical necessity for apnea monitoring.

Home Assessment and Monitoring

Assessment of the home situation should begin in the neonatal unit, newborn nursery, or pediatric unit. Psychosocial problems should be identified and addressed long before the infant is ready for discharge. Not all families can cope with the stress and responsibility of home monitoring. Many family situations are not appropriate for release of an infant into the home setting, and alternative arrangements must be made before caregiver training begins.

Apnea monitoring is an added burden to the parents or caregivers of an infant that has experienced complications such as apnea and brady-

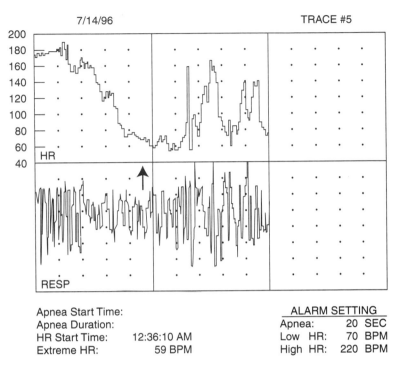

Waveform indicating bradycardia

7/14/96	TRACE #5

Apnea Start Time:		ALARM SETTING
Apnea Duration:		Apnea: 20 SEC
HR Start Time:	12:36:10 AM	Low HR: 70 BPM
Extreme HR:	59 BPM	High HR: 220 BPM

FIGURE 21-5   Data downloaded from an apnea monitor.

cardia or to parents that have suffered the loss of an infant to SIDS. Extensive education is the key to both reducing anxiety and lowering the risk of infant morbidity and mortality. Training should include proper use of the equipment and instruction on stimulation techniques and infant CPR. A step-by-step visual on CPR (posters are excellent) is a welcome reinforcement for any caregiver (Fig. 21-6).

"**Rooming in**" is a practice used by many hospitals to make parents more comfortable with caring for the infant's total needs. A private room simulating the home environment is made available for a day or two. The parents and infant are left alone unless they request assistance from hospital staff.

Parents should be questioned about the availability of a working telephone in the home. Emphasis should also be placed on outside lighting and proper identification of the home with house or apartment numbers. (Emergency personnel are frequently delayed by the inability to find the correct location.)

Written instruction should be readily available on equipment, including a manual and logs for charting apnea and heart rate alarms. Literature containing stories of other families who have monitored a child at home is also helpful at this time.

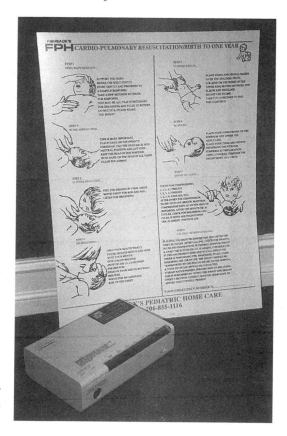

FIGURE 21-6 CPR poster for use in teaching parents and caregivers.

Ongoing monitoring of the apnea monitor patient should be extensive. Follow-up support reduces anxiety and increases compliance. A home program should include the following:

- Experienced respiratory care practitioners capable of providing initial and ongoing education
- A follow-up visit in the home within 24 to 48 hours following hospital discharge
- 24-hour telephone assistance
- Written notification of the presence of the apnea monitor to the appropriate 911 system, telephone company, and electrical company
- Monthly and PRN visits to the home
- Downloading and printing capabilities for delivery of monitor reports to physicians. Access to event recordings can result in shorter monitoring periods and lower overall cost of patient care.

Discontinuation of the monitor can be a difficult decision for parents even when the physician feels quite confident. The following are common criteria for discontinuation:

1. The infant has experienced no significant episodes for 2 to 3 months[2]
2. The infant has tolerated an external stress (illness, immunizations during the period) with no resultant episodes[2]

Families frequently require support and assistance during this period of transition. Further education on the indications for use and limitations of monitoring can be beneficial in relieving stress and reassuring the parents that their infant is no longer at medical risk.

Problems and Safety

Thorough education on the proper use of monitors will alleviate most problems. Incorporating a checklist on the initial set-up (Fig. 21-7) ensures that many of the following issues are addressed with parents and caregivers:

False and loose lead alarms. Are parents placing electrodes in the proper area? Does the infant move excessively and loosen electrodes? Do parents avoid the use of creams and lotions on the skin?

Responding to alarms appropriately. Can the monitor be heard throughout the house? Do parents understand stimulation techniques? Are parents always within 10 seconds of the monitor?

Skin irritation. Do parents use the monitor constantly without providing "time off" for the infant? Is any skin breakdown occurring? (Interactive time with the infant should be the time off since parents are observing the infant directly.)

Noncompliance. Do parents fully understand the need for monitoring during those periods when no one is interacting with the infant?

Adequate education. Do parents feel completely comfortable with the equipment? Was sufficient question and answer time provided during the set-up?

Medications. Is the infant being discharged on caffeine, Reglan, or another medication?

Physician Orders and Communication

As with other modalities, the physician must provide the home care provider with the appropriate referral information, including the following:

- Patient information (name, date of birth)
- Contact/caregiver information (parent's name)
- Monitor settings (apnea, slow heart, fast heart)
- Patient diagnosis
- Probable length of time monitoring is needed
- Third-party payer information
- Medications
- Psychosocial limitations affecting parents/caregivers
- Probable date of hospital discharge

Downloaded reports should be provided for the physician as necessary. An accompanying log of the infant's activities before, during, and after the alarms will prove beneficial to the physician in establishing the prob-

APNEA MONITOR CHECKLIST

Names of person(s) receiving instructions and primary caregiver(s):

_____

_____

Location _____   Date _____

General Information:

☐ Ensure appropriate person(s) in addition to patient are present during instruction.

☐ Provide patient/caregiver(s) with a Patient Instruction Manual and CPR poster. Advise all present to read it carefully.

☐ Monitor set with correct alarm settings per physician order. Caregiver(s) understands why the monitor was ordered and the purpose of alarm settings.

☐ Caregiver(s) instructed in proper CPR procedure per _____.

☐ Patient/caregiver(s) provided with Augusta Health Alliance 24-hour telephone number. Instructed to call for problems, concerns, additional service.

☐ Obtained billing information and explained any financial obligations that the family may incur.

☐ Caregiver(s) advised that the baby will be seen monthly in addition to PRN visits.

☐ Caregiver(s) advised that no one should attempt to make repairs or adjustments to equipment.

Safety Information and Precautions:

☐ Explain all warnings, cautions, and notes found in the Patient Guide concerning the operation of the equipment:
- proper placement to ensure that monitor cannot be pulled into the crib
- placement of monitor away from electrical appliances
- regular checks for proper positioning and connections of cables, lead wires, and electrodes
- placement of power cable into 3-prong outlet using no extension cords or plug modifications

☐ Explain the importance of a telephone in or close to baby's room.

☐ Stress the need for clearly marking the home with identification numbers and proper lighting for access by emergency personnel.

☐ Outlet checked for proper grounding.

☐ Verbalize understanding of electrical safety.

Apnea Monitor:

☐ Caregivers(s) familiarized with ON/OFF button, RESET button, and each light indicating an alarm function.

☐ Explain proper connection of patient cable, leads, electrodes, and proper placement of belt.

☐ Instruct caregiver(s) in the importance of using no oils, creams, etc. under the electrodes.

☐ Provide Sween Cream.

FIGURE 21-7   Equipment checklist for an apnea monitor. (*Continued.*)

☐ Explain the difference in alarm sounds:
- red lights—intermittent
- yellow light—continuous

☐ Explain the 30-second delay in the loose lead alarm.

☐ Two-point calibration procedure completed for alarms.

☐ Obtain information from caregiver(s) on notifying local emergency medical service, power company, and telephone company.

☐ Explain self-test procedure. Patient/caregiver(s) understand.

☐ Stress to caregivers(s) the monitor will alarm for many reasons and that they must evaluate the baby to determine true alarm.

Comments:

_____

_____

_____

_____

FIGURE 21-7   (Continued.)

able cause of the episode. Illnesses such as upper respiratory infections can result in apnea and bradycardia and should also be reported to the physician if the parents have not been in the office recently.

In summary, home monitoring requires a knowledgeable, dedicated, and sensitive person to provide for the needs of the family and infant. RCPs participating in infant monitoring must keep abreast of current literature, techniques, and technology. As monitoring continues to evolve, standards will also continue to change. Parents must be aware from the beginning that monitors will not cure the problem and that death cannot be prevented in every monitored infant. Home monitors are designed to assist the family through the period of medical risk.

▬ MECHANICAL VENTILATION

The quality of life issue is even more emotional when it involves a child. Home mechanical ventilation can provide many children with the opportunity to normalize their lifestyle and can also significantly reduce the cost of daily medical care. When discharge criteria are met, the option of going home should be made available to all families. Home care providers must have a proven and thorough home ventilation program before being considered for pediatric care.

Patient Selection

Good candidates for home ventilation include patients with congenital or birth-related disorders, neurologic/neuromuscular disorders, and trauma injuries.[4] Success with home ventilation depends on the proper selection of the patient. The following criteria are critical in the proper evaluation of each candidate:

Medical stability. The patient should have no acute medical problems that alter cardiopulmonary status. Other major organ systems must be functional. The patient should have had no major interventions in the previous month. Oxygen requirements should be as stable and as minimal as possible.

Family evaluation. The family must genuinely want to have the child at home and at least two individuals must be willing and knowledge-able enough to participate in training. Financial effects must be considered so parents can still provide for all other members of the family. Many times, at least one parent must give up employment. This compounds the burden of medical expenses and greatly increases stress on the family unit.

Selection of home health care company. Accreditation by JCAHO should be a major determination in the selection of a company. This will ensure the availability of qualified personnel, proper equipment, and 24-hour call. Other criteria should include the following:

- A reasonable geographic location
- The ability to supply all needs efficiently and economically
- Extensive experience in home ventilator care
- The ability to assist in reimbursement issues and financial matters

These patient selection criteria help determine whether home ventilation is a reasonable objective. At this point, the details of home assessment and discharge planning can begin.

Discharge Planning for Mechanical Ventilation Patients

As addressed previously, the important components of discharge planning for ventilation patients include the following:

Care plan. This clinical plan must address all areas of patient care. A common approach is to detail the patient's needs and then determine the personnel, equipment, and supplies required for adequate and safe treatment. This should be developed by both the hospital and home care teams. Selection of the appropriate ventilator should occur at this point. The ideal ventilator is "user friendly" and small in size. It must provide backup alarms for safety along with battery backup for power outages.[10]

Reimbursement. Before a patient is considered for home ventilation, payment for home services must be arranged. It is imperative that the care plan is inclusive of all equipment, supplies, and services so that funding is complete before release of the patient. The family must be given a clear picture of the financial impact before considering the patient's release. Home care is not feasible if the family cannot withstand the financial burden.

Parent teaching. The teaching process must begin weeks in advance. Parents and caregivers need adequate time to become familiar with the overall care of the child. An in-depth review of potential problems and goals for the patient is the best approach to initiation of the teaching process. This is accomplished also by the hospital and home care staff. Examples of goals include:

Maintain adequate respiratory status

Prevent respiratory infection

Increase the child's weight

Increase muscle strength

Improve cognitive and motor skills

Administer medications safely

Provide respite time for parents

Specific teaching programs should include:

Disease process related to patient's diagnosis

Tracheostomy care

Changing the tracheostomy tube

Suctioning techniques

CPR

Medication delivery and monitoring

Cardiac monitoring

Postural drainage and percussion

Nebulization of medicine

Mechanical ventilator use, circuit changes, trouble shooting, alarms, and humidifier use

Equipment cleaning

Nutrition

Physical therapy/range of motion exercises

Oral care

Emergency care

Evaluation of the parent's level of education and coping skills is important. The family must be capable of and prepared to absorb a great deal of information. Demonstrations of procedures and handouts of pertinent materials are valuable teaching tools.

Home assessment. Home assessment must be one of the first steps in the discharge process. Many times this assessment will result in a complete halt of the entire process due to identification of safety problems, inadequate space, or poor environmental conditions. The electrical system must have three-pronged outlets, proper grounding, and circuit breakers, and be adequate with respect to wattage consumption requirements. Additional electrical work is often required and is not covered by insurance. It is the responsibility of the family to arrange for and pay for these improvements. This is not always financially possible for overburdened family budgets.

Preparation of the home. Preparation includes notification to police, 911 system, apartment management, and utility companies that life support systems are in place and that priority status for services should be granted. This notification should be made by telephone and in writing (Fig. 21-8). Adequate storage space for supplies must be arranged with the parents. It is essential that all equipment and supplies are ordered and tested before placing them in the home.

Monitoring

Monitoring of patients on mechanical ventilatory support in the home depends on the needs of the patient and the capabilities of the family. Clinical monitoring of the patient and the equipment is essential and should include evaluation of the following signs and symptoms:

1. Physical signs such as color, sensorium, secretions, and respiratory patterns should be noted.
2. The weight of the child can give information relative to fluid balance and nutrition.
3. Vital signs such as heart rate, blood pressure, and respiratory rate must be checked.
4. Oxygenation may be checked periodically or continuously in certain situations.
5. Observation of chest excursion/ventilation is taught to the family. The health care providers should assess the chest during visits.

Detailed review of this clinical monitoring is taught to each parent and caregiver.

EMERGENCY RESCUE SQUAD

Notification of Home Monitoring

Date: _____

Name: _____

Address: _____

Phone: _____

Attention: Director of Emergency Services:

Our infant, _____, is under the care of Dr. _____ for apnea and/or bradycardia during sleep. In the event of an apneic or bradycardic episode, the infant may require resuscitation.

During sleep, the infant is on a home infant monitor to alert the parents to any episodes. We, the parents, have been trained in infant cardiopulmonary resuscitation (CPR). If the infant requires resuscitation, we will begin CPR and call for emergency help. If you receive a call, please respond immediately to transport the infant to the nearest emergency room. It will be necessary to contact Dr. _____ at phone # _____ concerning necessary treatment decisions.

The enclosed map will assist you in locating the home.

Thank you for your cooperation.

Sincerely,

FIGURE 21-8 Notification of home monitoring to be sent to local rescue squad or fire department.

Equipment monitoring performed by the home care company and the primary care providers includes the following points:

1. The circuit should be checked for leaks after emptying water from the tubing.
2. Overall function of the ventilator and accessory alarms must be checked to see that they are functioning properly.
3. Backup systems should function properly and be at the same settings as the primary system.
4. Oxygen concentration can be checked with an oxygen analyzer on a predetermined basis.
5. Review of the cleaning/disinfection procedures is important.
6. For transportation to the home, the proper equipment and personnel and coordination of care are imperative. This is an anxious time for the family and every effort should be made for the move to be timely and efficient.

The discharge planning process is important in creating a smooth transition to home and a mood conducive to a successful home stay. This, in turn, builds confidence for the family and their ability to handle the situation adequately. It is also necessary for the family to decide which medical institution they will use in an emergency situation. Will the discharging hospital and the reimburser agree to readmit the patient if home ventilator care is no longer possible or unsuccessful? Checking these details can prevent many potential problems.

Methods and Equipment

Home ventilation usually requires many types of equipment and supplies (Table 21-9). Simple written descriptions of assembly, function, and cleaning are important references for the family. Also, cleaning of filters, circuits, and humidifiers and maintenance of the equipment should be of prime concern.

Certain issues must be reviewed with parents: immediate, 24-hour-a-day services must be available from qualified professionals and the home health care companies must provide proper equipment maintenance and have backup equipment available.

It is important to remember that infants change significantly during the first year of life. When these changes occur, the equipment and supplies may require adjustment to meet new needs. As development occurs in older babies and children, similar changes must be made in the equipment and care plan.

Proper selection criteria, planned family education, and proper monitoring can result in a high probability for success in home ventilation. This approach can achieve the goals once thought to be impractical of providing a safe, cost effective alternative to hospitalization to the stabilized patient needing mechanical ventilation. A commitment to lower health care costs along with changes in technology will continue to encourage new advances in this area of home care.

Physician Orders and Communication

The complexity of the condition of the home ventilation patient usually requires more frequent communication with the physician. It is imperative

TABLE 21-9   Equipment Needed for Home Mechanical Ventilation

Ventilator with backup system	Ventilator circuits
Humidifiers	Tracheostomy tubes (at bedside)
Air compressor	Suction catheters and tubing
Oxygen system with backup	Sterile water
Oxygen analyzer	Sterile normal saline
Suction machine with backup system	Medication nebulizers
Manual resuscitation bag	Water-soluble lubricant
Hydrogen peroxide	Thermometer
Nebulizer	Oxygen and aerosol tubing
Gloves	Tracheostomy dressings and supplies
Syringes	Hospital crib/bed
Nebulizer heater	Medications
Stethoscope	External ventilator battery
Tape	Spirometer
Ventilator filters	Apnea monitor
Disinfectant solution	Oxygen adapters or accumulator
Blood pressure cuff	

that any changes in patient status be relayed to the appropriate physician and that changes in orders be documented just as thoroughly as in the hospital setting. It is always a wise decision to notify the physician even if the communication seems bothersome or trivial.

▬SUMMARY

Significant advances in pediatric and neonatal home health care have resulted in favorable outcomes. The home environment creates a quality of life for the infant and the family that is lost when hospitalization occurs. In addition, costs are reduced, which can extend insurance coverage.

This chapter has touched on many issues, the most important being that thorough education of families and caregivers is essential for successful home care and that families must be capable and willing to absorb the vast amounts of material that must be covered. Technology is improving and expanding, and funding issues are changing. Home care providers are growing in number and expertise. Detailed and adequate discharge planning is important and should consist of the care plan, reimbursement consideration, parent teaching, home assessment, and transportation to the home. Proper monitoring and safety measures will improve the chances of successful outcomes.

▬REFERENCES

1. Canadian Paediatric Society Position Statement: The infant home monitoring dilemma. Can Med Assoc J 147:1661, 1992.

2. Guntheroth WG: Crib Death: The Sudden Infant Death Syndrome, 2nd ed. Mt. Kisco, NY, Futura Publishing, 1989.
3. Hanna M: Traversing the reimbursement maze. Resp Ther 8:20, 1995.
4. Hilman BC: Pediatric Respiratory Disease: Diagnosis and Management. Philadelphia, WB Saunders, 1993.
5. Kacmarek RM, Hess D, Stoller JK: Monitoring in Respiratory Care. St. Louis, CV Mosby, 1993.
6. Koff PB, Eitzman D, Neu J: Neonatal and Pediatric Respiratory Care, 2nd ed. St. Louis, CV Mosby, 1993.
7. Lucas J, Golish JA, Sleeper G, O'Ryan JA: Home Respiratory Care. Norwalk, Appleton and Lange, 1988.
8. NIH Consensus Development Conference on Infantile Apnea and Home Monitoring. Pediatrics 79:292, 1987.
9. Tiep BL: Portable Oxygen Therapy: Including Oxygen Conserving Methodology. Mt. Kisco, NY, Futura Publishing, 1991.
10. Whitaker K: Comprehensive Perinatal and Pediatric Respiratory Care. Albany, NY, Delmar Publishers, 1992.
11. Whitaker S: The art and science of home monitoring in the 1990s. JOGNN 24:84, 1995.

■ SELF-ASSESSMENT QUESTIONS

1. List at least eight members of the discharge planning team.

2. The least expensive choice for short-term, low flow oxygen therapy in a child's home would most likely be
   a. liquid
   b. concentrator
   c. cylinder
   d. none of the above

3. Equipment management in the patient's home does not include
   a. delivery and change out of supplies
   b. tracking of equipment use
   c. psychosocial assessment
   d. environmental adequacy

4. Home oxygen does not require a physician's order.
   a. true
   b. false

5. List three potential problems that might affect the delivery of aerosol therapy in the home.

6. State the complete definition of SIDS.

7. List two common criteria for discontinuation of an apnea monitor.

8. Discuss the importance of each of the following when evaluating a patient for home ventilation:
   medical stability
   family evaluation
   selection of a home care company

Part 5
Special Procedures

Chapter 22

Transport of the Newborn and Child

GARTH RUBINS

OBJECTIVES

Having completed this chapter, the reader will be able to:

1 Explain the concept of regionalization as it applies to transport of the newborn.

2 Identify the indications for maternal transport.

3 Identify the members of a neonatal transport team and explain why they are selected.

4 Describe the stabilization of the newborn prior to transport.

5 Identify the equipment and supplies necessary for neonatal transport.

6 Describe the advantages and disadvantages of transport by ground, fixed-wing aircraft, and helicopter.

7 Describe conditions under which transport of the critically ill child should be considered.

8 Identify the equipment and supplies necessary for pediatric transport.

KEY TERMS

Boyle's Law
Dalton's Law
pediatric tertiary care center

perinatal center
regionalization
stabilization

▬ TRANSPORT OF THE NEWBORN

The Concept of Regionalization

Historically, the primary causes of death and disease during childbirth were poor sanitary conditions and the lack of proper education. During the 19th century, because of poor sanitary conditions, it was safer to deliver a child at home than in the hospital. By 1940, 56% of deliveries were still occurring at home. At this time, two thirds of the neonatal deaths were related to prematurity and its complications of pneumonia and congenital anomalies.

During the mid and late 1960s, great advances were being made in neonatal medicine. Drs. Gregory, Reynolds, and Bird were developing respirators capable of ventilating newborns, the theories of thermal regulation were better understood, and neonatal intensive care units were beginning to open in larger hospitals. Electronic cardiac monitors became standard equipment in most intensive care units. Blood gas measurement was available, although until recently, the volume of blood necessary made frequent analysis impossible. Finally, with the increased availability of antibiotics, many babies that would have died were being saved.

In 1966, the idea of **regionalization** was developed at the State University of New York Upstate Medical Center in Syracuse. Regionalization is a cooperative effort to share resources by centralizing facilities so that adequate medical care is available to all citizens in a large geographic area. The Upstate Medical Center program became the model for the regionalization system throughout the entire country.

In 1977, the Committee on Perinatal Health of the National Foundation of the March of Dimes made recommendations for the regional development of maternal and perinatal health services.[1] This report would serve as a guideline for the development of perinatal services based on geographical distribution of neonatal intensive care services supported by a cooperative arrangement among hospitals within a region. The concept of regionalization included a four-level grading system for hospitals that rated them according to technological capabilities, physical resources, and specialized medical personnel (Table 22-1).

Perinatal centers should provide outreach education and support for hospitals in their region. They should also provide a transportation service to move the mother or infant to the facility.

TABLE 22-1   Grading System for Regional Hospitals

LEVEL	CAPABILITIES
1	Provides services for uncomplicated deliveries and newborn patients. Because their number of deliveries is too low to provide adequate patient load, these institutions are unable to attract or support specialized staff.
2	Provide a full range of maternal and neonatal services for uncomplicated obstetrical problems and certain neonatal illnesses. These institutions vary in capabilities and are generally located in urban or suburban areas.
3	These institutions are able to care for all maternal/fetal and neonatal illnesses. These institutions should also provide strong leadership and continuing education for all institutions in their region.
Perinatal Center	These institutions provide intensive prenatal care for patients deemed high risk prior to delivery. They provide a wide range of both preventive and treatment services designed to provide a better pregnancy outcome. Medical care is determined by the patient's individual needs but includes nutritional support, education, and advanced medical care.

This concept of cooperation was very foreign to American health care, but came at the right time. Institutions were already battling with the problems of the cost of new technology and its limited use with a small patient population.

Maternal Transport

Within the concept of regionalization is the organization of high-risk perinatal centers. These centers specialize in the care of high-risk maternity patients and their infants. Patients with conditions deemed high risk by their physicians should be transported to these facilities.

More than half of infants that require resuscitation at birth can be identified prior to delivery, and many can even be identified prior to the onset of labor. Many of these mothers and their infants require intensive care prior to delivery and most, but not all, of the infants will require intensive care after delivery. If obstetric or neonatal intensive care is anticipated, it is best to refer the high-risk mother to a regional perinatal center.

It is impossible to predict with complete certainty which patients should be transported to perinatal centers. There are always cases in which high-risk infants are delivered and do just fine; but each patient should be assessed for possible problems or complications and considered for referral. Intrauterine transport is more desirable than neonatal transport because it utilizes the best incubator of all, the mother's uterus. Maternal transport also allows the mother and infant to be close together after delivery. It allows the cost-effective use of highly sophisticated, expensive medical resources that require high staff-to-patient ratios.

Maternal transport can be accomplished in many ways, depending on the woman's condition and local resources available. She may be transported by private car, local ambulance, or specialized transport service provided by the regional perinatal center. It is vitally important that each candidate considered for transport be carefully evaluated. Because labor is not always completely predictable, transport personnel should be prepared for any emergency. Transport members should carry equipment for the resuscitation of mother and infant. No mother who is in active labor should be transported.

Although candidates for maternal transport should be evaluated on an individual basis, general guidelines can be given for patients likely to require transfer to perinatal centers. These guidelines are listed in Table 22-2. It is important that any patient considered for transport be stabilized prior to transport. The essential requirements for **stabilization** are included in Table 22-3.

During transport, the mother should be accompanied by adequately trained personnel with the equipment available to treat any deterioration of her condition. Blood pressure monitoring, intravenous supplies, and oxygen delivery equipment should be readily available. If possible, fetal well being should be continuously assessed with a fetal heart rate monitor. Although transport should not be performed on an unstable patient, neonatal resuscitation equipment should also be available.

The Transport Team

The first discussion of neonatal transport appears long before the idea of regionalization was introduced. In 1900, Dr. Joseph Delee described a mobile transport incubator for the care of "weakly and premature born

---

TABLE 22-2　Conditions Requiring Maternal Transport

Maternal kidney disease with deteriorating renal function

Maternal drug dependency

Fetal malformation documented by ultrasound

Polyhydramnios

Oligohydramnios

Medical problems in the mother such as cardiovascular, thyroid, or neurological problems

Chronic or pregnancy-induced hypertension

Rh sensitization

Maternal diabetes mellitus

Abnormal results from fetal well-being test (non-stress test, contraction stress test, biophysical profile)

Third trimester bleeding

Premature rupture of membranes at less than 34 weeks gestation or less than 2000 grams estimated fetal weight

Multiple gestation

Intrauterine growth retardation

Post-term pregnancy

Severe maternal infection such as hepatitis, pyelonephritis, influenza, or pneumonia which may result in a preterm birth

---

(Adapted from Perinatal Continuing Education Program, Division of Neonatal Medicine, Department of Pediatrics, University of Virginia Health Sciences Center, 1993.)

---

infants." He envisioned that this incubator would be used to transport these delicate infants from distant parts of the city and suburbs.[2] With this insight, he described an understanding of the need for a device that simulated the in utero environment. It was not until the mid 1950s that a true neonatal transport organization was developed. With the development of regionalization in upstate New York came the first neonatal transport team. Long before the modern transport team was assembled, the New York Department of Health organized a team of dedicated nurses and physicians to go to outlying hospitals and transport newborns to the regional neonatal care facility. This team was very similar to present day

---

TABLE 22-3　Stabilization of the Mother Prior to Transport

Stable vital signs

Cessation of bleeding

Suppression of seizure activity

Control of metabolic status

Control of hypertension

---

transport teams. They were on-call 24 hours a day, used specialized vehicles, and had specialized equipment for the care of newborns. Over a 2-year period, they transported 1209 patients, with 194 of those patients weighing less than 1000 grams.[3] Modern transport crews have evolved into very organized teams using highly sophisticated equipment. The goals of neonatal transport teams are listed in Table 22-4.

When creating a transport team, a variety of personnel who participate in the hospital care of critically ill infants should be considered. Each transport program must choose their transport team based on their own unique situation. The participation of neonatologists, neonatal fellows, and residents on transport teams is desirable, but in perinatal centers that are responsible for a large number of transports, these physicians may not always be able to leave the intensive care unit for extended periods of time. Reimbursement policies also make physician participation in transport impractical and costly. Most centers have adopted teams using non-physician critical care personnel as care providers during transport. Since physicians are generally not present during transport, team members must be well trained in both assessment and specialized procedures that may or may not be performed by non-physician staff in the hospital.

Many centers choose nurse/nurse or nurse/respiratory therapist teams. These teams have been found to be very practical in terms of both cost effectiveness and the availability of staff. Although teams devoted solely to transport responsibilities who are stationed in the hospital at all times can respond quickly to the need for transport, this arrangement has been found to be too costly. Instead, many centers have converted teams to in-unit status, where they perform their regular responsibilities until the transport team is mobilized. This arrangement combines the advantage of a team that is ready to respond in a timely manner with the opportunity to maintain clinical skills in a critical care setting.

Many of the neonates transported suffer from respiratory distress; thus, respiratory care practitioners are a very important part of many transport teams. Their expertise in the use and maintenance of respiratory care equipment and their ability to maintain the patient's airway make the therapist's skills an important asset. The ability to adapt equipment to the unique environment of transport can be lifesaving, particularly when unexpected events occur. Another advantage that respiratory

---

TABLE 22-4 Goals of Neonatal Transport Teams

Provide quick response

Assess the status of the neonate

Stabilize the infant

Interface with referring staff members

Make transport quick and safe

Make independent clinical decisions

Function well in an unfamiliar environment

Provide the best care available

---

care practitioners bring to transport is that, in many states, licensing regulations for them are less restrictive and allow them to perform procedures not covered by some nursing practice laws, such as intubation and needle thoracentesis.

The absence of physicians during transport can create problems that must be anticipated. Many transport teams function with standing transport protocols. These protocols have been approved by physicians at the receiving hospital and allow the transport team to perform lifesaving and stabilization procedures without direct physician orders. In this way, a neonate can receive immediate lifesaving care without delay. These protocols require the team to be comfortable working independently and have confidence in their patient assessment skills.

In order for a transport team to function, all team members must know and understand their roles. When a request for transport is received from a referring hospital, all team members must respond quickly.

Stabilization of the Infant

Upon arrival at the referring hospital, a quick overall assessment of the patient should be performed. Evaluation of skin color, heart rate, and respiratory rate and effort should be quickly done. Team members should review with the referring staff the patient's history and what stabilization procedures have been done prior to the arrival of the team. A quick review of x-ray films and lab results can also be done at this time.

Stabilization of the infant is approached using three major categories: the respiratory system, temperature control, and metabolic/hemodynamic status. The first and second categories can be approached simultaneously and are closely related. Respiratory stabilization consists of evaluation of respiratory rate, breath sounds, and respiratory effort. Pulse oximetry and transcutaneous monitoring, as well as blood gas analysis, can be very helpful. The respiratory system must be stable before other stabilization procedures are performed. If necessary, intubation should be performed and the airway secured prior to vascular line placement. A secure airway is essential when transporting an infant. If a question arises about whether the infant needs to be intubated, it is probably better to perform the procedure in a controlled environment such as the nursery rather than in the back of the ambulance or helicopter. Oxygen should be provided at levels that keep the baby pink. At this point, it is helpful to monitor oxygenation with a transcutaneous monitor or pulse oximeter to prevent hyperoxia or hypoxia. Oxygen delivered to the infant should be warmed and humidified, since newborns are very sensitive to cold air around their face, potentially causing apnea.

When placing an infant on mechanical ventilation, the initial setting should be based on the amount of support desired. Because time-cycled, pressure-limited ventilators do not deliver a constant tidal volume, frequent physical assessment of the infant is important. The guidelines for initial settings are shown in Table 22-5. After placing the neonate on mechanical ventilation, follow-up blood gas analysis should be performed and appropriate adjustments made to the initial settings.

Temperature stabilization should be initiated immediately following the birth of the infant. The baby starts to cool immediately after birth because of evaporation of fluids from the skin. In order to prevent this

TABLE 22-5   Initial Ventilator Settings During Transport of the Newborn

PARAMETER	INITIAL SETTING
Respiratory rate	20–60 breaths per minute. Set according to the level of support desired.
Inspiratory time	0.3–0.8 sec. Longer inspiratory times may be hazardous.
Peak inspiratory pressure	20–25 cm H_2O. Excessive pressures may be hazardous to the lungs.
Positive end-expiratory pressure	3–5 cm H_2O. Low to moderate levels.

cooling effect, the baby should be dried with warm towels. Since the baby continues to lose heat to the environment by convection, the infant should be placed under a radiant warmer. The warmer should be pre-warmed so the infant does not lose heat to the blankets by conduction. The warmer should not be placed near windows or other cold objects to prevent cooling by radiation. Premature infants get cold-stressed very quickly and cold stress affects all other body systems. An infant cooled to 35° C body temperature doubles his or her oxygen consumption and carbon dioxide production. By allowing the infant to cool to 33° C, oxygen consumption and CO_2 production triples. If an infant requires 60% oxygen to maintain adequate saturation and becomes cold, it will be impossible to provide adequate oxygenation. As babies get cold-stressed, glucose consumption also increases. Premature infants have very little glucose reserve and can become hypoglycemic very quickly, leading to seizures and brain damage. It becomes easy to see why temperature stabilization is very important. The easiest way to prevent problems is to begin adequate temperature control immediately after birth. The infant should be warmed on a radiant warmer and, if necessary, a chemical warming mattress.

Once the infant's respiratory and temperature status has been stabilized, the team should begin hemodynamic and metabolic stabilization. All infants transported should have venous access. This can be accomplished through a peripheral intravenous line, an umbilical venous line, or an umbilical artery line. Blood glucose levels should be monitored and maintained within normal limits. The intravenous infusion should contain a sugar solution and be started at an initial rate of 80 to 100 cc/kg/day. Blood pressure should be frequently monitored, and if hypotension is present, the infant should be given a bolus of a nonsugar vascular expander, such as albumin or plasminate. Inotropic agents such as dopamine should only be started if intravenous solution boluses are not successful in restoring blood pressure to the normal range.

If time and the condition of the infant allow, the transport team should bring the baby to visit the parents before departing for the perinatal center. The mother's condition after delivery and the distance to the referring center may make it difficult for her to visit her newborn for several days. If family members wish to accompany the infant, they should be given directions to the center and instructed to travel in their own vehicle at a normal speed. Because of space limitations, family members do not usually ride with the infant and should be told not to follow directly behind the transport ambulance.

An equally important part of the transport process is the interaction between transport team members and staff from the referring hospital. The transport team has the opportunity to dramatically improve the relationship between the hospitals, or it can cause irreparable damage. The transport team members are the front-line ambassadors for the institution they represent, and the staff of the referring hospital are customers in the same way as the patient. Emotions are always high when dealing with sick infants who require transport. Referring staff members may be disappointed because they were unable to care for the infant, and team members must be careful not to criticize the care which has been provided to the patient. Transport team members should appreciate the contribution made by the referring staff. They should seek information about the patient history and ask for assistance when appropriate, explaining the need for performing all procedures. Nonphysician teams should avoid conflict with referring physicians over the need for different care procedures. If conflict should arise, this should be resolved by allowing the referring physician to speak directly to the consulting physician from the receiving hospital. Care and understanding by team members, not only for the patient but also the referring staff, can make transport a very rewarding experience for everyone.

Communication is very important throughout the entire transport procedure. Prior to arrival of the team, physician-to-physician and staff-to-staff communication is extremely important. This ensures that proper care is given to the child prior to arrival of the team and that the team has the proper equipment and is prepared to provide care. During the return trip to the perinatal center, the transport team members should stay in contact with their physicians by cellular phone or two-way radio. This enables the physicians to receive updated information and give additional directions for the care of the infant during transport.

Equipment and Supplies
The equipment and supplies required for transport of the neonate are listed in Table 22-6.

Modes of Transportation
Neonatal transport is performed in many different ways depending upon the geography of the area being covered. Ground transport is the simplest mode for a smaller region. An ambulance selected for transport of the newborn should have enough room for the transport staff and their equipment and should be equipped with a generator for supplying electrical power and back-up sources of compressed air and oxygen. Ambulance transport is convenient when referring facilities are within a 150-mile radius of the perinatal center. For centers with referring facilities farther than 150 miles, air transport is preferred and can be accomplished by either fixed-wing aircraft (airplanes) or helicopter. Air transport offers the convenience of quicker travel, but it is very expensive. Fixed-wing transport requires ground transportation for the infant and crew to and from

---

TABLE 22-6   Supplies for Neonatal Transport

Equipment

Incubator with AC and battery power supply	Oxygen and compressed air sources
Infant ventilator	Oxygen/air blender
Cardiac and BP monitor	IV pumps with external battery
Transcutaneous PO_2/CO_2 monitor	Portable suction pump
Pulse oximeter	Transillumination lamp
Stethescope	Manual resuscitation bag and masks
Laryngoscope	Endotracheal tubes (assorted sizes)
Umbilical catheter tray	

Medications / **IV Solutions (D1OW, D25W, NS)**

Atropine	Phenobarbitol
Epinephrine	THAM
Narcan (naloxone)	Sodium bicarbonate (4.6%)
Albumin	Heparin
Valium	Prostaglandins
Phenytoin	Ampicillin
Dopamine	Gentamycin

---

an airport or runway. Helicopter transport offers more versatility on landing and take-off but often compromises on cabin space. Airplanes and helicopters create considerable noise inside the patient care area, which makes patient assessment difficult. Air transport systems are also affected to a greater degree by weather conditions and may require ground transport back-up.

When transporting a patient by air, it is important to remember the effects of pressure on the patient and equipment. Although many aircraft used for medical transport are pressurized, some are not and this can have a profound effect on many medical modalities. Even pressurized aircraft generally only pressurize their cabins to approximately 6000 feet. **Boyle's law** states that the volume of a gas varies inversely with the pressure of that gas. As an aircraft ascends and the patient is moved from a sea level barometric pressure to an environment of reduced pressure, the volume of any pockets of trapped gas will expand. If a patient has a cuffed endotracheal tube with the cuff inflated, the cuff will expand and possibly damage the patient's trachea. Likewise, if the patient has a small pneumothorax that was asymptomatic at sea level, the trapped air will expand as the pressure decreases and may cause significant distress.

Dalton's law states that the total pressure of a gas is equal to the sum of all the individual pressures of gas in a mixture. As the aircraft ascends from sea level, the barometric pressure decreases and the partial pressure of oxygen also decreases. Careful monitoring is necessary to prevent hypoxia in patients receiving oxygen or at risk of hypoxemia.

▄ TRANSPORT OF THE CHILD

Pediatric transport is a new concept that has developed in the last few decades. Prior to that time, most hospitals had small pediatric units where they managed critically ill children. In many of these units, pediatric patients were treated like small adults, utilizing adult equipment and methods of adult medical practice. As pediatric medicine developed into a specialty, it became apparent that pediatric patients were very different and have different needs. Specialized pediatric practitioners and equipment are needed for the care of these critically ill patients. Pediatric tertiary care centers, specializing in emergency and critical pediatric care, opened in many larger hospitals. These centers, staffed by pediatric specialists, could provide better care and the newest technology for sick or injured pediatric patients. Many general care hospitals, unable to keep up with the challenges and expense, found it more economical to close their pediatric units and transfer their pediatric patients to regional pediatric centers. Pediatric transport teams were developed to transport these patients from referral hospitals to these specialized units.

Considerations for the composition of the transport team and the mode of transportation to be used are similar to those for transport of the infant.

Recognition of the Need to Transport

Unfortunately, most critical childhood illnesses or injuries do not occur in close proximity to a **pediatric tertiary care center**. Most pediatric patients are taken to the closest hospital and will then require transport. Identification of which patients are critical and which are not is very important. Conditions in which children should be considered for transport are listed in Table 22-7.

The decision to transport a patient should be made upon the basis of what is best for the child, according to the medical needs of the patient and the resources available on hand and in the tertiary care center. A standard rule to follow is that if the need for intensive care is a possibility, the child should be transported.

Stabilization of the Child

Stabilization of the pediatric patient is a shared responsibility between the referring facility and the transport team. The referring facility should begin stabilization procedures prior to team arrival and should follow the airway–breathing–circulation rules of basic life support (see Chap. 20).

TABLE 22-7   **Pediatric Conditions Requiring Transport**

Severe respiratory distress

Suspected airway obstruction

Need for intensive hemodynamic, metabolic, or neurologic monitoring

Severe trauma

Specialized diagnostic procedures

Any unstable child at risk for deterioration

Prior to transporting the patient, all intravenous lines, endotracheal tubes, and oral airways should be tightly secured. A patient who was previously stable can become very unstable if an important intravenous line or the endotracheal tube becomes dislodged. Prior to leaving the referring institution, the transport team should obtain copies of the patient's

---

TABLE 22-8 Equipment and Supplies for Pediatric Transport

Airway and Oxygen Delivery Supplies

Aerosol masks (pediatric and adult)	Nonrebreathing masks (pediatric and adult)
Medication nebulizers, albuterol, vaponefrin	Venturi masks
Nasal cannulas	Oropharyngeal airways (sizes 00–5)
Oxygen flowmeters	Nasopharyngeal airways

Intubation Supplies

Laryngoscope handle	Endotracheal tubes (sizes 2.5–8.0)
Laryngoscope blades (straight and curved)	Stylets
Extra laryngoscope batteries	Magill forceps
Extra laryngoscope light bulbs	Tape

Ventilation Supplies

Self-inflating manual resuscitation bags	Pressure manometers
Flow-inflating manual resuscitation bags	Oxygen tubing
Oxygen reservoirs	

IV Supplies and Solutions

Butterfly catheters (23 and 25 gauge)	Syringes
Angiocaths (18–25 gauge)	Tape
IV tubing	Armboards
IV pumps	Alcohol and Betadine swabs
IV solutions (D5NS, D10NS, NS, Ringer's)	Bedside glucose kit
Albumin	Dressings

Miscellaneous Supplies

Penlight	Blood pressure cuffs
Suction catheters (6–14 Fr)	Heimlich valves
Urinary catheters	Sterile gloves
Nasogastric tubes	

Medications

Sodium bicarbonate (4.2% and 8.4%)	Benadryl
25% dextrose	Phenobarbitol
Atropine	Solumedrol
Epinephrine (1:1000 and 1:10,000)	Dopamine
Aminophylline	Versed
Ativan	Norcuron
Narcan (naloxone)	Mivacron
Dilantin	

chart and x-ray films. Therapy in process should be continued during the return trip. Team members should contact the receiving physicians and inform them of the patient's condition and the equipment which may be needed upon their arrival.

Equipment and Supplies

The equipment and supplies required for transport of the child are listed in Table 22-8. The types of medications carried by the transport team will depend upon the protocol developed by each individual pediatric care center and transport team.

REFERENCES

1. Committee on Perinatal Health: Toward Improving the Outcome of Pregnancy. White Plains, NY, National March of Dimes Foundation, 1977.
2. Cone TE: History of the Care and Feeding of the Premature Infant. Boston, Little, Brown, 1985.
3. Wallace HM, Losty MA, Baumgartner L: Report of Two Years Experience in Transportation of Premature Infants in New York City. Pediatrics 22:439, 1952.

BIBLIOGRAPHY

American Heart Association: Textbook of Pediatric Advanced Life Support. Dallas, 1990.
Angelini DJ, Whelan-Knapp CM, Gibes RM: Perinatal Neonatal Nursing. Boston, Blackwell Scientific Publications, 1986.
Bose CL: Neonatal transport. In Avery GB, Fletcher MA, Gordon MG (eds): Neonatology: Pathophysiology and Management of the Newborn, 4th ed. Philadelphia, JB Lippincott, 1994.
Fleisher GR, Ludwig S: Textbook of Pediatric Emergency Medicine. Baltimore, Williams and Williams, 1993.
McCloskey K, Orr R: Pediatric Transport Medicine. St. Louis, Mosby-Year Book, 1995.
Reeder SJ, Martin LL, Koniak D: Maternity Nursing. Philadelphia, JB Lippincott, 1992.
Rudolph CS, Borker SR: Regionalization Issues in Intensive Care for High Risk Newborns and Their Families. New York, Praeger, 1987.

SELF-ASSESSMENT QUESTIONS

1. Define what is meant by the concept of regionalization.

2. Maternal transport can be accomplished by which of the following methods?
   a. private car
   b. specialized transport service
   c. local ambulance
   d. all of the above

3. Conditions that may require maternal transport include
   I. multiple gestation
   II. oligohydramnios
   III. maternal diabetes
   IV. primigravida
   a. I and II
   b. II and III
   c. I, II, and IV
   d. I, II, and III

4. Transport teams usually consist of the all of the following members *except*
   a. nurses
   b. respiratory care practitioners
   c. physicians

5. Goals of neonatal transport include
   I. facilitate early discharge of the infant
   II. make independent clinical decisions
   III. function well in an unfamiliar environment
   IV. reduce the cost of caring for the premature infant
       a. II and III   c. II, III, and IV
       b. I and IV   d. I and III

6. What is the simplest mode of transportation of the newborn within a small geographic region?
   a. helicopter   c. ambulance
   b. fixed-wing aircraft   d. private car

7. Conditions for which children may be transported include
   a. suspected airway obstruction   c. hemodynamic monitoring
   b. severe trauma   d. all of the above

8. _____ centers are able to care for all maternal/fetal and neonatal illnesses.
   a. Level 1   c. Level 3
   b. Level 2   d. Perinatal

9. What size endotracheal tubes should be carried in the pediatric transport vehicle?
   a. 2.0 to 5.5   c. 5.5 to 9.0
   b. 2.5 to 8.0   d. 6.0 to 10.0

10. Incubators used for neonatal transport must have both AC and battery power supplies.
    a. true
    b. false

Chapter 23

Surfactant Replacement Therapy

JACKIE L. LONG

OBJECTIVES

Having completed this chapter, the reader will be able to:

1 State the components of pulmonary surfactant.

2 State the physical law that governs the action of surfactant.

3 Describe the mechanism by which surfactant maintains end-tidal alveolar stability.

4 Compare and contrast the development of respiratory distress syndrome in the neonatal and pediatric patient.

5 Name two types of exogenous surfactant.

6 Name the two exogenous surfactant preparations currently approved by the Food and Drug Administration for use in the United States.

7 Compare and contrast prophylactic and rescue administration of exogenous surfactant.

8 Describe two methods commonly used for the administration of intratracheal administration of exogenous surfactant.

9 List three patient parameters that must be continuously monitored during the administration of exogenous surfactant.

10 Describe postadministration patient monitoring that must be conducted during the use of exogenous surfactant.

KEY TERMS

exogenous surfactant
Laplace's law
lecithin dipalmitoyl
  phosphatidylcholine

prophylactic surfactant
  administration
rescue surfactant administration

PHYSIOLOGIC PRINCIPLES

Pulmonary surfactant is a substance that occurs naturally in the mature mammalian lung. It is a phospholipid, consisting of approximately 90% lipids and 10% proteins.[11,20] The main lipid, a saturated fat, is called **lecithin dipalmitoyl phosphatidylcholine** (DPPC). In addition to the lipid, four proteins (SP-A, SP-B, SP-C, and SP-D) have been identified in pulmonary surfactant,[11,18-20] with three of these (SP-A, SP-B, and SP-C) thought to play significant roles in the ability of surfactant to exert its physiologic activity. The function of SP-D is not currently well defined.

Pulmonary surfactant is synthesized and secreted by type II alveolar cells. It is stored in lamellar bodies, which are secretory organelles found in the endoplasmic reticulum of the type II alveolar cell. During respiratory movements, surfactant is released from the lamellar bodies and spreads along the alveolar surface in a layer that is one molecule thick (a monolayer).[11,20,29] Once surfactant is present on the alveolar surface, it establishes an air–liquid interface and reduces surface tension, thus allowing the alveoli to remain inflated at end expiration when transpulmonary pressure is low.

The action of surfactant at the alveolar surface is explained by **Laplace's law**, which states that $P = 2ST/r$ (where P is distending pressure, ST is surface tension, and r is the radius of the alveoli). Surfactant's action is seen clinically when alveoli retain air at the level of the functional residual capacity and resist their natural inclination to collapse at end expiration (end tidal volume). The ability of surfactant to allow end-expiratory alveolar stability prevents the development of atelectasis, reduces the work of breathing associated with expansion of the alveoli during subsequent inspiratory efforts, allows more uniform distribution of ventilation by establishing and maintaining more consistent alveolar pressures in alveoli of differing radii, and reduces the driving pressure (hydrostatic pressures) across the alveolar–capillary membrane.

When any of these mechanisms fail, the patient is at risk for developing respiratory distress syndrome. In the neonate, the condition is called idiopathic respiratory distress syndrome (IRDS); in the pediatric and adult patient, it is called acute respiratory distress syndrome (ARDS). Although the precipitating factors for the development of IRDS and ARDS may differ, the primary pathophysiologic factor for both is the same: a deficiency of pulmonary surfactant. In newborns, especially in those born at less than 35 weeks' gestation, surfactant deficiency is related to a lower number of type II alveolar cells capable of secreting surfactant. In the pediatric and adult patient, surfactant deficiency is related to either a loss of type II cells or the presence of type II cells that malfunction as a result of injury or severe illness. Table 23-1 lists diseases and injuries that are associated with the development of ARDS in the pediatric patient.

SOURCES OF SURFACTANT

In 1959, Avery and Mead[1] documented the pathophysiologic events (Table 23-2) encountered in hyaline membrane disease (now known as RDS) and related the role of surfactant to those events. The work by Avery and Mead paved the way for clinical investigations in the use of **exogenous surfactants** as a replacement for the deficient endogenous surfactant. Despite

TABLE 23-1   **The Development of ARDS in Children: Precipitating Conditions**

Sepsis

Aspiration, including near drowning

Trauma, especially that which results in pulmonary contusions and long bone fractures

Smoke inhalation, with or without the presence of burns

Cardiopulmonary bypass

Any condition that requires massive transfusions

Organ transplantation

Sarnaik AP, Lieh-Lai M: Adult respiratory distress syndrome in children. Pediatr Clin North Am 41(2):337, 1994, and Eigen H. Adult respiratory distress syndrome. In Blumer JL: A Guide to Pediatric Intensive Care, 3rd ed. St. Louis, Mosby-Year Book, 1990.

early trials beginning in the 1960s and continuing through the 1970s,[21] the benefits of administering exogenous surfactant were difficult to demonstrate until 1980 when Fujiwara and colleagues first described positive outcomes of surfactant replacement therapy in a group of 10 infants who were born prematurely and were diagnosed with RDS.[7] Since that time, multiple center clinical trials have been conducted and are well documented in the literature.[4,8,15,16,21-23,25,28]

Exogenous surfactant preparations may be natural or artificial. Natural surfactant is secreted from the lungs of humans or other mammalians. Human surfactant is recovered from the amniotic fluid of a pregnant female when a cesarean section is used to deliver a term infant. Animal surfactant usually comes from cows or pigs. It is extracted from minced lung or from alveolar lavage fluid. Artificial surfactant, which is composed of DPPC and other agents that facilitate adsorption and spreading, is produced in a laboratory.[3,11] While only two exogenous surfactant preparations are currently approved by the Food and Drug Administration (FDA) for use in the United States, several others are either presently under investigation in the United States or are being used elsewhere, notably in Europe and Canada. Table 23-3 summarizes exogenous surfactant preparations.

ADMINISTRATION TECHNIQUES

Exogenous surfactant is administered either prophylactically or as rescue therapy. **Prophylactic surfactant administration** is administration in the

TABLE 23-2   **Pathophysiologic Events in RDS**

Atelectasis

Increased work of breathing

Uneven distribution of ventilation among alveolar units

Pulmonary edema

TABLE 23-3 Exogenous Surfactant Preparations: Source and Composition

PREPARATIONS	SOURCE	COMPOSITION
Synthetic Surfactants		
ALEC* (Pulmactant, Brittania, Red Hill, Surry, United Kingdom)	Synthetic	DPPC,* unsaturated phosphatidylglycerol
Colfosceril palmitate (Exosurf, Glaxo Wellcome, Research Triangle Park, NC)	Synthetic	DPPC, hexadecanol, tyloxapol
KL$_4$	Synthetic	DPPC, KL$_4$
Natural Human Surfactant		
Human	Amniotic fluid	Surfactant lipids, SP-A, SP-B, SP-C
Natural Animal Surfactants		
Alveofact (Thomae, Bilberach, Germany)	Lipid extract of cow lung lavage	Surfactant lipids, SP-B, SP-C
CLSE* (Infasurf, Forest Laboratories, St. Louis, MO)	Lipid extract of calf lung lavage	Surfactant lipids, SP-B, SP-C
Surosurf (Chiesi Farmaceutici, Parma, Italy)	Organic solvent of pig lung purified by chromatography	Lung phospholipids, SP-B, SP-C
Surfactant-TA (Surfacten, Tokyo Tanabe, Tokyo, Japan and beractant [Survanta] Ross Laboratories, Columbus, OH)	Lipid extract of cow lung and synthetic lipids	Lung lipids, DPPC, tripalmitin, palmitic acid

*ALEC, artificial lung expanding compounds; DPPC, dipalmitoyl phosphatidylcholine; CLSE, calf-lung-surfactant extract. Haas CF, Weg JG: Exogenous surfactant therapy: An update. Respir Care 41(5):397, 1996 (reproduced with permission).

delivery room immediately after birth for infants who are statistically at high risk for developing RDS. **Rescue surfactant administration** is used for infants who have begun to demonstrate early signs of RDS. Table 23-4 lists commonly used criteria for prophylactic and rescue protocols.

While many institutions have developed administration methods specific to their patient population, there are two commonly encountered administration modes. The first administration method involves the use of a *side-port adapter* on the endotracheal tube. When using this method, the practitioner administers the surfactant during the inspiratory cycle of the mechanical ventilator. This technique was used during the clinical trials for Exosurf and continues to be used with that preparation. The dose for Exosurf is 5 mL/kg, therefore, the practitioner prepares a syringe containing the appropriate amount of Exosurf solution. Approximately one-half of the solution is administered with the infant lying in the midline position. The infant is then turned 45 degrees to the right and held in that position for 30 seconds. The infant is returned to the midline position and the remainder of the Exosurf solution is administered, and the infant is then turned to the left side (again at 45 degrees) and held for 30 seconds in that position. A description of the procedure, including anatomic diagrams, is provided by the drug manufacturer as a package insert.

TABLE 23-4   Clinical Criteria for the Use of Exogenous Surfactant

PROPHYLACTIC THERAPY	RESCUE THERAPY
Gestational age < 30 weeks[2,21]	Clinical features of RDS, including:
Very low birth weight (<1,250 g)[2,21]	refractory hypoxemia[2,21,23]
Immature lecithin–sphingomyelin ratio[21]	decreased lung compliance and lung volumes that require mechanical ventilatory support[2,23]
Absence of phosphatidylglycerol in amniotic fluid[21]	diffuse alveolar infiltrates on chest radiograph[2,23]

Survanta is commonly administered by injecting the preparation through a *premeasured feeding tube* which has been attached to the syringe and inserted into the endotracheal tube. Survanta is administered in four aliquots. The infant is manually ventilated after each aliquot is administered, and postural positioning is used to disperse the medication throughout the lungs. This technique is also fully described as an insert in the Survanta package.

The optimal method for administering exogenous surfactant, particularly when more than one dose is required, continues to be debated in the literature.[6,9] Although most institutions and, indeed, most clinical researchers have focused on the administration of exogenous surfactant by intratracheal bolus, some investigators are exploring the use of aerosolization as a method of administration.[9-14,26,27,30] Aerosolization may have more utility in the treatment of older children and adults with ARDS. Each student or practitioner is encouraged to consult the department's policy and procedure manual for site-specific modifications of these general administration methods.

PATIENT MONITORING

During administration of exogenous surfactant, the practitioner must constantly monitor the patient for adverse reactions. Patient parameters to be monitored include oxygen saturation using pulse oximetry (maintain SpO_2 between 90% and 95%), heart rate, and blood pressure. In addition, the practitioner must carefully monitor the endotracheal tube for the presence of reflux of surfactant into the tube. If reflux into the endotracheal tube occurs during the administration of Exosurf, the practitioner should immediately reduce the rate at which the solution is being injected through the adapter. Mild bradycardia, hypotension, and hypoxemia may occur during the administration of surfactant. When any of these occur, the practitioner should immediately suspend administration of the solution and check the position and patency of the endotracheal tube, then stabilize the infant by increasing the FIO_2 and/or ventilating the infant, either by increasing the ventilatory support or by manual ventilation. Administration of any remaining surfactant should not be continued until the infant's SpO_2, heart rate, and blood pressure values have returned to baseline.

Immediately following the administration of surfactant, the practitioner must continue to monitor the infant closely. Oxygen requirements may decrease very quickly following the administration of surfactant; consequently, monitoring of the SpO_2 is essential. Because changes in compliance can also occur rapidly, either the respiratory care practitioner or nursing staff must continuously assess the infant for chest expansion, which can serve as a guide for the need to decrease the peak inspiratory pressure (PIP). Changes in the exhaled tidal volume can be monitored continuously by using in-line volume monitors.

In addition to the immediately observable adverse effects and complications of exogenous surfactant administration, at least two other clinically significant complications may occur. Pulmonary hemorrhage has been reported with the use of both Exosurf and Survanta.[2,21] The drop in pulmonary vascular resistance that occurs after the administration of exogenous surfactant is also linked to the development of left-to-right shunting through the ductus arteriosus.[21] The development of intraventricular hemorrhage in infants treated with exogenous surfactant is also being explored.[21]

■SUMMARY

The development of exogenous surfactant preparations has provided an effective means of treating infants who develop RDS. Today, the use of exogenous surfactant replacement therapy in premature newborns who demonstrate clinical evidence of RDS is the standard of care. While exogenous surfactant replacement therapy can be used in the delivery room, it should not be incorporated as a part of routine neonatal resuscitation.[21] The use of exogenous surfactant in the treatment of ARDS in children and adults is currently being investigated; however, the benefits seen in the neonatal population have not yet been realized in older patients.[5,17,24]

■REFERENCES

1. Avery ME, Mead J: Surface properties in relation to atelectasis and hyaline membrane disease. Am J Dis Child 97:517, 1959.
2. Bose CL, Wright MS: Surfactant replacement therapy. In Koff PB, Eitzman D, Neu J (eds): Neonatal and Pediatric Respiratory Care, 2nd ed. St. Louis, Mosby-Year Book, 1993.
3. Cottrell GP, Surkin HB: Pharmacology for Respiratory Care Practitioners. Philadelphia, F.A. Davis, 1995.
4. Dimitriou G, Greenough A, Giffin FJ, Karani J: The appearance of "early" chest radiographs and the response to surfactant replacement therapy. Brit J Rad 68(815):1177, 1995.
5. Eigen H: Adult respiratory distress syndrome. In Blumer JL: A Guide to Pediatric Intensive Care, 3rd ed. St. Louis, Mosby-Year Book, 1990.
6. Espinosa FF, Shapiro AH, Fredberg JJ, Kamm RD: Spreading of exogenous surfactant in an airway. J Appl Physiol 75:2028, 1993.
7. Fujiwara T, Maeta H, Chida S, et al: Artificial replacement therapy in hyaline membrane disease. Lancet 1:55, 1980.
8. Gibson AT, Primhak RA: Early changes in lung function and response to surfactant replacement therapy. Eur J Pediatr 153:495, 1994.
9. Grotberg JB, Halpern D, Jensen OE: Interaction of exogenous and endogenous surfactant: Spreading-rate effects. J Appl Physiol 78(2):750, 1995.
10. Haas CF, Folk LM, Weg JG, et al: A nebulizer system for administering synthetic surfactant (abstract). Respir Care 37(11):1367, 1992.

11. Haas CF, Weg JG: Exogenous surfactant therapy: An update. Respir Care 41(5):397, 1996.
12. Lewis J, Ikegami M, Higuchi R, et al: Nebulized vs. instilled exogenous surfactant in an adult lung injury model. J Appl Physiol 71:1270, 1991.
13. Long W, Thompson T, Sundell H, et al: Effects of two rescue doses of synthetic surfactant on mortality rate and survival without bronchopulmonary dysplasia in 700 to 1350 gram infants with respiratory distress syndrome. J Pediatr 118:595, 1991.
14. MacIntyre NR, Coleman RE, Schuller FS, et al: Efficiency of the delivery of aerosolized artificial surfactant to intubated patients with adult respiratory distress syndrome (abstract). Am J Respir Crit Care Med 149(4, Part 2):A125, 1994.
15. Pandit PB, Dunn MS, Kelly EN, Perlman M: Surfactant replacement in neonates with early chronic lung disease. Pediatrics 95(6):851, 1995.
16. Patel CA, Klein JM: Outcome of infants with birth weights less than 1000 g with respiratory distress syndrome treated with high-frequency ventilation and surfactant replacement therapy. Arch Pediatr Adolesc Med 149:317, 1995.
17. Perez-Benavides F, Riff E, Franks C: Adult respiratory distress syndrome and artificial surfactant replacement in the pediatric patient. Pediatr Emerg Care 11(3):153, 1995.
18. Persson A, Chang D, Rust K, et al: Purification and biochemical characterization of CP4(SP-D), a collagenous surfactant-associated protein. Biochemistry 28:6361 1989.
19. Possmayer F: A proposed nomenclature for pulmonary surfactant-associated proteins. Am Rev Respir Dis 138:990, 1988.
20. Poulain FR, Clements JA: Pulmonary surfactant therapy. West J Med 162:43, 1995.
21. Pramanik AK, Holtzman RB, Merritt TA: Surfactant replacement therapy for pulmonary disease. Pediatr Clin North Am 40(5):913, 1993.
22. Pulson TE, Spear RM, Peterson BM: New concepts in the treatment of children with acute respiratory distress syndrome. J Pediatr 127(2):163, 1995.
23. Ring JC, Stidham GL: Novel therapies for acute respiratory failure. Pediatr Clin North Am 41(6):1325, 1994.
24. Sarnaik AP, Lieh-Lai M: Adult respiratory distress syndrome in children. Pediatr Clin North Am 41(2):337, 1994.
25. Sinski A, Corbo J: Surfactant replacement in adults and children with ARDS—An effective therapy? Crit Care Nurse Dec:54, 1994.
26. Weg JG, Balk BA, Tharrat S, et al: Safety and potential efficacy of an aerosolized surfactant in human sepsis-induced adult respiratory distress syndrome. JAMA 272(18):1433, 1994.
27. Wiedemann H, Baughman R, DeBoisblanc E, et al, and the Exosurf ARDS Sepsis Study Group: A multicenter trial in human sepsis-induced ARDS of an aerosolized synthetic surfactant (Exosurf) (abstract). Am Rev Resp Dis 272(18):1433, 1992.
28. Woerndle S, Bartmann P: The effect of three surfactant preparations on in vitro lymphocyte functions. J Perinat Med 22:119, 1994.
29. Wright JR, Dobbs LG: Regulation of pulmonary surfactant secretion and clearance. Annu Rev Physiol 53:395, 1991.
30. Zelter M, Escudier J, Hoeffel JM, Murray JF: Effects of aerosolized artificial surfactant on repeated oleic acid injury in sheep. Am Rev Respir Dis 141:1014, 1990.

▬ SELF-ASSESSMENT QUESTIONS

1. Surfactant exerts its ability to decrease surface tension at the
   a. lamellar bodies
   b. type II alveolar cell
   c. alveolar–capillary membrane
   d. air–liquid interface in the alveolus

2. Which of the following exogenous surfactant preparations are currently approved by the FDA for use in the United States?
       I. Infasurf
      II. Survanta
     III. Exosurf
          a. I only   c. II and III only
          b. III only   d. I, II, and III

3. The most common route of administration for exogenous surfactant is
   a. aerosolization
   b. intratracheal bolus
   c. intravenous infusion
   d. instillation by side-port adapter

4. Which of the following patient parameters must be monitored during the administration of exogenous surfactant?
   I. heart rate
   II. oxygenation
   III. blood pressure
   IV. delivered tidal volume

   a. III only   c. II and IV only
   b. IV only   d. I, II, and III only

5. Reflux into the endotracheal tube can be identified by
   a. visual observation
   b. a sudden drop in SpO_2
   c. auscultation of the chest
   d. an increase in blood pressure

Chapter 24

High Frequency Ventilation

BARBARA G. WILSON

OBJECTIVES

Having completed this chapter, the reader will be able to:

1 Define terminology associated with high frequency ventilation.

2 Describe gas transport mechanisms during high frequency ventilation.

3 Understand physiologic principles for improving oxygenation and CO_2 elimination.

4 Describe patient management strategies for high frequency ventilation.

5 Demonstrate familiarity with high frequency ventilation equipment including the Bunnell Life Pulse, Sensormedics 3100A Oscillator, and Infrasonics InfantStar 950.

6 List common complications and hazards associated with high frequency ventilation.

KEY TERMS

airway pressure monitor
bulk convection
Bunnell Life Pulse
coaxial flow
convection streaming
electronic control and alarm

molecular diffusion
oscillator
patient circuit
pendelluft movement
pneumatic logic and control

High frequency ventilation (HFV) is a widely accepted mode of mechanical ventilation in neonatal and pediatric critical care. Often considered nonconventional ventilation, high frequency ventilation has become a conventional mode of ventilation in many pediatric centers for severe respiratory failure and for pulmonary barotrauma.[7,11] Researchers have also reported success with HFV in the treatment of respiratory distress syndrome,[5,22] air leak syndromes,[1,6,9,13,16,19] pulmonary hypoplasia secondary to congenital diaphragmatic hernia,[15,21] persistent pulmonary hypertension,[20] and congenital heart disease.[19] This early data is further supported by results of randomized, controlled clinical trials which demonstrate a significant reduction in chronic lung disease,[10] pulmonary interstitial emphysema, and other air leak syndromes.[12,17]

HFV is defined as positive pressure ventilation at breath rates in excess of 150 breaths per minute (bpm) and tidal volumes approximating anatomical dead space. It is important that the respiratory care practitioner be familiar with the use of HFV devices and the management strategies that govern the clinical application of these devices. This chapter will review the different forms of HFV available to neonates and children, offer clinical management strategies, and discuss complications and hazards associated with its use.

■ HIGH FREQUENCY VENTILATION TERMINOLOGY

All forms of HFV have three common characteristics: (1) breathing rates in excess of 150 bpm, (2) tidal volumes of 1 to 3 mL/kg, and (3) noncompliant ventilator circuitry. Manufacturers have selected various technical methods to produce this mode of ventilation. The four most common types of HFV are high frequency positive pressure (HFPPV), high frequency jet (HFJV), high frequency flow interrupter (HFFIV), and high frequency oscillatory (HFOV) (Table 24-1). Each ventilator platform has a unique principle of operation and will be reviewed separately. Perinatal/pediatric clinicians must understand each form of HFV thoroughly and be able to identify physiologic responses, clinical indications, limitations, and management strategies so that appropriate selection and application can be made for a given patient scenario.

HFPPV is the application of standard positive pressure ventilators at high breath rates (faster than 150 bpm) and small tidal volumes.[27] Inspiratory time is short to facilitate the fast breath rate and exhalation is passive. Increases in mean airway pressure achieved with this form of HFV should be monitored with external airway graphics (AG) systems to detect the presence or absence of incomplete exhalation and gas trapping as breathing rates increase. A minimum inhalation-to-exhalation ratio of 1:1 must be maintained to prevent the development of intrinsic positive end-expiratory pressure (PEEP). Continuous AG monitoring is recommended to prevent progression of pulmonary injury sequence as a result of volume overdistention of the lung. While HFPPV pioneered the high frequency concept, its use has declined with the availability of other HFV platforms developed in the 1970s and 1980s with higher breathing rates and better monitoring capabilities.

TABLE 24-1   Types of High Frequency Ventilation

High frequency positive pressure ventilation (HFPPV)

High frequency jet ventilation (HFJV)

High frequency flow interrupter ventilation (HFFIV)

High frequency oscillator ventilation (HFOV)

HFJV provides a high velocity pulse of blended gas through a side port at the tip of the endotracheal tube.[18,23,26] Additional fresh gas is entrained from a second time-cycled, pressure-limited ventilator which provides entrained tidal volume as well as warmed, humidified gas. The background ventilator also provides PEEP and intermittent bulk sigh volume breaths. Breath rates for HFJV are usually 100 to 600 bpm, and exhalation is passive and facilitated by extremely short inspiratory times (20–40 milliseconds).

High frequency flow interrupters deliver inspiratory flow to the patient in short bursts via a rotating ball valve or microprocessor-controlled solenoid valve. These ventilators produce breath rates of 2 to 22 Hz or 120 to 1320 bpm (1 Hz = 60 bpm). HFFIV is similar to HFOV in that inspiration and exhalation are both active processes. Active exhalation is defined as a mechanical drop in airway pressure during exhalation to accelerate exhaled gas flow. Conventional tidal volumes can also be administered intermittently as sigh breaths to prevent atelectasis and maintain end-expiratory lung volume.

HFOV can produce breath rates in excess of 3000 bpm with active inspiratory and expiratory phases and tidal volumes less than physiologic dead space.[2,4] This technology vibrates (oscillates) a volume of gas via a diaphragm, piston, or acoustic speaker to create a sinusoidal waveform throughout the conducting airways. A bias flow of fresh, humidified, and warmed gas intersects the oscillatory path to eliminate carbon dioxide (CO_2) from the circuit and prevent drying of respiratory mucosa and secretions. No bulk sigh breaths are available in HFOV.

■ MECHANISMS OF GAS TRANSPORT

The mechanism of gas exchange during HFV is not completely understood, as several individual mechanisms may be interacting at any one time.[8] Table 24-2 summarizes the mechanisms of gas exchange for HFV. **Bulk convection** is the bulk flow of gas down to the proximal alveoli with very low dead space volumes. **Coaxial flow** is produced as a result of the asymmetrical flow of high velocity gas, which mixes inspiratory and expiratory gases. Taylor's dispersion, or **convection streaming,** produces a mixing of gases as the high frequency breath is injected into the airway at high velocity. Gas transport then occurs as fresh gas molecules are injected down the center of conducting airways and exhaled gases passively curl upward along the outside edge of the airways. The exhaled

---

TABLE 24-2   Mechanisms of Gas Transport During HFV

Bulk flow

Coaxial flow

Taylor's dispersion

Pendelluft gas mixing

Molecular diffusion

gases travel at a lower velocity than the inspiratory gases, with a continuous exhalation of gases around the inspired gases being the net result. **Molecular diffusion** is the rapid kinetic motion of molecules (O_2 in and CO_2 out) which occurs in the terminal bronchioles and alveoli. **Pendelluft movement** mixes gas between lung regions that have different time constants via communications between neighboring lung units. Figure 24-1 diagrammatically demonstrates the regions of the lung where the various gas transport mechanisms are thought to operate.

PHYSIOLOGIC PRINCIPLES OF HIGH FREQUENCY VENTILATION

CO_2 Elimination

All gas transport mechanisms are thought to operate simultaneously during HFV. Therefore, the effects of specific ventilator interventions may be

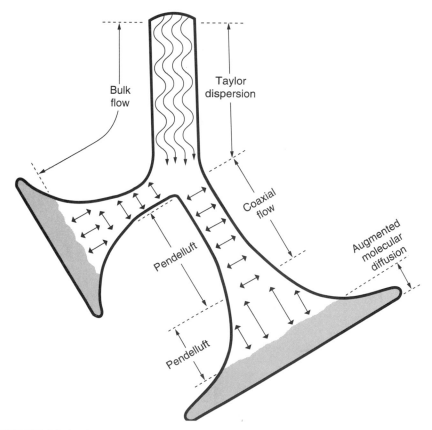

FIGURE 24-1   Areas of the tracheobronchial tree where various gas transport mechanisms of high frequency ventilation are thought to be operative. (Chang HK: Mechanisms of gas transport during ventilation by high frequency oscillation. J Appl Physiol Respir Environ Exercise Physiol 56:553, 1984.)

difficult to predict, as it is uncertain which ventilator parameter influences which gas transport mechanism. During traditional positive pressure ventilation, alterations in alveolar ventilation via changes in tidal volume or respiratory rate facilitate changes in CO_2 elimination.

CO_2 elimination during HFV is also determined by delivered alveolar ventilation. However, the minute ventilation delivered with HFV has a greater dependency on alterations in tidal volume than in breath frequency, with tidal volume most affected by changes in peak inspiratory pressure (PIP) or amplitude (increase PIP or amplitude, increase tidal volume). Ventilator frequency should ideally be set to achieve the resonant frequency of the lung. Resonant frequency is determined by the underlying lung structure and age of the patient. Premature infants with surfactant depletion have decreased compliance and short time constants, and, therefore, a higher resonant frequency of the lung. These patients require a higher set breathing frequency to match the time constant of the lung and produce ventilatory resonance (as structural time constants decrease, frequency should be increased).

Delivered HFV tidal volume is also frequency dependent; as set frequency increases, tidal volume decreases, resulting in decreased CO_2 elimination. For example, during HFJV, breathing frequency is initiated at rates of 350 to 450 bpm for premature infants, owing to the noncompliant premature lung, and maintained during the course of therapy. Small increases in HFV frequency in these babies may continue to alter alveolar ventilation and improve CO_2 elimination until the resonant frequency of the lung has been exceeded, tidal volume decreases, and alveolar ventilation actually begins to fall. In pediatric patients, however, the lungs are relatively more compliant than premature lungs and time constants are longer; lower breathing frequencies should be selected to match pediatric lung time constants. If breathing frequencies are increased within a predicted range for pediatric patients, delivered tidal volume and alveolar ventilation decrease, decreasing CO_2 elimination and increasing $Paco_2$.[14] Therefore, HFV is usually begun at 240 to 360 bpm (4–6 Hz) and maintained at that level for pediatric patients.

The conventional positive pressure ventilator used in some forms of HFV may be adjusted to provide periodic "sigh" breaths to recruit lung volume. When $Paco_2$ becomes elevated, increasing the tidal volume and rate of sigh breaths may be necessary to correct atelectasis and improve alveolar ventilation.

End-Expiratory Lung Volume

Mean lung volume during HFV is determined by the delivered mean airway pressure. Because delivered tidal volumes are small, mean lung volume does not change dramatically during inspiration. Therefore, end-expiratory lung volume remains static around the volume produced by the mean airway pressure and the compliance of the patient's lung.

Set PEEP is the primary contributor to mean airway pressure and end-expiratory lung volume during HFV. In many ways, HFV can be thought of as "vibrating" continuous positive airway pressure (CPAP). Applying this concept, end-expiratory lung volume is established via changes in mean airway pressure as a result of the PEEP setting and not bulk inflation of the lungs during a mechanical inspiration.

High frequency breaths remove CO_2 by multiple gas exchange mechanisms operating slightly above and below the end-expiratory lung volume. Ventilator-induced lung injury is reduced with this technique, as compared with traditional positive pressure ventilation, because the sustained high peak inflation pressures generated by bulk delivery of conventionally sized tidal volumes are eliminated and replaced by very rapid dead space-sized tidal volumes. Lung inflation is maintained by increased end-expiratory pressure and, as a result, ventilation–perfusion relationships are improved throughout the entire breathing cycle, not just during inspiration.

Oxygenation during HFV is dependent on restoring lung volume by increasing mean airway pressure until the critical opening and closing pressures of the lung have been exceeded. Collapsed alveoli are then "recruited" open and remain so throughout the ventilatory cycle. Ventilation–perfusion relationships improve as physiologic shunt is reduced.

Adequate end-expiratory lung volume may be determined clinically by observing incremental increases in arterial saturation (SpO_2) as FIO_2 is reduced, as well as lung expansion on chest radiograph (CXR). HFV neonatal and pediatric patients with respiratory failure should have a mean lung volume on chest x-ray film that places the diaphragms at the 8th to 9th rib level.[25] Patients with air leak syndromes or congenital heart disease should receive a lower lung inflation (*i.e.*, mean airway pressure) strategy.

Cardiovascular Effects

The cardiovascular effects of HFV vary with ventilatory strategy and the patient's pulmonary compliance. HFJV improves alveolar ventilation and CO_2 elimination at equivalent mean airway pressures as compared with conventional ventilation. Therefore, an initial change to HFJV should not compromise cardiovascular function, as intrathoracic pressure has not changed. As lung volume is recruited, mean airway pressure can be slowly reduced while maintaining adequate alveolar ventilation. This limits the adverse side effects of positive pressure ventilation on cardiovascular performance[28] and may result in increased systemic blood flow. However, if mean airway pressures greater than those used during conventional ventilation are required during HFV (as may be the case in HFOV or HFFIV), cardiovascular compromise may occur. Increases in intravascular volume and inotropic support (vasopressor) are useful in this scenario to preserve mean arterial blood pressure, cardiac output, and, thus, oxygen delivery (CaO_2 × cardiac output). Increases in central venous pressure or decreases in mean arterial pressure indicate decreases in systemic blood flow as a result of volume overdistention of the lung and inappropriately high mean airway pressure after adequate intravascular volume has been established. Table 24-3 summarizes the physiologic principles of HFV.

■MANAGEMENT STRATEGIES FOR HIGH FREQUENCY VENTILATION

Two management strategies exist for initiation of HFV: early intervention and rescue. Early intervention advocates view HFV as an equal, and often better, alternative to conventional mechanical ventilation.[8] Rescue advocates use HFV when maximal conventional ventilation fails to provide adequate gas exchange or contributes to lung injury.

TABLE 24-3 Physiologic Principles of HFV

Oxygenation goal: Restore end-expiratory lung volume via P_{aw}.

Respiratory disease: 9th rib lung expansion

Cardiac disease: 7th rib lung expansion

CO_2 elimination goal: Improve alveolar minute ventilation.

Frequency: determined by time constant of the lung; premature infants require higher frequencies (440–600 bpm), pediatric patients require lower frequencies (240–320 bpm).

Tidal volume: determined by PIP or amplitude; frequency dependent (↑ frequency, ↓ tidal volume)

Early intervention HFV attempts to achieve optimal lung inflation and reduce ventilator-induced lung injury by eliminating exposure to high inflation pressure, bulk-flow, conventional mechanical ventilation. HFV is initiated in critically ill premature infants at birth with mean airway pressures below the opening pressure of the lung (approximately P_{aw} 10 cm H_2O). P_{aw} is then increased slowly to achieve adequate lung inflation as visualized on chest x-ray film. In the early intervention strategy, babies who receive conventional mechanical ventilation at birth are converted to HFV within 2 hours at mean airway pressures 1 to 2 cm H_2O above that used during the trial of conventional ventilation.

HFV rescue advocates initiate HFV when critically ill children fail conventional ventilation, that is, maximal ventilator settings fail to produce adequate arterial oxygenation and CO_2 elimination, resulting in severe hypoxemia and respiratory acidosis. Air leak syndromes (pneumothorax, pulmonary interstitial emphysema, bronchopleural fistula, and pneumomediastinum) are also an indication for HFV rescue. Congenital heart disease complicated by respiratory failure has been shown to benefit from HFV rescue by reducing mean intrathoracic pressure and preserving cardiac function.[24]

The timing of initiating rescue HFV can alter clinical outcomes. Rescue patients have significantly more exposure to increased FIO_2 and peak inflation pressures than early intervention HFV patients. Therefore, when HFV fails in rescue patients, it may be that the trial of conventional ventilation was too long and that lung injury was irreversible, not that HFV failed. Institutions should establish clear criteria for initiation of rescue HFV to assist clinicians in determining when conventional ventilation has failed and to improve rescue HFV outcomes. A comparison of these early intervention versus rescue HFV management strategies is not possible, as entry criteria and patient populations are not similar.

▬ HFV EQUIPMENT

Bunnell Life Pulse
The **Bunnell Life Pulse** (Bunnell Corporation, Salt Lake City), Figure 24-2, is a microprocessor-controlled, constant-flow, time-cycled, pressure-limited jet ventilator for neonatal and pediatric patients. Jet pulses are delivered to

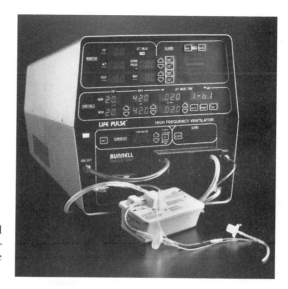

FIGURE 24-2 The Bunnell Life Pulse jet ventilator (Bunnell Incorporated, Salt Lake City, UT).

the patient via the jet port at the tip of a triple lumen endotracheal (ET) tube. Gas passes from the outlet of the ventilator through a heated humidification system into the patient box where the jet valve introduces inspiration as a sharp impulse that penetrates the resident dead space of the lung. The patient box also contains a pressure transducer for monitoring pressures at the tip of the ET tube and a valve for purging condensation and secretions from the pressure-monitoring tubing attached to the ET tube. A prototype Lifeport Adaptor may replace the need for reintubation with a triple lumen Hi-Lo ET tube, pending FDA approval (Fig. 24-3).[29] This adaptor would enable attachment to a conventional ventilator and delivery of HFJV using standard ET tubes.

All ventilator functions have computer-controlled responses to detect alterations in ventilation, such as those caused by tubing kinks, disconnects, increases in pressure, and mechanical and electrical failures. Ventilator controls include PIP, breathing frequency, and inspiratory time (valve on-time). PIP is servo-controlled via a reducing valve, which adjusts drive pressure to maintain PIP settings from 8 to 50 cm H_2O. This drive pressure is continuously reported as servo pressure on the front ventilator panel. Servo pressure changes as the patient-ventilator system changes, that is, increased servo pressure indicates improved lung compliance, air leak, or tubing disconnect/leak. Decreased servo pressure indicates worsening lung compliance, obstruction of the ET tube, pneumothorax, or tracheobronchial secretions. Table 24-4 summarizes the interpretation of servo pressure (automatically controlled drive pressure).

Frequency ranges are adjustable from 240 to 660 bpm (4–11 Hz). Inspiratory time, or valve-on time, is adjustable, but it is commonly set at 20 milliseconds. A separate air/oxygen blender must be used for regulation of FIO_2. PEEP is produced by the background conventional ventilator PEEP valve.

Monitoring the Bunnell jet requires thorough assessment of the tandem ventilator system. PIP, P_{aw}, PEEP, servo pressure, and frequency must be

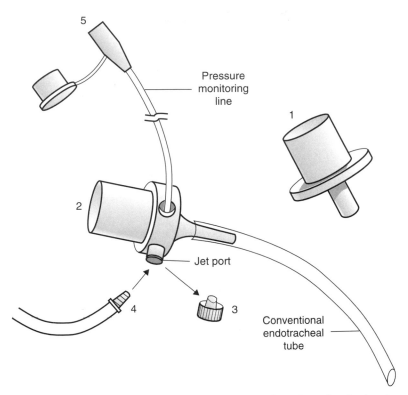

FIGURE 24-3   Bunnell Lifeport Adapter. The patient's endotracheal tube size will determine which size Lifeport to use. The conventional 15-mm ETT adapter (*1*) is replaced with the Lifeport adapter (*2*). The cap on the Jet Port (*3*) is removed and the luer fitting of the Life Pulse ventilator circuit (*4*) is attached to the Jet Port. The pressure monitoring connector from the jet's patient box is attached to the pressure monitoring line (*5*). The conventional ventilator circuit is attached to the 15-mm port of the Lifeport adapter. (Note: This adapter was not approved by the FDA at the time of publication.)

evaluated and recorded from the Life Pulse, as these parameters are functions of both ventilator systems and pressure measurements are performed at the tip of the ET tube. The set PIP and frequency of the conventional ventilator will determine the character of the sigh breaths. If the conventional mechanical ventilation PIP is greater than the jet PIP, jet breaths will be interrupted during the conventional ventilation inspiratory phase. Conventional ventilations are usually reduced to 0 to 10 bpm during jet ventilation to function as sigh breaths, and to reduce the risk of barotrauma. Table 24-5 describes the initial selection of jet ventilator settings.

Sensormedics 3100A

The 3100A (Sensormedics Critical Care, Yorba Linda, CA), Figure 24-4, is an electrically powered, microprocessor-controlled, piston-driven ventilator. The piston is rapidly displaced in forward and backward motion which moves a flexible diaphragm and produces a square-wave flow pattern. These oscillations are superimposed upon a baseline mean airway pres-

TABLE 24-4 The Importance of Servo Pressure During HFJV

INCREASED SERVO PRESSURE	DECREASED SERVO PRESSURE
Increased lung volume	Decreased lung volume
Increased lung compliance	Decreased lung compliance
Air leak	Obstruction of ETT
Tubing disconnect	Tension pneumothorax
	Suctioning required

Servo pressure = automatically controlled drive pressure.

sure. End-expiratory lung volume is determined by the P_{aw} and remains relatively constant during the respiratory cycle. HFOV can be achieved via traditional ET tubes, and reintubation is not required. The 3100A ventilator is composed of six ventilator subsystems: pneumatic logic and control, patient circuit, oscillator, airway pressure monitor, and electronic control and alarms. The **pneumatic logic and control** subsystems include four pneumatic controls: bias flow, mean pressure, mean pressure limit, and patient circuit calibration. The bias flow is blended gas that continuously moves through the patient circuit. Mean pressure adjustment determines the base pressure level on which the oscillatory waveform is produced via a control valve restriction on the expiratory limb of the circuit. The mean pressure limit determines the maximal proximal airway pressure developed within the patient circuit. The patient circuit calibration is a screwdriver adjustment used to set the mean pressure limit.

The **patient circuit** is the conducting path for humidified, blended, bias gas flow from the ventilator to the patient. Gas flows through the inspiratory limb of the circuit, to the patient Y connector, then into the expiratory

TABLE 24-5 Recommendations for Initial Jet Ventilator Settings

FIO_2	Same as CMV. May consider 1.0 FIO_2 during reintubation and establishment of HFJV, depending upon patient stability.
PIP	To maintain $Paco_2$, set PIP 1 to 2 cm H_2O lower than CMV. To reduce $Paco_2$ set PIP the same as CMV.
P_{aw}	Set PEEP at tandem ventilator to produce P_{aw} identical to that used during CMV. If increased oxygenation is desired, increase PEEP to increase P_{aw}.
Frequency	Depends upon age, weight, and underlying pulmonary disease. Premature infants, 440 to 600 bpm; full-term infants, 300 to 420 bpm; pediatric patients, 240 to 320 bpm. Adjust inspiratory time to .02 seconds (20 milliseconds).
PEEP	Adjusted at the tandem ventilator to produce the P_{aw} used during CMV. Record value from the Life Pulse.
CMV	As jet ventilation is initiated, observe progressive increase in jet PIP and PEEP. Slowly decrease CMV rate to 5 to 10 bpm, observing Spo_2 and transcutaneous CO_2 ($TCco_2$).

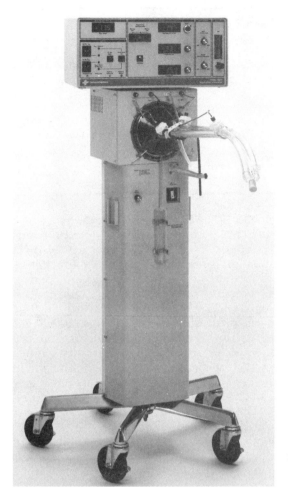

FIGURE 24-4 The Sensor-medics 3100A high frequency oscillator (Sensormedics Critical Care, Yorba Linda, CA).

limb and out the pressure control valve. This valve creates two paths for exhalation, one to a variable orifice restriction and another to a fixed orifice that monitors the presence of a minimal bias flow alarm system. The P_{aw} control and pressure limit valves are mushroom valves on the control valve assembly of the circuit. A dump valve, located at the midpoint of the circuit, can open the patient circuit to ambient air and allow the patient to breathe spontaneously at atmospheric pressure when predetermined pressure settings have been met (P_{aw} > 50 cm H_2O or P_{aw} < 20% of set maximum P_{aw}). Figure 24-5 illustrates the 3100A circuit as it appears attached to the ventilator.

The **oscillator** subsystem incorporates the electronic control circuit which drives the motor and piston assembly to produce the gas flow pattern. When the piston is driven forward, inspiration occurs; when the piston is driven backwards, expiration occurs. The percent (%) inspiratory time is the relative duration of the positive motion of the piston. As frequency decreases, the displacement amplitude of the piston increases, as

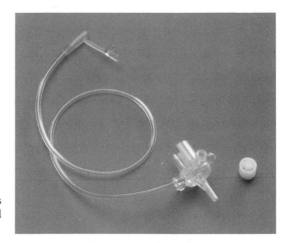

FIGURE 24-5 Sensormedics 3100A patient circuit attached to the ventilator.

does delivered tidal volume. The **airway pressure monitor** determines the instantaneous pressure measurements in the circuit via a pressure transducer to derive mean airway pressure and δ P (the oscillatory peak pressure minus the trough pressure).

The **electronic control and alarm** subsystem integrates information received from the other ventilator systems to orchestrate the activities of the ventilator according to preprogrammed algorithms to avoid patient injury and prevent equipment damage.

The user of this ventilator must provide an external heated humidifier and air/oxygen blender. The heated humidifier must be manufactured for neonatal/pediatric use and capable of performing in a 1 to 40 LPM flow range. Temperature is controlled via a proximal airway gas temperature probe on the patient circuit. A second gas flow source is required to cool the piston chamber and prevent overheating, but it does not require blended gas.

Initial ventilator settings should address FIO_2, mean airway pressure, amplitude, frequency, and inspiratory time. Table 24-6 suggests starting parameters for HFOV.

TABLE 24-6   Recommendations for Initial Oscillator Settings

FIO_2	Same as CMV. May consider 10% increase until stable.
P_{aw}	Set mean airway pressure 1 to 3 cm H_2O higher than that used during CMV. If SpO_2 does not progressively increase, increase in 1 cm H_2O increments every 15 to 30 minutes until SpO_2 rises.
Frequency	Depends upon age, weight, and underlying pulmonary disease. Premature infants, 12 to 15 Hz; full-term infants, 10 to 12 Hz; pediatric patients, 6 to 10 Hz.
% Inspiratory time	33% is most common starting point; 50% is considered maximum.
Amplitude	Adjust to the minimum setting. Slowly increase until the patient's chest visibly vibrates.
Bias flow	6 LPM for neonates, 12 LPM for pediatrics.

Infrasonics HFFIV

The Infrasonics Infant Star 950 (Infrasonics, Inc., San Diego, CA; see Fig. 16-18, Chap. 16) is classified as an electrically powered, time-cycled, pressure-limited, constant/demand flow ventilator. The high frequency flow interrupter option of the 950 produces high frequency pressure pulses during inspiration via the proportioning valves and a negative flow during expiration through an active jet venturi. It is recommended for infant use only. HFFIV can be administered with (HFV ± IMV) or without (HFV ONLY) intermittent mandatory pressure limited sigh breaths to recruit collapsed alveoli.

The HFFIV mode functions similar to that of the conventional ventilator, however the proportioning valves open and the exhalation valves close for a period of 18 milliseconds to generate each HFV pulse. The high frequency rate is adjustable from 2 to 22 Hz. The pulse intensity, or amplitude, is a function of the amount of flow allowed to exit the proportioning valves. Maximum flow is 120 LPM and minimum is 12 LPM during HFFIV. As the amplitude setting is increased, inspiratory flow is increased in increments of 2 LPM. At maximum flow, a volume of 36 mL is generated at the ventilator with each HFV pulse. The delivered tidal volume is considerably less than this volume, however, and is dependent upon compliance and resistance of the ventilator circuit and humidifier, ET tube size and length, and patient R_{aw} and lung compliance. Low compliance ventilator circuitry and the low volume humidifier canister are recommended to maximize tidal volume delivery.

During HFV, the exhalation venturi flow and diaphragm back pressure are adjusted to maintain the desired PEEP. The exhalation valve is simultaneously pulsed to create an increased expiratory resistance during the HFV pulse, to direct more energy toward the patient. PEEP/CPAP is maintained as the baseline pressure around which the inspiratory pulses occur. Therefore, the mean airway pressure and the PEEP/CPAP are commonly equal. Airway pressure measurements are sampled every 5 seconds; the computer averages these points over 30 seconds and displays this value as the mean airway pressure.

It is important to keep the ET tube in a straight line with the ventilator circuit during HFV. Clinicians should avoid bends and kinks in the ET tube to maximize waveform potential. HFV may loosen and mobilize respiratory secretions in the first several hours. It is important to perform tracheal suctioning to maintain a patent ET tube and airways. Table 24-7 presents initial HFFIV settings.

Table 24-8 compares the various HFV techniques.

▬COMPLICATIONS AND HAZARDS OF HFV

Complications associated with HFV include tracheal injury, segmental/lobar collapse, atelectasis, pulmonary overdistention, respiratory alkalosis, and patient instability if reintubation is required (Table 24-9). The earliest reported complication associated with HFV was tracheal injury as a result of the high velocity of gas as it is pulsed into the trachea. Inadequate humidification during HFV further contributed to the physical injury by drying tracheal mucosa.[3] Recent improvements in humidification systems have reduced this problem. Large areas of atelectasis have also been

TABLE 24-7   Recommendation for Initial Settings HFFIV Only

Change to noncompliant ventilator circuit, low deadspace humidifier canister, optimize water level in humidifier to minimize deadspace. Initiate $TCco_2$ monitoring.

Flo₂	Same as CMV. May consider 10% increase until stable.
P_aw	Set PEEP/CPAP at that used during CMV, to produce the pre-HFV Paw. If Spo₂ does not progressively increase, increase in 1 cm H₂O increments until Spo₂ rises.
Frequency	Depends upon age, weight, and underlying pulmonary disease. Premature infants, 12 to 15 Hz; Full-term infants, 10 to 12 Hz. Observe TCco₂, decrease frequency to decrease TCco₂
Amplitude	Adjust to the minimum setting. Slowly increase setting until the patient's chest visibly vibrates.
Pressure Relief	Set to fully closed.

HFFIV + IMV Ventilator Settings
  Select HFV + IMV mode. Disable flow synch option.

IMV rate	Set at 10 to 20 bpm, depending upon degree of atelectasis.
PIP	Set at pre-HFV level, unless > gestational age of infant. If so, decrease PIP to 1 cm H₂O per week of gestational age.
Inspiratory time	Adjust to provide adequate lung inflation during IMV breath, but minimize time to allow for maximum HFV pulse delivery.

observed as a result of mucus plugging or low airway pressures and resultant alveolar collapse. This can lead to worsening oxygenation and increased ventilatory requirements. Atelectasis can be prevented by maintaining adequate PEEP levels and sigh breaths large enough to allow for alveolar recruitment. Patients should be lavaged and suctioned per protocol at least every 12 hours to prevent retention of secretions. However, loss of lung volume during suctioning as patients are manually ventilated is a serious problem. Patients must be ventilated with PEEP bags which pro-

TABLE 24-8   Comparison of Various HFV Techniques

CATEGORY	HFJV	HFOV	HFFIV
Breath rates	1.5–10 Hz	6–50 Hz	2–22 Hz
Drive mechanisms	solenoid, pneumatic valves	piston, diaphragm	rotating ball valve
Gas delivery	delivered at tip of ETT	inspiratory limb of circuit, frequency and impedance dependent	inspiratory limb of ventilator circuit
Exhalation	passive	active	active
P_aw	≤ CMV	> HFJV	= HFOV
Pressure monitoring	distal ETT port	proximal	proximal
Humidification	built-in humidifier	user supplied	user supplied

TABLE 24-9   Hazards and Complications of HFV

Tracheal injury

Segmental/lobar collapse

Atelectasis

Pulmonary overdistention

Respiratory alkalosis

Patient instability (during change from CMV to HFV)

Note: Obtain chest x-ray film to assess end-expiratory lung volume.

vide a mean airway pressure similar to that used during HFV and elevated FIO_2 or closed system suction catheters.

Pulmonary overdistention and cardiac compromise can result from failure to wean excessive mean airway pressures as end-expiratory lung volume is restored during HFV. Overdistention can cause acute lung injury, pneumothorax, and further decreases in oxygenation as airway pressure is transmitted to the thorax and pulmonary blood flow is decreased, increasing the physiologic shunt. Increasing P_{aw} in this scenario is a common clinical error. For example, practitioners note the decrease in oxygenation without assessing lung expansion on CXR, and then increase P_{aw} in the hopes of increasing oxygenation. The combined physical signs of decreasing pulse oximetry with decreases in hemodynamics following a period of patient stability should stimulate respiratory care practitioners to examine the patient–ventilator system closely before making ventilator increases. Hyperventilation is also a common hazard of HFV. CO_2 elimination may be dramatically increased as HFV is initiated, causing rapid changes in arterial pH. It is common practice in many centers to initiate transcutaneous CO_2 monitoring before starting HFV to provide a more instantaneous measure of CO_2 elimination without the delay of arterial blood gas analysis. One final side effect is the risk of extubation and or destabilization during reintubation if a triple lumen jet tube is required. New adapters may reduce this risk.

▬SUMMARY

The role of HFV in neonatal/pediatric critical care is better defined than it is for the adult population. Management strategies are in place which provide adequate gas exchange with reduced risk of lung injury and cardiac compromise. Continued research and investigation is required to answer questions about the role of HFV versus conventional ventilation.

▬REFERENCES

1. Bishop MJ et al: Comparison of high-frequency ventilation with conventional mechanical ventilation for bronchopleural fistula. Anesth Analg 66:833, 1987.
2. Bohn DJ et al: Ventilation by high frequency oscillation. J Appl Physiol 48:710, 1980.

3. Boros SJ, Mammel MC, Lewallen PK et al: Necrotizing tracheobronchitis: A complication of high frequency ventilation. J Pediatr 109:95, 1986.
4. Butler WJ et al: Ventilation by high-frequency oscillation in humans. Anesth Anal 59:577, 1980.
5. Carlo WA, Chatburn RL, Martion RJ: Randomized trial of high-frequency jet ventilation versus conventional ventilation in respiratory distress syndrome. J Pediatr 110:275, 1987.
6. Carlon GC et al: High frequency positive pressure ventilation in management of a patient with bronchopleural fistulae. Anesthesiology 52:160, 1980.
7. Cavanagh K: High frequency ventilation of infants: An analysis of the literature. Respir Care 35:815, 1990.
8. Chang HK: Mechanisms of gas transport during ventilation by high frequency oscillation. J Appl Physiol 56:553, 1984.
9. Clark RH et al: Pulmonary interstitial emphysema treated by high-frequency oscillatory ventilation. Crit Care Med 14:926, 1986.
10. Clark RH et al: High-frequency oscillatory ventilation reduces the incidence of severe chronic lung disease in respirator distress syndrome. Am Rev Respir Dis 141:A686, 1990.
11. Coghill CJ et al: Neonatal and pediatric high-frequency ventilation: Principles and practice. Respir Care 36:596, 1991.
12. Courtney SE, HiFO Study Group: High frequency oscillation strategy decreases incidence of air leak syndrome in infants with severe respiratory distress syndrome. Pediatr Res 29:312A, 1991.
13. Dedrian SS et al: High frequency positive pressure jet ventilation in bilateral bronchopulmonary fistulae. Crit Care Med 19:119, 1982.
14. Fredberg JJ, Glass GM, Boynton BR et al: Factors influencing mechanical performance of neonatal ventilators. J Appl Physiol 62: 2485, 1987.
15. Fujino Y et al: High-frequency oscillation for persistent fetal circulation after repair of congenital diaphragmatic hernia. Crit Care Med 17:376, 1989.
16. Gayford MS, Quissel BJ, Lair ME: High-frequency ventilation in the treatment of infants weighing less than 1,500 grams with pulmonary interstitial emphysema: A pilot study. Pediatrics 79:915, 1987.
17. Keszler M, Donn SM, Bucciarelli RL: Multicenter controlled trial comparing high-frequency jet ventilation and conventional mechanical ventilation in newborn infants with pulmonary interstitial emphysema. J Pediatr 119:85, 1991.
18. Klain M, Keszler H, Brade E: High-frequency jet ventilation in CPR. Crit Care Med 9:421, 1981.
19. Kocis K, Meliones JN, Dekeon MK et al: High-frequency jet ventilation for respiratory failure after congenital heart surgery. Part 2. Circulation 86(2):127, 1992.
20. Kohelet D et al: High-frequency oscillation in the rescue of infants with persistent pulmonary hypertension. Crit Care Med 16:510, 1988.
21. Lassen GW et al: High frequency oscillatory ventilation in three cases of congenital diaphragmatic hernia. Respir Care 34:1023, 1989.
22. Marchak BE et al. Treatment of RDS by high-frequency oscillatory ventilation: A preliminary report. J Pediatr 99:287, 1981.
23. Meeuwis H, Vaes L, Klain M: Long term high-frequency ventilation in a 3-year-old child. Crit Care Med 11:309, 1981.
24. Meliones JN, Bove EL, Dekeon MK et al: High frequency jet ventilation improves cardiac function after the Fontan procedure. Circulation 84(suppl III):364, 1991.
25. Minton S, Gerstmann D, Stoddard R: Early intervention in respiratory distress syndrome. Cardiopulmonary Review: Current Applications and Economics. Yorba Linda, CA, Sensormedics Critical Care, 1995.
26. Schuster DP, Klain M, Synder JV: Comparison of high-frequency jet ventilation to conventional ventilation during severe acute respiratory failure in humans. Crit Care Med 10:625, 1982.
27. Sjostrand U: High-frequency positive pressure ventilation (HFPPV) techniques for artificial ventilation. In Stembera ZK, Polacek K, Sabata V (eds): Perinatal Medicine. Stuttgart, G Thieme, 1975.
28. Traverse JH, Korvenranta H, Adams EM et al: Cardiovascular effects of high frequency oscillatory and jet ventilation. Chest 96:1400, 1989.
29. Wood BL, Adams A, Richardson P: Double port endotracheal tube adapter for high frequency jet ventilation. 12th Conference on High Frequency Ventilation of Infants. Snowbird, Utah, 1995.

▬SELF-ASSESSMENT QUESTIONS

1. List three disease states that are successfully treated with high frequency ventilation in infants and children.

2. Compare and contrast the technical features of HFPPV, HFJV, HFFIV, and HFOV. Include breath rates, active or passive exhalation, and use of tandem ventilators in your descriptions.

3. Discuss CO_2 elimination during HFV. Include in your discussion a description of resonant frequency of the lung and HFV breath rates and how they affect CO_2 elimination.

4. Given the following patient descriptions, provide an initial high frequency breath range for each type of patient:
   a. premature infant with RDS
   b. term infant with pulmonary hypertension
   c. term infant with congenital diaphragmatic hernia
   d. pediatric patient with acute respiratory distress syndrome

5. Discuss the relationship between end-expiratory lung volume and oxygenation during HFV for respiratory disease. Include clinical and CXR indicators of adequate end-expiratory lung volume.

6. Compare and contrast the cardiovascular effects of HFJV and HFOV.

7. When is rescue HFV clinically indicated? Provide examples of diagnoses that respond to rescue HFV.

8. List examples of complications and hazards associated with HFV.

9. Describe a weaning method for HFV. Include target values for FIo_2, pH, $Paco_2$, and Pao_2.

10. Describe noninvasive monitors that can be used to evaluate CO_2 elimination and oxygenation during HFV. Discuss the benefits of this type of monitoring over serial blood gas measurements.

Chapter 25

Extracorporeal Membrane Oxygenation

DOUGLAS R. HANSELL

OBJECTIVES

Having completed this chapter, the reader will be able to:

1 Describe the principles of oxygen content and oxygen delivery as they relate to extracorporeal membrane oxygenation.

2 Describe the principle components of an extracorporeal membrane oxygenation circuit and their function.

3 Compare and contrast veno-arterial and veno-venous extracorporeal membrane oxygenation therapies.

4 Discuss the indications for and contraindications to extracorporeal membrane oxygenation in the neonatal and pediatric patient populations.

5 Describe the hazards and complications associated with neonatal and pediatric extracorporeal membrane oxygenation.

6 Discuss the appropriate monitoring techniques for the patient on extracorporeal membrane oxygenation.

7 Describe survival statistics for the various extracorporeal membrane oxygenation patient populations and discuss possible causes for the differences.

8 Discuss management of the patient on extracorporeal membrane oxygenation.

KEY TERMS

activated clotting time (ACT)
cardiac output
extracorporeal membrane
  oxygenation (ECMO)
membrane oxygenator

oxygen content
oxygen delivery
oxygen index
roller pump

Extracorporeal membrane oxygenation (ECMO) is an invasive treatment for cardiopulmonary failure. Also known as extracorporeal life support (ECLS), ECMO is a form of prolonged cardiopulmonary bypass. It is reserved for patients with an expected mortality of greater than 80% who are unresponsive to more conventional therapy. In the years since ECMO was introduced, what is considered to be conventional therapy has been redefined many times. High frequency jet ventilation (HFJV), high frequency oscillatory ventilation (HFOV), and surfactant replacement have become standards of care and are discussed elsewhere in this text. More recently, investigators of nitric oxide and liquid ventilation have begun trials to determine the safety, efficacy, and appropriateness of these modes of therapy for the patient unresponsive to conventional ventilation. The ability to study these new modalities, from HFJV to liquid ventilation, has, arguably, been enhanced with the availability of ECMO as a "bail out" therapy.

As an extension of the technology of cardiopulmonary bypass practiced in cardiothoracic surgery, ECMO has become a mainstay of support for neonates whose cardiac or pulmonary systems are no longer able to sustain life. The goal of ECMO is to provide temporary support or to replace the function of the heart, lungs, or both, to allow the patient's cardiopulmonary system time to recover. This system serves as an artificial heart and lungs. A thorough understanding of oxygen transport and **oxygen delivery** is, therefore, required to understand ECMO.

■ OXYGEN TRANSPORT/DELIVERY

The amount of oxygen available to the tissues is determined by two factors, the amount of oxygen per unit of blood (**oxygen content**) and the blood's availability to the tissues (**cardiac output**). O_2 content (CaO_2) is determined by three factors: the partial pressure of the oxygen dissolved in the blood plasma (PaO_2), the number of hemoglobin molecules available to carry oxygen (Hb level), and the actual amount of oxygen bound to those molecules (oxyhemoglobin saturation, SaO_2). These relationships are mathematically described in the oxygen content equation:

$$CaO_2 = (Hgb \times 1.34 \times SO_2) + (PO_2 \times 0.003)$$

Normal = 18-22 volume percent

As you examine the equation, it becomes obvious that PaO_2 plays a minor role in the amount of oxygen available in the blood; indeed, the majority of oxygen (97%) carried in the blood is bound to hemoglobin. It is imperative, not only in the ECMO patient, but in all critically ill patients, that the hemoglobin level be adequate to provide the transport medium for oxygen. Table 25-1 gives examples of oxygen content calculations under various conditions to demonstrate the relationship between PaO_2, saturation, and hemoglobin.

As seen in Table 25-1, the amount of hemoglobin available is the primary factor in determining the amount of oxygen the blood can carry. The importance of delivering that blood to the tissues cannot be understated, however, and it is the cardiovascular system that bears that responsibility. The relationship between the heart and the blood it pumps to the tissues is mathematically expressed in the following oxygen delivery equation:

TABLE 25-1   Relationship Between Pa_{O_2}, Saturation, and Hemoglobin

Pa_{O_2} (TORR)	HEMOGLOBIN (G)	O_2 SAT	Ca_{O_2} (VOL %)	STATUS
90.00	10.00	0.95	13.00	Low
60.00	15.00	0.85	17.27	Low (+/−)
40.00	18.00	0.70	18.09	Normal

$$D_{O_2} = \text{cardiac output} \times Ca_{O_2}$$

$$\text{Normal} = 225\text{-}330\text{mL } O_2/\text{kg}/\text{min}$$

Although the actual amount of oxygen delivered to the tissues varies with age, weight, stress, exercise, and illness, it is important to recognize the factors that will influence cardiac output. The critically ill patient suffering from heart disease, the neonate with pulmonary hypertension, a pediatric patient on ventilatory support requiring high mean airway pressures—each of these may be experiencing a reduced amount of oxygen being delivered to the tissues due to a decrease in cardiac output, even in the presence of a normal Pa_{O_2}. Table 25-2 summarizes several processes that may diminish cardiac output.

When cardiac output diminishes, oxygen delivery is compromised. The result is anaerobic metabolism and a rise in lactic acid. Serum lactic acid levels have been used to determine the need for ECMO and are a good indicator of the effectiveness of therapies applied for hypoxemic respiratory failure.[7,17] If serum lactic acid levels continue to rise in spite of maximal conventional therapy, ECMO should be considered.

THE ECMO SYSTEM

The ECMO system has been designed to provide temporary cardiac and pulmonary support to patients incapable of maintaining adequate tissue oxygen delivery. This is done by pumping blood through the patient's vas-

TABLE 25-2   Causes of Decreased Cardiac Output

Myocardial Dysfunction
  Decreased heart rate

  Myocardial hypoxia

  Structural abnormalities (cardiac and vascular)

  Increased intrathoracic pressure

  Pericardial effusion/tamponade

Hypovolemia
  Blood loss

  Vasodilation

culature, delivering oxygen, and removing carbon dioxide. Figure 25-1 shows the typical ECMO circuit.

The ECMO circuit is made from PVC tubing, typically with a $1/4$ inch inside diameter for the neonatal patient. This circuit is attached to a venous drain or cannula. The cannula is surgically inserted into the superior vena cava through the right internal jugular vein. The tip of this cannula is advanced to the level of the tricuspid valve. As large a cannula as possible is placed to ensure that adequate flows are provided. Pump flows are typically maintained at 100 mL/kg/min. Cannula size and resistance can adversely affect the ability to provide adequate support.

From the cannula, blood drains passively into a small venous reservoir, known as a bladder (Fig. 25-2). The bladder serves as a "right atrium" from which the ECMO pump draws blood. This reservoir also keeps negative pressure from pulling the vessel wall into the cannula and reduces the likelihood of trauma to the vena cava. The bladder is attached to a servo regulation mechanism, either a pressure sensitive switch or a pressure regulation mechanism, which reduces or stops pump flow in the event venous return drops to unsafe levels. If venous return is inadequate and the roller pump continues, enough negative pressure can be exerted on the blood to cause cavitation, which is the action of air being pulled out of a solution.

From the bladder a section of tubing leads to the ECMO pump. Two types of pumps are used, the centrifugal pump (Fig. 25-3) or, more commonly, the occlusive or **roller pump** (Fig. 25-4). Both pump systems have their advantages and disadvantages. Both pumps are capable of functioning as the "heart" of the ECMO system, providing blood flow to the patient. The type of tubing used in the pump varies with the pump used. While the centrifugal pump requires no special tubing, the roller pump applies direct and repeated pressure on the tubing. This action can occur as frequently as

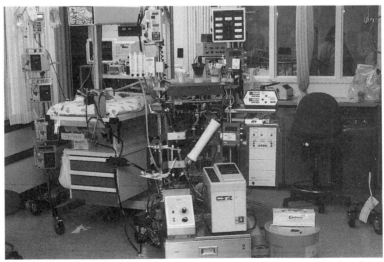

FIGURE 25-1 The ECMO system in use. This system is the Sorin Computer Aided Perfusion System.

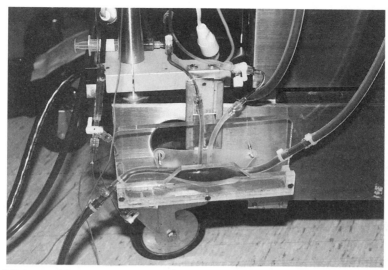

FIGURE 25-2 The ECMO circuit venous reservoir or "bladder."

120 or more times a minute for periods of 300 or more hours in larger patients. Therefore, a special Tygon tubing that is resistant to creasing and erosion that can occur with stress is used. The pump pulls blood from the bladder and pushes it through the remainder of the circuit.

As the blood leaves the pump, it enters the **membrane oxygenator** (Fig. 25-5). Currently, Avecor manufactures the only oxygenator approved for long-term use in the United States (Fig. 25-6). The oxygenator is a membrane lung made of a thin silicon rubber sheath with a plastic screen spacer inside. This silicon sheet is wound around a polycarbonate core. Encased in a silicon rubber sleeve, the configuration allows blood to pass on one side of the membrane and "sweep gas" to flow in the opposite direction on the other side. This maximizes gas exchange across the membrane.

The membrane is so efficient that it is not unusual to add CO_2, either as a carbogen mixture or as pure CO_2, to the sweep gas to raise the circuit Pco_2 to normal physiologic levels (35–45 torr). With the addition of these gases, continuous monitoring of the blood gases of the postoxygenator blood is recommended to ensure that pH and Pco_2 are within physiologic parameters. This oxygenator is available in sizes ranging from 0.4 m^2 to 4.5 m^2. The size selected is based upon the patient size and the total blood flow requirements anticipated. The maximal blood flow through the oxygenator is equal to 1.5 times the oxygenator size, and the maximal sweep gas flow is limited to 3 times the size. Therefore, a 0.8 m^2 oxygenator has a maximal rated blood flow of 1.2 LPM and a maximal rated sweep gas flow of 2.4 LPM (Table 25-3).

Most newborn ECMO patients are supported with the 0.8 m^2 oxygenator. Given the tremendous surface area that the blood is exposed to as it moves through the circuit, it is of no surprise that a great deal of heat is lost in extracorporeal circulation. While hypothermia is routinely used in the operating room, normothermia is usually the goal in ECMO. All ECMO systems use a heat exchanger, either postoxygenator or integrated

Inlet

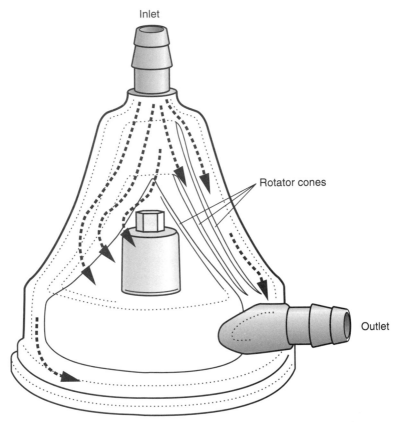

Rotator cones

Outlet

FIGURE 25-3   The centrifugal pump. The rotator cones spin causing a vortex which pulls the blood into the inlet and drives the blood through the outlet. Reprinted courtesy of Surgimedics, Inc.

in the oxygenator. Again, Avecor manufactures the heat exchangers most commonly applied in the ECMO setting. The ECMO Therm (Fig. 25-7) heat exchanger consists of stainless steel tubes enclosed in a clear, hollow polycarbonate core. The blood runs inside the stainless steel tubes and water warmed to 37° to 40° C flows around the outside of the tubes, warming the blood. It should be noted that stainless steel is used in ECMO applications because of the tendency of aluminum to corrode with long-term exposure to blood products. The heat exchanger also serves a secondary purpose. When placed after the oxygenator, it serves as a bubble trap, one last point for any stray air to be caught before the circuit returns blood to the patient.

From the heat exchanger, the blood returns to the patient. The return access can be via one of two methods. In veno-arterial (VA) ECMO, the arterial limb is attached to a cannula inserted into the right common carotid artery. This cannula is advanced along the carotid to the brachiocephalic artery and advanced so that the tip of the cannula is just proximal to the junction of the brachiocephalic artery and the aorta. This prac-

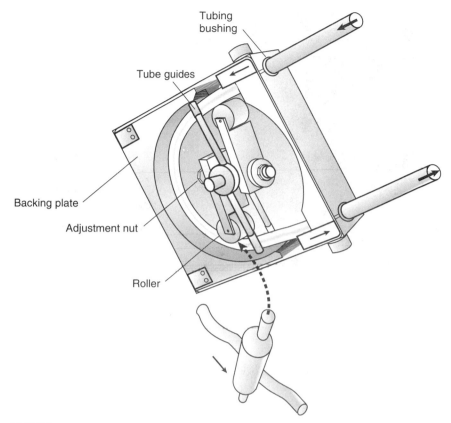

FIGURE 25-4 The roller pump. Blood is pushed through the tubing with an occlusive roller. The tubing is refilled owing to the negative pressure created as the roller progresses. Reprinted courtesy of Surgimedics, Inc.

tice may vary from center to center, based on the personal preference of the surgeon performing the cannulation. With this method of cannulation, ECMO becomes, in essence, cardiopulmonary bypass since the pump blood has bypassed the heart and lungs. The advantages and disadvantages of this technique will be discussed later.

In veno-venous (VV) ECMO, the arterial return may occur in several ways. In the neonate, a double lumen cannula is often used so that only one vessel is ligated. The oxygenated blood is directed into the right atrium when this special cannula is used (Fig. 25-8). Other VV access methods include arterial return via the right femoral vein. This technique is more common in patients too large (larger than 4 to 4.5 kg) for the dual lumen VV cannula. Again, the advantages and disadvantages of this technique will be discussed later.

The final component of the circuit is a bridge between the circuit's arterial and venous limbs (Fig. 25-9). This bridge provides a bypass if the patient requires isolation from the circuit for any reason, allowing flow to continue through the circuit and minimizing the risk of the circuit clotting. The bridge remains clamped unless required. The bridge is

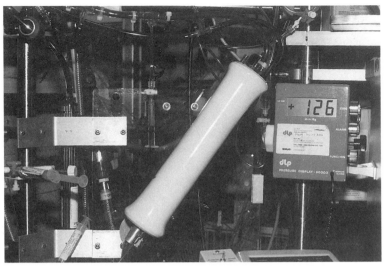

FIGURE 25-5   The "lung" of the ECMO system—the membrane oxygenator. This one is a 0.8 m² model typically used in the neonatal population.

unclamped for brief periods of time each hour to ensure that the line remains patent.

Additional equipment attached to the ECMO system consists of monitors and safety devices. Monitoring of the ECMO patient has been described as hours of boredom punctuated by moments of terror. As with cardiopulmonary bypass in the operating room, equipment failure or operator error can quickly lead to the demise of the patient. These monitoring and safety devices reduce the risk associated with the application of this therapy.

Pressure monitors (Fig. 25-10) are used to determine the pressure of blood returning to the bladder and serve as an indicator of the patient's volume status. Additionally, pressure monitors are placed before and after the oxygenator and help the ECMO specialist evaluate the functioning of the oxygenator. The pressure drop across the membrane is normally 100 to 200 mm Hg; pressure exceeding this level indicates that the blood flow through the oxygenator is meeting higher resistance (often due to clotting of blood) and that the oxygenator may require replacement. In pressure regulated systems like the Sorin CAPS pump system, the bladder and pre-oxygenator pressures may serve to regulate the pump, decreasing pump speed as bladder pressure drops below or premembrane pressure rises above operator-set limits. An audible alarm also sounds to alert the specialist of the problem.

Bubble detectors are often used to warn the operator that air has entered the system. This is a critical problem, especially in VA ECMO where the air will enter directly into the arterial system and flow directly to the patient's brain. Therefore, a rapid response to this alarm is required. The CAPS system quickly stops the pump. A unique device by Rocky Mountain Research uses electrically controlled clamps to isolate the patient from the pump by clamping off the arterial and venous lines and

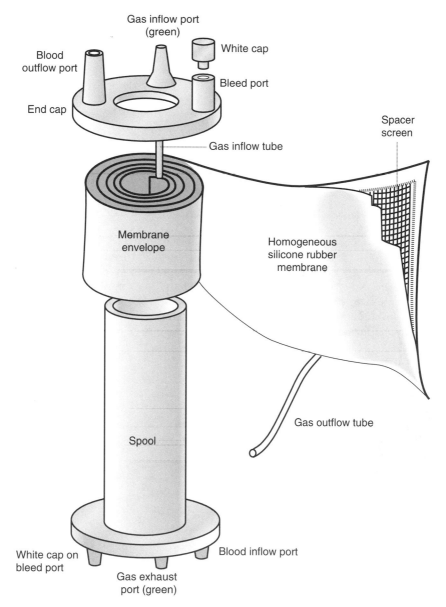

FIGURE 25-6 A schematic of the membrane oxygenator. The gas flows along the screen spacer countercurrent to blood flowing along the outside of the membrane.

opening the bridge, allowing the bubble to circulate down to the bladder where it can be removed. The patient can then be placed back on ECMO.

Blood gas sensors and blood oxygen sensors are used to monitor the values in blood returning from the patient as well as being delivered to the patient. Monitoring the oxygen saturation of the patient's venous blood is a reliable indicator of oxygen delivery and utilization during VA ECMO. Monitoring the blood gas levels of the postmembrane output allows the

TABLE 25-3   Specifications of Membrane Oxygenators

MODEL	0800	1500	2500	3500	4500
Surface area (M)	0.80	1.50	2.50	3.50	4.50
Prime Volume (mL)	100	175	455	575	665
Max gas flow (LPM)	2.40	4.50	7.5	10.50	13.50
Max blood flow (LPM)	1.2	2.25	4.50	5.50	6.50
Max patient weight (kg)	11.00	19.00	70.00	95.00	>95

specialist to ensure that appropriate levels of O_2 and CO_2 are delivered to the patient. Several monitors are available for use in ECMO applications, including the Gish StatSat (Fig. 25-11) and the CDI (Fig. 25-12).

Since blood that is in contact with a nonendothelialized surface will tend to clot, heparin is infused to reduce the coagulability of that blood. To insure that the clotting time is maintained within an acceptable range (usually 180–220 seconds), a small sample of blood is withdrawn from the circuit hourly and an **activated clotting time** (ACT) analysis is performed. Heparin therapy is adjusted based on the results of that study. The ACT is performed at the bedside using a device such as the Hemochron 801 (Fig. 25-13).

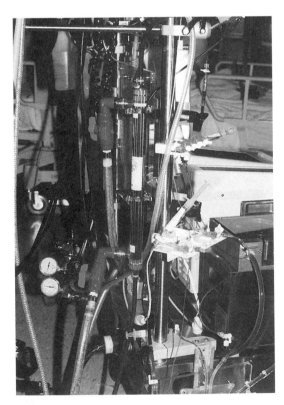

FIGURE 25-7 The ECMO-Therm Heat Exchanger. Blood temperature is restored to normothermia prior to returning to the patient.

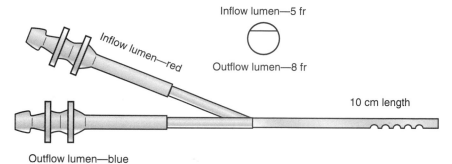

FIGURE 25-8 The dual lumen veno–venous cannula.

Priming the ECMO Circuit

ECMO is rarely a planned therapeutic intervention. The patients are often transferred to the ECMO center acutely ill, near death, and quite unstable. Preparation of the ECMO circuit for use on a patient must be performed quickly, safely, and with the utmost regard for sterile procedure. This is accomplished only with the support of multiple members of the health care team. Physicians, surgeons, lab technicians, transfusion services, unit clerks, nurses, perfusionists, and respiratory care practitioners must function cohesively as a team. Priming the circuit is performed by a select group, specially trained in the procedure to ensure that the process is completed as safely as possible.

The ECMO circuit is primed with blood to ensure that the patient's hematocrit remains normal. All the steps taken in the priming procedure are intended to ensure that the patient has a biologically compatible cir-

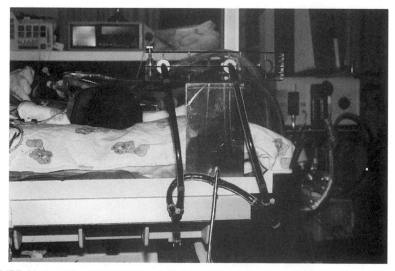

FIGURE 25-9 The ECMO Circuit Bridge. This component allows the patient to be isolated from the ECMO System.

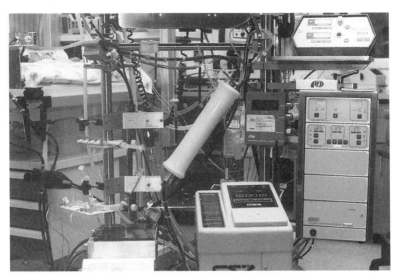

FIGURE 25-10   The CAPS and DLP pressure monitors. The CAPS Pressure Monitors (*far right*) provide servo regulation of the roller pump.

cuit, meaning that the system is free of air and particulate matter and has physiologically normal electrolyte and blood component concentrations. The team usually takes the following steps in the priming process:

1. The circuit pack is opened in a sterile fashion and assembled. All connections are checked and tie banded to reduce the risk of leaking. A priming set is attached to the circuit to facilitate recirculation of the prime products and air removal during the priming process (Fig. 25-14). The circuit is now hung on the ECMO pump stand and 100% CO_2 is flushed through the circuit, replacing all of the air. Doing this will help remove all bubbles from the circuit once fluids are added.

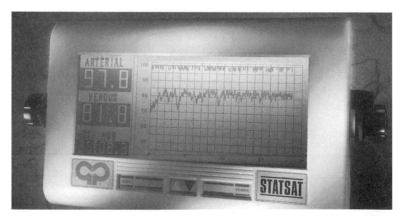

FIGURE 25-11   The STATSAT in-line oxygen saturation monitor. Continuous monitoring of the venous oxygen saturation provides an estimate of oxygen consumption.

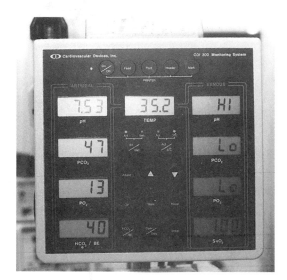

FIGURE 25-12 Continuous circuit arterial and venous blood gas monitoring assists in both patient and ECMO system monitoring.

2. Once the CO_2 sweep has been completed (usually approximately 5 minutes), the gas line is removed from the prime circuit, all stopcocks are closed, and a crystalloid solution is added to the circuit. This is done in a sequential manner to reduce the occurrence of air bubbles. Once the circuit is filled with crystalloid, the solution is circulated through the circuit to ensure that any particulate material is filtered and all air is removed.

3. Next, 25 to 50 mL of 25% albumin is added. The circuit has a large surface area, all of it foreign to the patient's immune system. Albumin is added to the circuit to form a biologic coating on the circuit to reduce the likelihood of clotting. The addition of albumin also ensures that appropriate protein levels are maintained in the blood that will become part of the patient's circulation.

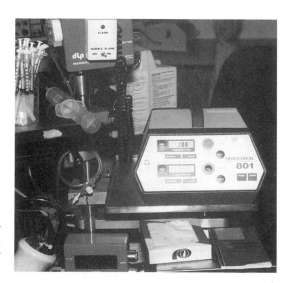

FIGURE 25-13 The Hemochron 801 is one of several devices used in ECMO to monitor the blood clotting time.

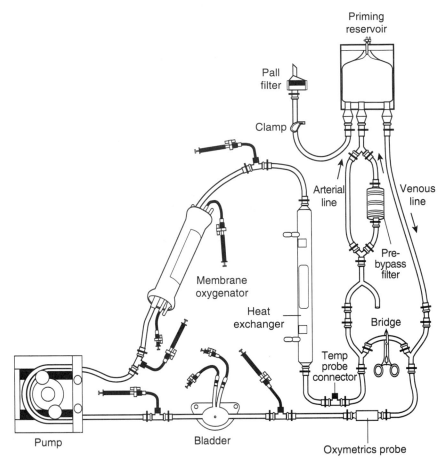

FIGURE 25-14   A schematic of the ECMO circuit with priming reservoir.

4. Once the albumin has circulated for 5 to 10 minutes, the priming reservoir is drained to nearly empty and packed red blood cells (PRBCs) are added to the circuit. The total amount of blood products required for the circuit will vary with the circuit and patient size. Blood product requirements are shown in Table 25-4. In addition, 100 units of porcine heparin can routinely be added to each unit of PRBCs to prevent clotting while ECMO is initiated. This amount may be decreased if the patient is at increased risk for bleeding. The crystalloid/albumin solution is slowly "chased" out of the circuit and allowed to drain into an intravenous bag attached to the priming circuit. Approximately 100 mL of fresh frozen plasma is then introduced to the circuit, in essence recreating whole blood with a hematocrit of 40% to 45%.

5. The next several steps are performed to "fine tune" the circuit, preparing the pump blood for contact with the patient's blood. Sodium bicarbonate is added to normalize the base deficit, sweep gases are adjusted to normalize the Pco_2, and calcium gluconate is added to normalize the ionized calcium in the circuit. This last addi-

TABLE 25-4 Blood Requirements for Priming the ECMO Circuit

	PATIENT WEIGHT			
BLOOD PRODUCT	*2–8 Kg*	*8–12 Kg*	*12–20 Kg*	*>20 Kg*
PRBCs	2 units	2 units	2 units	3 units
FFP	1 unit	1 unit	1 unit	1 unit

tive is quite important as calcium is essential for myocardial contraction. Meliones and associates demonstrated that reduced ionized calcium concentrations in the ECMO prime leads to hypotension.[13] Further studies revealed that normalized ICa^{++} in the circuit prevents the calcium-induced hypotension previously noted.[13]

Once the circuit is fully primed, laboratory studies are performed to ensure that the blood is ready for the patient. Arterial blood gas, potassium, hematocrit, and ionized calcium are checked. Once these values are within physiologic limits, ECMO is initiated.

Although priming techniques may vary slightly from center to center, most follow this basic procedure. If the patient is so unstable that delaying initiation of ECMO could result in death, a skilled team may hurry this process, omit obtaining laboratory studies, and initiate ECMO. In extreme situations, a circuit can be primed safely and ECMO initiated in 15 minutes. This requires the utmost in skill and practice and, quite fortunately, is rarely required.

ECMO TECHNIQUES

The therapeutic goal of ECMO is to provide adequate oxygen delivery to the tissues. Depending on the pathology of the disease, one of two techniques for accomplishing this goal is used:

Veno-arterial (VA)—blood is drained from the venous return and infuses to the aorta.

Veno-venous (VV)—blood is drained from and returned to the venous circulation.

Veno-Arterial ECMO

Long the mainstay of ECMO, VA ECMO is a true cardiopulmonary bypass procedure. With the venous outflow cannula inserted in the vena cava, the ability to completely drain the right side of the heart is limited only by the cannula size. With the arterial inflow provided to the aorta, the heart and lungs are bypassed (Fig. 25-15). The advantages of this method of support are listed in Table 25-5.[12]

Simply stated, since the VA ECMO system functions as the heart and lungs, the clinician can control patient oxygen delivery by controlling the ECMO pump.

The ability to provide direct cardiac support is important for those cardiac patients in the postoperative period who experience cardiac failure.

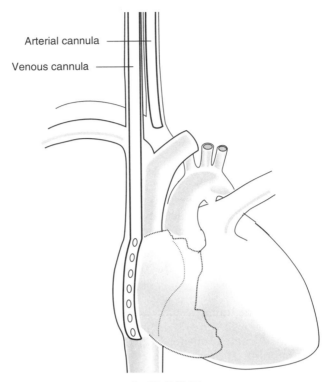

FIGURE 25-15   Cannula position in VA ECMO.

However, these patients do not fare well, as reflected by the current survival rates of about 50%.

Providing supernormal oxygenated blood to the patient who has been hypoxic and poorly perfused can help provide rapid stabilization and quick correction of oxygen debt and lactic acidosis. One must proceed with care to avoid the so-called "reperfusion injury" brought on by the rapid dilation of vessels in hypoxic vasoconstriction when they are suddenly exposed to high levels of oxygen in the blood. Once on ECMO, flow should be increased slowly to keep the patient stable yet not induce this injury. The speed with which one increases ECMO flow will vary depending on the con-

TABLE 25-5   Advantages and Disadvantages of VA ECMO

ADVANTAGES	DISADVANTAGES
Direct cardiac support	Ligation of the carotid artery
Supernormal oxygenation	Non-pulsatile blood flow
Minimized ventilatory support	Reduced pulmonary blood flow
Extensive clinical experience	Potential systemic embolization
	Decreased myocardial O_2 delivery

dition of the patient; for example, a postoperative cardiac patient in cardiac failure may require that flows be increased to 100 to 120 mL/kg/min almost instantly, whereas a baby with meconium aspiration syndrome may require increasing the flow gradually over a period of 1 hour or more.

Once the patient is on full VA ECMO support, the ventilator support can be decreased to "rest settings." The ability to turn the ventilator off during VA ECMO is helpful for those patients whose lung condition could benefit from minimal or no pressure. Patients with severe barotrauma or those requiring therapeutic bronchoscopy may require VA ECMO. Typically, the ventilator is turned down to a peak inspiratory pressure (PIP) of 20 to 25 cm H_2O, positive end-expiratory pressure (PEEP) of 5 to 10 cm H_2O, rate of 5 to 10 bpm, and FIo_2 of 0.21. The goal is to allow the lung to rest and heal from the damage sustained either from the pathologic process or from the ventilatory support required before ECMO.

There is extensive clinical experience in cardiopulmonary bypass and critical care management. Many cardiothoracic surgeons manage bypass patients several times per day. The intuitive ability to view the ECMO system as an artificial heart and lungs make management quite simple for surgeons and critical care physicians alike. If oxygen delivery is low, the cardiac output (pump flow) should be increased. If the lungs are better and contributing more to CO_2 removal, the sweep gas CO_2 should be decreased, and so on.

VA ECMO is not without disadvantages, which must be considered when evaluating the ECMO candidate (see Table 25-5).[1]

Ligation of the carotid artery is a theoretical disadvantage of VA ECMO. Although it would be advantageous to keep the carotid artery patent, there are no real data that show that cerebral blood flow is critically altered or that the long-term effects of ligation are detrimental. Indeed, studies by Chai and colleagues on newborn pigs revealed that intracranial and jugular venous pressure did not increase, but cerebral blood flow and cerebral metabolism did increase. They conclude that the cerebral vascular system is capable of rerouting cerebral blood flow when the artery is ligated.[4] Given that the oldest neonatal survivor is just now entering her 20s, it will be decades before we know the long-term effects of carotid artery ligation.

The effect of nonpulsatile blood flow on end organs is disputed. However, C. Walton Lillehei, a pioneer of cross-circulation for cardiac surgery, states that he "can find no convincing evidence in the extensive literature on this subject that pulsatile flow is a physiologic necessity or even advantageous."[11] There is no doubt, however, that the blood that does make it through the heart must now pump into the aorta against a constant afterload, which may lead to increased left ventricular pressures, increased myocardial wall pressure, and decreased coronary perfusion. These factors, combined with the lack of oxygenated blood returning from the pulmonary blood flow, lead to poorly oxygenated blood being pumped into poorly perfused coronary vessels. The end result may be a phenomenon known as myocardial stun, in which the myocardium suffers a transient depression of contractility. Fortunately, this stun is usually self-limiting and resolves within 24 to 48 hours.

Ninety percent or more of the cardiac output is run through the ECMO system in VA ECMO. This means that the pulmonary blood flow is greatly reduced. This is not inconsequential. The pulmonary capillary bed serves other functions besides gas exchange, most notably as a filter for the microemboli that we shower from damaged vessels on a routine basis. Given that clot formation in the circuit is a common complication, the loss of that sieve is of concern. Air, clot, and particulate emboli in the circuit are infused directly into the arterial system and then to the cerebral vasculature. The reduction of pulmonary blood flow appears to resolve somewhat as the pulmonary insult resolves.

Remember that the ECMO system has a fixed volume. It will circulate that volume at the set pump speed. The patient's blood volume is in a dynamic container. As the pulmonary vessels return to normal tone, the volume returning to the right atrium will diminish. More of the total blood volume will be contained in the pulmonary vasculature. As long as the ventilator remains on rest settings and ECMO pump flow is unchanged, the increased volume of blood from the pulmonary vasculature that is ejected into the aorta will lead to a reduction in PaO_2. In short, as a patient improves, the blood gases may actually get worse.

Patients most likely to require VA ECMO include postoperative cardiac surgery patients and patients with profound cardiomyopathy in cardiac failure—including those patients awaiting cardiac transplant, those patients with cardiopulmonary failure requiring high inotropic support, and those patients with jugular veins that are too small or too large for the 14 French dual lumen veno-venous cannula.

VA ECMO remains a favorite technique at many ECMO centers but has lost favor at others as VV ECMO has become recognized as a safe and effective approach.

Veno-Venous ECMO

The veno-venous ECMO circuit is identical to the VA ECMO circuit. The difference in these two techniques begins with the method of cannulation. As the name implies, blood is drained from and returned to the venous system, specifically, the right atrium. There are two main methods of VV cannulation: either jugular vein drainage to femoral vein inflow or cannulation of the jugular vein only with a double lumen cannula that provides both drainage and inflow at the right atrium.

The method of jugular vein drainage to femoral vein inflow is used in patients larger than 4.5 kg if it is determined that the advantage of providing VV ECMO is greater than the disadvantage of having two cannulation sites. Besides the problems of two surgical sites, the inflow cannula is much longer than an arterial inflow cannula inserted through the common carotid. This creates higher resistance to flow and, potentially, more hemolysis of the red blood cells. This technique is most often applied to pediatric patients larger than 10 to 15 kg and to adults.

Currently, the most common method of providing VV ECMO in the neonatal patient is with the Kendal 14 French dual lumen ECMO cannula.[15] This cannula has an outflow track of 8 French and an inflow track of 5 French. As one would suspect, the resistance to flow is much higher. In spite of this, the clinical experience with these cannulae remains generally positive and this method continues to gain in popularity.

Given the configuration of this cannulae, proper placement is paramount (Fig. 25-16). The tip of this cannula is placed in the right atrium with

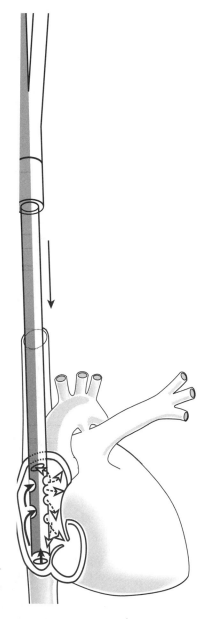

FIGURE 25-16 Cannula position in VV ECMO with the dual lumen cannula. Note the direction of blood flow.

the inflow directed toward the tricuspid valve and the outflow holes positioned toward the lateral wall of the right atrium. The surgeon will manipulate the cannula to get the best combination of adequate venous return, lowest arterial line pressure, and minimal recirculation. Once the cannula is sutured in place, a chest x-ray film is obtained to verify the cannula position.

The advantages of VV ECMO are listed in Table 25-6.[12]

We have addressed the issue of ligation of the carotid artery; although there is no evidence that ligation is harmful, to maintain normal anatomy must be advantageous in the long run.

TABLE 25-6   Advantages and Disadvantages of VV ECMO

ADVANTAGES	DISADVANTAGES
No ligation of the carotid artery	No direct cardiac support
Pulsatile blood flow	Blood recirculation in ECMO system
Avoids reperfusion injury	Lower systemic PaO_2
Heart and lungs receive oxygenated blood	Less intuitive than VA ECMO
Preservation of pulmonary "filter"	Limited cannulation options

The need for pulsatile blood flow remains questionable. The ability to preserve normal cardiac dynamics and systemic perfusion without hyperoxygenation decreases the likelihood of reperfusion injury in the cerebral vasculature as well as other end organs.

The perfusion of the lungs with oxygenated blood may speed the healing process in the lungs and helps maintain the lymphatic and secretory functions of the lung. The function of the vascular bed as a filter cannot be overemphasized. From this standpoint, VV ECMO is safer than VA ECMO.

The disadvantages of VV ECMO are listed in Table 25-6.

This circuit does not provide direct cardiac support, but it is capable of providing indirect cardiac support. As noted earlier, one of the disadvantages of VA ECMO is that the heart must pump against a constant afterload leading to increased left ventricular pressures, increased myocardial wall pressure, and decreased coronary perfusion. The SpO_2 of the blood entering the coronary vessels in VA ECMO is approximately 40%. In VV ECMO, the inflow blood has a saturation of 100% and combines with the patient venous return SvO_2 of 50% in the right atrium. At appropriate ECMO flow, this results in SpO_2 in the right ventricle of approximately 80%. Calculations demonstrate that the oxygen content of the blood in the right ventricle is thus approximately 16.5 volumes percent—a more than adequate supply of oxygen for the myocardium, indeed for cellular metabolism for the rest of the body. In this way, VV ECMO does provide indirect cardiac support.

Centers frequently report that inotropic support is rapidly weaned in those patients placed on VV ECMO. It is important to monitor other indicators of oxygen delivery and cardiac output, such as lactic acid levels, to ensure that the patient's oxygen debt is diminishing. Conversion to VA ECMO may be indicated if serum lactic acid levels are not returning to normal.

The position of the VV cannula is quite important. The oxygenated inflow must be directed into the right ventricle to minimize the phenomena known as recirculation. Recirculation occurs when the oxygenated inflow mixes with the venous outflow and returns to the ECMO system without entering the RV. The monitors on the venous return line will reflect a falsely high oxygen saturation if the oxygenated blood is mixing with the blood returning to the pump. Therefore, patient venous blood gas monitoring and serial lactic acid levels should be performed to ensure that adequate oxygen delivery is maintained. Appropriate regulation of pump flow as well as cannula positioning helps to minimize recirculation.

While lower systemic PaO_2 levels are provided in VV ECMO, in most instances adequate oxygen delivery is maintained. Again, as long as cardiac output and arterial oxygen content are appropriate, PaO_2 is of minor concern. However, if cardiac output is not adequate, then conversion to VA ECMO may be required.

Since VV ECMO is not cardiopulmonary bypass, the management of the patient is less intuitive for those used to VA ECMO. Indeed, the technique used in VA ECMO to increase oxygen delivery (increase flow) may cause a decrease in delivery on VV ECMO due to increased recirculation. This fact, coupled with the difficulty associated with cannulation techniques (a "one size fits all" cannula versus two cannulation sites), suggests that the team must develop expertise in management of VV ECMO. Accepting the limitations of VV ECMO in providing the high PaO_2 levels commonly seen in VA ECMO patients, remembering the importance of CaO_2, and watching indicators of tissue oxygenation (lactic acid) must be learned.

Ventilator management in VV ECMO is slightly different than in VA ECMO. It is not unusual to maintain higher vent settings to allow the lungs to contribute to gas exchange. Indeed, if oxygenation is inadequate, increasing the FIO_2 on the ventilator often will allow the patient to be maintained on VV ECMO. Typical ventilator settings on VV ECMO are as follows: PIP, 30 to 35 cm H_2O; PEEP, 10 to 15 cm H_2O; rate, 10 to 15 bpm; and FIO_2, 0.4 to 0.6.

NEONATAL ECMO

Since 1975, over 10,000 newborn patients have been supported with ECMO. This is a much larger group than either pediatric (982) or adult (197) patients.[6] This group also maintains the highest overall survival rate: nearly 80% of the entire population of neonates placed on ECMO survive to leave the hospital. Given that this population has an expected mortality rate of at least 80%, that figure becomes even more remarkable. The actual survival rate is dependent upon diagnosis, as shown in Figure 25-17.

The question that presents itself is why neonates fare so much better with ECMO than either pediatric or adult patients. There are many reasons that combine to increase the probability of survival, including the reversibility of the disease process, the lack of chronic injury, the greater experience in shear numbers, and the acceptance of the therapy in that population, allowing for earlier initiation of support.

Neonatal Diseases Treated With ECMO

The experience of the past 20 years has allowed practitioners to identify those disease processes that respond to ECMO, that is, those diseases in which recovery is possible within the time that ECMO can be provided. Patients who remain on ECMO for more than 300 hours seem to have a very poor chance of survival. At some centers, therefore, ECMO may be provided to those patients whose disease process is reversible within 10 to 12 days. Other centers have reported survival in patients who received ECMO for as long as 4 weeks or more.[8]

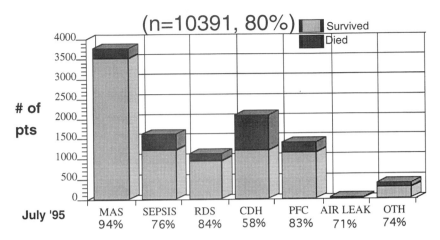

FIGURE 25-17   Neonatal ECMO survival statistics by diagnosis (ELSO Registry).

Given the need for reversibility, the primary indication for ECMO in the nonsurgical, noncardiac neonatal patient is persistent pulmonary hypertension of the newborn (PPHN) of any etiology that is unresponsive to other modes of therapy. A review of PPHN is, therefore, appropriate.

In utero, most of the blood leaving the right ventricle is shunted away from the pulmonary vasculature through the foramen ovale (FO) and the ductus arteriosis (DA). This occurs because the fluid in the fetal lung provides a high hydrostatic pressure gradient and hypoxic vasoconstriction in the pulmonary bed. At birth, as the infant takes the first several breaths, the fluid in the lungs is displaced, removing the hydrostatic pressure. Additionally, the PaO_2 increases, causing a rapid reversal of the pulmonary vasoconstriction. As the pressure in the right atrium and right ventricle decreases, the FO and DA close. This allows the entire blood flow leaving the right side of the heart to move through the pulmonary bed.

The closure of the DA usually occurs within 10 to 12 hours; normally, anatomic closure occurs within 2 to 4 days. However, any event that leads to hypoxemia or acidosis may cause the pulmonary vasculature to constrict, re-opening the FO and DA and shunting blood away from the lungs. This, in turn, causes further desaturation of the blood, as it is no longer coming in contact with the pulmonary bed. The result is hypoxemia, anaerobic metabolism, acidosis, and more pulmonary constriction.

Therapeutic interventions at this point include oxygen, mechanical ventilation, and alkalinization therapy. When successful, these therapies relax the pulmonary vasculature. If they are not successful, escalation of therapy may lead to barotrauma and further deterioration. Often, multiple modes of ventilation are attempted, including HFJV and HFOV. When these modes are unsuccessful, ECMO is, quite often, the only alternative.

Meconium aspiration syndrome occurs in approximately 0.8% of all live births in the United States.[9] Only a small fraction (0.16%) of these infants require mechanical ventilation; fewer require ECMO. Yet this population responds better to ECMO than any other population. While the disease can be quite severe, it is self-limiting and exquisitely reversible.

Meconium aspiration syndrome occurs when the near-term to post-term fetus is exposed to stress and hypoxia (umbilical venous oxygen saturation < 30%) in utero, usually around the time of delivery.[2] In response to this stress, the fetus begins to gasp, aspirating the meconium into the pulmonary tree. The meconium migrates to the small airways causing a ball valve obstruction. These babies present with air trapping, hypoxemia, and mixed respiratory and metabolic acidosis. In severe cases, pulmonary hypertension may result. If this occurs, the treatments for PPHN are initiated along with vigorous pulmonary toilet. Quite often, simple oxygen administration is sufficient. Occasionally, mechanical ventilation is required. Only in the most severe cases is ECMO required.

Respiratory distress syndrome, also called hyaline membrane disease, is a result of surfactant deficiency or deactivation. Although these patients are usually premature or small for gestation age, respiratory distress syndrome can occur in a term infant with other pathologic processes. For example, the infant with sepsis often experiences surfactant deactivation and requires increased pulmonary support, including surfactant replacement.

Sepsis and pneumonia in the neonate are frequently causes of respiratory distress. Often acquired perinatally, the infant may present after premature or prolonged rupture of the membranes or prolonged labor. A type of pneumonia that seems to be most likely to result in the need for ECMO is the group B beta hemolytic streptococci (GBS). GBS often leads to PPHN, and infants with this condition are severely and acutely compromised. The infant with suspected GBS pneumonia and sepsis should be treated, even without a positive culture. The infant who fails to get better on conventional therapy should be transferred to an ECMO center because such infants often deteriorate rapidly and may die or suffer severe intracranial hemorrhage before ECMO can be initiated.

Barotrauma, or pulmonary interstitial emphysema (PIE), occurs when the pressures required to move air into the chest cause gas to leak out of the alveolar bed. In some cases, pneumothorax can cause an acute decompensation that is rapidly corrected by needle aspiration. In more insidious cases, the air can leak into the pericardium (pneumopericardium), causing a decrease in cardiac output. In PIE, the air dissects into the interstitial space surrounding the alveoli, leading to collapsed alveoli and increasingly noncompliant lungs. In each of these processes, the goal is to reduce delivered airway pressure to minimize the continuance of the air leak. If gas exchange cannot be maintained at the pressures required to minimize the air leak, then ECMO can be used to support the patient while the ventilator settings are reduced to noninjurious levels. On occasion, a patient can be placed on a PEEP of 0 and a rate of 0 to facilitate sealing of the air leak.

Congenital diaphragmatic hernia (CDH) occurs in utero. The abdominal contents are pushed upwards through a defect in the diaphragm. Depending on the point in gestation in which the defect occurs and the severity of the defect, the patient may present with symptoms ranging from poor feeding to severe asphyxia at birth. The degree of pulmonary hypoplasia on both the ipsilateral and contralateral sides of the defect will determine the survivability of the patient. The care of the highly complex lesions associated with CDH is beyond the scope of this text. The use of ECMO to support these patients remains a controversial subject. The ability to determine which patients will do well has escaped the ECMO community, at least on a national level. While there are centers with acceptable success rates with these patients, others have such poor survival that it becomes hard to justify attempting ECMO in their CDH population.

Patients with cardiac malformations that require ECMO are grouped into two categories: those requiring stabilization prior to surgery and those requiring stabilization after surgery. The decision to place a child on ECMO before surgery must be made with a clear understanding of the lesion and the potential for surgical correction. In those patients who will require cardiac transplant, the open-ended nature of awaiting a suitable donor has led many centers to refrain from providing ECMO as a bridge to transplant. Multiple studies have shown survival for patients placed on ECMO in the operating room to be less than 30%. The use of ECMO postoperatively is often limited to those patients who have been successfully weaned from cardiopulmonary bypass in the operating room but have developed myocardial dysfunction in the postoperative period.

Criteria for Neonatal ECMO

The criteria for ECMO in the neonatal population continue to evolve. At issue is determining when all other more conventional therapies have failed and ECMO is required. Since ECMO is invasive and not without risk, it is important that it be used only when absolutely necessary. However, the desire to avoid ECMO must be balanced with the knowledge that to delay this therapy may lead to further decompensation, prolonged acidosis, end organ dysfunction and failure, intracranial hemorrhage, and death.

Each center that provides ECMO has been encouraged to identify the criteria that define 80% mortality in their patient population. This will vary from institution to institution, as not all centers have had access to HFOV, HFJV, nitric oxide, and other modalities. Additionally, the level of experience of the practitioners using those modalities will vary. Most importantly, the level of acuity of the patient population referred to each center will have a profound effect upon the survival statistics of an institution.

The diaphragmatic hernia patient population can be considered as an example to illustrate this point. Centers that receive CDH patients early, even before birth, will usually have much higher survival statistics than centers that have patients referred only after repair is attempted or when the child has failed conventional management and is in a pulmonary hypertensive crisis. This stands to reason: the first center has a wide range of patients, from the acutely ill to the stable, from the patient requiring ECMO to stay alive to the patient that does not even require mechanical ventilation. That center may have an 80% survival for all CDH patients referred. The second center receives only the sickest patients, those at death's door. While a few may survive, the acuity of the majority of those patients means their probability of survival is quite low. Indeed, only 20% of those CDH patients referred may survive.

Is the first center in this example "better" at treating CDH patients than the second? Quite possibly: they will have learned how to manage the CDH patient and prevent the PPHN crises that often lead to death. Is the first center better than the second? Not necessarily: the patient populations are so different that it is impossible to compare the success rates between the two centers. The first center would have a different set of criteria for placing the CDH patient on ECMO (hours on mechanical ventilation, highest peak inspiratory pressure, highest PaO_2) than the second center (made it here alive).

In sum, the criteria for ECMO are the inability to provide adequate oxygen delivery or CO_2 removal on maximal medical support. In spite of the variability from center to center in specifics, most centers follow the criteria listed in Table 25-7. The goal of these criteria is to assist the practitioner in knowing when maximal medical therapy is failing.

Hypoxia for Longer Than 4 Hours. There are several ways to define hypoxia. The **oxygen index** (OI) is a calculation that accounts for the amount of ventilatory support required to provide the level of oxygenation obtained. If a patient is on an FIO_2 of 1.0 and requires a mean airway pressure of 20 cm H_2O to obtain a PaO_2 of 50 torr, the OI equals 40. An OI of greater than 40 has been associated with mortality rates of 80% and is a common criterion for ECMO. It should be noted that the OI has been based upon the use of conventional ventilation. It is more difficult to know the impact of mean airway pressure in the HFOV and HFJV ventilatory modes and the significance of mean airway pressure as an indication for ECMO.

Other indicators of hypoxia for a period of greater than 4 hours are evidence that maximal medical support to provide oxygenation is failing. Regardless of the method used for determining failure, OI will tend to equal 40.

A pH of less than 7.20 in the patient with persistent pulmonary hypertension indicates a failure of maximal medical therapy. There are several methods used to correct this acidosis. The first is to hyperventilate the patient. Caution must be used with this method, as barotrauma, high mean airway pressures, reduced cardiac output, and reduced cerebral blood flow secondary to low $PaCO_2$ are potential detrimental side effects. Infusions of sodium bicarbonate or tromethamine may be used as alkalinizing agents. The additional fluid and sodium load received with sodium bicarbonate may make this therapy less than optimal.

Neonates who have been treated with high ventilatory support are quite prone to experiencing air leak syndromes. This is especially true with dis-

---

TABLE 25-7 Criteria for Neonatal ECMO

Hypoxia > 4 hours

    OI > 40 [OI = ((FIO_2 × MAP)/PaO_2) × 100]

    (A-a)DO_2 > 400 mm Hg

    PaO_2 < 50 mm Hg on vent with PIP > 35 or MAP > 20

Persistent acidosis

    pH < 7.20 in spite of alkalinization therapy, hyperventilation, $NaHCO_3$ infusion

    rising lactic acid levels

Barotrauma

Congenital diaphragmatic hernia

Cardiac dysfunction

eases with air trapping (meconium aspiration syndrome) or poor compliance (respiratory distress syndrome). Additionally, the use of surfactant may lead to air trapping and barotrauma. The common manifestations of this air leak include persistent pneumothoracies, tension pneumothoracies, pulmonary interstitial emphysema, and pneumomediastinum. Pneumomediastinum is a particularly insidious problem, leading to a rapidly falling cardiac output. However, any of the air leak syndromes may cause a rapid and life-threatening decompensation and, after treatment, may indicate the need for initiation of ECMO.

The criterion for initiation of ECMO in patients with congenital diaphragmatic hernia is center dependent. The indication to initiate ECMO in these patients seems less important than the absence of contraindications. Many centers require evidence that there is enough pulmonary vasculature to support life. Therefore, at least one blood gas with a PaO_2 greater than 100 torr and a $PaCO_2$ less than 50 torr is required to initiate support.

ECMO is used to stabilize the cardiac patient in either the preoperative or postoperative phase. Again, patients awaiting palliative or corrective surgical procedures may benefit from ECMO support. Those patients who fail to wean from cardiopulmonary support in the operating room remain poor ECMO candidates. Patients with myocardiopathies are also candidates for ECMO support. The requirement for temporary support for a self-limiting disease remains the indication for ECMO. Myocardiopathies may debilitate the myocardium to the point that heart transplantation is required. Once the decision to support the patient has been made, all efforts to continue support until a suitable donor is found should be made. Often, without a donor, complications associated with long-term ECMO support lead to the removal of support and the death of the patient. This is an unfortunate fact of ECMO "life." We do not always succeed.

Contraindications to Neonatal ECMO

In the more than 20 years that ECMO has been available as a treatment for respiratory and cardiac failure, practitioners have learned to identify the patient population that not only survives but has minimal morbidity associated with the use of ECMO. The goal is to apply the technology to the appropriate patient population. Just as there are indications for ECMO, there are also reasons to avoid this therapy. These contraindications are, for the most part, relative. There may be incidents where, in spite of a specific contraindication, the team elects to place a patient on ECMO. In the end, the application of ECMO is the decision of the physicians in charge.

The contraindications to ECMO in the neonatal patient are noted in Table 25-8 and are described in detail later.

The newborn cerebral vasculature is quite sensitive to changes in pH and PaO_2. Acidosis and increased PaO_2 lead to vasodilation, whereas alkalosis and hypoxemia lead to vasoconstriction. Additionally, the cerebral vasculature in the neonate is poorly formed and prone to leak with rapid changes in pH and PaO_2. This risk increases the younger the infant is and is greatest in the premature infant. Infants meeting the criteria for ECMO are already at risk for suffering an intraventricular hemorrhage (IVH) because of their profound hypoxemia and acidosis. Furthermore, the therapeutic interventions before ECMO carry an inherent risk of IVH.

TABLE 25-8   Contraindications for Neonatal ECMO

Intraventricular hemorrhage (IVH) > Grade 1

Mechanical ventilation for >7–10 days

Weight < 2.0 kg and/or gestation age < 34 weeks

Mechanical ventilation at high pressures increases the mean intrathoracic pressure, leading to reduced venous return, and may increase intracranial vascular pressure. The infusion of alkaline agents to increase the pH may cause rapid shifts in pH that lead to vascular leak. Sudden increases in blood PaO_2 may have the same result.

Because of these risks, it is a standard of practice that an ultrasound evaluation of the brain be performed before initiation of ECMO. The view of the brain is taken through the "soft spot" on the infant's head—the unfused anterior fontanelle. The presence and amount of blood in the brain can be determined. Using a scale the radiologist grades the severity of the bleed. An IVH of greater than grade 1 indicates that the patient is likely to continue to bleed. Given that the ECMO circuit is heparinized to reduce the possibility of clotting, introducing the patient to this additional insult would greatly increase the chance of a fatal or devastating neurologic insult. Patients with suspected IVH of grade 1 may receive ECMO. The ACTs are usually maintained at lower limits (160–180 seconds) and support, especially VA ECMO, is increased more slowly to minimize the rapid shifts in pH and PaO_2.

The contraindication of prolonged mechanical ventilation remains the most subjective of all. Patients who have been supported on mechanical ventilation for prolonged periods of time often have chronic fibrotic changes in the pulmonary parenchyma due to the baro-stress and high oxygen concentrations. Chest x-ray films may show hyaline membranes and fibrotic changes, but there is some question as to how much of that is caused by respiratory distress syndrome and how much is irreversible. Remembering that ECMO is a temporary support, it is difficult to justify its use in the face of lung damage that may take months or years to overcome. However, the extent of the fibrosis is quite difficult, if not impossible, to determine.

Since it is difficult to predict the extent of lung injury based on physical examination, a relative contraindication based on days of "maximal ventilatory support" can be used. *Maximal ventilatory support* is the length of time that the patient has been on "toxic" ventilator settings. Those settings have been defined as an FIO_2 of 1.0 and mean airway pressures greater than 20 cm H_2O. Infants who have required ventilatory support on these settings for more than 7 days are deemed to have a high probability of chronic lung disease and would be unlikely candidates for ECMO. However, if the patient had been on mechanical ventilation at low settings, such as an FIO_2 of 0.50 and mean airway pressures of 12 to 15, for several days or weeks and had a sudden decompensation, he or she would be a candidate for ECMO. It is a judgment to be made by the physician and ECMO team.

Birth weight and gestation age are closely related, both as functions of intrauterine development and eligibility for ECMO. It is unlikely that an infant of less than 34 weeks' gestation would weigh more than 2.0 kg, though it is not impossible. In spite of the weight, there are developmental considerations that must be recognized.

The patient whose weight is less than 2.0 kg is likely to have extremely small vessels for cannulation. Remember that adequate ECMO is dependent upon the ability to provide adequate pump flow. The resistance of the cannulae that would be required in the patient of that size would be too great for the ECMO system to overcome and the ability to provide support would be compromised.

Infants of less than 34 weeks' gestation age have passed many developmental milestones in their intrauterine growth. However, they are still premature and several systems are not well developed. The one that most concerns the ECMO practitioner is the cerebral vasculature. In these infants the region of the brain known as the germinal matrix is quite poorly developed and very sensitive to changes in intracranial pressure, pH, and Pao_2. Rapid changes, even subtle ones, are quite likely to lead to leakage in this region.

The use of ECMO in the neonatal population has been well proven, and is generally accepted, as a life-saving intervention for patients with PPHN unresponsive to conventional therapy. The use of unconventional therapies such as liquid ventilation and nitric oxide has been enhanced by the ability to use ECMO as the bail-out therapy. One could argue that recent reductions in neonatal survival rates on ECMO can be attributed to the delay in initiation while these therapies are attempted. However, the primary goals for practitioners are to find the least invasive, most successful, most cost effective means to treat patients. Neonatal ECMO is, simply, another method to support these patients and is not the best method. Practitioners must continue to define the best method for each patient.

▄ PEDIATRIC ECMO

As expertise in neonatal ECMO has grown, many centers have looked to expand the patient population for ECMO. Many facilities now have declared themselves *pediatric ECMO centers*, indicating that they have the equipment, circuits, and oxygenators to provide ECMO for pediatric patients. One of the difficulties associated with this nomenclature is defining when the neonatal period ends and the pediatric period begins. For the sake of classification, a child more than 2 weeks old is defined as a pediatric patient, even though, at that age, the equipment used to provide ECMO is identical to that used for neonatal ECMO. Furthermore, if a 195-pound, 14-year-old high school football player with acute respiratory distress syndrome after an automobile accident can be treated (clearly a pediatric patient), why can't a 195-pound, 41-year-old in the same circumstances (clearly not a pediatric patient)? These are paradoxes of the classification criterion that present an enigma to all who provide "pediatric ECMO."

Equipment Considerations

The pediatric ECMO patient may range in size from the 3.5 kg 2-week-old to the 100 kg 16-year-old. Although the ECMO circuit used for the 100 kg patient is larger, it is very similar in design to the neonatal circuit. The following are the differences in specific circuit components.

Oxygenators. The characteristics of the silicone membrane oxygenator and the various sizes available were discussed earlier in this chapter. In many ways, the size of the oxygenator required will influence the selection of many of the other components used. In patients up to 6 kg, the 0.8 m^2 oxygenator will be used, and in patients up to 10 kg, the 1.5 m^2 oxygenator is used. Other than the varying size of the oxygenator, the circuit remains identical. For patients larger than 10 kg, the 2.5 m^2 to 4.5 m^2 oxygenators will be used. These oxygenators require a circuit with larger tubing than the $^1/_4$ inch neonatal ECMO circuit. The internal diameter of the pediatric ECMO circuit is $^3/_8$ inch. This allows a greater volume of blood to be pumped with each pump revolution.

Raceway Tubing. The use of Tygon in the raceway was described earlier. The raceway tubing internal diameter is altered to provide the maximal blood flow to the patient at the lowest pump speed possible. For patients up to 20 kg, a $^3/_8$-inch internal diameter raceway is used. The $^3/_8$-inch internal diameter tubing holds approximately 25 mL in a 12-inch section, whereas the $^1/_2$-inch internal diameter tubing contains 50 mL. This compares with the 12.5 mL contained in the $^1/_4$-inch tubing of the neonatal raceway. As you can see, the volume of blood pumped per revolution doubles with each increase in tubing size. The reduction in revolutions per minute required helps to prolong the useful life of the ECMO raceway.

Bladder Bridge. The bladder of the ECMO circuit serves as a reservoir as well as a point for servo regulating flow. As the flow rates are increased in pediatric ECMO, the bladder may become a point of high resistance in the circuit. Incorporating a $^3/_8$-inch bridge around the bladder shunts approximately 80% of the flow around this high-resistance point without compromising servo regulation.[10]

Heat Exchanger. Although the 2.5 m^2 or larger oxygenators have integral heat exchangers, these are made of aluminum alloys. As discussed previously, aluminum heat exchangers are thought by many to be unacceptable for long-term ECMO applications. The Omni Therm heat exchanger by Avecor is one of several used on those patients requiring a $^3/_8$-inch circuit.

Criteria for Pediatric ECMO

The experience gained through more than 20 years and 10,000 patients has made it possible to identify the neonatal population of patients most likely to benefit from ECMO. The experience with pediatric patients is much more limited. As of July 1995, only 982 pediatric patients had been reported to the Extracorporeal Life Support Organization's Pediatric Registry, with an overall survival of 53%.[6] Developing criteria for supporting the pediatric patient in respiratory failure has been as difficult as developing criteria for the neonate 20 years ago.

The methods used to establish criteria for any therapeutic intervention consist of analysis of the current practice (retrospective analysis) and evaluation of the new modality (prospective analysis). Both of these methods were employed in the later 1980s and early 1990s. The retrospective studies were completed by Drs. Butt and McDougall in 1989. In reviewing the therapy for acute respiratory distress syndrome in the pediatric population, they found an 80% mortality rate among patients requiring mechanical ventilation with PIPs of greater than 40 cm H_2O and an alveolar–arterial oxygen difference (P[A-a]O_2) of greater than 580 torr.[3] A review by Tamburro and colleagues in 1990 further refined the data, showing that the amount of time on high support was predictive of mortality. Tamburro found that a P(A-a)o_2 of greater than 450 torr for 16 hours predicted mortality.[16]

Based in part on this data, Mohler and others at the University of Michigan performed a prospective study of 25 pediatric ECMO patients to determine predictors of survival in that population. They included 220 patients in their study and looked at multiple data points including age, length on mechanical ventilation before ECMO, maximal mean and peak airway pressure, time on ECMO, and time to extubation after ECMO. In their study, Mohler and colleagues concluded that mean airway pressures of greater than 25 cm H_2O and PIPs greater than 50 cm H_2O were associated with higher mortality rates. They also found that younger patients fared better than older patients.[14]

Given this information, most centers have devised their own criteria for pediatric ECMO. These criteria are, not surprisingly, quite similar to the criteria for neonatal ECMO and are listed in Table 25-9. As each of the approximately 85 centers now performing pediatric ECMO continues to gain experience, they revise their criteria to ensure that this modality is performed on patients who may benefit.

The indications for the use of ECMO in the pediatric population were perhaps most eloquently summarized by Drs. Bob Arensman and Vincent Adolph from the University of Chicago:

> If a child has developed fulminant respiratory failure and maximal, conventional therapy is failing to result in improvement, the care providers should ask the question: "Should ECMO therapy be considered as a possible therapeutic modality in this individual?" Most patients under consideration will be rejected because other therapeutic choices are available that are less invasive, less dangerous, and less costly. Still other patients will be rejected because of clear cut contraindications to undertaking vascular cannulation or systemic anticoagulation, but no child should die

---

TABLE 25-9   Criteria for Pediatric ECMO

Hypoxia > 4 hours

  (A-a)DO_2 > 400 mm Hg

  PaO_2 < 50 mm Hg on vent with PIP > 50 or MAP > 20

Persistent acidosis

  pH < 7.20 in spite of alkalinization therapy, hyperventilation, NaHCO_3 infusion

  rising lactic acid levels

Barotrauma

Cardiac dysfunction

from isolated respiratory failure in the last decade of the twentieth century without at least a brief consideration of using ECMO therapy.[1]

The diseases treated with pediatric ECMO are noted in Figure 25-18.

As with neonatal ECMO, there are relative contraindications to providing ECMO in the pediatric population. They are listed in Table 25-10 but warrant further discussion.

Patients whose long-term prognosis will remain unchanged in spite of ECMO should not be placed on this form of support. However, the Extracorporeal Life Support Organization (ELSO) registry data reveal that patients with pneumocystis pneumonia are placed on ECMO with a 38% survival. Since pneumocystis pneumonia is most commonly associated with the AIDS virus, there would seem to be a contraindication for the use of ECMO in its treatment. The issue is, however, complex. If the patient has been asymptomatic or has not had previous infections, the expected life span could be 5 to 10 years. In that instance, ECMO can and should be provided.

The level and duration of ventilation required before the initiation of ECMO may limit the ability of the lung to recover in spite of ECMO. Prolonged support at high pressures may lead to pulmonary fibrosis and the conventional wisdom is that ECMO cannot be prolonged to allow the lungs to recover. However, if the patient has been on mechanical ventilation on relatively benign settings for several days and has required increased support for only the past 3 to 4 days, the lung damage associated with mechanical ventilation may not be as profound. It is important that the level as well as the length of mechanical ventilation be considered.

Although immunosuppression as a contraindication applies to those patients who have received organ transplants, the immune suppression drugs that they receive do not make them ineligible for ECMO. Indeed, cardiac transplant patients have an overall survival of 41%.[6] However, patients with malignant disease, bone marrow transplant, and pulmonary transplant have been reported to have only a 12% survival in one study.[5] Those patients should not be offered ECMO.

The use of ECMO in the pediatric population remains less popular than in the neonatal population. It does remain a viable and effective mode of therapy for those pediatric patients in fulminant respiratory failure.

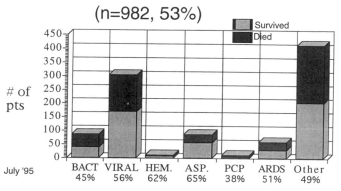

FIGURE 25-18 Pediatric ECMO survival statistics by diagnosis (ELSO Registry).

TABLE 25-10   **Contraindications for Pediatric ECMO**

Irreversible disease

Mechanical ventilation > 10 days

Immune compromised

■MANAGEMENT OF THE PATIENT ON ECMO

The patient on ECMO is both critically ill and more stable than most other patients in the intensive care unit. Although the patient may have been dying from sepsis, he or she is now completely supported with a well-controlled cardiac output and oxygen delivery is normal to above normal. All the medical maladies that were killing the patient are now left to run their course. We have provided the ultimate support. As one ECMO specialist has observed, "You can't die on VA ECMO."

Once the patient is on ECMO, the work of getting the patient off ECMO begins. Ideally, a team should be able to have the patient ready for decannulation within 5 to 10 days. Of course, the patient will dictate this to a large extent. Appropriate management will help to speed the process. In this section we will discuss systematic management of the ECMO patient.

Anticoagulation. Unless the patient is at high risk for bleeding, heparin is infused to maintain ACTs of 180 to 220 seconds. Heparin is titrated as required to maintain appropriate anticoagulation. The clotting times will be altered if the patient is more likely to suffer a hemorrhage or may be increased as the circuit shows signs of clot formation. In pediatric ECMO, the ACTs may be reduced because of the increased flow through the circuit.

Antibiotics. Antibiotics are used as indicated. Many centers continue to administer prophylactic antibiotics to prevent infection; however, others have reduced or discontinued these medications in patients without known or suspected sepsis and have seen no increase in culture-proven infections.

Sedation. The neonate on ECMO does not require paralysis. Indeed, some prefer that the patients remain only lightly sedated and able to be aroused with minimal stimulation. In this way, chemical dependency is avoided, the child is more awake for parental visits, and mobilization of extravascular fluid is enhanced. Levels are monitored and, unless the infant appears uncomfortable or his or her movement restricts the staff's ability to safely provide support, the child is given as little sedation as possible. The older child requires a different strategy. These children are quite aware of their surroundings. The unfamiliarity of the intensive care unit; the loss of parental contact; and the discomfort of the cannulae, chest tubes, endotracheal tube, and every other tube that might be in place may cause a high level of anxiety. These children may require complete sedation to ensure that they do not cause themselves harm. It is important that the sedation level be reduced on a daily basis to allow for a neurologic evaluation.

Nutrition. Although a full discussion of the topic is outside the scope of this chapter, healing from any disease process requires adequate nutrition. Neonates and pediatric patients alike are started on parenteral nutrition within 24 hours of initiation of ECMO. These fluids may have very high concentrations to reduce the free water given to the patient. In this case, total parenteral nutrition may be given through the ECMO circuit.

Respiratory Care. The majority of patients placed on ECMO are in respiratory failure. The first 24 to 72 hours on ECMO are often hallmarked by a profound increase in extravascular lung water. The chest x-ray film may reveal complete "white out," also known as "ECMO lung." With the improvement in renal function, the use of diuretics, and appropriate ventilatory strategies, this edema is absorbed into the vascular space and excreted over the next 24 to 48 hours, with a subsequent improvement in the chest x-ray film.

The goal of the pulmonary team is to avoid total collapse of the lung while minimizing barotrauma. Appropriate continuous positive airway pressure or PEEP levels can be determined by bedside pulmonary graphics monitors. In those patients with pneumonia and secretions, chest physiotherapy may be performed as long as the platelet counts are adequate to prevent bleeding. The patient may be rolled from side to side as needed. Daily lung compliance studies are useful in determining the recovery of the lung tissue as well as optimizing the ventilatory support required. In some patients, bronchoscopy may be required to clear secretions and may be used to deliver surfactant to specific areas of the lung.

Psychosocial Issues. For the neonate, parental visitation may not be as critical as for the pediatric patient. The ECMO team should provide as much support as possible to help the parents of these critically ill patients cope. Especially early in the ECMO course, the parents should be encouraged to rest. Their child is now more stable than they have been, and the parents will need to be well rested to cope with the days and weeks to come as their child recovers. The is especially true of the postpartum mother. The pediatric patient will have a much higher level of anxiety. Besides appropriate sedation and anxiolytics, parental and sibling visits should be encouraged when possible. Visits by child life specialists and even television should be provided as distractions.

▬SUMMARY

The use of ECMO in both neonatal and pediatric populations appears to be on a downward trend. In fact, since 1993 the number of ECMO cases per year has continued to drop. Interestingly, as the number of cases has decreased, so has overall survival. This may indicate the increased use of alternate therapies such as HFJV, HFOV, and nitric oxide. It may also indicate that patients who were once being saved on ECMO are not getting the chance or are being placed on support too late to have a positive outcome. ECMO is a temporary therapeutic intervention for profound cardiorespiratory failure. When provided to the appropriate patient population, it can reduce morbidity and increase survival in those patients most likely to die. The keys to success in the delivery of ECMO are early identification of those patients likely to require this support, referral to an ECMO center, and appropriate but early initiation of ECMO.

▬REFERENCES

1. Arensman RM, Adolph VR: Extracorporeal life support in children. In Arensman RM, Cornish JD (eds): Extracorporeal Life Support. Boston, Blackwell Scientific, 1993, p. 275.
2. Burchfield D, Neu J: Neonatal parenchymal diseases. In Koff PB, Eitzman D, Neu J (eds): Neonatal and Pediatric Respiratory Care. St. Louis, Mosby, 1993.
3. Butt W, McDougall P. What is the role of pediatric ECMO in Australia? Aust Paediatr J 25:189, 1989.
4. Chai PJ, Skaryack LA, Ungerleider RM et al: Jugular ligation does not increase intracranial pressure but does increase bihemispheric cerebral blood flow and metabolism. Crit Care Med 23:1864, 1995.
5. Chevalier JY: Extracorporeal respiratory assistance for pediatric acute respiratory failure. Crit Care Med 21: S382, 1993.
6. ECMO Registry Report of the Extracorporeal Life Support Organization. Ann Arbor, University of Michigan Hospitals, July 1995.
7. Grayck EN, Meliones JN, Kern FH, Hansell DR, Ungerleider RM, Greeley WJ: Elevated serum lactate correlates with intracranial hemorrhage in neonates treated with extracorporeal life support. Pediatrics 96:914, 1995.
8. Green TP, Moler FW, Goodman DM: Probability of survival after prolonged extracorporeal membrane oxygenation in pediatric patients with acute respiratory failure. Crit Care Med 23:1132, 1995.
9. Gregory GA et al: Meconium aspiration in infants: A prospective study. J Pediatr 85:848, 1974.
10. Hansell DR, Kirchoff J et al: Modification of the Ochsner bridge in the pediatric extracorporeal life support circuit. Breckenridge, CO, Proceedings from the Eighth Annual ECMO Symposium of Children's National Medical Center, 1992.
11. Lillehei CW: History of the development of extracorporeal circulation. In Arensman RM, Cornish JD (eds): Extracorporeal Life Support. Boston, Blackwell Scientific, 1993, p. 26.
12. Meliones JN, Hansell DR: Extracorporeal membrane oxygenation: The role of blood components. In Chambers LA, Issett LA (eds): Supporting the Pediatric Transfusion Recipient. Bethesda, MD, American Association of Blood Blanks, 1994.
13. Meliones JN, Mohler FW et al: Hemodynamic instability after the initiation of extracorporeal membrane oxygenation: Role of ionized calcium. Crit Care Med 10:1247, 1991.
14. Mohler FW et al: Extracorporeal life support for pediatric respiratory failure: Predictors of survival from 220 patients. Crit Care Med 21:1604, 1993.
15. Shearer I, Darling E: Venovenous extracorporeal life support: Clinical experience with a dual lumen cannula. Proc of Am Acad Cardiovasc Perf 13:36, 1992.
16. Tamburro R, Chyka D, Bungnitz M: The use of alveolar arterial oxygen gradient to predict mortality from severe respiratory failure in pediatrics. Breckenridge, CO, Proceedings from the Sixth Annual ECMO Symposium of Children's National Medical Center, 1990.
17. Toffaletti J, Hansell D: Interpretation of blood lactate measurements in pediatric open heart surgery and extracorporeal membrane oxygenation. Scand J Clin Lab Invest 55:301, 1995.

▬SELF-ASSESSMENT QUESTIONS

1. A 4.5-kg patient on ECMO has the following laboratory data: ABC; pH 7.45; $PaCO_2$ 39 torr; PaO_2 90 torr; HCO_3^- 24 mEq/L; SaO_2 0.95; Hgb 12. Calculate the oxygen content.

2. The above patient is on ECMO flows of 0.450 LPM. Calculate oxygen delivery.

3. The membrane oxygenator is made of what material?

4. The ECMO system has been designed to provide temporary cardiopulmonary support to patients incapable of maintaining ____?

5. The two indications for the use of VA ECMO over VV ECMO are
   _____ and _____?

6. Which of the following statements about VV ECMO are true?
   I. Pulmonary blood flow is maintained.
   II. Full cardiac support is provided.
   III. Pulsatile blood flow is maintained.
   IV. High systemic Pao_2 is provided.
      a. I, II, III, IV   c. II, IV only
      b. I, III, IV only   d. I, III only

7. Which of the following statements about VA ECMO are true?
   I. The heart and lungs are "bypassed."
   II. Full cardiac support is provided.
   III. The potential for system embolization is increased.
   IV. High systemic Pao_2 is provided.
      a. I, II, III, IV   c. II, IV only
      b. I, III, IV only   d. I, III only

8. The primary indication for ECMO in the neonatal nonsurgical patient
   is
     a. PPHN   c. acidosis
     b. hypoxia   d. CDH

9. Contraindications to ECMO include
   I. Uncontrolled bleeding
   II. An OI > 40
   III. ICH > Grade 1
   IV. Weight < 2.0 kg
      a. I, II, III, IV   c. I, III, IV only
      b. II, IV only   d. I, III only

10. The patient population with the highest overall survival on ECMO is
    the
      a. neonatal   c. cardiac
      b. adult   d. pediatric

Part 6
Psychosocial Interactions

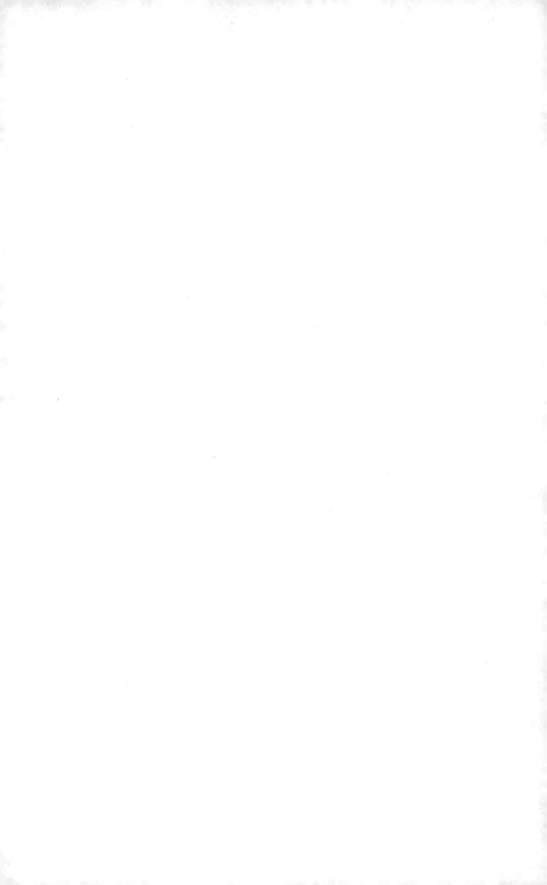

Chapter 26

Psychosocial Aspects

RUTH J. MESSINGER

OBJECTIVES

Having completed this chapter, the reader will be able to:

1 Describe common family reactions to having a child who requires respiratory care.

2 Discuss how culture affects families' health beliefs and behavior.

3 Identify commonly expressed needs of families who have a child who requires respiratory care.

4 Cite specific times in the course of the disease, the developmental stage of the child, and the life of the family when there might be increased stress.

5 Name coping resources which promote adaptation to the child's illness.

6 List essential roles for the respiratory care practitioner in the management of newborns and children who require respiratory care and their families.

KEY TERMS

conspiracy of silence
culturally competent services
family transitions

grief
self-advocacy skills

▬THE IMPACT OF ILLNESS ON THE FAMILY

With the advent of dramatic improvements in medical technology, fragile infants have increased survival rates. Pediatric health care providers are seeing more families who have extremely low–birth-weight babies, infants who require medical technology to live, infants exposed prenatally to drugs, and infants who have HIV. Most of these infants require the services of an interdisciplinary team, which may include a respiratory care practitioner.

When providing respiratory care to newborns or children, it is essential to acknowledge that the family is the constant in the child's life, while health care providers come and go. The child's illness and care are family affairs. Yet many of the families who have medically fragile infants also have other stresses. They may lack experience with health care providers or have difficulty dealing with them or gaining access to health care. They may be from minority backgrounds. They may live in poverty and have poor nutrition, inadequate education, and few social supports.[13]

No two families react exactly alike when they have a child who is ill. Within a family, each member may react differently. Factors that determine family reactions include characteristics associated with the illness itself, the age and developmental stage of the child and the family at onset, the family's resources, and the way the family and child have typically dealt with past stress.

It has been suggested that families go through several predictable stages when given bad medical news. Initially there is shock and denial, followed sequentially by anger, bargaining, depression, and adaptation.[4] However, practitioners dealing with a young population have found that this stage theory lacks applicability for several reasons. Many families report that they do not necessarily experience all the stages in a linear fashion. Such stages are rarely "time bound." One cannot state whether a family has been in one stage "too long," since these things are difficult to measure and judge. Families also indicate that stage theory tends to focus on the negative aspects of adjustment.

Increasingly, rather than utilize stage theory to help us understand families' experiences, practitioners apply theories associated with grief and loss.[5] In this paradigm, **grief** is seen as an unlearned, spontaneous process in reaction to significant loss. Each grief state is seen as having a purpose. Denial, anxiety, fear, guilt, depression, and anger collectively help the griever to find strength and support to separate from the lost, idealized child and to deal with the child they now have. Some mental health therapists and family members believe that if people do not openly express feelings associated with grieving, they may get "stuck" in a grief state. Using this model to explain common family reactions, it follows that all health care providers can assist families by acknowledging grief states and their normality and allowing each family member to grieve in his or her own unique way.

Other reactions felt or expressed include fatigue, a sense of failure, fear of the future coupled with a desire to live in the present or past, and feeling overwhelmed by care responsibilities. All of these feelings are normal responses to stressful events, and the respiratory care practitioner can expect to encounter them.

When the child's condition has placed an unremitting burden of care on a parent who has little family or other support and concomitant stresses, the parent may become incapacitated and unable to provide adequate care. Identification of the potential for parent "burn-out" prior to its happening and referral to informal community supports, respite,[12] or a mental health provider may be an important preventive service to the child and the family.

Cultural Determinants

The occurrence of a serious illness in a child can have a profound effect on a family. A child with an illness requiring the services of a respiratory care provider can be difficult for acculturated families who live in the mainstream. Our dominant culture has few rituals to assist us in caring for a seriously ill or dying child.

By the year 2010, it is estimated that nearly one quarter of all children in the United States will be children from minority backgrounds; we are becoming an increasingly diverse society. For families from a different culture, the diagnosis and treatment of a serious childhood illness can be especially difficult. One mother from Haiti wanted to sign her daughter out of the hospital against medical advice when a male respiratory therapist gave her treatments. Another child's Cambodian family agreed to administer aerosolized medication. However, it was subsequently discovered that this family never intended to be compliant with the physician's orders, but was merely being respectful to an authority figure.

These two examples demonstrate how cultural background and degree of acculturation to the dominant culture determine our view of illness, disability, and treatment; the role of family members in support and care; coping patterns; acceptance of Western medical methods; and communication with health care professionals.[9] In many first-generation immigrants' cultural traditions, folk medicine techniques are the first choice of treatment, care by non-family members of the opposite sex may be prohibited, and some medicines may be viewed as being incompatible with traditional beliefs about what is healing for respiratory ailments.

Providing **culturally competent services**, at the most basic level, means that service providers need to know about and be sensitive to their own and the patient's culturally prescribed beliefs about health and illness. When the family is not English speaking, it also means learning the communication skills that are required when working with an interpreter. For example, the speaker should look at and speak directly to the patient or family, not to the interpreter. To check for understanding, the practitioner should always ask that the patient and family repeat back material that was covered through the interpreter at the end of the session. Finally, respiratory care practitioners need to inquire about the family's ability to read instructions written in English.

■FAMILY NEEDS

Families' needs change over time. During the initial hospital admission, the family members may focus on fear about the child's dying if the condition is believed to be life threatening. However, if the child's survival chances increase, the family members begin to focus on how everyone will manage. They need to learn the specialized care the infant may require. Learning such skills and then performing them on their child may be very time consuming and conflict with other parental functions, such as attending to the needs of other children in the family or working outside the home.

If the child has been home with a demanding home-care regimen, the parent may have become socially isolated and need assistance in arranging personal time or in paying attention to the sick child's siblings. Indeed, the sick child's siblings are often the overlooked family members who feel abandoned or neglected over the long term. Also, once the family caretakers become proficient in their child's care, a struggle for control may occur between some health care providers and parents.

The extent to which families have certain needs depends on their circumstances and assets prior to the child's diagnosis in a number of areas including money, housing, education, support, and a feeling of belonging in the community.[6] Typical needs expressed by families in research studies include the following:[1,14]

1. Information about the condition: cause, treatment, prognosis
2. Equipment: how to get it, use it properly, get it repaired, pay for it
3. Financial assistance for medical and associated bills
4. Family supports: rights and entitlements, respite (time for themselves), parent-to-parent support networks for sharing, advocacy skills
5. Care coordination
6. Communication help: how to keep track of medication and treatment regimens, how to talk to doctors, what to tell family and friends and, most importantly, the sick child
7. Confidentiality about personal family or patient information

▬TRANSITIONS

Family members may reexperience the grief states discussed earlier at times of change. Transitions either in the life of the child or in the life of the family can be such times of change. For the child, transitions include discharge to home or hospital readmission, every medical appointment, birthdays, entry into special programs, alteration in type of therapy needed, or abrupt changes in the course of the illness.

Family transitions begin when the members are informed of the diagnosis or condition.[8] Other times of transition include when a younger sibling surpasses the sick child in some accomplishment or when the family is considering having another child. The respiratory care practitioner can provide support to family members by forewarning them that anger, anxiety, and guilt are typical responses to many transitions and that the grief process is a necessary, ongoing life function.

A child's dying is considered an unnatural event in our culture and is one that offers many challenges to health care professionals and the child's family. This special transitional time has great potential for conflict, especially when there is no clear agreement about the best course of action. Although parental choice and their role as central caretakers are usually acknowledged, conflict can occur within a family, among health care providers, and between health care providers and the family.

If the child is old enough, involving the child in making decisions about care and the management of pain, or at least informing the child, is optimal.[7] However, sometimes parents engage in a **conspiracy of silence** to shield the child from bad news. Parental lack of disclosure rarely protects the child; instead, it increases isolation and often shuts off important opportunities for intimate sharing.

Because of the intense emotional pressures on health care providers, a child who is dying is best cared for by an interdisciplinary team whose members can support each other. Team members, including the respiratory care practitioners, should be aware of their own feelings and comfort level about death and dying in general and about children's dying. The child or family members may feel most comfortable sharing personal questions or pain with a professional rather than further burdening another family member. Being a nonjudgmental listener to a family member is one important way a respiratory care practitioner can offer support.

COPING

Although caring for a severely ill infant or child can be an extraordinary burden on a family, many families facing numerous stresses demonstrate remarkable resilience.[2] Each family responds uniquely and there is no single recipe for successful adaptation.

The following are common elements of families who cope well:

1. They know that transitions can be stressful and that grief is normal.
2. They are not isolated. They seek out new social networks or work at maintaining old ones.
3. They have a system of beliefs, religious or otherwise, that helps them accept their burden of care.
4. They do not see themselves as passive victims. Rather, they ask for information or help when they need it and actively problem solve.
5. They can identify and utilize resources: money, transportation, helpers.
6. They have health and energy.

ROLE OF THE RESPIRATORY CARE PRACTITIONER

In addition to providing direct respiratory care to the infant or child, the respiratory care practitioner can do much to prevent increased mental health problems in sick children by promoting the highest quality of care possible for the patient and family, whether the care is provided in a hospital, a community program, or a home-based setting.[10]

Respiratory care can be most difficult to integrate into a family's life. If the family is the unit of care and there is a belief in the value of family-centered care, then each family's strengths, needs, and cultural background should be identified by all team members, including the respiratory care practitioner. The respiratory care practitioner can utilize a team approach, enhance communication and collaboration among and between providers and family, and assist families to learn **self-advocacy skills**. Self-advocacy can be taught by the respiratory care practitioner by encouraging family members to voice grievances directly to the appropriate health care provider (*e.g.*, the primary nurse, hospital unit director, home care equipment vendor, nursing agency supervisor or doctor).

While assessing strengths and needs, the respiratory care practitioner can identify and resolve potential compliance issues and provide assistance to the family by offering suggestions on how the home can be organized to ensure efficient, safe care while minimizing family disruptions and still providing other family members some personal, private space.

Respiratory care practitioners can also be supportive by warning the family about possible problems they might anticipate with equipment and supplies, how such problems can be resolved, and who should be contacted (with the correct telephone number) to assist in problem resolution relating to equipment and supplies. Stress the importance of keeping good written records.

When family members begin to care for their sick child, few feel comfortable or competent to provide skilled, technically demanding, and possibly painful or uncomfortable respiratory therapy procedures. During family education sessions, the respiratory care practitioner can recognize the family's and child's accomplishments in these important activities.[11]

Strengths and concerns identified during work with the family either in the hospital or at home should be reported by the respiratory care practitioner to the appropriate health care team member or service coordinator. Although most families want the best for their child and do provide excellent care, the respiratory care practitioner may observe behavior that could injure the child or place the child at risk.[3] It is, therefore, important to know the state's child abuse and neglect laws and the agency or hospital policies and procedures about dealing with possible child protective issues.

Finally, providing respiratory care to a sick or dying infant or child can be very difficult for the practitioner. Identifying health promotion and stress reduction techniques that are personally helpful and using them is an important professional responsibility.

▬SUMMARY

Current trends in our country's population, the health status of children, and the rapidly changing health care system will have a major effect on the future direction of respiratory care practice. Despite the fragility of infants and children with complex medical problems requiring respiratory care, many of them and their families can be helped in their adaptation and coping by coordinated services and support. Important care components for children and families include identifying and building on family members' strengths; providing appropriate education; respecting ethnic, religious, and cultural backgrounds; and promoting self-advocacy. The respiratory care practitioner, with the appropriate knowledge and skills, can be an invaluable team member who provides coordinated care in a variety of settings.

The following are resources to assist the practitioner or family to obtain more information:

National Network for Children with Special Needs
Georgetown University Child Development Center
3800 Reservoir Road N.W.
Bles Building, Room CG-52
Washington, DC 20007
(202) 687-8635

National Resource Center for Community-Based Systems of Service for Children with Special Health Care Needs and Their Families
University of Iowa
National Maternal and Child Health Resource Center
Boyd Law Building
Melrose and Byington
Iowa City, IA 52242
(319) 335-9067

National Center for Family-Centered Care
Association for the Care of Children's Health
7910 Woodmont Avenue, Suite 300
Bethesda, MD 20814
(301) 654-6549

REFERENCES

1. Bailey DB, Blasco PM, Simmeonsson RJ: Needs expressed by mothers and fathers of young children with disabilities. American Journal on Mental Retardation 97:1, 1992.
2. Barbero GF: Adverse life events and exacerbations of cystic fibrosis. Pediatric Pulmonology 18:73, 1994.
3. Benedict MI, Wulff LM, White RB: Current parental stress in maltreating and nonmaltreating families of children with multiple disabilities. Child Abuse and Neglect 16:155, 1992.
4. Blacher J: Sequential stages of parental adjustment to the birth of a child with handicaps: Fact or artifact. Mental Retardation 22:55, 1984.
5. Briskin H, Liptak GS: Helping families with children with developmental disabilities. Pediatric Annals 24:262, 1995.
6. Dyson L: Families of young children with handicaps: Parental stress and family functioning. American Journal on Mental Retardation 95:623, 1991.
7. Fleischman AR, Nolan K, Dubler NN, Epstein MF, Gerben MA, Jellinek MS, Litt IF, Miles MS, Oppenheimer S, Shaw A, Van Eys J, Vaughn VC: Caring for gravely ill children. Pediatrics 94:433, 1994.
8. Messinger R, Davidson P, Hoekelman R: Communication with parents and patients. In Hoekelman R (ed): Primary Pediatric Care. St. Louis, Mosby-Year Book, 1992.
9. Pachter LM, Weller SC: Acculturation and compliance with medical therapy developmental and behavioral pediatrics 14:163, 1993. J Dev Behav Pediatr 14:163, 1993.
10. Patterson JM, Geber G: Preventing mental health problems in children with chronic illness or disability. Childrens Health Care 20:150, 1991.
11. Petr CG, Barney DD: Reasonable efforts for children with disabilities: The parents' perspective. Social Work 38:247, 1993.
12. Rimmerman A: Provision of respite care for children with developmental disabilities: Changes in maternal coping and stress over time. Mental Retardation 27:99, 1989.
13. Siefert K: Future directions for social work practice in maternal and child health. Unpublished manuscript, 1995.
14. Walker DK, Epstein SG, Taylor AB, Crocker AC, Tuttle, GA: Perceived needs of families with children with chronic health conditions. Childrens Health Care 18:196, 1989.

SELF-ASSESSMENT QUESTIONS

1. What are three social trends that influence families' reactions to having a child with a special health care need?

2. How does grief theory help us understand families' reactions to having a child with a special health care need?

3. How do families' cultural backgrounds influence their reactions to a child with special health care needs?

4. What are four common needs expressed by families?

5. What are four transition times in the life of the child or the family when they are likely to reexperience some grief states?

6. When a child is gravely ill or dying, what are three special issues that challenge health care providers?

7. What are three attributes of families who cope well with having a child with special health care needs?

8. What are five functions, in addition to direct provision of care to the infant or child, that the respiratory care practitioner can provide to optimize care?

Chapter 27

Ethical Issues in Patient Care

OBJECTIVES

Having completed this chapter, the reader will be able to:

1 Describe how the fundamental ethical principles relate to care of the patient.

2 Describe how fidelity, veracity, confidentiality, and uncertainty affect the professional–patient relationship.

3 Identify steps to be taken in decision making.

4 Identify the ethical issues involved in the cases of Baby Doe and Baby Jane Doe, fetal cell implantation, and organ transplantation.

KEY TERMS

autonomy	fidelity
beneficence	nonmaleficence
benevolent deception	paternalism
ethics	veracity

Ethics is defined as the study of rational processes for determining the most morally desirable courses of action in view of conflicting moral choices.[5] Respiratory care practitioners may find themselves faced with a clinical situation in which the right choice for the patient is not obvious and several of the available options are reasonable, depending upon a particular point of view. When real choices exist between possible courses of action, we have an ethical dilemma.

Patient care decisions in these situations are never easy. They are influenced by the individual beliefs and values of not only the patient and family members but often the health care providers involved in caring for the patient. The ways in which a person views the preservation of life, the avoidance of death, and the relief of pain and suffering will have an effect on the choices they make when faced with an ethical dilemma. Religious beliefs, cultural views of life and death, and opinions about science and technology also influence decision making.

When we take all of these issues and factors into consideration, it is apparent that when decisions must be made about initiation or termination of life-supporting therapy, there is often no clearly right or clearly wrong choice. Most of this book addresses respiratory care of the newborn and child from a purely scientific perspective. The purpose of this final chapter is to provide a different perspective for making decisions about the treatment of infants and children with respiratory or cardiac disease, particularly when there may be disagreement about what course of action is in the best interest of the patient.

▬FUNDAMENTAL ETHICAL PRINCIPLES

Autonomy

The first fundamental principle to be considered in an ethical dilemma is individual **autonomy**. This principle states that the patient has the right to make decisions regarding his or her medical care.[1] In an ideal situation, the physician and other members of the health care team provide all of the information necessary for the patient to make informed decisions. In order for this to occur, the patient must be capable of understanding a certain amount of scientific information and be willing to ask questions about what he or she does not fully understand. This is possible when the patient is an adult, but what happens when the patient is an infant or child? These patients cannot express or exercise their right to autonomy, and medical decision making becomes the responsibility of surrogates—the parents, legal guardians, medical teams, hospital ethics committees, or, in some instances, the courts.

Autonomy has two basic requirements.[3] The first is the freedom to decide. This requirement depends upon complete, accurate information and the comprehension of that information by the patient. The second requirement is the freedom to act without coercion. This implies that health care professionals and family members must respect the personal autonomy of the patient. The principle of autonomy includes the provision that a patient has the right to decide against treatment, even when it is medically indicated and effective. When a well-informed patient chooses to refuse treatment, despite the advice of the physician and other health care practitioners, we are ethically bound to respect those wishes.

The essential right of the patient's individual autonomy may be overridden by paternalism, which is the tendency of health care professionals to assume that they know what is best for the patient.

Beneficence

Individual **beneficence** dictates that all medical decisions must be made so as to do good for the patient. Above and beyond all other considerations, health care practitioners must do what is best for the patient at all times. The interest of the patient should be the primary criterion by which decisions are reached. Challenges arise when there is disagreement among the patient, the family, and the medical team about which treatment option is truly in the best interest of the patient.

The principle of beneficence includes not only the importance of preserving life but also the realization that sometimes it is necessary to stop preserving life, if it is in the best interest of and consistent with the wishes of the patient. Medical treatment is not mandated if (1) it is not medically indicated; (2) it merely prolongs the process of dying; (3) it is futile; (4) it fails to ameliorate all of the patient's life-threatening condition; or (5) it is virtually futile and under the circumstances inhumane.[1]

Nonmaleficence

The principle of **nonmaleficence** holds that the health care practitioner must also do no harm to the patient. This includes avoiding certain acts that may potentially inflict harm, injury, or suffering on the patient.[5] The principle of nonmaleficence may conflict with the principle of beneficence at times. It may be necessary for the practitioner to inflict some pain and suffering in the process of providing beneficial treatment or preventing a more significant harm. The act of drawing blood from an infant or child in order to perform diagnostic tests or evaluate the patient's response to therapy may inflict temporary pain, yet the surrogates (parents and health care team) decide that the value of the information obtained from testing the blood overrides the momentary harm done to the patient. Table 27-1 shows examples of "goods" and "harms" that conflict in the provision of medical care.

Justice

This principle directs a sense of fairness to all, that all patients should receive equal consideration in matters of medical care.[1] It implies that scarce resources should be allocated for the maximum common good and not be consumed by a favored majority. The issue of how scarce and expensive medical resources are distributed has challenged the medical profession for decades. We provide intensive care for sick infants but no support to families who provide a lifetime of care to handicapped children. Billions of dollars are spent on neonatal intensive care rather than adequate prenatal care. Can we justify spending millions of dollars for an extremely premature infant who may not survive when millions of Americans do not have medical insurance and access to basic medical care which could prevent serious disease? Again, it becomes clear that in an ethical dilemma, there is not a clear and obvious answer.

▬ PROFESSIONAL–PATIENT RELATIONSHIPS

In dealing with neonatal and pediatric patients and their families, certain principles should govern the behavior of health care practitioners.

TABLE 27-1 Clinical Interpretation of "Goods" and "Harms"

GOODS	HARMS
Health	Illness
Prevention, elimination, or control of disease or injury	Disease (morbidity and injury)
Relief from unnecessary pain and suffering	Unnecessary pain and suffering
Amelioration of handicapping conditions	Handicapping conditions
Prolonged life	Premature death

(Beauchamp T, Childress J: Principles of Biomedical Ethics, 2nd ed. New York, Oxford University Press, 1983.)

Fidelity

Fidelity is the duty of the practitioner to keep promises made to the patient, whether they were clearly stated (explicit) or implied (implicit). This includes a responsibility not to abandon or neglect the patient during the period that they require medical care. Practitioners should be careful not to make inappropriate promises to a child, such as agreeing to stay at the bedside throughout the night or until the child feels better. Breaches of fidelity can also destroy the level of trust that has been built up between the patient and caregiver. Practitioners should also avoid conflicting duties to patients and their families. The practitioner's primary obligation is always to the patient.

Veracity (Truth-Telling)

The principle of **veracity** holds that practitioners have an ethical obligation to be truthful in all dealings with the patient and the patient's family. There is an implicit contract between the parties that the truth will be told, and this also helps to establish a trusting relationship.[5] In some cases, health care professionals withhold the truth from the patient for his or her own good. This is called **benevolent deception** and is related to the concept of **paternalism**, in which the practitioner assumes to know what is best for the patient.

Confidentiality

The principle of confidentiality has been an important tenet in medicine for centuries. Even within the Oath of Hippocrates is the promise to hold sacred that which the patient reveals. Practitioners have an obligation to maintain the confidentiality of any information regarding a patient and his or her condition. There are, however, circumstances in which confidentiality is justifiably breached, such as when failure to reveal information can harm others. In these instances, the practitioner is faced with an ethical dilemma that he or she must personally resolve.

Uncertainty

One of the most difficult ethical considerations is that of uncertainty, because even with all of the progress made in the treatment of infants and children, we are never 100% certain what the outcome will be. Our predictions of the outcome are simply that—our best guess about what will happen. Practitioners may cite statistics on incidences and survival rates and share their own experiences in treating children with similar problems, but in reality they cannot know what will happen. In the end, therefore, parents are left to make decisions about the care and future of their children with a degree of uncertainty.

■ DECISION MAKING IN AN ETHICAL DILEMMA

Several authors have proposed a list of essential steps to decision making in cases where an ethical dilemma exists:[2,4,5]

1. **Consider who is involved in making and implementing the decision.** It is important to identify both who can make the decision and who will be responsible for implementing the decision. A conflict may exist if these are different individuals.

2. Determine who shall make the decision, whether it will be the parents and family, physician and health care team, hospital ethics committee, or legal system. The decision makers should receive as much assistance and support as possible but must realize that they must ultimately make the choice.

3. Establish and evaluate all of the medical facts and information available and make it available to the decision makers in a manner in which they can comprehend it.

4. Identify and understand the significant human factors and values in the case. Families who are inexperienced in dealing with medical crises may need assistance in understanding everything that is involved.

5. Identify all major theoretical and value conflicts in the case, clarifying which ethical principles (autonomy, beneficence, nonmaleficence, and justice) are at odds.

6. Make a decision. While this is often the most difficult step in the process, it is inevitable. Family members, although fearful of the ramifications of the decision, may feel some small sense of relief that a decision has been made.

7. Review each step to determine the moral and rational defensibility of the action taken.

The decision-making process may vary, depending upon the patient, his or her family, and the circumstances surrounding the dilemma.

▬ETHICAL ISSUES IN NEWBORN CARE
The following issues are presented briefly to illustrate the types of dilemmas facing practitioners who care for critically ill newborns and children. Definitive answers are not available, and discussion can raise more questions than solutions.

Baby Doe
Baby Doe was a full-term infant born with esophageal atresia and relatively severe Down syndrome. After much discussion and agonizing, the parents refused to grant permission for the doctors to perform a life-saving operation, and the infant received only supportive care, dying of starvation approximately 2 weeks later. In 1983, the federal government acting paternalistically passed regulations requiring notification of cases in which life-saving treatment was withheld. Posters appeared in neonatal intensive care units inviting anonymous phone calls to a central reporting agency. Many investigations followed, but no instances of treatment withholding were identified or corrected. The federal regulations were later found to have been promulgated illegally.[1]

Baby Jane Doe
This case involved a child with spina bifida in which the parents denied consent for a life-saving operation. A lawyer, unknown to the family of the child, pursued the case through the New York State court system and ultimately to the U.S. Supreme Court in order to force the corrective surgery. The hospital that treated the child refused to provide the medical records, stating that a cause for action did not exist and that the patient's right to

confidentiality had priority.[1] Without access to the medical records, the Surgeon General could not make a judgment about the credibility of the case, and it was dismissed.

Fetal Cell Implantation

The practice of taking cells from unviable fetuses for research and implantation into healthy patients has stimulated much discussion, particularly of ethical considerations. The questions raised range from the issue of how far medical research should be allowed to go in the name of experimentation to questions about our moral obligations to the fetus and the mother. Do the potential benefits to the recipient have priority over the rights of the fetus and mother? If consent is required, can the mother provide that consent on behalf of her unborn child?

Organ Transplantation

The final ethical issue to be raised relates to the use of anencephalic infants (babies born without brain tissue) as organ donors. Organ transplantation is a very difficult issue when the wishes of the adult donor are known, and greatly complicated when the potential donor is an unborn child whose wishes cannot be expressed or determined. This issue raises the question of whether these infants are technically alive or dead at birth and whether the definition of brain death applies in these cases. The criteria for brain death are harder to agree on in infants than in adults.[1] Are such infants to be considered persons? If so, who should act as their surrogate in making medical decisions? At what point does death occur in order to allow harvesting of the organs?

▬SUMMARY

This chapter introduced the reader to the basic principles to be considered when confronted with ethical dilemmas. The notions of autonomy, beneficence, nonmaleficence, and justice are essential to the manner in which health care is provided to preserve the rights and privileges of the patient. When more than one choice is morally and medically appropriate, an ethical dilemma exists. The fundamental principles of the professional—patient relationship are fidelity, veracity, confidentiality, and uncertainty. The practitioner must keep these principles in mind in all dealings with patients and their families. A model for making decisions in an ethical dilemma was presented and can serve as a framework for approaching difficult medical decisions. Finally, several ethical issues involving the care of newborn infants were presented to illustrate the types of circumstances in which practitioners may find themselves. Resolution of such dilemmas calls into question the moral values, religious beliefs, and customs of not only the patient and family but the caregivers as well.

▬REFERENCES

1. Avery GB: The morality of drastic intervention. In Avery GB, Fletcher MA, MacDonald MG (eds): Neonatology: Pathophysiology and Management of the Newborn, 4th ed. Philadelphia, JB Lippincott, 1994.
2. Brody H: Ethical decisions in medicine. Boston, Little, Brown, 1981.

3. Edge R: Ethical and legal implications of practice. In Scanlon CL, Spearman C, Sheldon RL (eds): Egan's Fundamentals of Respiratory Care, 6th ed. St. Louis, Mosby-Year Book, 1995.
4. Francoeur RT: From then to now. In Harris CC, Snowden F (eds): Bioethical Frontiers in Perinatal Intensive Care. Natchitoches, LA, Northwestern State University Press, 1985.
5. Sandling J, Carter B, Moore C, Sparks JW: Ethics in neonatal intensive care. In Merenstein GB, Gardner SL (eds): Handbook of Neonatal Intensive Care, 2nd ed. St. Louis, CV Mosby, 1989.

▬SELF-ASSESSMENT QUESTIONS

1. Explain what is meant by the term *ethical dilemma*.

2. List the factors that influence the manner in which individuals approach decisions regarding medical care.

3. How does the principle of autonomy apply to a newborn infant?

4. Give an example of a situation in which the principles of beneficence and nonmaleficence are in conflict.

5. Describe a situation in which a health care provider might justifiably breach the principle of confidentiality.

6. How does uncertainty influence the way in which we approach medical decisions?

7. List the decision-making steps to be taken in cases in which an ethical dilemma exists.

8. Identify the ethical principles that conflict in the Baby Doe and Baby Jane Doe cases.

Index

Page numbers followed by *f* indicate figures; those followed by *t* indicate tables.

557

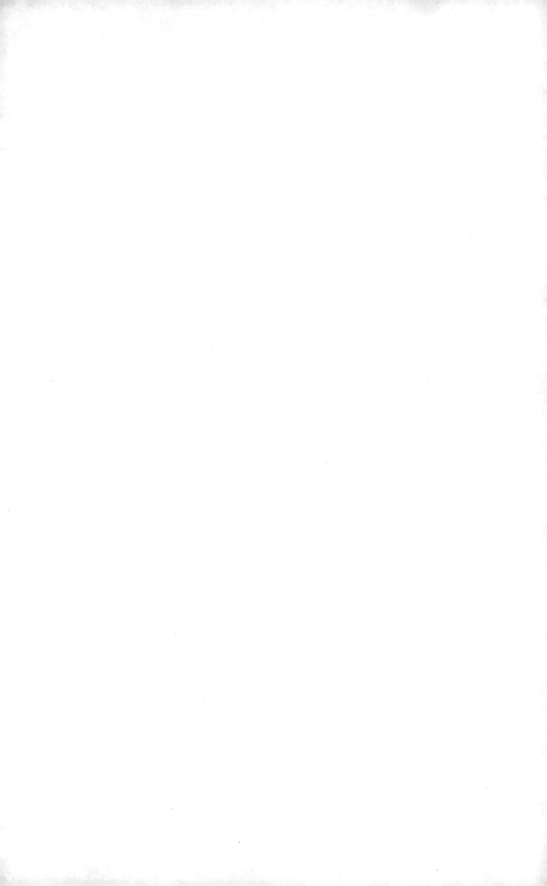

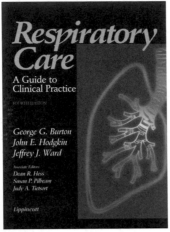
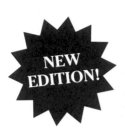
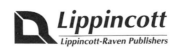